Bioactive Compounds Derived from Plants and Their Medicinal Potential

Bioactive Compounds Derived from Plants and Their Medicinal Potential

Guest Editors

Maria de Lourdes Pereira
Veeranoot Nissapatorn
Ana Paula Girol
Sonia M. R. Oliveira

MDPI

Basel • Beijing • Wuhan • Barcelona • Belgrade • Novi Sad • Cluj • Manchester

Guest Editors
Maria de Lourdes Pereira
CICECO-Aveiro Institute of
Materials and Department of
Medical Sciences
University of Aveiro
Aveiro
Portugal

Veeranoot Nissapatorn
School of Science and World
Union for Herbal Drug
Discovery (WUHeDD)
Walailak University
Nakhon Si Thammarat
Thailand

Ana Paula Girol
Pro-Rector of Research and
Post-Graduation
UNIFIPA
Catanduva, SP
Brazil

Sonia M. R. Oliveira
CICECO—Aveiro Institute of
Materials
University of Aveiro
Aveiro
Portugal

Editorial Office
MDPI AG
Grosspeteranlage 5
4052 Basel, Switzerland

This is a reprint of the Special Issue, published open access by the journal *Pharmaceuticals* (ISSN 1424-8247), freely accessible at: https://www.mdpi.com/journal/pharmaceuticals/special_issues/65WHQ1BRU9.

For citation purposes, cite each article independently as indicated on the article page online and as indicated below:

Lastname, A.A.; Lastname, B.B. Article Title. *Journal Name* **Year**, *Volume Number*, Page Range.

ISBN 978-3-7258-8171-0 (Hbk)
ISBN 978-3-7258-8172-7 (PDF)
https://doi.org/10.3390/books978-3-7258-8172-7

Cover image courtesy of Ana Paula Girol

Contents

About the Editors . . . . **vii**

Preface . . . . **ix**

Sónia M. R. Oliveira, Ana Paula Girol, Veeranoot Nissapatorn and Maria de Lourdes Pereira
Bioactive Compounds Derived from Plants and Their Medicinal Potential
Reprinted from: *Pharmaceuticals* **2025**, *18*, 1732, https://doi.org/10.3390/ph18111732 . . . . **1**

Mateusz Kciuk, Nitika Garg, Sanchit Dhankhar, Monika Saini, Somdutt Mujwar, Sushma Devi, et al.
Exploring the Comprehensive Neuroprotective and Anticancer Potential of Afzelin
Reprinted from: *Pharmaceuticals* **2024**, *17*, 701, https://doi.org/10.3390/ph17060701 . . . . **5**

Syed Mohammed Basheeruddin Asdaq, Abdulaziz Ali Almutiri, Abdullah Alenzi, Maheen Shaikh, Mujeeb Ahmed Shaik, Sultan Alshehri and Syed Imam Rabbani
Unveiling the Neuroprotective Potential of Date Palm (*Phoenix dactylifera*): A Systematic Review
Reprinted from: *Pharmaceuticals* **2024**, *17*, 1221, https://doi.org/10.3390/ph17091221 . . . . **26**

Vinícius Lopes Lessa, Gustavo Gonçalves, Beatriz Santos, Victoria Cruz Cavalari, Rafael Felipe da Costa Vieira and Fabiano Borges Figueiredo
In Vitro Evaluation of the Combinatorial Effect of Naringenin and Miltefosine against *Leishmania amazonensis*
Reprinted from: *Pharmaceuticals* **2024**, *17*, 1014, https://doi.org/10.3390/ph17081014 . . . . **41**

Fekandine V. Douti, Gnatoulma Katawa, Kathrin Arndts, Fagdéba D. Bara, Essimanam R. Awesso, Simplice D. Karou, Achim Hoerauf and Manuel Ritter
Potential of *Aframomum melegueta* and *Xylopia aethiopica* Against *Taenia* spp.: Plant Based Remedies as Novel Anthelmintics
Reprinted from: *Pharmaceuticals* **2025**, *18*, 749, https://doi.org/10.3390/ph18050749 . . . . **49**

Jue Wang, Linlin Zhang, Lu Fu and Zheng Pang
Kaempferol Mitigates *Pseudomonas aeruginosa*-Induced Acute Lung Inflammation Through Suppressing GSK3β/JNK/c-Jun Signaling Pathway and NF-κB Activation
Reprinted from: *Pharmaceuticals* **2025**, *18*, 322, https://doi.org/10.3390/ph18030322 . . . . **68**

Reem Binsuwaidan, Thanaa A. El-Masry, Maysa M. F. El-Nagar, Enas I. El Zahaby, Mohamed M. S. Gaballa and Maisra M. El-Bouseary
Investigating the Antibacterial, Antioxidant, and Anti-Inflammatory Properties of a Lycopene Selenium Nano-Formulation: An In Vitro and In Vivo Study
Reprinted from: *Pharmaceuticals* **2024**, *17*, 1600, https://doi.org/10.3390/ph17121600 . . . . **94**

Meng-Ting Zeng, Li-Yue Huang, Xiao-Hui Zheng, Yan-Qi Fu and Ching-Feng Weng
Ethanolic Extracts of Cupressaceae Species Conifers Provide Rapid Protection against Barium Chloride-Induced Cardiac Arrhythmia
Reprinted from: *Pharmaceuticals* **2024**, *17*, 1003, https://doi.org/10.3390/ph17081003 . . . . **122**

Yasmen F. Mahran, Amira M. Badr, Layla A. Al-Kharashi, Hanaa N. Alajami, Nouf T. Aldamry, Nervana Moustafa Bayoumy, et al.
Thymol Protects against 5-Fluorouracil-Induced Hepatotoxicity via the Regulation of the Akt/GSK-3β Pathway in In Vivo and In Silico Experimental Models
Reprinted from: *Pharmaceuticals* **2024**, *17*, 1094, https://doi.org/10.3390/ph17081094 . . . . **141**

Jun Yang, Kai Luo, Ziliang Guo, Renjie Wang, Qingyuan Qian, Shuhe Ma, Maoxing Li and Yue Gao
Evaluation of Crocetin as a Protective Agent in High Altitude Hypoxia-Induced Organ Damage
Reprinted from: *Pharmaceuticals* **2024**, *17*, 985, https://doi.org/10.3390/ph17080985 . . . . **160**

Lucas Sylvestre Silva, Eduardo Cavallini, Rafael André da Silva, Monielle Sant'Ana, Ariane Harumi Yoshikawa, Thiago Salomão, et al.
Garcinia brasiliensis Leaves Extracts Inhibit the Development of Ascitic and Solid Ehrlich Tumors
Reprinted from: *Pharmaceuticals* **2025**, *18*, 24, https://doi.org/10.3390/ph18010024 . . . . **182**

Md Shamshir Alam, Md Jamir Anwar, Manish Kumar Maity, Faizul Azam, Mariusz Jaremko and Abdul-Hamid Emwas
The Dynamic Role of Curcumin in Mitigating Human Illnesses: Recent Advances in Therapeutic Applications
Reprinted from: *Pharmaceuticals* **2024**, *17*, 1674, https://doi.org/10.3390/ph17121674 . . . . **206**

Ionela Daniela Popescu, Elena Codrici, Sevinci Pop, Tudor Emanuel Fertig, Maria Dudău, Iliuta Laurentiu Anghelache, et al.
Potential of Newly Synthesized Sea Buckthorn Phytocarriers as Anti-Inflammatory Active Agents
Reprinted from: *Pharmaceuticals* **2025**, *18*, 212, https://doi.org/10.3390/ph18020212 . . . . **236**

Yuliana García-Martínez, Amparo Celene Razo-Estrada, Ricardo Pérez-Pastén-Borja, Candelaria Galván-Colorado, Germán Chamorro-Cevallos, José Jorge Chanona-Pérez, et al.
Protective Effects of Phycobiliproteins from *Arthrospira maxima* (Spirulina) Against Cyclophosphamide-Induced Embryotoxicity and Genotoxicity in Pregnant CD1 Mice
Reprinted from: *Pharmaceuticals* **2025**, *18*, 101, https://doi.org/10.3390/ph18010101 . . . . **252**

Gabriela Castañeda-Corral, Mayra Cedillo-Cortezano, Magdalena Aviles-Flores, Misael López-Castillo, Juan José Acevedo-Fernández and Vera L. Petricevich
Antinociceptive and Anti-Inflammatory Activities of Acetonic Extract from *Bougainvillea x buttiana* (var. Rose)
Reprinted from: *Pharmaceuticals* **2024**, *17*, 1037, https://doi.org/10.3390/ph17081037 . . . . **271**

Caren Naomi Aguero Ito, Elisangela dos Santos Procopio, Natália de Matos Balsalobre, Lucas Luiz Machado, Saulo Euclides Silva-Filho, Taíse Fonseca Pedroso, et al.
Analgesic and Anti-Arthritic Potential of Methanolic Extract and Palmatine Obtained from *Annona squamosa* Leaves
Reprinted from: *Pharmaceuticals* **2024**, *17*, 1331, https://doi.org/10.3390/ph17101331 . . . . **293**

Salud Pérez-Gutiérrez, Nimsi Campos-Xolalpa, Sofía A. Estrada-Barajas, Alan Carrasco-Carballo, Angel Mendoza and Ernesto Sánchez-Mendoza
Anti-Inflammatory Activity of Two Labdane Enantiomers from *Gymnosperma glutinosum*: An *In Vivo*, *In Vitro*, and *In Silico* Study
Reprinted from: *Pharmaceuticals* **2025**, *18*, 516, https://doi.org/10.3390/ph18040516 . . . . **310**

Natália de M. Balsalobre, Elisangela dos Santos-Procopio, Cristhian S. Oliveira, Silvia C. Neves, Maria H. Verdan, Saulo E. Silva-Filho, et al.
The Anti-Arthritic Potential of the Ethanolic Extract of *Salvia Lachnostachys* Benth. Leaves and Icetexane Dinor-Diterpenoid Fruticuline B
Reprinted from: *Pharmaceuticals* **2025**, *17*, 1226, https://doi.org/10.3390/ph17091226 . . . . **326**

About the Editors

Maria de Lourdes Pereira

Maria de Lourdes Pereira is an Associate Professor with Habilitation at the Department of Medical Sciences, University of Aveiro, Portugal, with foundational training in Biology and decades of experience in biomedical research. Her scientific work encompasses biomaterials, natural products, toxicology, reproduction, and cellular biology, with numerous peer-reviewed publications and leadership in international scientific meetings. She has supervised many doctoral and master's students and contributed to collaborative projects linking natural compounds to biomedical applications. Her role as Guest Editor reflects her commitment to advancing evidence-based research on medicinal plant bioactivity and therapeutic development.

Veeranoot Nissapatorn

Veeranoot Nissapatorn is an Associate Professor at the School of Allied Health Sciences, Walailak University, Thailand, with medical training and advanced qualifications in clinical tropical medicine. She is an internationally recognized parasitologist with research interests in infectious parasitic diseases, waterborne parasites, epidemiology, and natural products, and plays active roles in international research networks such as the Southeast Asia Water Team and the World Union for Herbal Drug Discovery. Dr. Nissapatorn has published extensively, serves on editorial boards, and contributes as a reviewer and speaker in global scientific forums, bringing depth in infectious disease and pharmacological research.

Ana Paula Girol

Ana Paula Girol serves as Pro-Rector of Research and Post-Graduation at the Padre Albino University Center (UNIFIPA) in Catanduva, Brazil, and holds extensive academic experience in morphology, cell biology, histology, embryology, and molecular biology. She has developed research on herbal medicines and biomaterials in inflammatory and tumoral processes, including studies on mast cells and the annexin A1 protein, and coordinates experimental and translational projects involving medicinal plant extracts and bioactive compounds. In addition to her leadership roles in research and postgraduate training, she collaborates internationally and fosters multidisciplinary scientific development.

Sónia M. R. Oliveira

Sónia M. R. Oliveira is a researcher at CICECO - Aveiro Institute of Materials (Aveiro, Portugal) and affiliated with HMRI – Hunter Medical Research Institute (Newcastle, Australia). Her scientific interests encompass neurophysiology, cancer biology, reproductive and developmental biology, cellular and molecular biology, biomimetic systems, rare diseases, biomedicine, infectious diseases, and public health. Her interdisciplinary research bridges fundamental cellular mechanisms with translational biomedical applications, with particular emphasis on the therapeutic potential of bioactive compounds. She has contributed to several peer-reviewed publications and collaborative research projects focusing on neuroprotective and anticancer natural products. As Guest Editor of this Special Issue, she provides expertise in pharmacological evaluation and integrative approaches to plant-derived bioactive compounds.

Preface

This Reprint brings together selected research and review articles from the Special Issue 'Bioactive Compounds Derived from Plants and Their Medicinal Potential.' The collection emphasizes the multifaceted therapeutic properties of plant-derived compounds, including neuroprotection, anti-inflammation, anticancer activity, antimicrobial effects, and organ protection. Featuring experimental, computational, and review studies, the Reprint provides a comprehensive resource for understanding the pharmacological applications of natural products. It is intended for researchers, clinicians, and students seeking insights into the development of plant-based therapeutics and advances in bioactive compound research.

Maria de Lourdes Pereira, Veeranoot Nissapatorn, Ana Paula Girol, and Sonia M. R. Oliveira
Guest Editors

pharmaceuticals
MDPI

Editorial

Bioactive Compounds Derived from Plants and Their Medicinal Potential

Sónia M. R. Oliveira [1,*], Ana Paula Girol [2,*], Veeranoot Nissapatorn [3,*] and Maria de Lourdes Pereira [1,4,*]

1 CICECO-Aveiro Institute of Materials, University of Aveiro, 3810-193 Aveiro, Portugal
2 Experimental and Clinical Research Center (CEPEC), Padre Albino University Center (UNIFIPA), Catanduva 15809-144, SP, Brazil
3 Futuristic Science Research Center, School of Science, World Union for Herbal Drug Discovery and Research Excellence Center for Innovation and Health Products (RECIHP), Walailak University, Nakhon Si Thammarat 80160, Thailand
4 Department of Medical Sciences, University of Aveiro, 3810-193 Aveiro, Portugal
* Correspondence: sonia.oliveira@ua.pt (S.M.R.O.); anapaula.girol@unifipa.com.br (A.P.G.); veeranoot.ni@wu.ac.th (V.N.); mlourdespereira@ua.pt (M.d.L.P.)

The inaugural edition of the Special Issue "Bioactive compounds derived from plants and their medicinal potential" offers a comprehensive exploration of the therapeutic promise inherent in plant-based compounds. This collection of 17 studies highlights the diverse bioactivities of medicinal plants, including antimicrobial, anti-inflammatory, anti-cancer, and immunomodulatory effects, and their potential to address current therapeutic challenges. As previously established, plants are a source of bioactive compounds that play vital roles in pharmacotherapy, and serve as a foundation for emerging therapeutics and nutraceutical agents [1,2]. Together, these contributions employ a range of research methodologies, from in vitro assays to in vivo models, reflecting the dynamic and multidisciplinary nature of natural products pharmacology.

While technological advancements, including data science applications, are refining the study of plant-derived bioactive compounds, significant challenges remain. Among these is the difficulty of translating preclinical findings into clinical applications—the "bench-to-bedside" gap. Inconsistent efficacy and safety profiles observed in clinical trials often arise from the inherent complexity of plant extracts, variability in composition, and quality control issues.

This Special Issue addresses these gaps by presenting studies that not only examine the bioactivity of plant-derived compounds, but also investigate their mechanisms of action, explore synergistic effects, and evaluate opportunities for formulation and delivery improvements.

For example, Mateusz Kciuk et al. (2024) [3] provide a narrative synthesis on afzelin (kaempferol-3-O-rhamnoside), a flavonoid glycoside, highlighting its diverse bioactivities. Their review emphasizes afzelin's neuroprotective effects in neurodegenerative diseases and its anti-cancer properties, including the induction of apoptosis and inhibition of cancer cell proliferation. A systematic review by Syed Mohammed Basheeruddin Asdaq et al. (2024) [4] comprehensively analyzes in vitro and clinical studies on date palm extracts (*Phoenix dactylifera*), detailing their antioxidant, anti-inflammatory, and neurogenic effects. This work positions date palm extracts as promising natural therapies for neurodegenerative conditions.

Our Special Issue also includes novel research.

Vinícius Lopes Lessa et al. (2024) [5] investigated the citrus flavonoid naringenin using in vitro promastigote assays, fractional inhibitory concentrations, and isobologram in combination with miltefosine against *Leishmania amazonensis* (a cutaneous leishmaniasis pathogen), reporting advantages of this combination strategy. The combinatorial effect of naringenin and miltefosine against *Leishmania amazonensis* exemplifies the potential of integrating natural compounds into existing pharmaceutical drugs to enhance therapeutic efficacy.

Similarly, Fekandine V. Douti et al. (2025) [6] explored the effects of spices such as *Aframomum melegueta* and *Xylopia aethiopica* on taeniasis/cestoda. Through docking analyses of known phytochemicals—such as pungent phenolics and terpenoids—they identified promising interactions with helminth targets. Although in vivo validation and constituent isolation are needed, this study highlights the need for alternative treatments to combat parasitic infections.

In an in vivo study conducted by Meng-Ting Zeng (2024) [7], ethanolic extracts from the leaves and branches of several Cupressaceae conifer species (e.g., *Chamaecyparis lawsoniana, Cupressus sempervirens,* and *Platycladus orientalis*), demonstrated systemic protection. The extracts rapidly prevented arrhythmias in a barium chloride ($BaCl_2$)-induced arrhythmia model, an effect mediated through M2/M3 muscarinic receptors. This work represents the first in vivo demonstration of this rapid protective mechanism, elucidated with muscarinic antagonists.

Yasmen F. Mahran et al. (2024) [8] evaluated thymol (from *Thymus* spp.) in a rat model of 5-FU-induced liver injury (IP 150 mg/kg). Administering oral thymol at 60/120 mg/kg and using in silico analysis for pathway identification, the study revealed that thymol effectively reduces oxidative stress and apoptosis while modulating Akt/GSK-3beta and ERK1/2 pathways. These findings support thymol's potential as a therapeutic agent for chemotherapy-induced hepatotoxicity.

Additionally, Jun Yang et al. (2024) [9] investigated crocetin, a saffron carotenoid, in an animal model of high-altitude hypoxia. Their results showed that crocetin mitigates oxidative stress and inflammation, protecting organs from hypoxia-induced damage.

The scope of research extends to cancer and toxicity models as well.

In an Ehrlich tumor-bearing mouse model (ascitic and solid), Lucas Sylvestre Silva et al. (2025) [10] demonstrated that leaf extracts of *Garcinia brasiliensis* inhibited tumor growth and improved survival, suggesting antitumor bioactivity.

Targeting pain and inflammation, other authors used classic rodent models to investigate crude extracts of other valuable plant species.

Gabriela Castañeda-Corral et al. (2024) [11] demonstrated that an acetonic extract of *Bougainvillea x buttiana* has potent anti-nociceptive and anti-inflammatory effects, supporting its traditional medicinal use.

Caren Naomi Aguero Ito et al. (2024) [12] further demonstrated significant analgesic and anti-arthritic activities of methanolic extract and palmatine, an alkaloid derived from *Annona squamosa* leaves, substantiating their potential in pain and inflammation management.

Finally, Salud Pérez-Gutiérrez et al. (2025) [13] identified two labdane enantiomers from *Gymnosperma glutinosum* with anti-inflammatory activity through comprehensive in vivo, in vitro, and in silico studies. This research provides insights into these active enantiomers' mechanisms and potential therapeutic applications.

Infectious disease applications were also well represented.

Reem Binsuwaidan et al. (2024) [14] developed a lycopene–selenium nano-formulation exhibiting potent antibacterial, antioxidant, and anti-inflammatory properties. Characterized by FTIR, zeta potential, and particle size (~126 nm), the nanoparticles showed significant in vitro antioxidant and antibacterial effects and enhanced healing in a rat wound infection model. These findings suggest the formulation's promise as a multifunctional therapeutic agent against infection and inflammation.

Looking ahead, advancing plant-based therapeutics will require bridging the gap between laboratory research and clinical applications. This will require rigorous clinical trials, improved standardization of extraction and formulation methods, and advances in pharmacokinetics and pharmacodynamics modeling. At the same time, integrating machine learning and data science can accelerate compound discovery, support sustainable synthesis, and predict clinical outcomes.

Achieving these goals will require interdisciplinary collaboration, equitable access to funding, and responsible stewardship of natural resources. We are reminded that some of the most transformative and lucrative therapies today, such as paclitaxel (from *Taxus brevifolia, Pacific yew* tree), morphine (from *Papaver somniferous*, the *Opium poppy*), and artemisinin (from *Artemisia annua*, sweet wormwood), originated from persistence in investigating plant-based compounds—often against conventional expectations or in the face of skepticism—and today save millions of lives.

The contributions in this Special Issue reaffirm that same spirit of perseverance in reporting the untapped potential of plant-derived bioactive compounds in addressing pressing health challenges.

Funding: This research was funded by the Plant Genetic Conservation Project under Royal Initiative of Her Royal Highness Princess Maha Chakri Sirindhorn-Botanical Garden of Walailak University (Grant No. RSPG-WU-24/2568), and Project CICECO-Aveiro Institute of Materials UID/50011/2025 (DOI 10.54499/UID/50011/2025) & LA/P/0006/2020 (DOI 10.54499/LA/P/0006/2020), financed by national funds through the FCT/MCTES (PIDDAC).

Conflicts of Interest: The authors declare no conflict of interest.

References

1. Sanjai, C.; Gaonkar, S.L.; Hakkimane, S.S. Harnessing Nature's Toolbox: Naturally Derived Bioactive Compounds in Nanotechnology Enhanced Formulations. *ACS Omega* **2024**, *9*, 43302–43318. [CrossRef] [PubMed] [PubMed Central]
2. Dincheva, I.; Badjakov, I.; Galunska, B. New Insights in the Research on Bioactive Compounds from Plant Origins with Nutraceutical and Pharmaceutical Potential II. *Plants* **2025**, *14*, 500. [CrossRef] [PubMed]
3. Kciuk, M.; Garg, N.; Dhankhar, S.; Saini, M.; Mujwar, S.; Devi, S.; Chauhan, S.; Singh, T.G.; Singh, R.; Marciniak, B.; et al. Exploring the Comprehensive Neuroprotective and Anticancer Potential of Afzelin. *Pharmaceuticals* **2024**, *17*, 701. [CrossRef] [PubMed]
4. Asdaq, S.M.B.; Almutiri, A.A.; Alenzi, A.; Shaikh, M.; Shaik, M.A.; Alshehri, S.; Rabbani, S.I. Unveiling the Neuroprotective Potential of Date Palm (*Phoenix dactylifera*): A Systematic Review. *Pharmaceuticals* **2024**, *17*, 1221. [CrossRef] [PubMed]
5. Lessa, V.L.; Gonçalves, G.; Santos, B.; Cavalari, V.C.; da Costa Vieira, R.F.; Figueiredo, F.B. In Vitro Evaluation of the Combinatorial Effect of Naringenin and Miltefosine against *Leishmania amazonensis*. *Pharmaceuticals* **2024**, *17*, 1014. [CrossRef] [PubMed]
6. Douti, F.V.; Katawa, G.; Arndts, K.; Bara, F.D.; Awesso, E.R.; Karou, S.D.; Hoerauf, A.; Ritter, M. Potential of *Aframomum melegueta* and *Xylopia aethiopica* Against *Taenia* spp.: Plant-Based Remedies as Novel Anthelmintics. *Pharmaceuticals* **2025**, *18*, 749. [CrossRef] [PubMed]
7. Zeng, M.-T.; Huang, L.-Y.; Zheng, X.-H.; Fu, Y.-Q.; Weng, C.-F. Ethanolic Extracts of Cupressaceae Species *Conifers* Provide Rapid Protection against Barium Chloride-Induced Cardiac Arrhythmia. *Pharmaceuticals* **2024**, *17*, 1003. [CrossRef] [PubMed]
8. Mahran, Y.F.; Badr, A.M.; Al-Kharashi, L.A.; Alajami, H.N.; Aldamry, N.T.; Bayoumy, N.M.; Elmongy, E.I.; Soliman, S. Thymol Protects against 5-Fluorouracil-Induced Hepatotoxicity via the Regulation of the Akt/GSK-3β Pathway in In Vivo and In Silico Experimental Models. *Pharmaceuticals* **2024**, *17*, 1094. [CrossRef] [PubMed]
9. Yang, J.; Luo, K.; Guo, Z.; Wang, R.; Qian, Q.; Ma, S.; Li, M.; Gao, Y. Evaluation of Crocetin as a Protective Agent in High Altitude Hypoxia-Induced Organ Damage. *Pharmaceuticals* **2024**, *17*, 985. [CrossRef] [PubMed]
10. Silva, L.S.; Cavallini, E.; da Silva, R.A.; Sant'Ana, M.; Yoshikawa, A.H.; Salomão, T.; Huang, B.; Craice, P.; de Souza Ferreira, L.P.; Della Matta, H.P.; et al. *Garcinia brasiliensis* Leaves Extracts Inhibit the Development of Ascitic and Solid Ehrlich Tumors. *Pharmaceuticals* **2025**, *18*, 24. [CrossRef] [PubMed]
11. Castañeda-Corral, G.; Cedillo-Cortezano, M.; Aviles-Flores, M.; López-Castillo, M.; Acevedo-Fernández, J.J.; Petricevich, V.L. Antinociceptive and Anti-Inflammatory Activities of Acetonic Extract from *Bougainvillea x buttiana* (var. Rose). *Pharmaceuticals* **2024**, *17*, 1037. [CrossRef] [PubMed]

12. Ito, C.N.A.; Santos Procopio, E.d.; Balsalobre, N.d.M.; Machado, L.L.; Silva-Filho, S.E.; Pedroso, T.F.; Lourenço, C.C.d.; Oliveira, R.J.; Arena, A.C.; Salvador, M.J.; et al. Analgesic and Anti-Arthritic Potential of Methanolic Extract and Palmatine Obtained from *Annona squamosa* Leaves. *Pharmaceuticals* **2024**, *17*, 1331. [CrossRef] [PubMed]
13. Pérez-Gutiérrez, S.; Campos-Xolalpa, N.; Estrada-Barajas, S.A.; Carrasco-Carballo, A.; Mendoza, A.; Sánchez-Mendoza, E. Anti-Inflammatory Activity of Two Labdane Enantiomers from *Gymnosperma glutinosum*: An In Vivo, In Vitro, and In Silico Study. *Pharmaceuticals* **2025**, *18*, 516. [CrossRef] [PubMed]
14. Binsuwaidan, R.; El-Masry, T.A.; El-Nagar, M.M.F.; El Zahaby, E.I.; Gaballa, M.M.S.; El-Bouseary, M.M. Investigating the Antibacterial, Antioxidant, and Anti-Inflammatory Properties of a Lycopene Selenium Nano-Formulation: An In Vitro and In Vivo Study. *Pharmaceuticals* **2024**, *17*, 1600. [CrossRef] [PubMed]

pharmaceuticals

Review

Exploring the Comprehensive Neuroprotective and Anticancer Potential of Afzelin

Mateusz Kciuk [1,†], Nitika Garg [2,†], Sanchit Dhankhar [2], Monika Saini [3,4], Somdutt Mujwar [2,*], Sushma Devi [2], Samrat Chauhan [2,*], Thakur Gurjeet Singh [2], Randhir Singh [5], Beata Marciniak [1], Adrianna Gielecińska [1,6] and Renata Kontek [1]

1 Department of Molecular Biotechnology and Genetics, Faculty of Biology and Environmental Protection, University of Lodz, 12/16 Banacha St., 90-237 Lodz, Poland; mateusz.kciuk@biol.uni.lodz.pl (M.K.); beata.marciniak@biol.uni.lodz.pl (B.M.); adrianna.gielecinska@edu.uni.lodz.pl (A.G.); renata.kontek@biol.uni.lodz.pl (R.K.)
2 Chitkara College of Pharmacy, Chitkara University, Rajpura 140401, Punjab, India; nitikagarg1609@gmail.com (N.G.); sanchitdhankhar@gmail.com (S.D.); sushma.mehla@gmail.com (S.D.); gurjeet.singh@chitkara.edu.in (T.G.S.)
3 M. M. College of Pharmacy, Maharishi Markandeshwar (Deemed to be) University, Mullana, Ambala 133207, Haryana, India; monika210692@gmail.com
4 Swami Vivekanand College of Pharmacy, Ramnagar, Banur 140601, Punjab, India
5 Department of Pharmacology, Central University of Punjab, Bathinda 151401, Punjab, India; randhirsingh.dahiya@gmail.com
6 Doctoral School of Exact and Natural Sciences, University of Lodz, 90-237 Lodz, Poland
* Correspondence: somduttmujwar@gmail.com (S.M.); samrat.chauhan11@gmail.com (S.C.)
† These authors contributed equally to this work.

Abstract: Neurodegenerative diseases (Alzheimer's disease, Parkinson's disease, Huntington's disease, and others) and cancer, seemingly disparate in their etiology and manifestation, exhibit intriguing associations in certain cellular and molecular processes. Both cancer and neurodegenerative diseases involve the deregulation of cellular processes such as apoptosis, proliferation, and DNA repair and pose a significant global health challenge. Afzelin (kaempferol 3-O-rhamnoside) is a flavonoid compound abundant in various plant sources. Afzelin exhibits a diverse range of biological activities, offering promising prospects for the treatment of diseases hallmarked by oxidative stress and deregulation of cell death pathways. Its protective potential against oxidative stress is also promising for alleviating the side effects of chemotherapy. This review explores the potential therapeutic implications of afzelin, including its capacity to mitigate oxidative stress, modulate inflammation, and promote cellular regeneration in neurodegenerative and cancer diseases.

Keywords: afzelin; neurodegeneration; neuroinflammation; Alzheimer's disease; Parkinson's disease; cancer

1. Introduction

Neurodegenerative diseases are complex conditions that share the characteristics of cell death and malfunctioning of neurons. These conditions, sometimes referred to as geriatric diseases, are primarily characterized by a gradual degeneration of neurons, ultimately leading to the decline of crucial cognitive, motor, and sensory skills [1–3]. The defining features of Alzheimer's disease, a prevalent neurodegenerative disorder, involve the development of aberrant protein aggregates in the brain, including beta-amyloid plaques and tau tangles. The presence of these aggregates hinders the transmission of brain signals and induces an inflammatory response, both of which are implicated in the development of cognitive dysfunction [4,5]. Similarly, Parkinson's disease is defined by the degeneration of dopaminergic neurons in the substantia nigra, which ultimately leads to the death of these neurons. The depletion of neurons leads to motor dysfunctions characterized by tremors, rigidity, and bradykinesia [6]. In contrast, Huntington's disease arises as a consequence of a genetic mutation that results in the misfolding of proteins. This phenomenon results in a progressive deterioration of cognitive and physical functions. The neuronal cell loss implicated in amyotrophic lateral sclerosis (ALS), colloquially referred to as Lou Gehrig's disease, is accountable for muscle atrophy, culminating in eventual paralysis [7]. Various types of neurodegeneration, including multiple sclerosis (MS) [8] and frontotemporal dementia (FTD) [9], are characterized by specific patterns of neuronal degeneration and exhibit diverse manifestations across the brain and spinal cord [10]. Despite their intended objectives of symptom relief and disease progression cessation, conventional therapies often fail to provide comprehensive solutions. The examination of diverse natural compounds has arisen as a feasible avenue to harness the potential of nature's abundant medicinal properties to treat these intricate disorders. Natural chemicals are derived from diverse sources, encompassing plants, herbs, fungi, and marine life [11]. Within the research area of neurodegenerative disorder treatments, some naturally occurring compounds have garnered interest because of their inherent neuroprotective, anti-inflammatory, antioxidative, and modulatory properties. For example, curcumin (a compound extracted from turmeric), resveratrol (derived from red grapes), and flavonoids (isolated from citrus fruits) have all demonstrated neuroprotective properties in various studies. These compounds are believed to provide neuroprotection due to their impact on inflammation and toxic protein aggregation-induced neuronal injury. Furthermore, it was shown that naturally derived compounds possess the capacity to regulate cellular pathways that play a critical role in the survival and proliferation of cells [12–14].

The increasing prevalence of cancer and the limitations of conventional therapies have spurred a growing interest in exploring alternative treatment modalities, particularly the use of natural products. Bioactive compounds such as polyphenols, alkaloids, terpenoids, and flavonoids have exhibited potent anti-proliferative, anti-angiogenic, and pro-apoptotic effects across a spectrum of cancer types. Moreover, the potential synergistic interactions between natural products and conventional anti-cancer therapies are explored. Evidence suggests that natural products can enhance the efficacy of chemotherapy and radiotherapy while mitigating their adverse effects. The modulation of drug resistance mechanisms and the promotion of sensitization to standard therapies underscore the promising role of natural products in combination regimens [15].

Oxidative stress, which is caused by an imbalance between reactive oxygen species (ROS) and antioxidants, is also an essential factor in the pathophysiology of neurodegenerative diseases [16–19] and cancer [20–22]. Natural compounds, such as vitamin E [23,24], vitamin C [25,26], or flavonoids, can scavenge dangerous free radicals, thereby minimizing the amount of oxidative damage that is caused to neurons. This antioxidative capability goes beyond only protecting cells; it also has the potential to influence the signaling cascades and gene expression inside the cells [27,28].

Flavonoids represent a class of polyphenolic compounds that are widely distributed across the plant kingdom. Afzelin (Figure 1), also known as kaempferol 3-O-rhamnoside, is a flavonoid compound that can be found in high concentrations in a wide variety of plant sources. The diverse range of biological activities, including the antioxidative properties exhibited by afzelin, holds a significant translational potential of this compound in the prevention and therapy of cancer and neurodegenerative diseases manifested by oxidative stress and deregulation of cell death pathways [29–32]. Moreover, intrinsic links have been discovered between oxidative stress and inflammation. Therefore, the ROS-scavenging effects of afzelin could mitigate neuroinflammation, which constitutes a characteristic feature of neurodegenerative disorders such as Alzheimer's disease and Parkinson's disease [33,34].

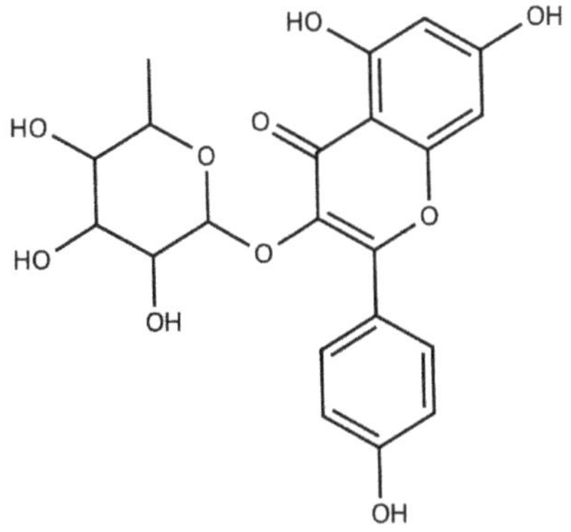

Figure 1. Chemical structure of kaempferol 3-O-rhamnoside (Afzelin).

2. Sources and Pharmacological Profile of Afzelin

The anti-bacterial, anti-inflammatory, antioxidant, and cytoprotective effects of afzelin have been supported by numerous studies [29–32].

Afzelin come from a variety of different places, including but not limited to the following:

Houttuynia cordata: The plant under consideration is native to Southeast Asia and possesses a rich historical background in its utilization within traditional medicinal practices. Its applications encompass a diverse array of diseases, such as cancer, inflammation, infection, and fever. The main flavonoids found in the *Houttuynia cordata* plant include afzelin, quercetin, and hyperoside [35,36].

Nymphaea odorata: The plant is native to North America and is alternatively referred to as the American white waterlily. This botanical remedy has a long-standing medicinal history, as it was historically used for the treatment of skin conditions, wounds, inflammation, and cancer. Afzelin, kaempferol, quercetin, myricetin, and gallic acid represent abundant phenolic compounds found in this plant [37,38].

Kalanchoe pinnata: This plant is commonly known as an 'air plant' or 'miracle leaf' and is native to regions in Africa and Asia. The *Kalanchoe pinnata* plant has been employed in traditional medicinal practices for the treatment of various diseases, including ulcers, asthma, coughing, and diarrhea. Afzelin represents one of the flavonoids present in this plant. Others include quercitrin, quercetin, kaempferol, and rutin. The hepatoprotective benefits of afzelin, derived from *Kalanchoe pinnata*, have been demonstrated, indicating its potential to mitigate liver damage induced by carbon tetrachloride [39–42].

Quercus spp. (Oak Trees): Oak trees are renowned for their impressive stature in woodland areas and natural environments. Additionally, they offer a wide array of biologically active secondary metabolites, including afzelin. Afzelin is present in several anatomical components of oak trees, encompassing their foliage, bark, and reproductive structures, such as acorns. *Quercus* species exhibit a wide range of climatic and geographical distributions. Variability in the concentration of afzelin in *Quercus* plants can be attributed to several factors, including species differences, the conditions under which the plant is growing, and the age of the plant [43,44].

Filipendula ulmaria (Meadowsweet): This perennial herbaceous plant is native to both Europe and Asia. It has a rich history of application in the practice of herbal medicine. Afzelin found in meadowsweet is responsible for the pain-relieving and anti-inflammatory effects of the herb [45].

Hawthorn (*Crataegus* spp.): This plant belongs to the *Rosaceae* family and is well-known for its beneficial effects on the cardiovascular system. The antioxidative and vasorelaxant properties of hawthorn can be partially attributed to the presence of afzelin in the plant [46,47].

The natural sources of afzelin were summarized in Figure 2.

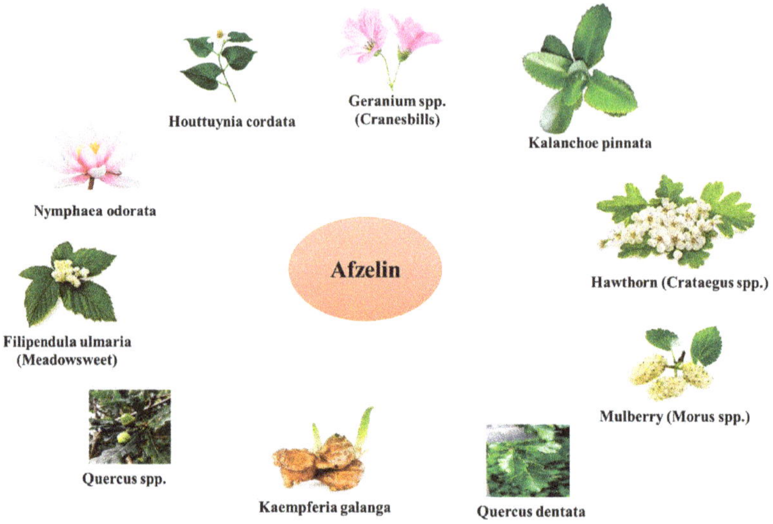

Figure 2. Natural sources of afzelin.

3. Biological Activity of Afzelin

3.1. Antioxidative Effects of Afzelin

Oxidative stress arises from a state of disequilibrium between the generation and buildup of ROS within cells and tissues, as well as the capacity of a biological system to effectively neutralize these reactive byproducts. ROS fulfill various physiological functions, such as cell signaling, and are typically produced as byproducts of oxygen metabolism. However, exposure to environmental stressors like UV radiation, ionizing radiation, pollutants, and heavy metals, as well as the presence of xenobiotics, significantly enhance ROS production. Consequently, this imbalance results in oxidative stress, leading to cellular and tissue damage [48]. Afzelin's potential therapeutic applications in the context of neurodegenerative illnesses and cancer could be mainly attributed to the chemical's ability to alter redox signaling pathways and prevent oxidative stress [30,49–51] through the following:

- Scavenging of free radicals: Highly reactive chemicals, such as free radicals and ROS, can oxidatively damage biological components like DNA, proteins, and lipids [52]. Afzelin has been found to possess ROS-scavenging characteristics, suggesting it can neutralize the effects of dangerous compounds through interaction with them [53,54].
- Metal chelation: Afzelin also possesses metal chelation capabilities, making it possible for it to bind to metal ions such as those of iron and copper. These metal ions are well-known to have a role in the generation of free radicals via the Fenton and Haber-Weiss reactions. Afzelin is effective in blocking the generation of ROS because of its binding affinity for these metals [55–57].
- Activation of nuclear factor erythroid 2-related factor 2 (NRF2) pathway: The NRF2 pathway plays a significant role in the regulation of the antioxidant response in cells via transcriptional control of many target genes involved in the maintenance of oxidation-reduction homeostasis inside the cell. The antioxidative actions of kaempferol and its derivatives, including afzelin, extend to the protection of cellular components like cell membranes and mitochondria from the destructive effects of oxidation. Thereby, afzelin may contribute to the maintenance of proper cellular function by preserving the structural integrity of these components [58].

Mitochondria are crucial for the various biochemical activities that are fundamental to the survival of cells. The morphology of mitochondria undergoes alterations in response to external stimuli and metabolic fluctuations through the processes of fission and fusion, collectively known as mitochondrial dynamics. The elimination of impaired mitochondria is facilitated through a cellular mechanism referred to as mitophagy, wherein these damaged organelles undergo breakdown via a distinct autophagosomal pathway. In recent years, significant endeavors have been undertaken to examine the influence of mitochondrial dysfunction manifested by excessive production of ROS, disturbances in mitochondrial calcium homeostasis, depletion of adenosine triphosphate (ATP), impairments in mitochondrial dynamics and transport, and deficiencies in mitophagy on the development of Alzheimer's disease [59,60], Parkinson's disease [61,62], other neurodegenerative diseases [63], and cancer [64,65].

Lee et al. investigated the cytoprotective mechanisms of afzelin against D-galactosamine (GalN)/lipopolysaccharide (LPS)-induced fulminant hepatic failure (FHF), with a specific emphasis on mitochondrial quality control and dynamics. The findings of the study demonstrated that the administration of the flavonoid compound resulted in enhanced survival rates and decreased levels of alanine aminotransferase and pro-inflammatory cytokines in mice that were treated with GalN/LPS. Afzelin contributed to a reduction in mitochondrial damage in mice treated with GalN/LPS, as evidenced by a decrease in mitochondrial swelling and a reduction in the mitochondrial glutamate dehydrogenase activity. The administration of afzelin resulted in an augmentation of mitochondrial biogenesis, as evidenced by elevated levels of PPAR-γ coactivator 1α (PGC-1α), nuclear respiratory factor 1 (NRF1), and mitochondrial transcription factor A (TFAM) [31].

PGC-1α has been shown to exert a protective effect on neuroblastoma cells by mitigating neuronal mortality and neuroinflammation produced by amyloid-beta (Aβ). Additionally, the neuroprotective impact of PGC-1α is governed by the nuclear factor kappa B (NF-κB) pathway [66]. There is evidence to suggest that PGC-1α plays a crucial role in the preservation of neuronal viability and the facilitation of synaptic transmission. Changes in the levels of PGC-1α expression were observed in patients with neurodegenerative disorders, including Alzheimer's [67]. The down-regulation of PGC-1α in various brain regions, such as the hippocampus, substantia nigra (SN), cortex, striatum, and spinal cord, has been observed in animal and cellular models of neurodegenerative diseases. This down-regulation is associated with neurological damage, including oxidative stress, neuronal loss, and motor disorders. The existing body of evidence suggests that the overexpression of PGC-1α may offer a promising therapeutic strategy in mitigating the onset and advancement of neuronal damage [68]. Changes and adjustments in cellular metabolism are distinctive characteristics of cancer cells; therefore, it is unsurprising that PGC-1α has a function in cancer. Recent papers have demonstrated that the expression of PGC-1α is changed in metastatic tumors because of alterations in cellular metabolism, as recently reviewed [69].

TFAM is an important protein for genome maintenance as it binds to and stabilizes mitochondrial DNA (mtDNA). Multiple neurodegenerative diseases exhibit alterations in mtDNA and TFAM protein levels. In studies of neurodegenerative models, it has been observed that the levels of mtDNA exhibit a reduction of approximately 30%. In both cellular and animal models of neurodegeneration, the overexpression of TFAM and the administration of TFAM replacement therapy demonstrated significantly enhanced brain function and composition [70].

Furthermore, afzelin use was associated with the reduction in the expression of mitophagy-associated proteins, namely parkin (PARKIN) and PTEN-induced putative kinase 1 (PINK1) [31]. The signaling pathways involving PINK1 and PARKIN are crucial in regulating mitophagy. PINK1 exhibits an accumulation at the outer mitochondrial membrane (OMM) as a result of a decrease in mitochondrial membrane potential ($\Delta\Psi$m) due to injury or malfunction. Consequently, this process induces the translocation of PARKIN from the cytosol to the OMM, where its E3 enzymatic activity facilitates mitophagy by ubiquitinating mitochondrial proteins, ultimately resulting in the degeneration of mitochondria. Neurodegenerative disorders such as Alzheimer's disease and Parkinson's disease [71] or cancer [72,73] often exhibit the presence of defective mitophagy and aberrant

PINK1/PARKIN signaling pathways. In addition, it was observed that the administration of GalN/LPS resulted in a substantial elevation in the expression of dynamin-related protein 1 (DNM1L), a protein associated with fission processes, while concurrently causing a reduction in the expression of mitofusin 2 (MFN2), a protein involved in fusion processes. However, the impact of GalN/LPS on these protein levels was mitigated by the presence of afzelin [31].

It has been shown that kaempferol-3-O-β-D-glucuronate or afzelin inhibits neuroinflammation by preventing the phosphorylation of mitogen-activated protein kinases (MAPKs) [74,75] and also boosts antioxidant defenses by increasing the activity of the NRF2/heme oxygenase-1 (HO-1) signaling pathway possibly via glycogen synthase kinase-3β (GSK-3β) inhibition [50]. NRF2 constitutes a pivotal transcription factor that is of significant importance in the cellular response to oxidative stress and the maintenance of redox equilibrium in cells. The fundamental role of this NRF2 is to control the activation of several antioxidant and detoxification proteins in reaction to oxidative stress and other stressors present in the environment. NRF2 facilitates the transcriptional activation of a diverse array of genes that encode antioxidant enzymes, phase II detoxification enzymes, and other proteins that safeguard cellular integrity. The genes encompassed in this set include HO-1, NAD(P)H quinone oxidoreductase 1 (NQO1), glutathione S-transferases (GSTs), and superoxide dismutase (SOD). Several studies have shown that activation of the NRF2 signaling pathway can protect neuronal cells against oxidative stress, as reviewed by many authors [76–78], and its activation could constitute an important approach to the treatment of Alzheimer's disease [79], Parkinson's disease [78], ALS [80], and other movement disorders [81]. On the other hand, the NRF2 signaling pathway can act as a double-edged sword in cancer. The NRF2 pathway protects against exogenous chemical-induced oxidative damage. It regulates downstream cytoprotective genes to preserve redox equilibrium and has anti-inflammatory and anti-cancer actions, ensuring cell survival. Aberrant NRF2 activity is related to poor prognosis in cancer patients. Constitutive NRF2 activation in malignancies increases cancer cell proliferation by metabolic reprogramming, suppression of apoptosis, and enhanced self-renewal potential of cancer stem cells. Furthermore, NRF2 is linked to cancer cell chemoresistance and radioresistance [82]. HO-1 is an enzyme that performs a pivotal function in the process of heme catabolism, which entails the degradation of heme into biliverdin, carbon monoxide (CO), and iron [83]. HO-1 is a member of the heme oxygenase enzyme family, alongside another isoform—heme oxygenase-2 (HO-2). However, HO-2 differs from HO-1 in terms of its tissue distribution and regulatory function [84]. Biliverdin undergoes conversion into bilirubin by the catalytic action of an enzyme known as biliverdin reductase. Bilirubin possesses antioxidant capabilities that contribute to cellular protection against oxidative stress through its ability to scavenge free radicals [85]. HO-1 also plays a crucial role in the modulation of the immune response and the regulation of inflammation. It can inhibit the synthesis of pro-inflammatory molecules and enhance the synthesis of anti-inflammatory cytokines, thereby facilitating the mitigation of inflammation [86,87]. The phenomenon of HO-1 overexpression has been linked to the recovery of numerous ailments, such as cardiovascular diseases, neurodegenerative disorders, and different inflammatory conditions. The stimulation of HO-1 activity has the potential to ameliorate tissue damage and facilitate tissue regeneration. The potential therapeutic targeting of HO-1 and its associated targets have been extensively investigated due to their protective and anti-inflammatory effects across a range of disorders. Efforts are currently undertaken to pharmacologically stimulate the expression of HO-1 or regulate its functionality as a potential therapeutic approach for illnesses that are characterized by the presence of oxidative stress and inflammation [88–91].

Anti-Inflammatory Effects of Afzelin

Neuroinflammation, a complex immune response that occurs within the central nervous system (CNS), is an underlying factor that is shared by many of these conditions. Neuroinflammation plays a significant role in neuronal damage and the unrelenting pro gression of these diseases when it is dysregulated. The activation of glial cells, namely microglia and astrocytes, in pathological states such as Alzheimer's disease, Parkinson's disease, and MS initiates an intricate cascade of events leading to the secretion of pro-inflammatory mediators, cytokines, chemokines, and ROS. The aberrant immune response contributes to the perpetuation of neurotoxicity and intensifies neuronal cell death. This topic was covered in excellent review papers by multiple authors and will not be discussed here in detail [92–97]. Chronic inflammation has emerged as a pivotal contributor to cancer initiation, progression, and metastasis, representing a dynamic and intricate interplay between the immune system and tumorigenesis. Inflammatory responses, intended as protective mechanisms against infections or tissue damage, can become persistently activated, fostering a microenvironment conducive to carcinogenesis [98].

Focusing on afzelin, its anti-inflammatory properties are believed to stem from its interactions at the molecular level with several cellular processes and components associated with the inflammatory response [30,35,99]. Elevated concentrations of nitric oxide (NO), mostly generated by the synthesis of inducible nitric oxide synthase (iNOS) in glial cells, have been discovered to induce neuronal cell death by inhibiting neuronal mitochondrial cytochrome oxidase. Therefore, targeting NO signaling with natural compounds can constitute a feasible approach. Afzelin was shown to act as an inhibitor of NO production with an IC_{50} value of 42.8 μg/mL with comparable efficacy to nitric oxide inhibitor L-NMMA used in the experiment as a positive control (IC_{50} of 42.1 μg/mL) [100]. Furthermore, interleukin-1 beta (IL-1), interleukin-6 (IL-6), and tumor necrosis factor-alpha (TNF-α) production were shown to be down-regulated by afzelin treatment suggesting that this compound can dampen the inflammation in the human skin for effective prevention of skin cancers [101,102]. The administration of flavonoids, specifically quercitrin, isoquercitrin, and afzelin, to human neuroblastoma SH-SY5Y cells have demonstrated advantageous outcomes via modulating inflammation, apoptosis (through inhibition of caspase activation), and ROS-scavenging [103,104]. In contrast, the pro-apoptotic properties of afzelin in cancer cells may account for its anti-cancer effects [105,106], as described in the following sections of this work (Figure 3).

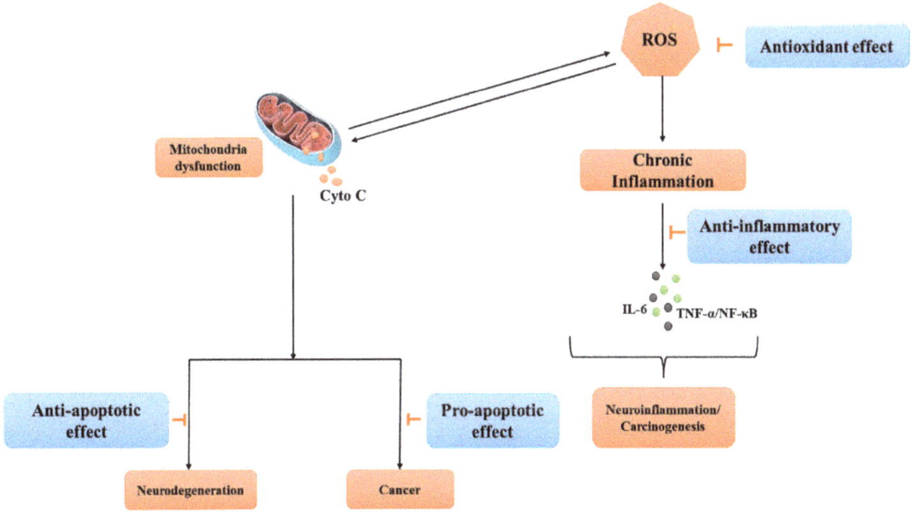

Figure 3. Antioxidative, anti-inflammatory, and anti/pro-apoptotic effects of afzelin.

3.2. *Neuroprotective and Neurogenic Effects*

Brain-derived neurotrophic factor (BDNF) is a member of the neurotrophin protein family and works as a pivotal growth factor required for the integrity, individuality, and adaptability of neuronal populations [107]. BDNF is broadly expressed in the mammalian brain, with especially high levels in the hippocampus and parahippocampal regions, both of which are involved in memory formation. Its expression is modulated dynamically in response to external cues and internal states, which at the molecular level involves the cooperation of multiple events, including transcriptional control, epigenetic processes, and post-translational modifications. BDNF interacts with its receptors, tropomyosin kinase B (TRKB) and P75 neurotrophin receptor (P75NTR), to play an important role in synaptic transmission and activity-dependent plasticity [108]. By interacting with these proteins, BDNF triggers a cascade of signaling events that control gene expression, synaptic strength, neuronal shape, and neurogenesis. In addition, BDNF is involved in a wide variety of physiological and pathological processes, including nutritional control, stress response, aging, neurodegeneration, and neuropsychiatric diseases. Changes in BDNF expression levels are associated with Alzheimer's disease, Parkinson's disease, Huntington's disease, and other forms of neurodegeneration [109,110]. As a consequence of this, BDNF is being investigated as a potential therapeutic target for neurological conditions. An increase in the synthesis of BDNF has been suggested as a therapeutic avenue for neurodegenerative disease treatment [109,111].

The introduction of afzelin into the mice brains on a chronic schedule resulted in the improvement of synaptic plasticity and cognitive/memory functions in animals that were administered scopolamine. Research conducted on the hippocampi of mice has demonstrated that the restorative effects observed in the cholinergic systems and molecular signal transduction through cyclic AMP response element-binding protein (CREB)-BDNF pathways can be attributed to the response elicited by afzelin. It was demonstrated that the administration of afzelin resulted in enhanced neurocognitive and neuroprotective effects on synaptic plasticity and behaviors, partially attributed to the up-regulation of CREB-BDNF signaling [112]. Moreover, the increased BDNF production may promote neuroprotective activity in hippocampal neurons through the stimulation of phosphatidylinositol 3-kinase (PI3K) and RAS/MAPK pathways and consequent abrogation of apoptotic cell death as evidenced by reduced caspase activity and increased B-cell lymphoma 2 (BCL2) protein expression [113]

Aldose reductase (AR) is an enzymatic protein responsible for the conversion of glucose into sorbitol within the NADPH-dependent polyol pathway of glucose metabolism. AR plays a pivotal role in the activation of microglia and the progression of retinal neurodegeneration. The activation of surveillance microglia occurs with the application or deposition of β-amyloid, subsequently leading to the formation of ROS, increased release of TNF-α, and enhanced phagocytosis. These processes collectively contribute to the death of neurons. The enhanced migratory capacity of microglia may result in cerebral injury. The inhibition of AR activity has the potential to impede the activation and migration of microglia, hence offering a potential therapeutic strategy for mitigating neuronal cell death and decelerating the progression of Alzheimer's disease [114]. Afzelin was shown to act as an AR inhibitor with an IC_{50} concentration of 1.91 μM compared with 12.87 μM estimated for kaempferol and could constitute one of the underlying causes of down-regulation of inflammatory mediators expression observed during the study [115], as shown for other AR inhibitors. These effects can be attributed to the modulation of MAPK and NF-κB-mediated pathways [116].

The areas inside the brain that are responsible for the production of significant quantities of neuromelanin (NM), a dark cytoplasmic pigment, are limited to the SN and locus coeruleus (LC). Evidence suggests that NM serves an initial protective function by isolating toxic catecholamine metabolites and heavy metals. However, it is posited that this protective role may transition into a destructive one during the aging process, especially in the context of Parkinson's disease. This transition occurs as the aforementioned toxic substances accumulate to a point where they overpower cellular recovery machinery and are subsequently released during the process of neurodegeneration. The accumulation of NM was linked to the occurrence of neurodegeneration, as well as a strong neuroinflammatory response [117]. The process of synthesizing human NM is considered to be analogous to the generation of melanin in melanocytes. In the skin, melanin synthesis occurs through the conversion of DOPAquinone (DQ) by the enzyme tyrosinase. On the other hand, NM synthesis in neurons takes place through the conversion of dopamine quinone (DAQ) by the enzymes tyrosine hydroxylase (TH) and aromatic L-amino acid decarboxylase (AADC). Dopamine within the cytoplasm exhibits a high level of reactivity and is thought to undergo spontaneous oxidation or be oxidized by an undiscovered tyrosinase enzyme, resulting in the formation of DAQ. Subsequently, DAQ is converted into NM. The buildup of intracellular NM over a certain threshold has been documented to be linked to the death of dopaminergic neurons and the manifestation of symptoms associated with Parkinson's disease. Therefore, tyrosinase inhibition could constitute a potential therapeutic approach in this neurodegenerative disease [118].

Rho et al. aimed to assess the tyrosinase inhibitory activity of the ethanolic extract derived from the leaves of kenaf (*Hibiscus cannabinus* L.) both before and after exposure to far-infrared (FIR) irradiation. No inhibitory activity of the extract was seen in a tyrosinase enzymatic activity experiment before FIR irradiation. Nevertheless, when subjecting it to FIR, a noteworthy degree of tyrosinase inhibitory activity (IC_{50} = 3500 ppm) was detected. The high-performance liquid chromatography (HPLC) examination revealed the presence of derhamnosylation products, specifically kaempferol, afzelin, and α-rhamnoisorobin. The observed inhibitory activity could perhaps be attributed to the presence of derhamnosylation products [119].

Afzelin is one of 28 metabolites revealed by liquid chromatography–tandem mass spectrometry (LC-MS/MS) in the ethanolic extract of *Polygonum minus*. Studies of neuroprotection against H_2O_2-induced oxidative stress performed on differentiated SH-SY5Y cells revealed activation of NRF2/antioxidant response element (ARE), NF-κB/IκB, and MAPK signaling pathways. A 48 h pre-incubation of cells with PMEE extract resulted in a significant up-regulation of *NRF2, NQO1, SOD1, SOD2,* and catalase gene expression levels compared to both PMEE extract and H_2O_2 treatments. A similar effect was observed for *MAPK8* (JNK), *MAPK14* (p38), and *PPP2CA* (PP2A) genes. Also, there are various in silico and molecular docking studies that showed that afzelin was one of the compounds present in the *Polygonum minus* extract with the highest stability and docking score [120].

Acetylcholine (ACH) is a neurotransmitter that may play a positive role in modulating the cellular response to oxidative stress by regulating antioxidant processes, mitochondrial function, and protection against negative effects resulting from excess ROS. In some neurodegenerative diseases like Alzheimer's disease, low levels of ACH are observed. Acetylcholinesterase (AChE) is an enzyme responsible for metabolizing the ACH into acetic acid and choline, which allow for the termination of the signal transmission at the synapses. AChE inhibitors have beneficial effects in certain neurological conditions by temporarily enhancing cholinergic neurotransmission [121]. Under conditions of H_2O_2-induced oxidative stress, prior administration of PMEE increased ACH concentration in differentiated SH-SY5Y cells supernatant. Molecular docking results showed that afzelin was one of the three compounds present in the *Polygonum minus* ethanolic extract with the highest docking score to AChE [120].

3.3. *Anti-Cancer Effects of Afzelin*

Flavonoids, which include flavonol glycoside, have long been studied for their anti-cancer effects. In the case of afzelin, recent years have yielded the results of the few studies to date that indicate the potential to induce cell death and inhibit tumor proliferation in an in vitro model. Androgen-sensitive LNCaP and androgen-independent PC-3 cell lines were used in one of the anti-cancer activity studies on afzelin. The investigation revealed that afzelin, at a concentration of 1 μg/mL, caused a significant decrease in prostate cancer cell proliferation after 24 h incubation. Flow cytometry cell cycle evaluation showed accumulation of PC-3 and LNCaP cells in the G_0 phase (27.6% and 19.4% of the population, respectively) after 10 μg/mL afzelin exposure and indicated the occurrence of extensive apoptosis or an ongoing cytotoxic response. At the molecular level, afzelin suppressed Rho GTPase family proteins such as LIM domain kinase 1 (LIMK1), myotonic dystrophy kinase-related Cdc42-binding kinase α (MRCKα), and Rho-associated coiled-coil-containing protein kinase (ROCK1) expression. The Rho GTPase family is intricately linked to the modulation of actin cytoskeleton arrangement, mediation of the focal adhesions, stress fiber formation, and regulation of cell proliferation and differentiation via activation of different proteins. Expression of LIMK1 is observed to be elevated in prostate cancer cells, while ROCK1 and MRCKα are involved in its activation. In examined prostate cancer cells, a reduction in the phosphorylation level of the aforementioned proteins was detected dependent on the concentration of afzelin tested [38].

Suppression of cell migration of highly invasive MDA-MB-231 triple-negative breast cancer (TNBC) cells following afzelin treatment was shown to be mediated by focal adhesion kinase (FAK) and Ras-related C3 botulinum toxin substrate 1 (RAC1) deregulation. FAK and RAC1 proteins interact in signaling pathways that control the organization of the cytoskeleton and the dynamics of focal adhesions, which in turn affect cell migration processes. Afzelin induced moderate cytotoxicity of MDA-MB-231 cells (IC_{50} = 992 μg/mL); however, at the same time, it actively reduced focal adhesion formation in a concentration-dependent manner. Because FAK and RAC1 are often excessively activated in numerous tumor types, they increase the likelihood of invasion and metastasis, which correlates with a worse prognosis for patients. Afzelin at 400 and 800 μg/mL significantly reduced RAC1 GTPase activation by 60% compared to the negative control, while the highest concentration also reduced FAK and phosphorylated FAK (pFAK) expression [122]. Additionally, Rachimi et al., using the reverse docking method, confirmed the inhibitory potential of afzelin toward molecular targets relevant to TNBC, including FAK, ERK2, and KRAS [123].

The pro-apoptotic efficacy of afzelin has been assessed in vitro in a variety of cancer cell types. For instance, kaempferol-3-O-rhamnoside isolated from leaves of *Schima wallichii* Korth was able to reduce the proliferation of MCF-7 human breast cancer cells. The findings demonstrated that afzelin triggers apoptotic mechanisms through activation of the caspase signaling pathway [124]. Afzelin was found to induce apoptotic cell death in gastric cancer cells (AGS) [105] as well as lung cancer cells (A549 and H1299) [106]. In the case of A549 cells, exposure to 60 and 120 μM afzelin resulted in an increase in the mRNA levels (an increase of 30% and 80%, respectively) of the pro-apoptotic factor BAX in comparison with non-treated cells. Increased afzelin concentrations resulted in stimulation of the caspase cascade, with the involvement of both caspase 8 and caspase 9 [105]. In a study using a model of lung cancer, characteristic indicators of immunogenic cell death, such as calreticulin exposure or high-mobility group box 1 (HMGB1) and ATP release, were observed [106].

4. ADMET Properties of Afzelin

Afzelin was shown to reach a maximal concentration of 211.02 ± 27.97 μg/L at a t_{max} = 0.83 ± 0.26 h, following administration of the inflorescence of *Polygonum orientale* at a concentration of 0.3 g/mL, which is comparable to a crude herb dosage of 86 g/kg or an extract dosage of 3 g/kg. This dosage constituted six times the recommended daily dose for an adult [125].

The study conducted by Alves et al. provided evidence indicating that hydroalcoholic extract of *Copaifera lansdorffii* Desf. (CLE) did not exhibit genotoxic effects in the mouse micronucleus experiment. The administration of CLE plus doxorubicin to animals resulted in a considerable reduction in the number of micronuclei, as compared to animals that were treated only with doxorubicin [126]. The protective effects of afzelin and quercitrin against the cytotoxicity induced by doxorubicin or methyl methanesulfonate (MMS) in V79 and HepG2 cell lines were investigated using the same extract. Moreover, it was observed that CLE did not elicit a statistically significant alteration in the occurrence of chromosomal abnormalities and micronuclei in the tested cells. Additionally, the number of revertants in the Ames test remained the same, indicating the absence of its mutagenic effects. On the other hand, it was observed that CLE exhibited anti-genotoxic properties in mammalian cells. The administration of afzelin and quercitrin showed a reduction in genotoxicity generated by MMS in HepG2 cells. The observed antigenotoxic impact of CLE in this study could potentially be ascribed, at least in part, to the antioxidative activity of the combined main components, namely afzelin and quercitrin [127].

Afzelin is widely recognized for its antioxidative characteristics [128], which can be seen from its capacity to scavenge various oxidative species. Despite its beneficial properties, it was found to induce cytotoxic effects that can be beneficial for the treatment of cancer. Afzelin was found to have a promotional effect on neutrophil death, particularly when the oxidative burst was induced by phorbol myristate acetate. Hence, while its widely recognized ability to scavenge free radicals and oxidants, this molecule can inflict side effects in living organisms by exerting its effects on erythrocytes and neutrophils [129].

Given the importance of assessing other toxicological endpoints for new promising molecules like afzelin, future research could focus on expanding the evaluation of its ADMET properties beyond the scope of its genotoxicity and cytotoxicity. Investigating the metabolic fate of pure afzelin in vivo could provide insights into its biotransformation pathways and the formation of metabolites. This information is crucial for understanding its pharmacokinetic profile and potential interactions with other drugs or compounds. Assessing the distribution of afzelin in various tissues after administration could help determine its target organs and potential accumulation in specific tissues. Understanding its tissue distribution profile is essential for predicting its efficacy and potential toxicity. Studying the excretion pathways of afzelin, including renal and biliary excretion, could provide valuable information about its elimination kinetics and potential for accumulation. This knowledge is important for determining appropriate dosing regimens and potential risks associated with long-term exposure. Conducting comprehensive toxicity studies to evaluate the acute and chronic effects of afzelin at various doses and duration of exposure in animal models could help assess its safety profile. This includes assessing its effects on organ function, histopathological changes, and overall systemic toxicity. In summary, by systematically evaluating these additional toxicological endpoints, researchers could gain a more comprehensive understanding of the safety profile of afzelin, which is essential for its further development as a potential therapeutic agent.

5. Conclusions and Future Prospects

Plants possess the ability to manufacture a diverse range of chemical compounds, which exhibit potential significance in various biological contexts. Numerous phytochemicals have the potential to effectively address various human illnesses and enhance long-term well-being. [15,29]. Neurodegenerative diseases and cancer are of significant concern in the medical field due to the absence of efficacious therapeutic interventions and the alarming increase in the number of individuals affected by these conditions. Despite the varied clinical presentations of various illnesses, they all exhibit a shared cellular stress response. The cellular stress responses encompass various physiological processes, such as oxidative stress and inflammation. In recent years, there has been a significant focus on the potential of small molecules, specifically flavonoids, to mitigate cellular stress [130].

Afzelin (kaempferol 3-O-rhamnoside) is a representative of the flavonoid class of compounds. It has been observed to occur in a diverse range of plant sources. The potential benefits it may give to human health are beginning to be recognized. Afzelin demonstrates a wide array of biological activities, such as antioxidative, anti-inflammatory, anti-cancer, and neuroprotective properties. These characteristics make it a promising candidate for the prevention and treatment of neurodegenerative diseases that are characterized by oxidative stress and disruptions in cell death pathways (Figure 4).

The utilization of botanical extracts and isolated compounds in the management of neurodegenerative disorders and cancers encompasses diverse methodologies and presents inherent advantages and drawbacks. Plant extracts frequently consist of intricate combinations of diverse chemicals that are present in a given plant. These extracts have the potential to encompass a diverse array of phytochemicals, including polyphenols, alkaloids, and flavonoids. The intricate nature of these extracts presents difficulty in precisely determining the mechanisms of action and distinguishing the specific components accountable for therapeutic benefits. On the contrary, the obtaining of isolated substances involves the extraction and purification of particular components from plants. This methodology enables the examination of specific compounds and their impact on disorders, hence facilitating the identification of the exact bioactive component responsible for the therapeutic outcome. Furthermore, plant extracts contain substances that can increase the bioavailability of active ingredients or demonstrate synergistic effects. Nevertheless, the existence of additional chemicals may also potentially impede the processes of absorption, distribution, metabolism, and excretion (ADME) of bioactive constituents. In contrast, isolated substances frequently exhibit distinct pharmacokinetic characteristics, facilitating a comprehension process of ADME inside the human body. Understanding this information is of utmost importance when determining appropriate dose and treatment approaches. The safety characteristics of plant extracts can differ based on their specific composition. They may contain chemicals that have the potential to induce adverse effects or interact with other pharmaceutical substances. Isolated chemicals exhibit a greater degree of predictability in terms of safety. Nevertheless, it is important to note that even isolated substances can potentially exhibit adverse consequences. The ADME and toxicity profiling of afzelin and various plant extracts containing this flavonoid has not been performed (except for genotoxic studies) and constitutes one of the remaining issues that will determine the therapeutic usefulness of this compound. Furthermore, its blood–brain barrier (BBB) permeability has not been examined. The BBB serves as a crucial protective factor that effectively limits the permeability of medicines and therapeutic agents, hence impeding their access to the brain. The development of pharmaceutical agents capable of efficiently traversing the BBB to achieve precise localization within CNS is a major challenge. Strategies aimed at improving the bioavailability of these substances, such as the utilization of nanoformulations or prodrugs, have the potential to increase their pharmacokinetic characteristics and ultimately optimize their therapeutic efficacy.

The diverse composition of plant extracts may provide a wider range of activity, rendering them appropriate for addressing various targets in the context of neurodegenerative disorders. This can confer advantages in the context of diseases characterized by complex pathologies. In the context of therapeutic interventions, the utilization of isolated chemicals enables the precise targeting of a single molecular target or pathway. This approach is advantageous in cases where a comprehensive understanding of the illness mechanism exists and necessitates a highly focused strategy.

Afzelin has been shown to elicit a complex cellular response involving its suppressive effects on NF-κB or MAPK pathway conferring reduced expression of pro-inflammatory mediators or down-regulation of NO synthesis, inhibition of tyrosinase activity or up-regulation of molecular signaling pathways involving CREB-BDNF or influence on mitochondrial quality control and function. Moreover, it showed significant oxidative stress mitigating effects associated with ROS scavenging, metal chelation, and the influence of the NRF2 signaling pathway.

In the context of neurodegenerative diseases, current therapies often focus on symptomatic management rather than addressing the underlying disease mechanisms. For example, in Alzheimer's disease, acetylcholinesterase inhibitors such as donepezil and memantine are commonly prescribed to alleviate cognitive symptoms, but they do not halt disease progression [131]. Similarly, in Parkinson's disease, dopamine replacement therapy with levodopa is a mainstay treatment for managing motor symptoms, but it does not prevent the degeneration of dopaminergic neurons [132]. In contrast, afzelin offers a multifaceted approach to addressing neurodegenerative diseases by targeting oxidative stress, inflammation, mitochondrial dysfunction, and neuroprotection, as outlined in the manuscript. Its ability to modulate redox signaling pathways, scavenge free radicals, and inhibit inflammatory mediators suggests a potential neuroprotective effect that may complement existing therapies. According to a recent study of afzelin in Parkinson's disease, the cataleptic behaviors and locomotor activity of rats were greatly improved when administered with a combination of reserpine at a dose of 1 mg/kg and afzelin at doses of 5 mg/kg, 10 mg/kg, and 20 mg/kg. Furthermore, the administration of afzelin alone resulted in the induction of BCL-2 expression, suggesting potential neuroprotective characteristics. This study yielded valuable insights into the efficacy of afzelin in managing catalepsy and other degenerative neurological illnesses. Therefore, further investigations are required to ascertain the causes of the reactions and ascertain the enduring impacts of Afzelin on these situations [133].

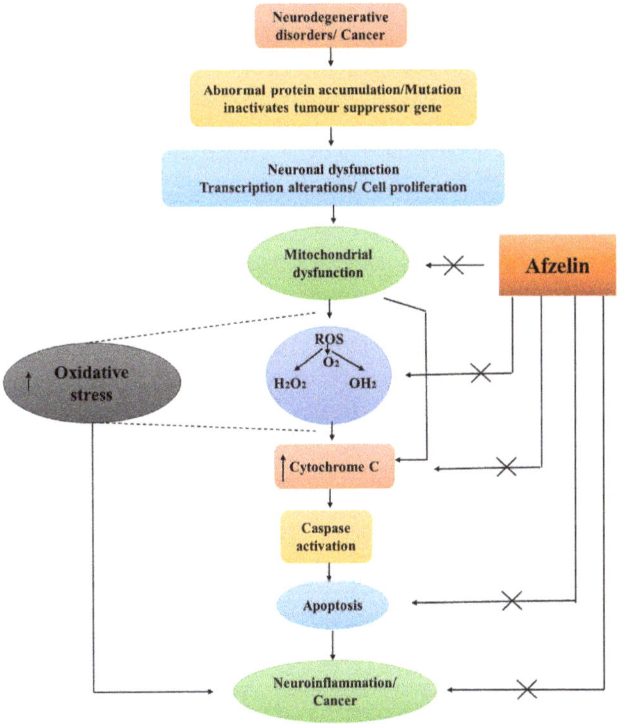

Figure 4. Therapeutic potential of afzelin in neurodegenerative diseases.

Similarly, in the context of cancer, current treatments such as chemotherapy, radiation therapy, and targeted therapies often have significant side effects and may lead to drug resistance [134,135]. Afzelin's anti-cancer properties, including its ability to induce apoptosis and inhibit inflammatory pathways, offer a novel approach to cancer treatment that may have fewer adverse effects compared to conventional therapies and may help prevent the development of treatment resistance or constitute a novel scaffold for drug discovery endeavors.

Furthermore, Wu et al. presented a method that is both ecologically sustainable and efficient in terms of speed and productivity for the extraction and purification of four bioactive components from *Zanthoxylum bungeanum* leaves, including afzelin. The findings can be employed for the incorporation of *Z. bungeanum* leaves as a dietary supplement in an industrial context, offering an accessible source of afzelin for therapeutical use [136]. Similarly, de Sousa et al. provided a validated chromatographic method for the detection of afzelin in *Copaifera langsdorffii* extracts by HPLC, providing another method suitable for the detection and isolation of this flavonoid [137]. The process of standardizing plant extracts to assure constant quantities of bioactive chemicals is of particular importance as it might present challenges, primarily stemming from inherent variances in plant material. Quality control can be more difficult compared to isolated substances. Isolated compounds can be synthesized or purified to a high degree of purity, enabling precise dosing and consistent therapeutic effects. Furthermore, the ease and cost-effectiveness of the afzelin isolation and purification procedure are of importance. In order to provide care to a diverse patient population, it is imperative that the treatment is made readily available and economically feasible, taking into account the socioeconomic obstacles encountered by those afflicted with neurodegenerative disorders and cancers.

In summary, the future prospects for utilizing plant-derived compounds like afzelin in the treatment of neurodegenerative diseases and cancer are promising. Afzelin, a flavonoid with multifaceted properties, holds potential as a therapeutic agent due to its anti-inflammatory, antioxidative, anti-cancer, and neuroprotective effects. Additionally, recent advancements in extraction and purification methods, such as those demonstrated by Wu et al. and de Sousa et al., offer sustainable and efficient means of obtaining afzelin and other bioactive compounds from natural sources. While challenges remain, including standardization of plant extracts and addressing bioavailability and BBB issues, the continued exploration of plant-derived compounds, including afzelin, represents a valuable avenue for developing novel treatments for neurodegenerative diseases.

While this paper extensively covers in vitro and animal studies, it is crucial to acknowledge the necessity of transitioning these findings into clinical settings to ascertain the efficacy and safety of afzelin in humans. As of the current literature review, there are no clinical trials or human studies available for afzelin. Therefore, the focus of this review paper has been on detailing the results from preclinical studies, which provide valuable insights into the potential mechanisms of action and therapeutic effects of afzelin.

Author Contributions: Conceptualization: S.C., S.D. (Sanchit Dhankhar) and S.M.; writing—original draft preparation: M.S., M.K., N.G. and S.D. (Sushma Devi); writing—review and editing: A.G., B.M. and R.K.; supervision: T.G.S. and R.S. All authors have read and agreed to the published version of the manuscript.

Funding: This research did not receive any specific grant from funding agencies in the public, commercial, or not-for-profit sectors.

Conflicts of Interest: The authors declare no conflicts of interest.

Abbreviations

Aβ	amyloid-beta
AADC	aromatic L-amino acid decarboxylase
ACH	acetylcholine
AChE	acetylcholinesterase
ADMET	absorption, distribution, metabolism, excretion, and toxicity
ALS	amyotrophic lateral sclerosis
AR	aldose reductase
ARE	antioxidant response element
ATP	adenosine triphosphate
BBB	blood–brain barrier
BCL2	B-cell lymphoma 2
BDNF	brain-derived neurotrophic factor
CLE	hydroalcoholic extract of *Copaifera lansdorffii* Desf.
CNS	central nervous system
CO	carbon monoxide
CREB	cyclic AMP response element-binding protein
DAQ	dopamine quinone
DNM1L	dynamin-related protein 1
DQ	DOPAquinone
ERK	extracellular signal regulated kinase

FAK	focal adhesion kinase
FHF	fulminant hepatic failure
FIR	far-infrared
FTD	frontotemporal dementia
GalN	D-galactosamine
GSK-3β	glycogen synthase kinase-3β
GSTs	glutathione S-transferases
HMGB1	high-mobility group box 1
HO-1/HO-2	heme oxygenase-1/2
HPLC	high-performance liquid chromatography
IL-1/IL-6	interleukin-1/6
iNOS	inducible nitric oxide synthase
JNK	c-Jun N-terminal kinase
LC	locus coeruleus
LC-MS/MS	liquid chromatography–tandem mass spectrometry
LIMK1	LIM domain kinase 1
LPS	lipopolysaccharide
MAPK	mitogen-activated protein kinase
MFN2	mitofusin 2
MRCKα	myotonic dystrophy kinase-related Cdc42-binding kinase α
MS	multiple sclerosis
MtDNA	mitochondrial DNA
NF-κB	nuclear factor kappa B
NM	neuromelanin
NQO1	NAD(P)H quinone dehydrogenase 1
NRF1	nuclear respiratory factor 1
NRF2	nuclear factor erythroid 2-related factor 2
OMM	outer mitochondrial membrane
P75NTR	P75 neurotrophin receptor
PARKIN	parkin protein
pFAK	phosphorylated focal adhesion kinase
PGC-1α	PPAR-γ coactivator 1α
PI3K	phosphatidylinositol 3-kinase
PINK1	PTEN-induced putative kinase 1
PMEE	*Polygonum minus* ethanolic extract
RAC1	Ras-related C3 botulinum toxin substrate 1
ROCK1	Rho-associated coiled-coil-containing protein kinase
ROS	reactive oxygen species
SOD1/SOD2	superoxide dismutase 1/2
SN	substantia nigra
TFAM	mitochondrial transcription factor A
TH	tyrosine hydroxylase
TNBC	triple-negative breast cancer
TNF-α	tumor necrosis factor-alpha
TRKB	tropomyosin kinase B

References

1. Dugger, B.N.; Dickson, D.W. Pathology of Neurodegenerative Diseases. *Cold Spring Harb. Perspect. Biol.* **2017**, *9*, a028035. [CrossRef] [PubMed]
2. Jellinger, K.A. Basic Mechanisms of Neurodegeneration: A Critical Update. *J. Cell. Mol. Med.* **2010**, *14*, 457. [CrossRef] [PubMed]
3. Lamptey, R.N.L.; Chaulagain, B.; Trivedi, R.; Gothwal, A.; Layek, B.; Singh, J. A Review of the Common Neurodegenerative Disorders: Current Therapeutic Approaches and the Potential Role of Nanotherapeutics. *Int. J. Mol. Sci.* **2022**, *23*, 1851. [CrossRef] [PubMed]
4. Gulisano, W.; Maugeri, D.; Baltrons, M.A.; Fà, M.; Amato, A.; Palmeri, A.; D'Adamio, L.; Grassi, C.; Devanand, D.P.; Honig, L.S.; et al. Role of Amyloid-β and Tau Proteins in Alzheimer's Disease: Confuting the Amyloid Cascade. *J. Alzheimer's Dis.* **2018**, *64*, S611–S631. [CrossRef] [PubMed]
5. Murphy, M.P.; LeVine, H. Alzheimer's Disease and the β-Amyloid Peptide. *J. Alzheimer's Dis.* **2010**, *19*, 311. [CrossRef] [PubMed]

6. Maiti, P.; Manna, J.; Dunbar, G.L. Current Understanding of the Molecular Mechanisms in Parkinson's Disease: Targets for Potential Treatments. *Transl. Neurodegener.* **2017**, *6*, 28. [CrossRef] [PubMed]
7. Hardiman, O.; Al-Chalabi, A.; Chio, A.; Corr, E.M.; Logroscino, G.; Robberecht, W.; Shaw, P.J.; Simmons, Z.; van den Berg, L.H. Amyotrophic Lateral Sclerosis. *Nat. Rev. Dis. Prim.* **2017**, *3*, 17071. [CrossRef] [PubMed]
8. Ghasemi, N.; Razavi, S.; Nikzad, E. Multiple Sclerosis: Pathogenesis, Symptoms, Diagnoses and Cell-Based Therapy. *Cell J.* **2017**, *19*, 1–10. [PubMed]
9. Young, J.J.; Lavakumar, M.; Tampi, D.; Balachandran, S.; Tampi, R.R. Frontotemporal Dementia: Latest Evidence and Clinical Implications. *Ther. Adv. Psychopharmacol.* **2018**, *8*, 33–48. [CrossRef] [PubMed]
10. Ajmal, M.R. Protein Misfolding and Aggregation in Proteinopathies: Causes, Mechanism and Cellular Response. *Diseases* **2023**, *11*, 30. [CrossRef]
11. Kennedy, D.O.; Wightman, E.L. Herbal Extracts and Phytochemicals: Plant Secondary Metabolites and the Enhancement of Human Brain Function. *Adv. Nutr.* **2011**, *2*, 32–50. [CrossRef] [PubMed]
12. Mohd Sairazi, N.S.; Sirajudeen, K.N.S. Natural Products and Their Bioactive Compounds: Neuroprotective Potentials against Neurodegenerative Diseases. *Evid.-Based Complement. Altern. Med.* **2020**, *2020*, 6565396. [CrossRef] [PubMed]
13. Sharifi-Rad, M.; Lankatillake, C.; Dias, D.A.; Docea, A.O.; Mahomoodally, M.F.; Lobine, D.; Chazot, P.L.; Kurt, B.; Tumer, T.B.; Moreira, A.C.; et al. Impact of Natural Compounds on Neurodegenerative Disorders: From Preclinical to Pharmacotherapeutics. *J. Clin. Med.* **2020**, *9*, 1061. [CrossRef] [PubMed]
14. Srivastava, P.; Yadav, R.S. Efficacy of Natural Compounds in Neurodegenerative Disorders. *Adv. Neurobiol.* **2016**, *12*, 107–123. [CrossRef] [PubMed]
15. Gielecińska, A.; Kciuk, M.; Mujwar, S.; Celik, I.; Kołat, D.; Kałuzińska-Kołat, Ż.; Kontek, R. Substances of Natural Origin in Medicine: Plants vs. Cancer. *Cells* **2023**, *12*, 986. [CrossRef] [PubMed]
16. Chen, X.; Guo, C.; Kong, J. Oxidative Stress in Neurodegenerative Diseases. *Neural Regen. Res.* **2012**, *7*, 376–385. [CrossRef] [PubMed]
17. Liu, Z.; Zhou, T.; Ziegler, A.C.; Dimitrion, P.; Zuo, L. Oxidative Stress in Neurodegenerative Diseases: From Molecular Mechanisms to Clinical Applications. *Oxid. Med. Cell. Longev.* **2017**, *2017*, 2525967. [CrossRef] [PubMed]
18. Niedzielska, E.; Smaga, I.; Gawlik, M.; Moniczewski, A.; Stankowicz, P.; Pera, J.; Filip, M. Oxidative Stress in Neurodegenerative Diseases. *Mol. Neurobiol.* **2016**, *53*, 4094–4125. [CrossRef] [PubMed]
19. Singh, A.; Kukreti, R.; Saso, L.; Kukreti, S. Oxidative Stress: A Key Modulator in Neurodegenerative Diseases. *Molecules* **2019**, *24*, 1583. [CrossRef] [PubMed]
20. Arfin, S.; Jha, N.K.; Jha, S.K.; Kesari, K.K.; Ruokolainen, J.; Roychoudhury, S.; Rathi, B.; Kumar, D. Oxidative Stress in Cancer Cell Metabolism. *Antioxidants* **2021**, *10*, 642. [CrossRef] [PubMed]
21. Klaunig, J.E. Oxidative Stress and Cancer. *Curr. Pharm. Des.* **2018**, *24*, 4771–4778. [CrossRef] [PubMed]
22. Hayes, J.D.; Dinkova-Kostova, A.T.; Tew, K.D. Oxidative Stress in Cancer. *Cancer Cell* **2020**, *38*, 167–197. [CrossRef] [PubMed]
23. da Cunha Germano, B.C.; de Morais, L.C.C.; Idalina Neta, F.; Fernandes, A.C.L.; Pinheiro, F.I.; do Rego, A.C.M.; Araújo Filho, I.; de Azevedo, E.P.; de Paiva Cavalcanti, J.R.L.; Guzen, F.P.; et al. Vitamin E and Its Molecular Effects in Experimental Models of Neurodegenerative Diseases. *Int. J. Mol. Sci.* **2023**, *24*, 11191. [CrossRef] [PubMed]
24. Trela-Makowej, A.; Leśkiewicz, M.; Kruk, J.; Żądło, A.; Basta-Kaim, A.; Szymańska, R. Antioxidant and Neuroprotective Activity of Vitamin E Homologues: In Vitro Study. *Metabolites* **2022**, *12*, 608. [CrossRef] [PubMed]
25. Bonnet, U. The Sour Side of Vitamin C Might Mediate Neuroprotective, Anticonvulsive and Antidepressant-like Effects. *Med. Hypotheses* **2019**, *131*, 109320. [CrossRef] [PubMed]
26. Kangisser, L.; Tan, E.; Bellomo, R.; Deane, A.M.; Plummer, M.P. Neuroprotective Properties of Vitamin C: A Scoping Review of Pre-Clinical and Clinical Studies. *J. Neurotrauma* **2021**, *38*, 2194–2205. [CrossRef] [PubMed]
27. Hasan, S.; Khatri, N.; Rahman, Z.N.; Menezes, A.A.; Martini, J.; Shehjar, F.; Mujeeb, N.; Shah, Z.A. Neuroprotective Potential of Flavonoids in Brain Disorders. *Brain Sci.* **2023**, *13*, 1258. [CrossRef] [PubMed]
28. Putteeraj, M.; Lim, W.L.; Teoh, S.L.; Yahaya, M.F. Flavonoids and Its Neuroprotective Effects on Brain Ischemia and Neurodegenerative Diseases. *Curr. Drug Targets* **2018**, *19*, 1710–1720. [CrossRef] [PubMed]
29. Akter, M.; Parvin, M.S.; Hasan, M.M.; Rahman, M.A.A.; Islam, M.E. Anti-Tumor and Antioxidant Activity of Kaempferol-3-O-Alpha-L-Rhamnoside (Afzelin) Isolated from *Pithecellobium dulce* Leaves. *BMC Complement. Med. Ther.* **2022**, *22*, 169. [CrossRef] [PubMed]
30. Kim, J.H.; Kim, M.; Kim, J.M.; Lee, M.-K.; Seo, S.J.; Park, K.Y. Afzelin Suppresses Proinflammatory Responses in Particulate Matter-Exposed Human Keratinocytes. *Int. J. Mol. Med.* **2019**, *43*, 2516–2522. [CrossRef] [PubMed]
31. Lee, S.-B.; Kang, J.-W.; Kim, S.-J.; Ahn, J.; Kim, J.; Lee, S.-M. Afzelin Ameliorates D-Galactosamine and Lipopolysaccharide-Induced Fulminant Hepatic Failure by Modulating Mitochondrial Quality Control and Dynamics. *Br. J. Pharmacol.* **2017**, *174*, 195–209. [CrossRef] [PubMed]
32. Lotha, R.; Sundaramoorthy, N.S.; Shamprasad, B.R.; Nagarajan, S.; Sivasubramanian, A. Plant Nutraceuticals (Quercetrin and Afzelin) Capped Silver Nanoparticles Exert Potent Antibiofilm Effect against Food Borne Pathogen *Salmonella enterica* Serovar Typhi and Curtail Planktonic Growth in Zebrafish Infection Model. *Microb. Pathog.* **2018**, *120*, 109–118. [CrossRef] [PubMed]
33. Cherbuin, N.; Walsh, E.; Baune, B.T.; Anstey, K.J. Oxidative Stress, Inflammation and Risk of Neurodegeneration in a Population Sample. *Eur. J. Neurol.* **2019**, *26*, 1347–1354. [CrossRef]

34. Simpson, D.S.A.; Oliver, P.L. ROS Generation in Microglia: Understanding Oxidative Stress and Inflammation in Neurodegenerative Disease. *Antioxidants* **2020**, *9*, 743. [CrossRef] [PubMed]
35. Lee, J.H.; Ahn, J.; Kim, J.W.; Lee, S.G.; Kim, H.P. Flavonoids from the Aerial Parts of Houttuynia Cordata Attenuate Lung Inflammation in Mice. *Arch. Pharm. Res.* **2015**, *38*, 1304–1311. [CrossRef] [PubMed]
36. Zhang, X.; Cheng, B.; Liu, X.; Li, Y.; Hou, J.; Chen, S.; Chen, J.; Li, S. Screening of α-Glucosidase Inhibitors from Houttuynia Cordata and Evaluation of the Binding Mechanisms. *ChemistrySelect* **2020**, *5*, 8440–8446. [CrossRef]
37. Zhang, Z.; ElSohly, H.N.; Li, X.-C.; Khan, S.I.; Broedel, S.E.; Raulli, R.E.; Cihlar, R.L.; Burandt, C.; Walker, L.A. Phenolic Compounds from Nymphaea Odorata. *J. Nat. Prod.* **2003**, *66*, 548–550. [CrossRef] [PubMed]
38. Zhu, K.-C.; Sun, J.-M.; Shen, J.-G.; Jin, J.-Z.; Liu, F.; Xu, X.-L.; Chen, L.; Liu, L.-T.; Lv, J.-J. Afzelin Exhibits Anti-Cancer Activity against Androgen-Sensitive LNCaP and Androgen-Independent PC-3 Prostate Cancer Cells through the Inhibition of LIM Domain Kinase 1. *Oncol. Lett.* **2015**, *10*, 2359–2365. [CrossRef] [PubMed]
39. Hernández-Caballero, M.E.; Sierra-Ramírez, J.A.; Villalobos-Valencia, R.; Seseña-Méndez, E. Potential of Kalanchoe Pinnata as a Cancer Treatment Adjuvant and an Epigenetic Regulator. *Molecules* **2022**, *27*, 6425. [CrossRef]
40. Mejía-Méndez, J.L.; Bach, H.; Lorenzo-Leal, A.C.; Navarro-López, D.E.; López-Mena, E.R.; Hernández, L.R.; Sánchez-Arreola, E. Biological Activities and Chemical Profiles of Kalanchoe Fedtschenkoi Extracts. *Plants* **2023**, *12*, 1943. [CrossRef]
41. Nascimento, L.B.d.S.; Casanova, L.M.; Costa, S.S. Bioactive Compounds from Kalanchoe Genus Potentially Useful for the Development of New Drugs. *Life* **2023**, *13*, 646. [CrossRef]
42. Yadav, N.P.; Dixit, V.K. Hepatoprotective Activity of Leaves of Kalanchoe Pinnata Pers. *J. Ethnopharmacol.* **2003**, *86*, 197–202. [CrossRef] [PubMed]
43. Mady, M.S.; Ibrahim, R.R.; El-Sayed, E.K.; El-Shazly, M.; Chen, L.-Y.; Lai, K.-H.; El Shaarawy, F.S.; Moharram, F.A. UHPLC-MS Profiles and Antidiarrheal Activity of *Quercus coccinea* Münchh. and *Quercus robur* L. Employing In Vivo Technique. *Front. Pharmacol.* **2023**, *14*, 1120146. [CrossRef] [PubMed]
44. Oliveira, P.A.; Medeiros-Fonseca, B.; Vasconcelos-Nóbrega, C.; Alvarado, A.; Pires, M.J.; Vala, H.; Barros, A.I.R.N.A.; Faustino-Rocha, A.I. *Quercus* spp. Extract as a Promising Preventive or Therapeutic Strategy for Cancer: A Systematic Review. *Mol. Med. Rep.* **2023**, *28*, 175. [CrossRef] [PubMed]
45. Jung, J.; Kim, H.; Lee, S.; Hong, M.; Hwang, D. Antioxidant and Anti-Inflammatory Activity of Filipendula Glaberrima Nakai Ethanolic Extract and Its Chemical Composition. *Molecules* **2022**, *27*, 4628. [CrossRef] [PubMed]
46. Marčetić, M.; Samardžić, S.; Ilić, T.; Božić, D.D.; Vidović, B. Phenolic Composition, Antioxidant, Anti-Enzymatic, Antimicrobial and Prebiotic Properties of *Prunus spinosa* L. Fruits. *Foods* **2022**, *11*, 3289. [CrossRef] [PubMed]
47. Soares, S.S.; Bekbolatova, E.; Cotrim, M.D.; Sakipova, Z.; Ibragimova, L.; Kukula-Koch, W.; Giorno, T.B.S.; Fernandes, P.D.; Fonseca, D.A.; Boylan, F. Chemistry and Pharmacology of the Kazakh *Crataegus almaatensis* Pojark: An Asian Herbal Medicine. *Antioxidants* **2019**, *8*, 300. [CrossRef] [PubMed]
48. Pizzino, G.; Irrera, N.; Cucinotta, M.; Pallio, G.; Mannino, F.; Arcoraci, V.; Squadrito, F.; Altavilla, D.; Bitto, A. Oxidative Stress: Harms and Benefits for Human Health. *Oxid. Med. Cell. Longev.* **2017**, *2017*, 8416763. [CrossRef] [PubMed]
49. Cechinel-Zanchett, C.C.; Bolda Mariano, L.N.; Boeing, T.; da Costa, J.d.C.; Da Silva, L.M.; Bastos, J.K.; Cechinel-Filho, V.; de Souza, P. Diuretic and Renal Protective Effect of Kaempferol 3-O-Alpha-l-Rhamnoside (Afzelin) in Normotensive and Hypertensive Rats. *J. Nat. Prod.* **2020**, *83*, 1980–1989. [CrossRef] [PubMed]
50. Jung, E.; Kim, J.H.; Kim, M.O.; Lee, S.Y.; Lee, J. Melanocyte-Protective Effect of Afzelin Is Mediated by the Nrf2-ARE Signalling Pathway via GSK-3β Inactivation. *Exp. Dermatol.* **2017**, *26*, 764–770. [CrossRef] [PubMed]
51. Kim, M.; Shin, S.; Ryu, D.; Cho, E.; Yoo, J.; Park, D.; Jung, E. Evaluating the Sun Protection Factor of Cosmetic Formulations Containing Afzelin. *Chem. Pharm. Bull.* **2021**, *69*, 1039–1044. [CrossRef] [PubMed]
52. Juan, C.A.; de la Lastra, J.M.P.; Plou, F.J.; Pérez-Lebeña, E. The Chemistry of Reactive Oxygen Species (ROS) Revisited: Outlining Their Role in Biological Macromolecules (DNA, Lipids and Proteins) and Induced Pathologies. *Int. J. Mol. Sci.* **2021**, *22*, 4642. [CrossRef] [PubMed]
53. Liu, Y.; Chen, P.; Zhou, M.; Wang, T.; Fang, S.; Shang, X.; Fu, X. Geographic Variation in the Chemical Composition and Antioxidant Properties of Phenolic Compounds from *Cyclocarya paliurus* (Batal) Iljinskaja Leaves. *Molecules* **2018**, *23*, 2440. [CrossRef] [PubMed]
54. Ma, L.; Li, K.; Wei, D.; Xiao, H.; Niu, H.; Huang, W. High Anti-Oxidative and Lipid-Lowering Activities of Flavonoid Glycosides-Rich Extract from the Leaves of *Zanthoxylum bungeanum* in Multi-System. *J. Food Nutr. Res.* **2015**, *3*, 62–68. [CrossRef]
55. Aldana, J.A.; De Grandis, R.A.; Nicolella, H.; Guissoni, A.P.P.; Squarisi, I.; Arruda, C.; Ribeiro, V.P.; Tavares, D.C.; Barcelos, G.R.M.; Antunes, L.M.G.; et al. Evaluation of Cytoprotective Effects of Compounds Isolated from *Copaifera langsdorffii* Desf. against Induced Cytotoxicity by Exposure to Methylmercury and Lead. *Nat. Prod. Res.* **2020**, *34*, 2528–2532. [CrossRef] [PubMed]
56. Fernandez, M.T.; Mira, M.L.; Florêncio, M.H.; Jennings, K.R. Iron and Copper Chelation by Flavonoids: An Electrospray Mass Spectrometry Study. *J. Inorg. Biochem.* **2002**, *92*, 105–111. [CrossRef] [PubMed]
57. Merino, J.J.; Parmigiani-Izquierdo, J.M.; Toledano Gasca, A.; Cabaña-Muñoz, M.E. The Long-Term Algae Extract (*Chlorella* and *Fucus* sp.) and Aminosulphurate Supplementation Modulate SOD-1 Activity and Decrease Heavy Metals (Hg++, Sn) Levels in Patients with Long-Term Dental Titanium Implants and Amalgam Fillings Restorations. *Antioxidants* **2019**, *8*, 101. [CrossRef] [PubMed]

58. Kashyap, D.; Sharma, A.; Tuli, H.S.; Sak, K.; Punia, S.; Mukherjee, T.K. Kaempferol—A Dietary Anticancer Molecule with Multiple Mechanisms of Action: Recent Trends and Advancements. *J. Funct. Foods* **2017**, *30*, 203. [CrossRef] [PubMed]
59. Alqahtani, T.; Deore, S.L.; Kide, A.A.; Shende, B.A.; Sharma, R.; Dadarao Chakole, R.; Nemade, L.S.; Kishor Kale, N.; Borah, S.; Shrikant Deokar, S.; et al. Mitochondrial Dysfunction and Oxidative Stress in Alzheimer's Disease, and Parkinson's Disease, Huntington's Disease and Amyotrophic Lateral Sclerosis—An Updated Review. *Mitochondrion* **2023**, *71*, 83–92. [CrossRef] [PubMed]
60. Misrani, A.; Tabassum, S.; Yang, L. Mitochondrial Dysfunction and Oxidative Stress in Alzheimer's Disease. *Front. Aging Neurosci.* **2021**, *13*, 617588. [CrossRef] [PubMed]
61. Bose, A.; Beal, M.F. Mitochondrial Dysfunction and Oxidative Stress in Induced Pluripotent Stem Cell Models of Parkinson's Disease. *Eur. J. Neurosci.* **2019**, *49*, 525–532. [CrossRef] [PubMed]
62. Hauser, D.N.; Hastings, T.G. Mitochondrial Dysfunction and Oxidative Stress in Parkinson's Disease and Monogenic Parkinsonism. *Neurobiol. Dis.* **2013**, *51*, 35–42. [CrossRef] [PubMed]
63. Lin, M.T.; Beal, M.F. Mitochondrial Dysfunction and Oxidative Stress in Neurodegenerative Diseases. *Nature* **2006**, *443*, 787–795. [CrossRef] [PubMed]
64. Księżakowska-Łakoma, K.; Żyła, M.; Wilczyński, J.R. Mitochondrial Dysfunction in Cancer. *Prz. Menopauzalny* **2014**, *13*, 136–144. [CrossRef] [PubMed]
65. Luo, Y.; Ma, J.; Lu, W. The Significance of Mitochondrial Dysfunction in Cancer. *Int. J. Mol. Sci.* **2020**, *21*, 5598. [CrossRef] [PubMed]
66. Zhang, Y.; Chen, C.; Jiang, Y.; Wang, S.; Wu, X.; Wang, K. PPARγ Coactivator-1α (PGC-1α) Protects Neuroblastoma Cells against Amyloid-Beta (Aβ) Induced Cell Death and Neuroinflammation via NF-κB Pathway. *BMC Neurosci.* **2017**, *18*, 69. [CrossRef] [PubMed]
67. Mota, B.C.; Sastre, M. The Role of PGC1α in Alzheimer's Disease and Therapeutic Interventions. *Int. J. Mol. Sci.* **2021**, *22*, 5769. [CrossRef] [PubMed]
68. Panes, J.D.; Wendt, A.; Ramirez-Molina, O.; Castro, P.A.; Fuentealba, J. Deciphering the Role of PGC-1α in Neurological Disorders: From Mitochondrial Dysfunction to Synaptic Failure. *Neural Regen. Res.* **2021**, *17*, 237–245. [CrossRef] [PubMed]
69. Bost, F.; Kaminski, L. The Metabolic Modulator PGC-1α in Cancer. *Am. J. Cancer Res.* **2019**, *9*, 198–211. [PubMed]
70. Kang, I.; Chu, C.T.; Kaufman, B.A. The Mitochondrial Transcription Factor TFAM in Neurodegeneration: Emerging Evidence and Mechanisms. *FEBS Lett.* **2018**, *592*, 793–811. [CrossRef] [PubMed]
71. Quinn, P.M.J.; Moreira, P.I.; Ambrósio, A.F.; Alves, C.H. PINK1/PARKIN Signalling in Neurodegeneration and Neuroinflammation. *Acta Neuropathol. Commun.* **2020**, *8*, 189. [CrossRef] [PubMed]
72. Wang, M.; Luan, S.; Fan, X.; Wang, J.; Huang, J.; Gao, X.; Han, D. The Emerging Multifaceted Role of PINK1 in Cancer Biology. *Cancer Sci.* **2022**, *113*, 4037–4047. [CrossRef] [PubMed]
73. Denisenko, T.V.; Gogvadze, V.; Zhivotovsky, B. Mitophagy in Carcinogenesis and Cancer Treatment. *Discov. Oncol.* **2021**, *12*, 58. [CrossRef] [PubMed]
74. Lee, D.; Kim, J.-Y.; Qi, Y.; Park, S.; Lee, H.L.; Yamabe, N.; Kim, H.; Jang, D.S.; Kang, K.S. Phytochemicals from the Flowers of *Prunus persica* (L.) Batsch: Anti-Adipogenic Effect of Mandelamide on 3T3-L1 Preadipocytes. *Bioorg. Med. Chem. Lett.* **2021**, *49*, 128326. [CrossRef] [PubMed]
75. Lim, H.J.; Prajapati, R.; Seong, S.H.; Jung, H.A.; Choi, J.S. Antioxidant and Antineuroinflammatory Mechanisms of Kaempferol-3-O-β-d-Glucuronate on Lipopolysaccharide-Stimulated BV2 Microglial Cells through the Nrf2/HO-1 Signaling Cascade and MAPK/NF-κB Pathway. *ACS Omega* **2023**, *8*, 6538–6549. [CrossRef] [PubMed]
76. Calkins, M.J.; Johnson, D.A.; Townsend, J.A.; Vargas, M.R.; Dowell, J.A.; Williamson, T.P.; Kraft, A.D.; Lee, J.-M.; Li, J.; Johnson, J.A. The Nrf2/ARE Pathway as a Potential Therapeutic Target in Neurodegenerative Disease. *Antioxid. Redox Signal.* **2009**, *11*, 497–508. [CrossRef] [PubMed]
77. Johnson, J.A.; Johnson, D.A.; Kraft, A.D.; Calkins, M.J.; Jakel, R.J.; Vargas, M.R.; Chen, P.-C. The Nrf2-ARE Pathway: An Indicator and Modulator of Oxidative Stress in Neurodegeneration. *Ann. N. Y. Acad. Sci.* **2008**, *1147*, 61–69. [CrossRef] [PubMed]
78. Wang, Y.; Gao, L.; Chen, J.; Li, Q.; Huo, L.; Wang, Y.; Wang, H.; Du, J. Pharmacological Modulation of Nrf2/HO-1 Signaling Pathway as a Therapeutic Target of Parkinson's Disease. *Front. Pharmacol.* **2021**, *12*, 757161. [CrossRef] [PubMed]
79. Kaur, K.; Narang, R.K.; Singh, S. Role of Nrf2 in Oxidative Stress, Neuroinflammation and Autophagy in Alzheimer's Disease: Regulation of Nrf2 by Different Signaling Pathways. *Curr. Mol. Med.* **2023**, in press. [CrossRef]
80. Minj, E.; Yadav, R.K.; Mehan, S. Targeting Abnormal Nrf2/HO-1 Signaling in Amyotrophic Lateral Sclerosis: Current Insights on Drug Targets and Influences on Neurological Disorders. *Curr. Mol. Med.* **2021**, *21*, 630–644. [CrossRef] [PubMed]
81. Soni, D.; Kumar, P. GSK-3β-Mediated Regulation of Nrf2/HO-1 Signaling as a New Therapeutic Approach in the Treatment of Movement Disorders. *Pharmacol. Rep.* **2022**, *74*, 557–569. [CrossRef] [PubMed]
82. Wu, S.; Lu, H.; Bai, Y. Nrf2 in Cancers: A Double-edged Sword. *Cancer Med.* **2019**, *8*, 2252–2267. [CrossRef] [PubMed]
83. Consoli, V.; Sorrenti, V.; Grosso, S.; Vanella, L. Heme Oxygenase-1 Signaling and Redox Homeostasis in Physiopathological Conditions. *Biomolecules* **2021**, *11*, 589. [CrossRef] [PubMed]
84. Wegiel, B.; Nemeth, Z.; Correa-Costa, M.; Bulmer, A.C.; Otterbein, L.E. Heme Oxygenase-1: A Metabolic Nike. *Antioxid. Redox Signal.* **2014**, *20*, 1709–1722. [CrossRef] [PubMed]

85. Jansen, T.; Daiber, A. Direct Antioxidant Properties of Bilirubin and Biliverdin. Is There a Role for Biliverdin Reductase? *Front. Pharmacol.* **2012**, *3*, 30. [CrossRef] [PubMed]
86. Dutra, F.F.; Bozza, M.T. Heme on Innate Immunity and Inflammation. *Front. Pharmacol.* **2014**, *5*, 115. [CrossRef] [PubMed]
87. Pae, H.-O.; Chung, H.-T. Heme Oxygenase-1: Its Therapeutic Roles in Inflammatory Diseases. *Immune Netw.* **2009**, *9*, 12–19. [CrossRef] [PubMed]
88. Cuadrado, A.; Rojo, A.I. Heme Oxygenase-1 as a Therapeutic Target in Neurodegenerative Diseases and Brain Infections. *Curr. Pharm. Des.* **2008**, *14*, 429–442. [CrossRef] [PubMed]
89. Neis, V.B.; Rosa, P.B.; Moretti, M.; Rodrigues, A.L.S. Involvement of Heme Oxygenase-1 in Neuropsychiatric and Neurodegenerative Diseases. *Curr. Pharm. Des.* **2018**, *24*, 2283–2302. [CrossRef] [PubMed]
90. Wu, M.-L.; Ho, Y.-C.; Lin, C.-Y.; Yet, S.-F. Heme Oxygenase-1 in Inflammation and Cardiovascular Disease. *Am. J. Cardiovasc. Dis.* **2011**, *1*, 150–158. [PubMed]
91. Wu, Y.-H.; Hsieh, H.-L. Roles of Heme Oxygenase-1 in Neuroinflammation and Brain Disorders. *Antioxidants* **2022**, *11*, 923. [CrossRef] [PubMed]
92. Ahmad, M.A.; Kareem, O.; Khushtar, M.; Akbar, M.; Haque, M.R.; Iqubal, A.; Haider, M.F.; Pottoo, F.H.; Abdulla, F.S.; Al-Haidar, M.B.; et al. Neuroinflammation: A Potential Risk for Dementia. *Int. J. Mol. Sci.* **2022**, *23*, 616. [CrossRef]
93. DiSabato, D.J.; Quan, N.; Godbout, J.P. Neuroinflammation: The Devil Is in the Details. *J. Neurochem.* **2016**, *139* (Suppl. S2), 136–153. [CrossRef] [PubMed]
94. Kaur, N.; Chugh, H.; Sakharkar, M.K.; Dhawan, U.; Chidambaram, S.B.; Chandra, R. Neuroinflammation Mechanisms and Phytotherapeutic Intervention: A Systematic Review. *ACS Chem. Neurosci.* **2020**, *11*, 3707–3731. [CrossRef] [PubMed]
95. Kwon, H.S.; Koh, S.-H. Neuroinflammation in Neurodegenerative Disorders: The Roles of Microglia and Astrocytes. *Transl. Neurodegener.* **2020**, *9*, 42. [CrossRef] [PubMed]
96. Onyango, I.G.; Jauregui, G.V.; Čarná, M.; Bennett, J.P.; Stokin, G.B. Neuroinflammation in Alzheimer's Disease. *Biomedicines* **2021**, *9*, 524. [CrossRef] [PubMed]
97. Shabab, T.; Khanabdali, R.; Moghadamtousi, S.Z.; Kadir, H.A.; Mohan, G. Neuroinflammation Pathways: A General Review. *Int. J. Neurosci.* **2017**, *127*, 624–633. [CrossRef] [PubMed]
98. Greten, F.R.; Grivennikov, S.I. Inflammation and Cancer: Triggers, Mechanisms and Consequences. *Immunity* **2019**, *51*, 27–41. [CrossRef] [PubMed]
99. Rho, H.S.; Ghimeray, A.K.; Yoo, D.S.; Ahn, S.M.; Kwon, S.S.; Lee, K.H.; Cho, D.H.; Cho, J.Y. Kaempferol and Kaempferol Rhamnosides with Depigmenting and Anti-Inflammatory Properties. *Molecules* **2011**, *16*, 3338. [CrossRef] [PubMed]
100. Kim, S.K.; Kim, H.J.; Choi, S.E.; Park, K.H.; Choi, H.K.; Lee, M.W. Anti-Oxidative and Inhibitory Activities on Nitric Oxide (NO) and Prostaglandin E2 (COX-2) Production of Flavonoids from Seeds of *Prunus tomentosa* Thunberg. *Arch. Pharm. Res.* **2008**, *31*, 424–428. [CrossRef] [PubMed]
101. Shin, S.W.; Jung, E.; Kim, S.; Kim, J.-H.; Kim, E.-G.; Lee, J.; Park, D. Antagonizing Effects and Mechanisms of Afzelin against UVB Induced Cell Damage. *PLoS ONE* **2013**, *8*, e0061971. [CrossRef] [PubMed]
102. Yoon, C.-S.; Lee, H.; Liu, Z.; Lee, H.-K.; Lee, D.-S. Effects of Compounds Isolated from Lindera Erythrocarpa on Anti-Inflammatory and Anti-Neuroinflammatory Action in BV2 Microglia and RAW264.7 Macrophage. *Int. J. Mol. Sci.* **2022**, *23*, 7122. [CrossRef] [PubMed]
103. Kim, J.H.; Quilantang, N.G.; Kim, H.Y.; Lee, S.; Cho, E.J. Attenuation of Hydrogen Peroxide-Induced Oxidative Stress in SH-SY5Y Cells by Three Flavonoids from Acer Okamotoanum. *Chem. Pap.* **2019**, *73*, 1135–1144. [CrossRef]
104. Kim, J.H.; Lee, S.; Cho, E.J. Acer Okamotoanum Protects SH-SY5Y Neuronal Cells against Hydrogen Peroxide-Induced Oxidative Stress. *Food Sci. Biotechnol.* **2019**, *28*, 191–200. [CrossRef] [PubMed]
105. Radziejewska, I.; Supruniuk, K.; Czarnomysy, R.; Buzun, K.; Bielawska, A. Anti-Cancer Potential of Afzelin towards AGS Gastric Cancer Cells. *Pharmaceuticals* **2021**, *14*, 973. [CrossRef] [PubMed]
106. Xia, L.; Xu, X.; Li, M.; Zhang, X.; Cao, F. Afzelin Induces Immunogenic Cell Death against Lung Cancer by Targeting NQO2. *BMC Complement. Med. Ther.* **2023**, *23*, 381. [CrossRef]
107. Colucci-D'Amato, L.; Speranza, L.; Volpicelli, F. Neurotrophic Factor BDNF, Physiological Functions and Therapeutic Potential in Depression, Neurodegeneration and Brain Cancer. *Int. J. Mol. Sci.* **2020**, *21*, 7777. [CrossRef] [PubMed]
108. Garcia, N.; Tomàs, M.; Santafé, M.M.; Besalduch, N.; Lanuza, M.A.; Tomàs, J. The Interaction between Tropomyosin-Related Kinase B Receptors and Presynaptic Muscarinic Receptors Modulates Transmitter Release in Adult Rodent Motor Nerve Terminals. *J. Neurosci.* **2010**, *30*, 16514–16522. [CrossRef] [PubMed]
109. Song, J.H.; Yu, J.T.; Tan, L. Brain-Derived Neurotrophic Factor in Alzheimer's Disease: Risk, Mechanisms, and Therapy. *Mol. Neurobiol.* **2015**, *52*, 1477–1493. [CrossRef] [PubMed]
110. Mittal, P.; Dhankhar, S.; Chauhan, S.; Garg, N.; Bhattacharya, T.; Ali, M.; Chaudhary, A.A.; Rudayni, H.A.; Al-Zharani, M.; Ahmad, W.; et al. A Review on Natural Antioxidants for Their Role in the Treatment of Parkinson's Disease. *Pharmaceuticals* **2023**, *16*, 908. [CrossRef] [PubMed]
111. Azman, K.F.; Zakaria, R. Recent Advances on the Role of Brain-Derived Neurotrophic Factor (BDNF) in Neurodegenerative Diseases. *Int. J. Mol. Sci.* **2022**, *23*, 6827. [CrossRef] [PubMed]

112. Oh, S.-Y.; Jang, M.J.; Choi, Y.-H.; Hwang, H.; Rhim, H.; Lee, B.; Choi, C.W.; Kim, M.S. Central Administration of Afzelin Extracted from Ribes Fasciculatum Improves Cognitive and Memory Function in a Mouse Model of Dementia. *Sci. Rep.* **2021**, *11*, 9182. [CrossRef] [PubMed]
113. Almeida, R.D.; Manadas, B.J.; Melo, C.V.; Gomes, J.R.; Mendes, C.S.; Grãos, M.M.; Carvalho, R.F.; Carvalho, A.P.; Duarte, C.B. Neuroprotection by BDNF against Glutamate-Induced Apoptotic Cell Death Is Mediated by ERK and PI3-Kinase Pathways. *Cell Death Differ.* **2005**, *12*, 1329–1343. [CrossRef] [PubMed]
114. Huang, Y.-R.; Liu, C.-C.; Wang, S.; Cheng, H.-C.; Meadows, C.; Chang, K.-C. The Role of Aldose Reductase in Beta-Amyloid-Induced Microglia Activation. *Int. J. Mol. Sci.* **2022**, *23*, 15088. [CrossRef] [PubMed]
115. Lee, D.G.; Lee, J.S.; Quilantang, N.G.; Jacinto, S.D.; Lee, S. Determination of Afzelin and Astragalin from Lespedeza Cuneata on Aldose Reductase Inhibition. *J. Chromatogr. Sci.* **2021**, *59*, 381–387. [CrossRef] [PubMed]
116. Song, X.-M.; Yu, Q.; Dong, X.; Yang, H.O.; Zeng, K.-W.; Li, J.; Tu, P.-F. Aldose Reductase Inhibitors Attenuate β-Amyloid-Induced TNF-α Production in Microlgia via ROS-PKC-Mediated NF-κB and MAPK Pathways. *Int. Immunopharmacol.* **2017**, *50*, 30–37. [CrossRef] [PubMed]
117. Iannitelli, A.F.; Segal, A.; Pare, J.-F.; Mulvey, B.; Liles, L.C.; Sloan, S.A.; McCann, K.E.; Dougherty, J.D.; Smith, Y.; Weinshenker, D. Tyrosinase-Induced Neuromelanin Accumulation Triggers Rapid Dysregulation and Degeneration of the Mouse Locus Coeruleus. *bioRxiv* **2023**. [CrossRef] [PubMed]
118. Nagatsu, T.; Nakashima, A.; Watanabe, H.; Ito, S.; Wakamatsu, K. Neuromelanin in Parkinson's Disease: Tyrosine Hydroxylase and Tyrosinase. *Int. J. Mol. Sci.* **2022**, *23*, 4176. [CrossRef]
119. Rho, H.S.; Ahn, S.M.; Lee, B.C.; Kim, M.K.; Ghimeray, A.K.; Jin, C.W.; Cho, D.H. Changes in Flavonoid Content and Tyrosinase Inhibitory Activity in Kenaf Leaf Extract after Far-Infrared Treatment. *Bioorg. Med. Chem. Lett.* **2010**, *20*, 7534–7536. [CrossRef] [PubMed]
120. Sayuti, N.H.; Zulkefli, N.; Tan, J.K.; Saad, N.; Baharum, S.N.; Hamezah, H.S.; Bunawan, H.; Ahmed, Q.U.; Parveen, H.; Mukhtar, S.; et al. Ethanolic Extract of Polygonum Minus Protects Differentiated Human Neuroblastoma Cells (SH-SY5Y) against H2O2-Induced Oxidative Stress. *Molecules* **2023**, *28*, 6726. [CrossRef] [PubMed]
121. Işık, M.; Beydemir, Ş. AChE mRNA Expression as a Possible Novel Biomarker for the Diagnosis of Coronary Artery Disease and Alzheimer's Disease, and Its Association with Oxidative Stress. *Arch. Physiol. Biochem.* **2022**, *128*, 352–359. [CrossRef] [PubMed]
122. Rachmi, E.; Purnomo, B.B.; Endharti, A.T.; Fitri, L.E. Afzelin Inhibits Migration of MDA-MB-231 Cells by Suppressing FAK Expression and Rac1 Activation. *J. Appl. Pharm. Sci.* **2020**, *10*, 77–82. [CrossRef]
123. Rachmi, E.; Purnomo, B.B.; Endharti, A.T.; Fitri, L.E. Identification of Afzelin Potential Targets in Inhibiting Triple-Negative Breast Cancer Cell Migration Using Reverse Docking. *Porto Biomed. J.* **2020**, *5*, e095. [CrossRef]
124. Diantini, A.; Subarnas, A.; Lestari, K.; Halimah, E.; Susilawati, Y.; Supriyatna, S.; Julaeha, E.; Achmad, T.H.; Suradji, E.W.; Yamazaki, C.; et al. Kaempferol-3-O-Rhamnoside Isolated from the Leaves of *Schima wallichii* Korth. Inhibits MCF-7 Breast Cancer Cell Proliferation through Activation of the Caspase Cascade Pathway. *Oncol. Lett.* **2012**, *3*, 1069–1072. [CrossRef] [PubMed]
125. Zheng, L.; Li, Y.; Zhou, Z.; Xiang, W.; Gong, Z.; Chen, S.; Wang, Y.; Wang, A.; Lan, Y.; Li, Y.; et al. Comparative Pharmacokinetics of Quercitrin, Astragalin, Afzelin and Taxifolin in Plasma after Oral Administration of Polygonum Orientale Inflorescence in Sham-Operated and Myocardial Ischemia-Reperfusion Injury Rats. *Xenobiotica* **2020**, *50*, 822–830. [CrossRef]
126. Alves, J.M.; Munari, C.C.; de Azevedo Bentes Monteiro Neto, M.; Furtado, R.A.; Senedese, J.M.; Bastos, J.K.; Tavares, D.C. In Vivo Protective Effect of *Copaifera langsdorffii* Hydroalcoholic Extract on Micronuclei Induction by Doxorubicin. *J. Appl. Toxicol.* **2013**, *33*, 854–860. [CrossRef] [PubMed]
127. Ozelin, S.D.; Senedese, J.M.; Alves, J.M.; Munari, C.C.; Costa, J.D.C.D.; Resende, F.A.; Campos, D.L.; Lima, I.M.D.S.; Andrade, A.F.; Varanda, E.A.; et al. Preventive Activity of *Copaifera langsdorffii* Desf. Leaves Extract and Its Major Compounds, Afzelin and Quercitrin, on DNA Damage in In Vitro and In Vivo Models. *J. Toxicol. Environ. Health A* **2021**, *84*, 569–581. [CrossRef] [PubMed]
128. Hong, C.-O.; Lee, H.A.; Rhee, C.H.; Choung, S.-Y.; Lee, K.-W. Separation of the Antioxidant Compound Quercitrin from *Lindera obtusiloba blume* and Its Antimelanogenic Effect on B16F10 Melanoma Cells. *Biosci. Biotechnol. Biochem.* **2013**, *77*, 58–64. [CrossRef]
129. Vellosa, J.C.R.; Regasini, L.O.; Belló, C.; Schemberger, J.A.; Khalil, N.M.; de Araújo Morandim-Giannetti, A.; da Silva Bolzani, V.; Brunetti, I.L.; de Faria Oliveira, O.M.M. Preliminary in Vitro and Ex Vivo Evaluation of Afzelin, Kaempferitrin and Pterogynoside Action over Free Radicals and Reactive Oxygen Species. *Arch. Pharm. Res.* **2015**, *38*, 1168–1177. [CrossRef] [PubMed]
130. Devi, S.; Kumar, V.; Singh, S.K.; Dubey, A.K.; Kim, J.-J. Flavonoids: Potential Candidates for the Treatment of Neurodegenerative Disorders. *Biomedicines* **2021**, *9*, 99. [CrossRef] [PubMed]
131. Passeri, E.; Elkhoury, K.; Morsink, M.; Broersen, K.; Linder, M.; Tamayol, A.; Malaplate, C.; Yen, F.T.; Arab-Tehrany, E. Alzheimer's Disease: Treatment Strategies and Their Limitations. *Int. J. Mol. Sci.* **2022**, *23*, 13954. [CrossRef] [PubMed]
132. Armstrong, M.J.; Okun, M.S. Diagnosis and Treatment of Parkinson Disease: A Review. *JAMA* **2020**, *323*, 548–560. [CrossRef]
133. Alharthy, K.M.; Rashid, S.; Yusufoglu, H.S.; Alqasoumi, S.I.; Ganaie, M.A.; Alam, A. Neuroprotective Potential of Afzelin: A Novel Approach for Alleviating Catalepsy and Modulating Bcl-2 Expression in Parkinson's Disease Therapy. *Saudi Pharm. J.* **2024**, *32*, 101928. [CrossRef] [PubMed]
134. Behranvand, N.; Nasri, F.; Zolfaghari Emameh, R.; Khani, P.; Hosseini, A.; Garssen, J.; Falak, R. Chemotherapy: A Double-Edged Sword in Cancer Treatment. *Cancer Immunol. Immunother.* **2022**, *71*, 507–526. [CrossRef] [PubMed]
135. Najafi, M.; Majidpoor, J.; Toolee, H.; Mortezaee, K. The Current Knowledge Concerning Solid Cancer and Therapy. *J. Biochem. Mol. Toxicol.* **2021**, *35*, e22900. [CrossRef] [PubMed]

136. Wu, Z.; Wang, W.; He, F.; Li, D.; Wang, D. Simultaneous Enrichment and Separation of Four Flavonoids from *Zanthoxylum bungeanum* Leaves by Ultrasound-Assisted Extraction and Macroporous Resins with Evaluation of Antioxidant Activities. *J. Food Sci.* **2018**, *83*, 2109–2118. [CrossRef] [PubMed]
137. de Sousa, J.P.B.; Brancalion, A.P.S.; Júnior, M.G.; Bastos, J.K. A Validated Chromatographic Method for the Determination of Flavonoids in *Copaifera langsdorffii* by HPLC. *Nat. Prod. Commun.* **2012**, *7*, 25–28. [CrossRef] [PubMed]

pharmaceuticals MDPI

Systematic Review

Unveiling the Neuroprotective Potential of Date Palm (*Phoenix dactylifera*): A Systematic Review

Syed Mohammed Basheeruddin Asdaq [1,*], Abdulaziz Ali Almutiri [1], Abdullah Alenzi [1], Maheen Shaikh [2], Mujeeb Ahmed Shaik [3], Sultan Alshehri [4] and Syed Imam Rabbani [5]

1 Department of Pharmacy Practice, College of Pharmacy, AlMaarefa University, Dariyah, Riyadh 13713, Saudi Arabia; 191120097@student.um.edu.sa (A.A.A.); 202120443@student.um.edu.sa (A.A.)
2 College of Medicine, Alfaisal University, Riyadh 11533, Saudi Arabia; maheensskh@gmail.com
3 Department of Basic Medical Science, College of Medicine, AlMaarefa University, Dariyah, Riyadh 13713, Saudi Arabia; smujeeb@um.edu.sa
4 Department of Pharmaceutical Sciences, College of Pharmacy, AlMaarefa University, Dariyah, Riyadh 13713, Saudi Arabia; sshehri@um.edu.sa
5 Department of Pharmacology and Toxicology, College of Pharmacy, Qassim University, Buraydah 51452, Saudi Arabia; s.rabbani@qu.edu.sa
* Correspondence: sasdaq@gmail.com or sasdag@um.edu.sa

Abstract: Background: Neurodegenerative diseases primarily afflict the elderly and are characterized by a progressive loss of neurons. Oxidative stress is intricately linked to the advancement of these conditions. This study focuses on *Phoenix dactylifera* (*P. dactylifera;* Family: *Arecaceae*), commonly known as "Ajwa," a globally cultivated herbal plant renowned for its potent antioxidant properties and reported neuroprotective effects in pharmacological studies. **Method:** This comprehensive systematic review delves into the antioxidant properties of plant extracts and their phytochemical components, with a particular emphasis on *P. dactylifera* and its potential neuroprotective benefits. Preferred reporting items for systemic reviews and meta-analysis (PRISMA) were employed to review the articles. **Results:** The study includes 269 articles published in the literature and 17 were selected after qualitative analysis. The growing body of research underscores the critical role of polyphenolic compounds found in *P. dactylifera*, which significantly contribute to its neuroprotective effects through antioxidant mechanisms. Despite emerging insights into the antioxidant actions of *P. dactylifera*, further investigation is essential to fully elucidate the specific pathways through which it confers neuroprotection. **Conclusions:** Like many other plant-based supplements, *P. dactylifera*'s antioxidant effects are likely mediated by synergistic interactions among its diverse bioactive compounds, rather than by any single constituent alone. Therefore, additional preclinical and clinical studies are necessary to explore *P. dactylifera*'s therapeutic potential comprehensively, especially in terms of its targeted antioxidant activities aimed at mitigating neurodegenerative processes. Such research holds promise for advancing our understanding and potentially harnessing the therapeutic benefits of *P. dactylifera* in neuroprotection.

Keywords: drug efficacy; *Pheonix dactylifera*; antioxidant; neuroprotection; oxidative stress; phenolic compounds

1. Introduction

The survival of living things depends heavily on oxygen, which also serves as the building block for cellular respiration, which results in aerobic respiration [1]. Numerous molecules and cellular structures can be harmed by oxidative stress (OS), which can alter how well organs and systems function. The body builds up OS through both internal and external mechanisms [2]. Chronic exposure to chemicals including medications may result in modifications to the host system functioning [3]. An overabundance of reactive oxygen species (ROS) can harm nucleic acids, membrane lipids, and cellular proteins, impairing normal cellular function [4,5]. Furthermore, NO· radicals produced by nitric oxide have also been reported to induce damaging effects on organs such as the endothelium [6].

According to the literature, several conventional medications used in the treatment of several diseases are losing their efficacy [7]. Today, though, the focus is shifting away from synthetic medications and toward natural medications derived from bacteria or plants to treat illnesses [8]. The potential pharmacological value of natural products is continuously being investigated, with a focus on their potential effects on amoebicidal, cytotoxic, antimicrobial, spasmolytic, bronchodilator, antioxidant, anti-diarrheal, anti-Parkinsonism, anti-inflammatory, hypotensive, hepatoprotective, and hypoglycaemic functions [9].

The use of various herbs and medicinal plants as supplements to maintain overall mental well-being has drawn a lot of interest, especially considering their potential to improve memory and protect against neurodegeneration through antioxidant properties [10]. These plants have been investigated for likely therapeutic use in neurodegenerative disorders, with Alzheimer's disease being the more prevalent type, followed by Parkinson's disease [11]. Ginsenosides, the primary active plant element of various Panax species, have been the subject of intensive research due to their potential protective effects against neurological illnesses [12]. This has led to the practice of ginsenosides as a general tonic for enhancing well-being and managing stress [13]. Similarly, increasing scientific data showing that *Ginkgo biloba* supplements are effective in treating a variety of neurological disorders, such as ischemic stroke and cognitive impairment, has led to their classification as high-claim products [14].

The *Arecaceae* family, sometimes called the "Palm" family, comprises 2000 genera and 4000 species. Major crops from this family include dates, coconuts, and African palm oil [15]. Five of the 12 species in the Phoenix genus, including *Phoenix dactylifera*, are edible. Worldwide, there are roughly 3000 growers of the palm family [16]. The date palm is indigenous to the Persian Gulf and North Africa; still, its exact origin is unknown. Iraq, Egypt, Saudi Arabia, Tunisia, Algeria, the United Arab Emirates, Oman, Libya, Saudi Arabia, Pakistan, Sudan, Europe, and the United States are the top 10 producers of date palms [17].

Phoenix dactylifera, also known as Ajwa, is a variety of dates that is grown in different countries, including Saudi Arabia. It is useful in the treatment of many disorders and has been shown to have a protective effect against liver toxicity [18]. Regarding the potential health risks of dates, several biological and folkloric activities based on in vitro and animal models have been reported. These comprise protecting the heart and circulatory system by lowering blood levels of triglycerides and LDL cholesterol, preventing atherosclerosis and heart problems, preventing anemia, and maintaining a healthy nervous system and energy production [19–22]. Figure 1 represents *Phoenix dactylifera* cultivated in Saudi Arabia. Due to their high degree of nutraceutical potential for boosting the power of resistance, *P. dactylifera* dates and their preparations may be used in the care of long-suffering patients with considerably weakened or suppressed immune systems [23].

Furthermore, it has been found that cyanidin inhibits the death of neurons caused by amyloid beta by reducing reactive oxygen species (ROS) and reactive nitrogen species (RNS), which are linked to the modification of the mitochondrial death pathway in SK-N-SH cells [24,25]. To the best of our knowledge, a widespread published literature review has not previously been conducted on the protective effects of this plant product or on preparation against neurodegeneration brought on by oxidative stress. To investigate the possible advantages of *Pheonix dactylifera* against ROS-mediated neurodegeneration, a comprehensive assessment of the literature's several scientific studies on the subject was planned for this study.

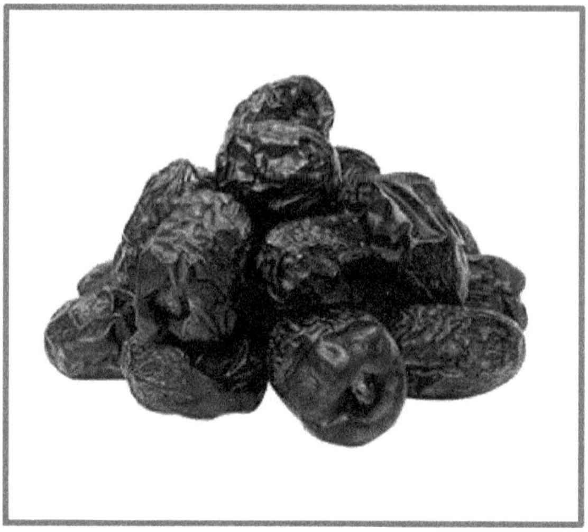

Figure 1. *Phoenix dactylifera* fruits cultivated in Madina province of Saudi Arabia [20,21].

2. Methodology

This systematic review was prepared following Preferred Reporting Items for Systematic Reviews and Meta-Analyses (PRISMA) standards (registration number IRB24-007). This study conducted the systemic review using the procedures outlined in the literature [26].

2.1. Literature Search Strategy

From December 2023 to March 2024, electronic literature searches of PubMed (n = 216), SCOPUS (n = 26), Web of Science (n = 15), and BIOSIS (n = 12) were conducted using keywords like *Pheonix dactylifera* OR *P. dactylifera* OR Ajwa OR Ajwa dates AND antioxidant OR oxidative stress OR free radicals OR reactive oxygen species AND neuroprotection OR neurodegeneration (Table S1).

2.2. Eligibility Criteria

Studies satisfying the following criteria were included in this review:

- Full-length, English-language articles that include detailed information, particularly details about the *P. dactylifera* research.
- Cross-sectional studies that were released in the previous two years, 2022–2023.
- Investigations that were conducted to ascertain the impact of *P. dactylifera* and oxidative stress on neurodegenerative disorders.
- Information about *P. dactylifera*'s pharmacological properties, including dose, duration, side reactions, and potential mechanisms of action.
- Investigated and evaluated publications from indexed journals that provide comprehensive details on statistics and their significance level.

Studies that failed to meet the eligibility criteria were excluded. Furthermore, data that overlapped or was duplicated, as well as information that could not be recovered, were not included in the analysis [27].

2.3. Study Selection

Two authors of this work independently reviewed the literature to determine *P. dactylifera*'s involvement in neurodegenerative illnesses. To decrease the chance of overlapping data, the authors segregated the diseases (e.g., Alzheimer's' disease, Parkinson's disease, Huntington's disease, amyotrophic lateral sclerosis, Lewy body disease, and spinal muscular atrophy) and analyzed the role of the plant on individual diseases. There were mainly two steps in the eligibility screening procedure. The author started by going over the titles and abstracts of the documents that were obtained. A thorough screening of the full-text articles chosen in the first phase was carried out in the second step. Any differences that emerged from the results were addressed and settled by the other authors of the study [28].

2.4. Data Extraction

Relevant data were separately retrieved using a pre-structured data extraction form. The retrieved data contained several crucial components, such as the study design, the parameters that were measured, and specifics on significant discoveries. Other elements that were crucial for evaluating the articles' content included the language used in the publication, study design, strain and quantity of animals, protocol, dosage, duration, and mode of administration, as well as ethical approvals, statistical approaches, and biomarker evaluations. Additionally, a review of the literature was conducted to determine the influence of phytoconstituents found in *P. dactylifera* on the host system's oxidative stress-mediated damages [29].

2.5. Quality Assessment

The Newcastle–Ottawa scale is a technique used to assess bias risk in cross-sectional studies. This tool covers multiple categories, with precise attention placed on elements like the study outcomes, statistical analysis description, and sample design. The author carried out a blind assessment of the study's quality, and any disagreements were settled through conversations with an authority on the topic [30]. Articles that are part of the study have to be eligible for it, which is determined by their Newcastle–Ottawa scale score, which cannot be less than 3.

2.6. Representation of Data

The population's data were gathered, documented, examined, and shown as either tabular data or figures. Figure 2 shows the results of the PRISMA search for scientific articles in the literature. Table 1 lists the significant phytoconstituents found in *P. dactylifera* that have been linked to antioxidant capacity. Figure 3 summarizes the potential mechanism for the neuroprotective impact.

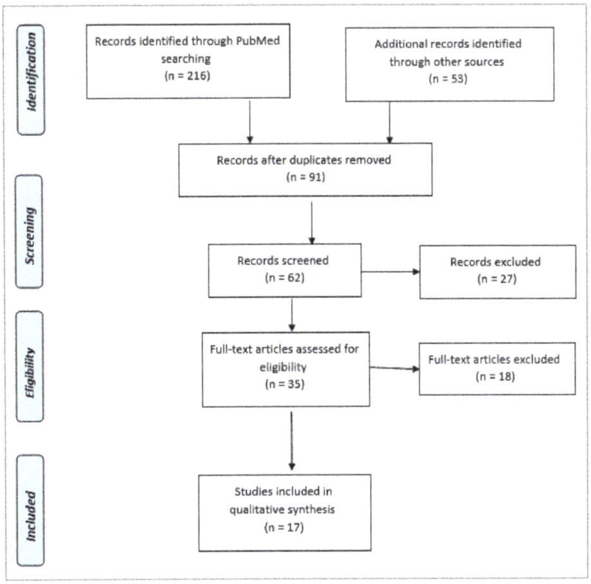

Figure 2. PRISMA flow diagram to select the scientific studies from the literature.

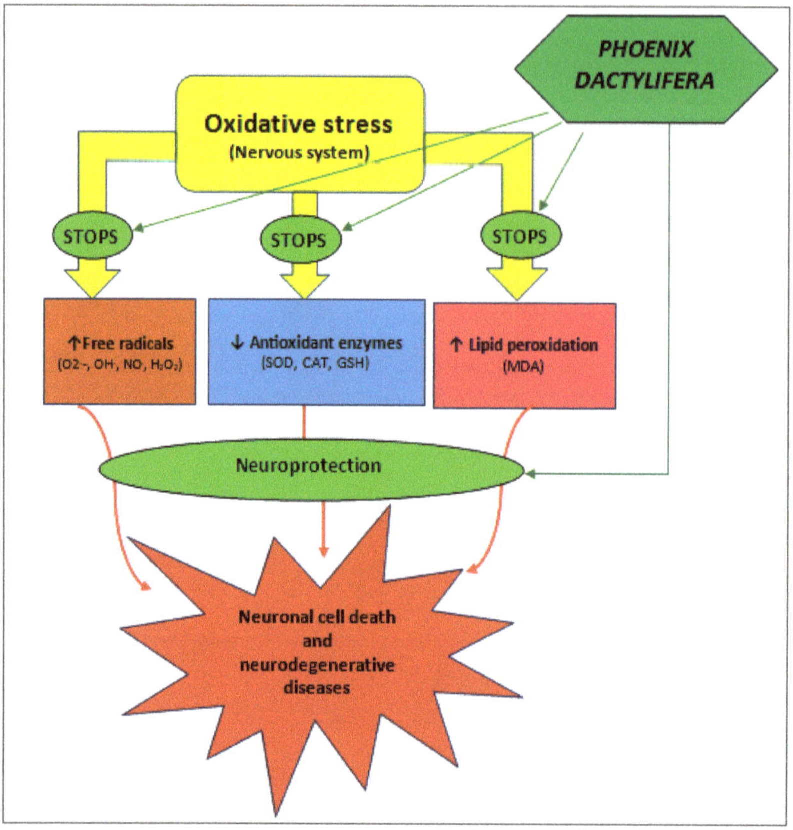

Figure 3. Potential mechanism for the neuroprotective effect of *Phoenix dactylifera*.

3. Oxidative Stress in Neurodegeneration

The redox reaction of oxidation involves the loss of electrons [31]. Reactive oxygen species (ROS), which are constantly produced throughout cell metabolism processes, are one byproduct of oxidation [32]. Free radicals from cell catabolism are thought to play a role in aging and other degenerative disorders [33]. Because of this, the human body contains built-in antioxidant defenses against free radicals, including glutathione (GSH), catalase, and superoxide dismutase (SOD) [34]. Oxidative stress is brought on by the build-up of ROS in a compromised antioxidant nerve system [35]. Pro-apoptotic Bcl-2 family members are involved in a neuronal cell death event that is triggered by oxidative stress [36].

The process of lipoperoxidation (LPO) is one way that OS damages lipids [37]. Hydroperoxides, including propanal, hexanal, 4-hydroxynonenal, isoprostane, and malondialdehyde (MDA), are the primary products of LPO [38]. Additionally, when ROS interact with guanine nucleotides, they can cause structural damage to DNA [39]. Under typical circumstances, these metabolites are restored by the oxoguanine glycosylase (hOGG1) enzyme and are collectively referred to as OS biomarkers [40].

Because of the high concentration of polyunsaturated fatty acids (PUFA), such as linoleic acid and arachidonic acid, the human brain is susceptible to oxidative stress [41]. In the neurological system, oxidized PUFA and ROS react to generate lipid peroxidation products, such as lipid peroxyl radical, which starts a chain reaction that further oxidizes PUFA [42]. Therefore, by scavenging peroxyl radicals, an antioxidant system is required to break the chain reaction of free radicals [41,43]

4. Major Phytochemicals of *Phoenix dactylifera* with Antioxidant Potential

Perhaps because of worries about the adverse effects of manmade chemicals, there has been a spike in interest in discovering novel antioxidants from plants. Many investigations have been carried out to clarify *P. dactylifera*'s naturally occurring chemicals and indicated the presence of several phenolic compounds [44].

P. dactylifera dates contain the following phenolic components: caffeic acid, catechin, and rutin. The ripening stage also affected *P. dactylifera*'s phenolic content, which ranged from 10 mg/100 g to 290 mg/100 g. The polyphenol content of *P. dactylifera* dates was found to be greatest at the kimri stage (290 mg/100 g), followed by the khalal (150 mg/100 g), rutab (20 mg/100 g), and tamr (10 mg/100 g) stages. The most prevalent phenolic compounds discovered in *P. dactylifera* dates were derivatives of gallic acid, ferulic acid, and p-coumaric acid [45–47].

Similar to this, it was discovered that *P. dactylifera*'s primary phenolic components and acids at various ripening stages included protocatechuic acid, hydroxybenzoic acid, vanillic acid, gallic acid, isovanillic acid, chlorogenic acid, ferulic acid, isoferulic acid, caffeic acid, hydroxycinnamic acid, and chlorogenic acid. Gallic acid, caffeic acid, chlorogenic acid, syringic acid, p-coumaric acid, m-coumaric acid, and ferulic acid were identified by many researchers as the main phenolics and acids in roasted *P. dactylifera* pits [48–52].

There are several subclasses of flavonoids, including anthocyanins, iso-flavones, flavones, and flavonols, identified in *P. dactylifera*. Active flavonoids, such as luteolin, rutin, isoquercetin, apgenin, and quercetin, are abundant in *P. dactylifera*. Within the kingdom of plants, flavonols are the most prevalent type of flavonoid. Flavonols, also known as oglycosides, are abundant in *P. dactylifera* flesh and pits. The amounts of these substances, however, differed significantly between the *P. dactylifera* fruit's meat and pits. Chrysoeriol-7-O-(2,6-dirhamnosyl)-glucoside has recently been found in *P. dactylifera* fruit. Using LC-MS/MS techniques, researchers examined the flavonoid composition of *P. dactylifera* at various ripening stages and discovered significant amounts of luteolin, kaempferol, myricetin, naringenin, apigenin, and quercetin [53–57].

Triterpenoids such as lupeol and lup-20(29)-en-3-one, steroids such as b-sitosterol, b-sitosteryl-3-O-b-glucoside, and b-sitosteryl-3b-glucopyranoside60-O-palmitate, and phthalates such as bis(2-ethylheptyl) phthalate and bis(2-ethylhexyl) terephthalate are among the other minor ingredients in *P. dactylifera* fruit. *P. dactylifera*'s bioactive components contribute to its antioxidant and anti-inflammatory qualities. An important quantity of anthocyanidins is also present in *P. dactylifera*, which is primarily found in the kimri stage. A few significant organic acids, such as succinic, oxalic, malic, citric, isobutyric, and formic acids, are present in *P. dactylifera*. These acids enhance *P. dactylifera*'s functionality even more [58–62]. Table 1 displays the chemical structures of the main phytochemicals that are present in *P. dactylifera*.

Table 1. Important phytoconstituents of *Phoenix dactylifera* identified for antioxidant properties, retrieved from the selected articles.

Sl. No.	Name	Chemical Structure	Reference (s)
1	Caffeic acid	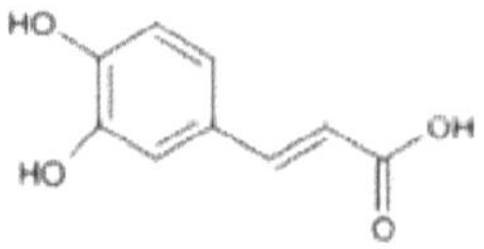	[47–49]
2	Ferulic acid	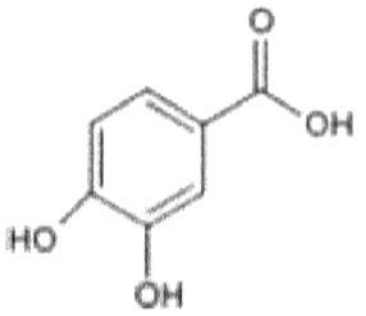	[46–48]
3	Catechin	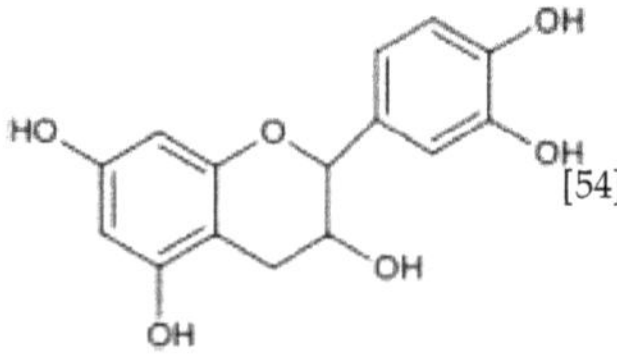	[54]
4	Gallic acid	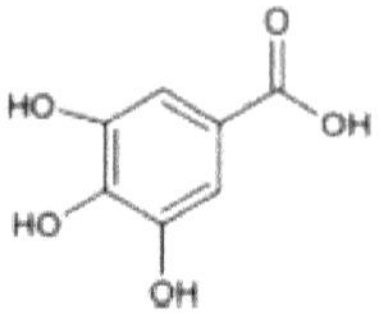	[53,55]
5	p-coumaric acid	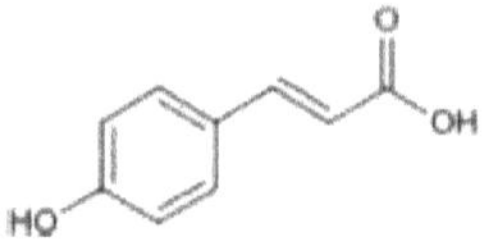	[49,51]
6	Resorcinol acid	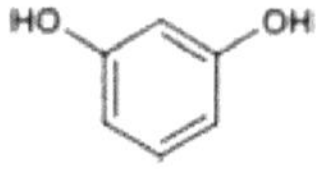	[59–61]
7	Quercetin	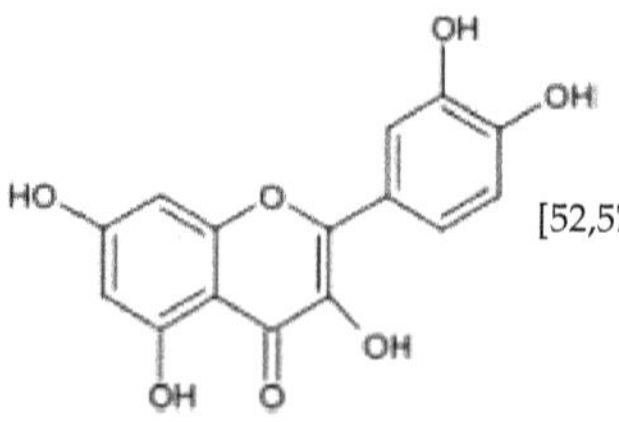	[52,57]

Table 1. *Cont.*

Sl. No.	Name	Chemical Structure	Reference (s)
8	Protocatechuic acid	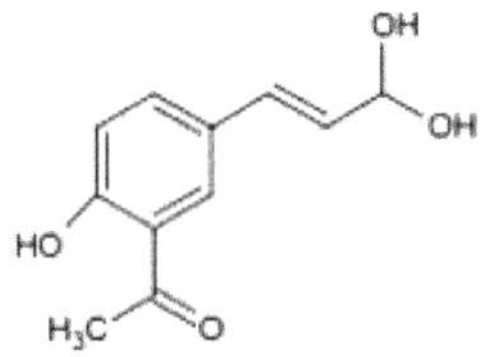	[49,62]
9	Rutin	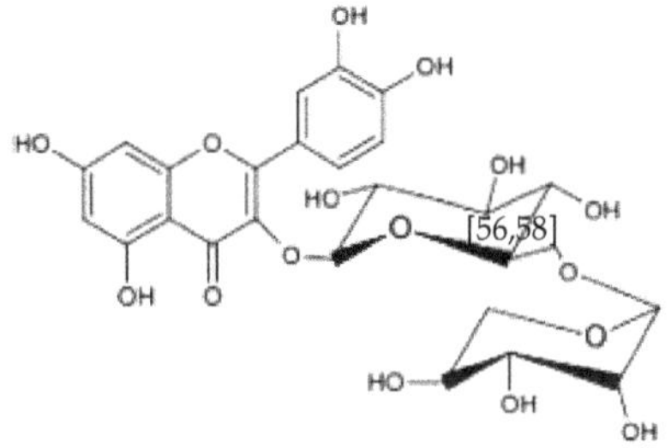	[56,58]
10	Apigenin	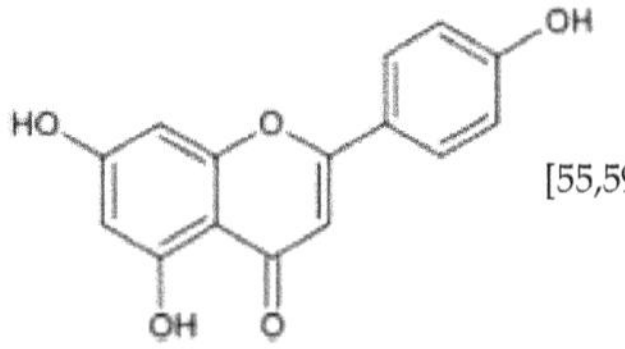	[55,59]

5. Antioxidant Properties of *P. dactylifera*

Because *P. dactylifera* fruits contain higher levels of phenolics, melatonin, carotenoids, and vitamins, they are used commonly in Arabian nations and have strong antioxidant potential [63]. Most studies on *P. dactylifera* fruit's antioxidant potential have used alcoholic and aqueous extracts. Most of the hydrophilic antioxidants in *P. dactylifera* fruit exhibit powerful antioxidant action in the lipid membrane system [64]. When compared to alcoholic extracts, it was found that the aqueous extract of *P. dactylifera* exhibited considerable antioxidant activity. Lipid peroxidation was prevented to an extent of up to 91% using different solvents such as ethyl acetate, methanolic, and aqueous for extraction of *P. dactylifera* in the MTT (3-(4,5-dimethylthiazol-2-yl)-2,5-diphenyltetrazolium bromide) assay [65]. Furthermore, the antioxidant potential of Phoenix dactylifera was found to be comparable to that of well-established herbal remedies such as *Panax notoginseng* and *Ginkgo biloba* [13,14].

In cadmium-intoxicated animals, the ethanolic extract of *P. dactylifera* resulted in a decrease in lipid hydroperoxides and an increase in blood antioxidant enzyme levels [66]. *P. dactylifera may exert* its antioxidant action by suppressing free radicals, which, in turn, slows down the spread of disease [67].

P. dactylifera has been shown to have potent antioxidant benefits by additional research. *P. dactylifera* extracts have been shown to stop the depletion of important antioxidants such glutathione peroxidase, superoxide dismutase, and carnitine acyltransferase [68]. Strong antioxidant activity was observed in an investigation using several *P. dactylifera* extracts, with methanolic extracts exhibiting equipotent with gallic acid [69]. Furthermore, they demonstrated potent radical scavenging ability in DPPH and lipid peroxidation tests using *P. dactylifera* date acetone extracts. In contrast to other solvents, they did note the exceptional radical scavenging activity of *P. dactylifera* aqueous extracts [70].

In vivo and in vitro studies on the neuroprotective properties of caffeic acid are reported in the literature. While the hybrid molecule of 20 mg/kg caffeic acid-syringic acid showed excellent neuroprotective effects on transient cerebral ischemia injury in the hippocampal CA1 area, caffeic acid in gerbils established only modest neuroprotection [71]. Due to its potent antioxidant properties, caffeine exhibited dose-dependent protection for neuronal cells against H_2O_2-induced cytotoxicity [72]. In a different study, caffeine reduced AChE activity in the cortex and striatum, which enhanced learning and memory in an inhibitory avoidance task [73].

6. Putative Mechanisms of Antioxidant Action of *P. dactylifera* in Neurodegenerative Diseases

The precise processes behind *P. dactylifera*'s scavenging action are still unknown, despite the organism's well-documented antioxidant properties. Based on prior research on the plant extract and its chief phytochemicals, which were covered above, we propose potential pathways for its therapeutic antioxidant actions (Figure 3). In summary, phenolic compounds can respond directly to ROS by scavenging free radicals and demonstrate antioxidant activity by preventing the death of neurons [74].

It is possible that their antioxidative effects were mediated by the polyphenol compounds' ability to transfer an electron to the free radicals, stabilizing them. The antioxidative activities of phenolic compounds were reported to reduce the Bax/Bcl-2 ratio and caspase-3 production, pro-apoptotic signals, and lipid peroxidation, thus preventing cell death [75]. On the other hand, SOD's antioxidant enzyme increased [76]. Meanwhile, *P. dactylifera* extract increased the levels of endogenous antioxidant GSH and catalase, which, in turn, decreased lipid peroxidation and demonstrated effects that protected cells [77]. The expression of the neuronal marker genes tyrosine hydroxylase (TH) and brain-derived neurotropic factor (BDNF), which are critical for cell survival because they are involved in neurotransmitter synthesis, also mediates the neuroprotective effects of phenols [78].

Moreover, selenium, which is known to have strong antioxidant properties, is present in *P. dactylifera* [79]. Numerous studies have shown that the main source of this essential trace element's antioxidant action is selenocysteine residues, which are an essential component of the ROS-detoxifying seleno-enzymes (GPx, thioredoxin reductases, and, maybe, selenoprotein P) [80–82]. The combination of selenium and other phenolic compounds seems to be the most plausible source of documented antioxidant and free radical scavenging properties [83].

Rats were given a methanolic extract of *P. dactylifera* fruits at doses of 30, 100, and 300 mg/kg for 15 days as part of a study on the neuroprotective effects of *P. dactylifera* against bilateral common carotid artery blockage. At dosages of 100 and 300 mg/kg, *P. dactylifera* extract significantly reduced the ischemia-induced diminution of GSH, SOD, and CAT expression; however, at lower dosages (30 mg/kg), no significant changes were seen [84]. The methanolic extract of *P. dactylifera* consequently showed brain damage and antioxidant protection that was dose-dependent [85].

In a different study, *P. dactylifera*'s compounds, which include ellagic acid, epicatechin, catechin, kaempferol, quercetin, and apigenin, were shown to have the capacity to function as dual inhibitors of acetylcholinesterase (AChE) and COX-2, potentially improving both cholinergic and inflammatory disorders. In contrast, the compounds cinnamic acid, hesperidin, hesperetin, narengin, and rutin were found to be solely responsible for improving cholinergic transmission. *P. dactylifera* provides neuroprotection against LPS-induced cognitive impairments in rats by preventing neuroinflammation and enhancing cholinergic function [86]. The results showed that extract therapy, probably because of its antioxidant properties, may shield cortical neurons from brain injury [87].

Date seed extract's potential to prevent cerebral ischemia in male rats was investigated. This study shows that seed extract greatly reduces neuronal damage [84]. The application of seed extracts also retained the ultra-structures of cortical neurons. The group that received seed extract treatment also displayed improvements in fall out latency times [88]. Additionally, the brain's oxidative stress decreased and its antioxidative enzymes were restored [89]. In addition to these advantages, *P. dactylifera* seed extract also lessens muscle weakness, which protects against the damage caused by ischemia-reperfusion [90]. *P. dactylifera* may have a cerebroprotective effect because of its antioxidant activity. According to this study, using *P. dactylifera* to treat cerebral ischemia may be advantageous [89,91].

The neuroprotective effect of *P. dactylifera* fruits has also been shown by another study, which used male rats in which aluminium chloride was used to induce experimental Alzheimer's disease. The results of this activity clearly show that *P. dactylifera* is a neuroprotective agent due to its antioxidative qualities, and this activity is attributed to the presence of polyphenolic components such as flavonoids, plant sterols, and ascorbic acid [92]. Furthermore, it has been found that caffeic acid inhibits the synthesis of AChE and the activation of Keap1-Nrf2 [93]. From these data, it is clear that *P. dactylifera* has neuroprotective qualities. This is mainly because the plant contains naturally occurring antioxidants such as phenols, which were previously mentioned.

7. Future Implications

Researchers have placed a lot of emphasis on phenolic chemicals that have been extracted from plants because of their strong antioxidant properties. The specificity in the etiology of neurodegenerative defects may contribute to the ongoing debate about the role of oxidative stress in neurodegeneration [94]. Antioxidant supplementation has been demonstrated to have no advantages in certain clinical trials, and in some cases, it has even had negative effects on the cognitive performance of people with Alzheimer's disease [95]. Nonetheless, the high oxygen consumption of the brain makes it clear that neuronal cells are extremely susceptible to oxidative stress [96]. Consequently, one of the possible causes of neurodegeneration may be compromised antioxidant defense systems, indicating the significance of antioxidants in halting or postponing the beginning of neurodegeneration [97]. Drugs derived from plants are reported to exhibit a balancing act in the suppression of oxidative stress-induced damages [25]. One of the reasons identified is due to the presence of different classes of phytochemicals that can produce multiple mechanisms [12]. Hence, there is growing interest in determining the potential of plant-based products in overcoming oxidative stress-mediated disorders including neurological defects.

A growing body of evidence indicates that *P. dactylifera*, and especially its polyphenolic components, exhibited potent antioxidant properties. The literature selected for this study identified the presence of vital phytocomponents in *P. dactylifera* that have antioxidant potential. *P. dactylifera*'s main active ingredients are polyphenols, which have strong antioxidant properties [98]. Even though *P. dactylifera* showed strong antioxidant activity, there is still a growing amount of preclinical evidence and no clinical literature to date to adequately support the neuroprotective capabilities of *P. dactylifera*. Although potential pathways for *P. dactylifera*'s antioxidant actions have been suggested, more research is needed to clarify these mechanisms to better understand how *P. dactylifera*'s antioxidant actions relate to its neuroprotective effects.

Alternatively, *P. dactylifera*'s antioxidant benefits may be due to the synergy of several different naturally occurring bioactive compounds in the plant, meaning that rather than products made from a single bioactive compound extracted from the plant, the putative effects would need to be produced by oral administration of the whole plant extract as a dietary supplement [99]. Thus, more preclinical and clinical research examining *P. dactylifera*'s medicinal potential, particularly in the prevention of neurodegeneration, is necessary due to its targeted targeting of neuroprotection through antioxidant activities.

8. Conclusions

According to the study's research, *P. dactylifera* may have antioxidant characteristics that have neuroprotective effects. By scavenging free radicals and enhancing the antioxidant defense system, the phenolic chemicals found in the plant may be the cause of the oxidative stress attenuation. The fruit is taken for its spiritual and therapeutic benefits and is well-liked throughout the world. Further investigation into the different phytoactive components may reveal a possible naturally derived medication option for the treatment of a range of conditions, including neurodegenerative illnesses.

Supplementary Materials: The following supporting information can be downloaded at: https://www.mdpi.com/article/10.3390/ph17091221/s1, Table S1: Electronic search thread used for *Phoenix dactylifera*.

Author Contributions: The manuscript writing, editing, and original draft preparation were performed by A.A.A., S.A., and A.A. The data and literature were extracted by M.S. and M.A.S. The conception and design were performed by S.M.B.A. and S.A. The review and final editing of the manuscript was carried out by S.M.B.A. and S.I.R. The supervision of the manuscript writing was performed by S.M.B.A. All authors have read and agreed to the published version of the manuscript.

Funding: The authors would like to express gratitude to AlMaarefa University, Riyadh, Saudi Arabia, for extending financial support to do this research project through grant number (UM-DSR-IG-2023-01).

Data Availability Statement: Data are contained within the article or Supplementary Materials.

Acknowledgments: The authors would like to acknowledge the funding support provided by AlMaarefa University through grant number (UM-DSR-IG-2023-01).

Conflicts of Interest: The authors declare no conflicts of interest.

References

1. Marín, R.; Abad, C.; Rojas, D.; Chiarello, D.I.; Alejandro, T.G. Biomarkers of oxidative stress and reproductive complications. *Adv. Clin. Chem.* **2023**, *113*, 157–233. [PubMed]
2. Matyas, C.; Haskó, G.; Liaudet, L.; Trojnar, E.; Pacher, P. Interplay of cardiovascular mediators, oxidative stress and inflammation in liver disease and its complications. *Nat. Rev. Cardiol.* **2021**, *18*, 117–135. [CrossRef] [PubMed]
3. Daenen, K.; Andries, A.; Mekahli, D.; Van Schepdael, A.; Jouret, F.; Bammens, B. Oxidative stress in chronic kidney disease. *Pediatr. Nephrol.* **2019**, *34*, 975–991. [CrossRef] [PubMed]
4. Bai, R.; Guo, J.; Ye, X.Y.; Xie, Y.; Xie, T. Oxidative stress: The core pathogenesis and mechanism of Alzheimer's disease. *Ageing Res. Rev.* **2022**, *77*, 101619. [CrossRef] [PubMed]
5. Hajam, Y.A.; Rani, R.; Ganie, S.Y.; Sheikh, T.A.; Javaid, D.; Qadri, S.S.; Pramodh, S.; Alsulimani, A.; Alkhanani, M.F.; Harakeh, S.; et al. Oxidative Stress in Human Pathology and Aging: Molecular Mechanisms and Perspectives. *Cells* **2022**, *11*, 552. [CrossRef]
6. Salvagno, M.; Sterchele, E.D.; Zaccarelli, M.; Mrakic-Sposta, S.; Welsby, I.J.; Balestra, C.; Taccone, F.S. Oxidative Stress and Cerebral Vascular Tone: The Role of Reactive Oxygen and Nitrogen Species. *Int. J. Mol. Sci.* **2024**, *25*, 3007. [CrossRef]
7. Njoroge, J.N.; Teerlink, J.R. Pathophysiology and Therapeutic Approaches to Acute Decompensated Heart Failure. *Circ. Res.* **2021**, *128*, 1468–1486. [CrossRef]
8. De Franciscis, P.; Colacurci, N.; Riemma, G.; Conte, A.; Pittana, E.; Guida, M.; Schiattarella, A. A Nutraceutical Approach to Menopausal Complaints. *Medicina* **2019**, *55*, 544. [CrossRef]
9. Tasneem, S.; Liu, B.; Li, B.; Choudhary, M.I.; Wang, W. Molecular pharmacology of inflammation: Medicinal plants as anti-inflammatory agents. *Pharmacol. Res.* **2019**, *139*, 126–140. [CrossRef]
10. Zhu, T.; Wang, L.; Wang, L.P.; Wan, Q. Therapeutic targets of neuroprotection and neurorestoration in ischemic stroke: Applications for natural compounds from medicinal herbs. *Biomed. Pharmacother.* **2022**, *148*, 112719. [CrossRef]
11. Chen, S.; Liu, H.; Wang, S.; Jiang, H.; Gao, L.; Wang, L.; Teng, L.; Wang, C.; Wang, D. The Neuroprotection of Verbascoside in Alzheimer's Disease Mediated through Mitigation of Neuroinflammation via Blocking NF-κB-p65 Signaling. *Nutrients* **2022**, *14*, 1417. [CrossRef] [PubMed]
12. Chen, Y.Y.; Liu, Q.P.; An, P.; Jia, M.; Luan, X.; Tang, J.Y.; Zhang, H. Ginsenoside Rd: A promising natural neuroprotective agent. *Phytomedicine* **2022**, *95*, 153883. [CrossRef] [PubMed]
13. Wu, L.; Song, H.; Zhang, C.; Wang, A.; Zhang, B.; Xiong, C.; Zhuang, X.; Zang, Y.; Li, C.; Fang, Q.; et al. Efficacy and Safety of Panax notoginseng Saponins in the Treatment of Adults with Ischemic Stroke in China: A Randomized Clinical Trial. *JAMA Netw. Open* **2023**, *6*, e2317574. [CrossRef] [PubMed]
14. Singh, S.K.; Srivastav, S.; Castellani, R.J.; Plascencia-Villa, G.; Perry, G. Neuroprotective and Antioxidant Effect of Ginkgo biloba Extract Against AD and Other Neurological Disorders. *Neurotherapeutics* **2019**, *16*, 666–674. [CrossRef]
15. Al-Okbi, S.Y. Date Palm as Source of Nutraceuticals for Health Promotion: A Review. *Curr. Nutr. Rep.* **2022**, *11*, 574–591. [CrossRef]
16. El-Far, A.H.; Oyinloye, B.E.; Sepehrimanesh, M.; Allah, M.A.G.; Abu-Reidah, I.; Shaheen, H.M.; Razeghian-Jahromi, I.; Alsenosy, A.E.A.; Noreldin, A.E.; Al Jaouni, S.K.; et al. Date Palm (*Phoenix dactylifera*): Novel Findings and Future Directions for Food and Drug Discovery. *Curr. Drug Discov. Technol.* **2019**, *16*, 2–10. [CrossRef]

17. Ahmed, O.S.; Sedraoui, S.; Zhou, B.; Reversat, G.; Rocher, A.; Bultel-Poncé, V.; Guy, A.; Vercauteren, J.; Selim, S.; Galano, J.M.; et al. Phytoprostanes from Date Palm Fruit and Byproducts: Five Different Varieties Grown in Two Different Locations As Potential sources. *J. Agric. Food Chem.* **2021**, *69*, 13754–13761. [CrossRef]
18. Saputri, R.D.; Usman, A.N.; Widaningsih, Y.; Jafar, N.; Ahmad, M.; Ramadhani, S.; Dirpan, A. Date palm (*Phoenix dactylifera*) consumption as a nutrition source for mild anemia. *Gac. Sanit.* **2021**, *35* (Suppl. 2), S271–S274. [CrossRef]
19. Alkhoori, M.A.; Kong, A.S.; Aljaafari, M.N.; Abushelaibi, A.; Erin Lim, S.H.; Cheng, W.H.; Chong, C.M.; Lai, K.S. Biochemical Composition and Biological Activities of Date Palm (*Phoenix dactylifera* L.) Seeds: A Review. *Biomolecules* **2022**, *12*, 1626. [CrossRef]
20. Ibiyeye, R.; Sulaimon, F.; Imam, A.; Adana, M.; Okesina, A.; Ajao, M. *Phoenix dactylifera* and polyphenols ameliorated monosodium glutamate toxicity in the dentate gyrus of Wistar rats. *Niger. J. Physiol. Sci.* **2023**, *38*, 73–78. [CrossRef]
21. Younas, A.; Naqvi, S.A.; Khan, M.R.; Shabbir, M.A.; Jatoi, M.A.; Anwar, F.; Inam-Ur-Raheem, M.; Saari, N.; Aadil, R.M. Functional food and nutra-pharmaceutical perspectives of date (*Phoenix dactylifera* L.) fruit. *J. Food Biochem.* **2020**, *44*, e13332. [CrossRef] [PubMed]
22. Al-Dashti, Y.A.; Holt, R.R.; Keen, C.L.; Hackman, R.M. Date Palm Fruit (*Phoenix dactylifera*): Effects on Vascular Health and Future Research Directions. *Int. J. Mol. Sci.* **2021**, *22*, 4665. [CrossRef] [PubMed]
23. Barakat, H.; Alfheeaid, H.A. Date Palm Fruit (*Phoenix dactylifera*) and Its Promising Potential in Developing Functional Energy Bars: Review of Chemical, Nutritional, Functional, and Sensory Attributes. *Nutrients* **2023**, *15*, 2134. [CrossRef] [PubMed]
24. Alberti, Á.; Riethmüller, E.; Béni, S. Characterization of diarylheptanoids: An emerging class of bioactive natural products. *J. Pharm. Biomed. Anal.* **2018**, *147*, 13–34. [CrossRef] [PubMed]
25. Hall, E.D.; Wang, J.A.; Miller, D.M.; Cebak, J.E.; Hill, R.L. Newer pharmacological approaches for antioxidant neuroprotection in traumatic brain injury. *Neuropharmacology* **2019**, *145 (Pt B)*, 247–258. [CrossRef]
26. Watson, N.; Diamandis, T.; Gonzales-Portillo, C.; Reyes, S.; Borlongan, C.V. Melatonin as an Antioxidant for Stroke Neuroprotection. *Cell Transpl.* **2016**, *25*, 883–891. [CrossRef]
27. Abu-Odeh, A.; Fino, L.; Al-Absi, G.; Alnatour, D.; Al-Darraji, M.; Shehadeh, M.; Suaifan, G. Medicinal plants of Jordan: Scoping review. *Heliyon* **2023**, *9*, e17081. [CrossRef]
28. Głąbska, D.; Guzek, D.; Groele, B.; Gutkowska, K. Fruit and Vegetable Intake and Mental Health in Adults: A Systematic Review. *Nutrients* **2020**, *12*, 115. [CrossRef]
29. Leisegang, K.; Finelli, R.; Sikka, S.C.; Panner Selvam, M.K. Eurycoma longifolia (Jack) Improves Serum Total Testosterone in Men: A Systematic Review and Meta-Analysis of Clinical Trials. *Medicina* **2022**, *58*, 1047. [CrossRef]
30. Awad, A.; Goh, M.S.; Trubiano, J.A. Drug Reaction with Eosinophilia and Systemic Symptoms: A Systematic Review. *J. Allergy Clin. Immunol. Pract.* **2023**, *11*, 1856–1868. [CrossRef]
31. Roy, J.; Galano, J.M.; Durand, T.; Le Guennec, J.Y.; Lee, J.C. Physiological role of reactive oxygen species as promoters of natural defenses. *FASEB J.* **2017**, *31*, 3729–3745. [CrossRef] [PubMed]
32. Yang, D.; Guo, X.; Xie, T.; Luo, X. Reactive oxygen species may play an essential role in driving biological evolution: The Cambrian Explosion as an example. *J. Environ. Sci.* **2018**, *63*, 218–226. [CrossRef] [PubMed]
33. Miwa, S.; Kashyap, S.; Chini, E.; von Zglinicki, T. Mitochondrial dysfunction in cell senescence and aging. *J. Clin. Investig.* **2022**, *132*, e158447. [CrossRef] [PubMed]
34. Roy, Z.; Bansal, R.; Siddiqui, L.; Chaudhary, N. Understanding the Role of Free Radicals and Antioxidant Enzymes in Human Diseases. *Curr. Pharm. Biotechnol.* **2023**, *24*, 1265–1276. [PubMed]
35. Di Meo, S.; Venditti, P. Evolution of the Knowledge of Free Radicals and Other Oxidants. *Oxid. Med. Cell Longev.* **2020**, *2020*, 9829176. [CrossRef]
36. Wang, K.; Liu, H.; Sun, W.; Guo, J.; Jiang, Z.; Xu, S.; Miao, Z. Eucalyptol alleviates avermectin exposure-induced apoptosis and necroptosis of grass carp hepatocytes by regulating ROS/NLRP3 axis. *Aquat. Toxicol.* **2023**, *264*, 106739. [CrossRef]
37. Mortensen, M.S.; Ruiz, J.; Watts, J.L. Polyunsaturated Fatty Acids Drive Lipid Peroxidation during Ferroptosis. *Cells* **2023**, *12*, 804. [CrossRef]
38. Jaganjac, M.; Milkovic, L.; Zarkovic, N.; Zarkovic, K. Oxidative stress and regeneration. *Free Radic. Biol. Med.* **2022**, *181*, 154–165. [CrossRef]
39. Chen, P.P.; Yang, P.; Liu, C.; Deng, Y.L.; Luo, Q.; Miao, Y.; Zhang, M.; Cui, F.P.; Zeng, J.Y.; Shi, T.; et al. Urinary concentrations of phenols, oxidative stress biomarkers and thyroid cancer: Exploring associations and mediation effects. *J. Environ. Sci.* **2022**, *120*, 30–40. [CrossRef]
40. Li, J.; Jia, B.; Cheng, Y.; Song, Y.; Li, Q.; Luo, C. Targeting Molecular Mediators of Ferroptosis and Oxidative Stress for Neurological Disorders. *Oxid. Med. Cell Longev.* **2022**, *2022*, 3999083. [CrossRef]
41. Ma, X.H.; Liu, J.H.; Liu, C.Y.; Sun, W.Y.; Duan, W.J.; Wang, G.; Kurihara, H.; He, R.R.; Li, Y.F.; Chen, Y.; et al. ALOX15-launched PUFA-phospholipids peroxidation increases the susceptibility of ferroptosis in ischemia-induced myocardial damage. *Signal Transduct. Target. Ther.* **2022**, *7*, 288. [CrossRef] [PubMed]
42. Liu, D.; Zhou, L.; Yang, M.; McIntyre, R.S.; Cao, B. Oxidative Stress Mediates the Association Between Dietary Fat Intake and Cognition in US Older Adults. *Am. J. Geriatr. Psychiatry* **2022**, *30*, 761–773. [CrossRef] [PubMed]
43. Videla, L.A.; Hernandez-Rodas, M.C.; Metherel, A.H.; Valenzuela, R. Influence of the nutritional status and oxidative stress in the desaturation and elongation of n-3 and n-6 polyunsaturated fatty acids: Impact on non-alcoholic fatty liver disease. *Prostaglandins Leukot. Essent. Fatty Acids* **2022**, *181*, 102441. [CrossRef] [PubMed]

44. Yasin, B.R.; El-Fawal, H.A.; Mousa, S.A. Date (*Phoenix dactylifera*) Polyphenolics and Other Bioactive Compounds: A Traditional Islamic Remedy's Potential in Prevention of Cell Damage, Cancer Therapeutics and Beyond. *Int. J. Mol. Sci.* **2015**, *16*, 30075–30090. [CrossRef] [PubMed]
45. Ahmad Mohd Zain, M.R.; Abdul Kari, Z.; Dawood, M.A.O.; Nik Ahmad Ariff, N.S.; Salmuna, Z.N.; Ismail, N.; Zainal Abidin, S.; Seong Wei, L.; Ahmed Shokri, A. Bioactivity and Pharmacological Potential of Date Palm (*Phoenix dactylifera* L.) Against Pandemic COVID-19: A Comprehensive Review. *Appl. Biochem. Biotechnol.* **2022**, *194*, 4587–4624. [CrossRef]
46. Gad El-Hak, H.N.; Mahmoud, H.S.; Ahmed, E.A.; Elnegris, H.M.; Aldayel, T.S.; Abdelrazek, H.M.A.; Soliman, M.T.A.; El-Menyawy, M.A.I. Methanolic *Phoenix dactylifera* L. Extract Ameliorates Cisplatin-Induced Hepatic Injury in Male Rats. *Nutrients* **2022**, *14*, 1025. [CrossRef]
47. Shivanandappa, T.B.; Alotaibi, G.; Chinnadhurai, M.; Dachani, S.R.; Ahmad, M.D.; Aldaajanii, K.A. *Phoenix dactylifera* (Ajwa Dates) Alleviate LPS-Induced Sickness Behaviour in Rats by Attenuating Proinflammatory Cytokines and Oxidative Stress in the Brain. *Int. J. Mol. Sci.* **2023**, *24*, 10413. [CrossRef]
48. Balasmeh, R.; Jarrar, Y.; Al-Sheikh, I.; Alshaiah, H.; Jarrar, Q.; Alani, R.; Abudahab, S. Effects of Fasting and *Phoenix dactylifera* on the Expression of Major Drug- Metabolizing Enzymes in the Mouse Livers. *Curr. Drug Metab.* **2022**, *23*, 666–676. [CrossRef]
49. Alkhalidy, H.; Al-Nabulsi, A.A.; Al-Taher, M.; Osaili, T.; Olaimat, A.N.; Liu, D. Date (*Phoenix dactylifera* L.) seed oil is an agro-industrial waste with biopreservative effects and antimicrobial activity. *Sci. Rep.* **2023**, *13*, 17142. [CrossRef]
50. Osman, K.M.; Kamal, O.E.; Deif, H.N.; Ahmed, M.M. *Phoenix dactylifera*, mentha piperita and montanide™ ISA-201 as immunological adjuvants in a chicken model. *Acta Trop.* **2020**, *202*, 105281. [CrossRef]
51. Alahyane, A.; ElQarnifa, S.; Ayour, J.; Elateri, I.; Ouamnina, A.; Ait-Oubahou, A.; Benichou, M.; Abderrazik, M. Date seeds (*Phoenix dactylifera* L.) valorization: Chemical composition of lipid fraction. *Braz. J. Biol.* **2022**, *84*, e260771. [CrossRef] [PubMed]
52. Gantait, S.; El-Dawayati, M.M.; Panigrahi, J.; Labrooy, C.; Verma, S.K. The retrospect and prospect of the applications of biotechnology in *Phoenix dactylifera* L. *Appl. Microbiol. Biotechnol.* **2018**, *102*, 8229–8259. [CrossRef] [PubMed]
53. Zein, N.; Elewa, Y.H.A.; Alruwaili, M.K.; Dewaard, M.; Alorabi, M.; Albogami, S.M.; Batiha, G.E.; Zahran, M.H. Barhi date (*Phoenix dactylifera*) extract ameliorates hepatocellular carcinoma in male rats. *Biomed. Pharmacother.* **2022**, *156*, 113976. [CrossRef] [PubMed]
54. Otify, A.M.; Hammam, A.M.; Aly Farag, M. *Phoenix dactylifera* L. date tree pollen fertility effects on female rats in relation to its UPLC-MS profile via a biochemometric approach. *Steroids* **2021**, *173*, 108888. [CrossRef] [PubMed]
55. Taleb, H.; Maddocks, S.E.; Morris, R.K.; Kanekanian, A.D. Chemical characterisation and the anti-inflammatory, anti-angiogenic and antibacterial properties of date fruit (*Phoenix dactylifera* L.). *J. Ethnopharmacol.* **2016**, *194*, 457–468. [CrossRef]
56. Ismail, H.; Khalid, D.; Ayub, S.B.; Ijaz, M.U.; Akram, S.; Bhatti, M.Z.; Yousef, F.M.; Waard, M. Effects of *Phoenix dactylifera* against Streptozotocin-Aluminium Chloride Induced Alzheimer's Rats and Their In Silico Study. *Biomed. Res. Int.* **2023**, *2023*, 1725638. [CrossRef]
57. Halabi, A.A.; Elwakil, B.H.; Hagar, M.; Olama, Z.A. Date Fruit (*Phoenix dactylifera* L.) Cultivar Extracts: Nanoparticle Synthesis, Antimicrobial and Antioxidant Activities. *Molecules* **2022**, *27*, 5165. [CrossRef]
58. Bettaieb, I.; Ali Benabderrahim, M.; Rodríguez Arcos, R.; Jose Jiménez Araujo, A.; Elfalleh, W. Date Seeds (*Phoenix dactylifera*): Antioxidant Potential and Profile of Free and Bound Polyphenols from Different Cultivars. *Chem. Biodivers.* **2023**, *20*, e202300179. [CrossRef]
59. Khan, M.A.; Singh, R.; Siddiqui, S.; Ahmad, I.; Ahmad, R.; Upadhyay, S.; Barkat, M.A.; Ali, A.M.A.; Zia, Q.; Srivastava, A.; et al. Anticancer potential of *Phoenix dactylifera* L. seed extract in human cancer cells and pro-apoptotic effects mediated through caspase-3 dependent pathway in human breast cancer MDA-MB-231 cells: An in vitro and in silico investigation. *BMC Complement. Med. Ther.* **2022**, *22*, 68. [CrossRef]
60. Djaoudene, O.; López, V.; Cásedas, G.; Les, F.; Schisano, C.; Bachir Bey, M.; Tenore, G.C. *Phoenix dactylifera* L. seeds: A by-product as a source of bioactive compounds with antioxidant and enzyme inhibitory properties. *Food Funct.* **2019**, *10*, 4953–4965. [CrossRef]
61. Athinarayanan, J.; Periasamy, V.S.; Alshatwi, A.A. *Phoenix dactylifera* lignocellulosic biomass as precursor for nanostructure fabrication using integrated process. *Int. J. Biol. Macromol.* **2019**, *134*, 1179–1186. [CrossRef] [PubMed]
62. Habib, H.M.; El-Fakharany, E.M.; El-Gendi, H.; El-Ziney, M.G.; El-Yazbi, A.F.; Ibrahim, W.H. Palm Fruit (*Phoenix dactylifera* L.) Pollen Extract Inhibits Cancer Cell and Enzyme Activities and DNA and Protein Damage. *Nutrients* **2023**, *15*, 2614. [CrossRef] [PubMed]
63. Boroujeni, S.N.; Malamiri, F.A.; Bossaghzadeh, F.; Esmaeili, A.; Moudi, E. The most important medicinal plants affecting sperm and testosterone production: A systematic review. *JBRA Assist. Reprod.* **2022**, *26*, 522–530. [CrossRef] [PubMed]
64. Abbassi, R.; Pontes, M.C.; Dhibi, S.; Duarte Filho, L.A.M.S.; Othmani, S.; Bouzenna, H.; Almeida, J.R.G.S.; Hfaiedh, N. Antioxidant properties of date seeds extract (*Phoenix dactylifera* L.) in alloxan induced damage in rats. *Braz. J. Biol.* **2023**, *83*, e274405. [CrossRef] [PubMed]
65. Subash, S.; Essa, M.M.; Al-Asmi, A.; Al-Adawi, S.; Vaishnav, R.; Guillemin, G.J. Effect of dietary supplementation of dates in Alzheimer's disease APPsw/2576 transgenic mice on oxidative stress and antioxidant status. *Nutr. Neurosci.* **2015**, *18*, 281–288. [CrossRef]
66. Al-Qurainy, F.; Khan, S.; Tarroum, M.; Nadeem, M.; Alansi, S.; Alshameri, A. Biochemical and Genetical Responses of *Phoenix dactylifera* L. to Cadmium Stress. *Biomed. Res. Int.* **2017**, *2017*, 9504057. [CrossRef]

67. Habib, H.M.; El-Fakharany, E.M.; Souka, U.D.; Elsebaee, F.M.; El-Ziney, M.G.; Ibrahim, W.H. Polyphenol-Rich Date Palm Fruit Seed (*Phoenix dactylifera* L.) Extract Inhibits Labile Iron, Enzyme, and Cancer Cell Activities, and DNA and Protein Damage. *Nutrients* **2022**, *14*, 3536. [CrossRef]
68. Ajiboye, B.O.; Oloyede, H.O.B.; Salawu, M.O. *Phoenix dactylifera* Linn fruit based-diets palliate hyperglycemia in alloxan-induced diabetic rats. *J. Basic. Clin. Physiol. Pharmacol.* **2020**, *17*, 180–185. [CrossRef]
69. Alqarni, M.M.M.; Osman, M.A.; Al-Tamimi, D.S.; Gassem, M.A.; Al-Khalifa, A.S.; Al-Juhaimi, F.; Mohamed Ahmed, I.A. Antioxidant and antihyperlipidemic effects of Ajwa date (*Phoenix dactylifera* L.) extracts in rats fed a cholesterol-rich diet. *J. Food Biochem.* **2019**, *43*, e12933. [CrossRef]
70. Shahbaz, K.; Asif, J.A.; Liszen, T.; Nurul, A.A.; Alam, M.K. Cytotoxic and Antioxidant Effects of *Phoenix dactylifera* L. (Ajwa Date Extract) on Oral Squamous Cell Carcinoma Cell Line. *Biomed. Res. Int.* **2022**, *2022*, 5792830. [CrossRef]
71. Zhang, M.; Wang, L.; Wen, D.; Ren, C.; Chen, S.; Zhang, Z.; Hu, L.; Yu, Z.; Tombran-Tink, J.; Zhang, X.; et al. Neuroprotection of retinal cells by Caffeic Acid Phenylethyl Ester (CAPE) is mediated by mitochondrial uncoupling protein UCP2. *Neurochem. Int.* **2021**, *151*, 105214. [CrossRef] [PubMed]
72. Ayna, A. Caffeic acid prevents hydrogen peroxide-induced oxidative damage in SH-SY5Y cell line through mitigation of oxidative stress and apoptosis. *Bratisl. Lek. Listy* **2021**, *122*, 120–124. [CrossRef] [PubMed]
73. Kulkarni, N.P.; Vaidya, B.; Narula, A.S.; Sharma, S.S. Caffeic Acid Phenethyl Ester (CAPE) Attenuates Paclitaxel-induced Peripheral Neuropathy: A Mechanistic Study. *Curr. Neurovasc Res.* **2022**, *19*, 293–302.
74. Domínguez-Avila, J.A.; Salazar-López, N.J.; Montiel-Herrera, M.; Martínez-Martínez, A.; Villegas-Ochoa, M.A.; González-Aguilar, G.A. Phenolic compounds can induce systemic and central immunomodulation, which result in a neuroprotective effect. *J. Food Biochem.* **2022**, *46*, e14260. [CrossRef] [PubMed]
75. Tavan, M.; Hanachi, P.; de la Luz Cádiz-Gurrea, M.; Segura Carretero, A.; Mirjalili, M.H. Natural Phenolic Compounds with Neuroprotective Effects. *Neurochem. Res.* **2024**, *49*, 306–326. [CrossRef]
76. Rojas-García, A.; Fernández-Ochoa, Á.; Cádiz-Gurrea, M.L.; Arráez-Román, D.; Segura-Carretero, A. Neuroprotective Effects of Agri-Food By-Products Rich in Phenolic Compounds. *Nutrients* **2023**, *15*, 449. [CrossRef]
77. Sahyon, H.A.; Al-Harbi, S.A. Antimicrobial, anticancer and antioxidant activities of nano-heart of *Phoenix dactylifera* tree extract loaded chitosan nanoparticles: In vitro and in vivo study. *Int. J. Biol. Macromol.* **2020**, *160*, 1230–1241. [CrossRef]
78. Moslemi, E.; Dehghan, P.; Khalafi, M. Effectiveness of supplementation with date seed (*Phoenix dactylifera*) as a functional food on inflammatory markers, muscle damage, and BDNF following high-intensity interval training: A randomized, double-blind, placebo-controlled trial. *Eur. J. Nutr.* **2023**, *62*, 2001–2014. [CrossRef]
79. Al-Farsi, M.; Alasalvar, C.; Morris, A.; Baron, M.; Shahidi, F. Compositional and sensory characteristics of three native sun-dried date (*Phoenix dactylifera* L.) varieties grown in Oman. *J. Agric. Food Chem.* **2005**, *53*, 7586–7591. [CrossRef]
80. Kiełczykowska, M.; Kocot, J.; Paździor, M.; Musik, I. Selenium—A fascinating antioxidant of protective properties. *Adv. Clin. Exp. Med.* **2018**, *27*, 245–255. [CrossRef]
81. Bjørklund, G.; Shanaida, M.; Lysiuk, R.; Antonyak, H.; Klishch, I.; Shanaida, V.; Peana, M. Selenium: An Antioxidant with a Critical Role in Anti-Aging. *Molecules* **2022**, *27*, 6613. [CrossRef] [PubMed]
82. Huang, J.; Xie, L.; Song, A.; Zhang, C. Selenium Status and Its Antioxidant Role in Metabolic Diseases. *Oxid. Med. Cell Longev.* **2022**, *2022*, 7009863. [CrossRef] [PubMed]
83. Groth, S.; Budke, C.; Weber, T.; Neugart, S.; Brockmann, S.; Holz, M.; Sawadski, B.C.; Daum, D.; Rohn, S. Relationship between Phenolic Compounds, Antioxidant Properties, and the Allergenic Protein Mal d 1 in Different Selenium-Biofortified Apple Cultivars (*Malus domestica*). *Molecules* **2021**, *26*, 2647. [CrossRef]
84. Pujari, R.R.; Vyawahare, N.S.; Kagathara, V.G. Evaluation of antioxidant and neuroprotective effect of date palm (*Phoenix dactylifera* L.) against bilateral common carotid artery occlusion in rats. *Indian. J. Exp. Biol.* **2011**, *49*, 627–633. [PubMed]
85. Salem, G.A.; Shaban, A.; Diab, H.A.; Elsaghayer, W.A.; Mjedib, M.D.; Hnesh, A.M.; Sahu, R.P. *Phoenix dactylifera* protects against oxidative stress and hepatic injury induced by paracetamol intoxication in rats. *Biomed. Pharmacother.* **2018**, *104*, 366–374. [CrossRef] [PubMed]
86. Mani, V.; Arfeen, M.; Dhaked, D.K.; Mohammed, H.A.; Amirthalingam, P.; Elsisi, H.A. Neuroprotective Effect of Methanolic Ajwa Seed Extract on Lipopolysaccharide-Induced Memory Dysfunction and Neuroinflammation: In Vivo, Molecular Docking and Dynamics Studies. *Plants* **2023**, *12*, 934. [CrossRef]
87. Xiao, Q.; Liu, H.; Yang, C.; Chen, Y.; Huang, Y.; Xiao, X.; Pan, Y.; He, J.; Du, Q.; Wang, Q.; et al. Bushen-Yizhi formula exerts neuroprotective effect via inhibiting excessive mitophagy in rats with chronic cerebral hypoperfusion. *J. Ethnopharmacol.* **2023**, *310*, 116326. [CrossRef]
88. Mallhi, T.H.; Qadir, M.I.; Ali, M.; Ahmad, B.; Khan, Y.H.; Rehman, A. Review: Ajwa date (*Phoenix dactylifera*)—An emerging plant in pharmacological research. *Pak. J. Pharm. Sci.* **2014**, *27*, 607–616.
89. Behl, C.; Moosmann, B. Antioxidant neuroprotection in Alzheimer's disease as preventive and therapeutic approach. *Free Radic. Biol. Med.* **2002**, *33*, 182–191. [CrossRef]
90. Moslemi, E.; Dehghan, P.; Khani, M.; Sarbakhsh, P.; Sarmadi, B. The effects of date seed (*Phoenix dactylifera*) supplementation on exercise-induced oxidative stress and aerobic and anaerobic performance following high-intensity interval training sessions: A randomised, double-blind, placebo-controlled trial. *Br. J. Nutr.* **2022**, *14*, 1151–1162. [CrossRef]

91. Al-Alawi, R.A.; Al-Mashiqri, J.H.; Al-Nadabi, J.S.M.; Al-Shihi, B.I.; Baqi, Y. Date Palm Tree (*Phoenix dactylifera* L.): Natural Products and Therapeutic Options. *Front. Plant Sci.* **2017**, *8*, 845. [CrossRef] [PubMed]
92. Zidan, N.S.; Omran, A.M.E.; Rezk, S.M.; Atteia, H.H.; Sakran, M.I. Anti-Alzheimer's disease potential of Arabian coffee versus Date palm seed extract in male rats. *J. Food Biochem.* **2022**, *46*, e14017. [CrossRef] [PubMed]
93. Khan, A.; Park, J.S.; Kang, M.H.; Lee, H.J.; Ali, J.; Tahir, M.; Choe, K.; Kim, M.O. Caffeic Acid, a Polyphenolic Micronutrient Rescues Mice Brains against Aβ-Induced Neurodegeneration and Memory Impairment. *Antioxidants* **2023**, *12*, 1284. [CrossRef] [PubMed]
94. Razak, A.M.; Tan, J.K.; Mohd Said, M.; Makpol, S. Modulating Effects of Zingiberaceae Phenolic Compounds on Neurotrophic Factors and Their Potential as Neuroprotectants in Brain Disorders and Age-Associated Neurodegenerative Disorders: A Review. *Nutrients* **2023**, *15*, 2564. [CrossRef] [PubMed]
95. Carrera, I.; Martínez, O.; Cacabelos, R. Neuroprotection with Natural Antioxidants and Nutraceuticals in the Context of Brain Cell Degeneration: The Epigenetic Connection. *Curr. Top. Med. Chem.* **2019**, *19*, 2999–3011. [CrossRef]
96. Uddin, M.S.; Al Mamun, A.; Kabir, M.T.; Ahmad, J.; Jeandet, P.; Sarwar, M.S.; Ashraf, G.M.; Aleya, L. Neuroprotective role of polyphenols against oxidative stress-mediated neurodegeneration. *Eur. J. Pharmacol.* **2020**, *886*, 173412. [CrossRef]
97. Hsueh, Y.J.; Chen, Y.N.; Tsao, Y.T.; Cheng, C.M.; Wu, W.C.; Chen, H.C. The Pathomechanism, Antioxidant Biomarkers, and Treatment of Oxidative Stress-Related Eye Diseases. *Int. J. Mol. Sci.* **2022**, *23*, 1255. [CrossRef]
98. AlFaris, N.A.; AlTamimi, J.Z.; AlGhamdi, F.A.; Albaridi, N.A.; Alzaheb, R.A.; Aljabryn, D.H.; Aljahani, A.H.; AlMousa, L.A. Total phenolic content in ripe date fruits (*Phoenix dactylifera* L.): A systematic review and meta-analysis. *Saudi J. Biol. Sci.* **2021**, *28*, 3566–3577. [CrossRef]
99. Singh, A.; Dhaneshwar, S.; Mazumder, A. Investigating Neuroprotective Potential of Berberine, Levetiracetam and their Combination in the Management of Alzheimer's Disease Utilizing Drug Repurposing Strategy. *Curr. Rev. Clin. Exp. Pharmacol.* **2023**, *18*, 182–190.

pharmaceuticals

Brief Report

In Vitro Evaluation of the Combinatorial Effect of Naringenin and Miltefosine against *Leishmania amazonensis*

Vinícius Lopes Lessa [1,2,*], Gustavo Gonçalves [1], Beatriz Santos [1], Victoria Cruz Cavalari [1], Rafael Felipe da Costa Vieira [3,4] and Fabiano Borges Figueiredo [1]

1 Carlos Chagas Institute, Oswaldo Cruz Foundation (Fiocruz), Curitiba 81310-020, PR, Brazil; ggustavogonsalves@gmail.com (G.G.); beatrizsantos.biobs@gmail.com (B.S.); viccavalari97@gmail.com (V.C.C.); fabiano.figueiredo@fiocruz.br (F.B.F.)
2 Graduate Program in Veterinary Sciences, Federal University of Paraná, Curitiba 80035-060, PR, Brazil
3 Department of Epidemiology and Community Health, College of Health and Human Services, University of North Carolina at Charlotte, Charlotte, NC 28223, USA; rvieira@charlotte.edu
4 Center for Computational Intelligence to Predict Health and Environmental Risks (CIPHER), University of North Carolina at Charlotte, Charlotte, NC 28223, USA
* Correspondence: vlessa19@gmail.com

Abstract: *Leishmania amazonensis* causes a clinical form called diffuse cutaneous leishmaniasis (DCL) with challenges to treatment, like low efficiency and drug toxicity. Therefore, it is necessary to investigate new therapies using less toxic leishmanicidal compounds, such as flavonoids like naringenin, and their combination with conventional drugs, such as miltefosine. Antileishmanial dose/response activity, isobologram, calculation of dose reduction index (DRI), and fractional inhibitory concentration index (FICI) tests were performed on in vitro assays using reference promastigote forms of *L. amazonensis* (IFLA/BR/67/PH8) to assess the combinatorial effect between naringenin and miltefosine. The in vitro results of isobologram, DRI, and FICI calculations showed that the combination of the compounds had an additive effect and was able to reduce the half maximal inhibitory concentration (IC_{50}) of miltefosine in the promastigote forms of the parasite compared to the treatment of the drug alone. This study demonstrated in vitro the viability of a combination action of the flavonoid with the treatment with miltefosine, opening space for further investigations on the association of natural compounds with the drugs used for the treatment of *L. amazonensis*.

Keywords: flavonoids; naringenin; n-hexadecylphosphonocholine; leishmaniasis; cutaneous leishmaniasis

1. Introduction

Leishmaniasis is a disease caused by single-celled protozoan of the genus *Leishmania*. The three main forms of the disease are visceral leishmaniasis (VL), mucocutaneous leishmaniasis (CML), and cutaneous leishmaniasis (CL). In the Americas, 18 countries are endemic to CL and CML, with Brazil, Colombia, Peru, Nicaragua, and Bolivia having the highest estimated case counts [1]. Among the species that cause CL in Brazil, *Leishmania amazonensis* has an incidence in primary and secondary forest areas of the legal Amazon (Amazonas, Pará, Rondônia, Tocantins, and Maranhão) and also in the northeastern (Bahia), southeastern (Minas Gerais and São Paulo), central–western (Goiás), and southern (Paraná) states. This species causes a wide spectrum of clinical forms, which are localized cutaneous leishmaniasis (LCL), CML, diffuse cutaneous leishmaniasis (DCL), and disseminated leishmaniasis (DL) [2].

Although DCL is relatively rare, it is extremely severe; diffuse skin infiltration and a large number of nodules and papules clinically characterize this form. Patients affected by DCL present lesions that cover the entire body, predominantly in the extremities, which rarely involve the nasopharyngeal mucous membranes [2]. Among the clinical forms caused by *L. amazonensis*, DCL is difficult to treat with conventional drugs; this clinical form has as its main characteristics the Th2 response with expression of interleukin-10, IL-4, and low expression of interferon gamma (IFN), leading to the patient's anergy to the parasite, high parasitic loads, and deforming lesions that generate physical stigmas and psychological impacts [3]. In addition to the ineffective immune response to DCL, the use of meglumine antimoniate and second-choice drugs like liposomal amphotericin B and pentamidine isethionate proved unsuccessful in cases of refractoriness [3]. Treatments with first- and second-choice drugs in the different clinical forms caused by *L. amazonensis* present some complications. These complications include toxic effects and restricted access of the population with economic vulnerability to medical care and follow-up, especially in the northern and northeastern Brazilian regions, due to the lack of resources and professionals. Additionally, drug resistance to treatment by meglumine antimoniate is an aggravating factor [4]. Miltefosine (n-hexadecylphosphonocholine), a phospholipid that is the hexdecyl monoester of phosphocholine with a molecular weight of 407.6 g/mol, shows a lower toxicity when compared with the meglumine antimoniate, easy oral administration, and an efficiency rate in the elimination of the parasite close to that of first- and second-choice drugs [5,6].

However, due to their teratogenic effect, new therapeutic alternatives demonstrating similar and less toxic efficacy have been explored. Efforts have been directed toward treatment based on plants and their metabolites, in particular the flavonoids, which have properties as preventive agents against cancer, antioxidant activity, and leishmanicidal activity [7,8]. Herein, we selected the flavonoid naringenin (5,7-Dihydroxy-2-(4-hydroxyphenyl) chroman-4-one), which is a trihydroxyflavanone, a flavanone substituted by hydroxyl groups at positions 5, 6, and 4 with molecular weight of 272.25 g/mol. In addition to its important immunomodulatory properties [5,9], naringerin has demonstrated potent in vitro activity against promastigotes and amastigotes of *Leishmania donovani* [10]. Considering the effects of naringenin and the fact that miltefosine is the drug with less toxic effects, we sought to associate these two compounds and investigate their therapeutic potential against *L. amazonensis*.

2. Results

2.1. In Silico Study

The physicochemical properties of naringenin and miltefosine were assessed to compare their predicted oral bioavailability using Lipinski's and Veber's criteria. Miltefosine presents one violation and naringenin none (Table 1). The structures of miltefosine and naringenin are represented in Figures 1a and 1b, respectively; for both substances, pan assay interference compounds (PAINS) were not identified by the SwissADME web tool.

Table 1. Molecular properties of naringenin and miltefosine according to Lipinski's and Veber's criteria and the number of pan assay interference compounds according to SwissADME. MW: molecular weight; Log Po/w: Log of partition coefficient (consensus LogP on SwissADME); RB: number of rotable bonds; H-Acc: number of hydrogen bond acceptors; H-Don: number of hydrogen bond donors; tPSA ($Å^2$): molecular polar surface area; PAINS: pan assay interference compounds.

	Naringenin	Miltefosine	Limit
MW	272.25 g/mol	407.57 g/mol	≤500
Log Po/w	1.84	3.35	≤5
RB	1	20	≤10
H-Acc	5	4	≤10
H-Don	3	0	≤5
tPSA ($Å^2$)	86.99 $Å^2$	68.4 $Å^2$	≤140
PAINS	0	0	-
Violations	0	1	-

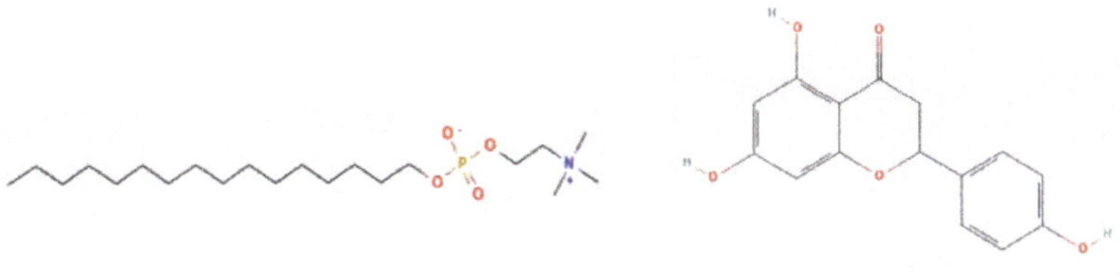

(a) (b)

Figure 1. The structures of miltefosine and naringenin. (**a**) Miltefosine presents a molecular formula of $C_{21}H_{46}NO_4P$ (PubChem CID: 3599). (**b**) Naringenin presents a molecular formula of $C_{15}H_{12}O_5$ (PubChem CID: 932). These structures were generated by PubChem [11].

2.2. Growth Curve

The growth of parasites presented an adaptation phase up to 48 h; after this period, the parasites reached their exponential growth phase in up to 96 h, reaching the stationary phase following 120 h of cultivation.

2.3. Antipromastigote Activity In Vitro

The mean IC_{50} obtained from the treatment with miltefosine alone was 13.20 μM, while naringenin had an IC_{50} of 219.86 μM. For the synergism tests, the IC_{50} values of the proportions 1:1, 2:1, 4:1, and 6:1 were first obtained, allowing the calculation of ΣFICI (Table 2) and enabling the construction of the isobologram (Figure 2). Calculating the average of the sum of FICI, we arrived at the value of χΣFICI, which was 0.803. It was observed that the interaction between the compounds is additive in all proportions tested.

Table 2. Representation of the IC_{50} values of miltefosine and naringenin in different proportions. FICI and DRI values were calculated using the formulas described in Section 4.3 of the Materials and Methods section. The IC_{50} values are represented with their mean and standard deviation; the FICI values are represented by the means extracted from the IC_{50} values. The DRI values are represented by means obtained by the calculation of the IC_{50} means of miltefosine in treatment alone and in combination with naringenin.

Proportion	IC_{50} Miltefosine (μM)	IC_{50} Naringenin (μM)	FICI	DRI
01:01	6.65 ± 0.9543	6.657 ± 0.9543	0.53	1.984277
02:01	6.73 ± 3.512	13.468 ± 7.029	0.57	1.961879
04:01	10.27 ± 3.832	41.08 ± 15.32	0.96	1.285955
06:01	11.12 ± 3.834	66.77 ± 23.00	1.14	1.186965
00:00	13.21 ± 3.125	219.9 ± 12.46		

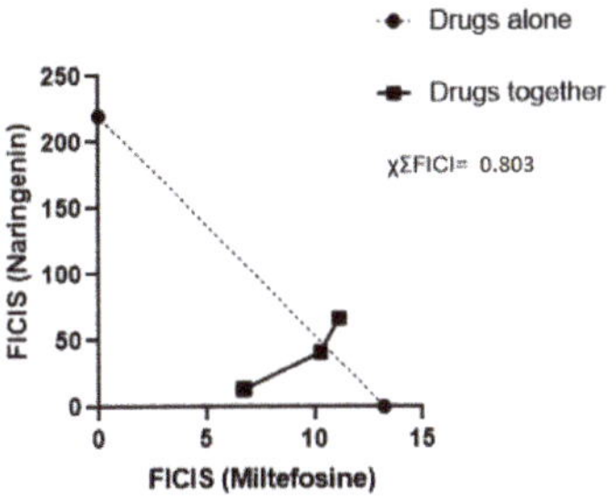

Figure 2. Isobologram analyzing the interaction of miltefosine and naringenin. Each point represents the FICI averages of the proportions 1:1, 2:1, 4:1, and 6:1 for naringenin and miltefosine; the points of the proportions 1:1 and 2:2 are overlapped due to the proximity of their FICI values. The dotted line represents the line of indifference. The result of χΣFICI is located at the top right.

3. Discussion

The compound combination strategy is adopted to optimize treatments for a wide range of diseases. Past studies have reported treatment regimens where antibiotics are combined to combat multidrug-resistant bacteria like *Acinetobacter baumannii*, reducing the mortality of infected patients [12], cancer cells such as breast cancer [13], and different types of viruses like HIV, HCV, and influenza [14]. The combination of compounds for treating leishmaniasis is also adopted to improve the effectiveness of treatments, diminishing their cost and time and reducing the likelihood of the emergence of resistant parasite strains. Compared to monotherapies, combined drug therapies present greater stimulation in the activity of leukocytes and their replication during infection, as well as increased production of cytokines that regulate the Th1 and ROS responses acting on the elimination of the parasite [15]. Faced with the challenges of monotherapies with first- and second-choice drugs, known by their side effects that hinder treatment, some efforts have been made to search for antiparasitic compounds in plants. In this sense, flavonoids stand out, which consist of a large group of phenolic compounds synthesized by the phenylpropanoid pathway in plants and have several antimicrobial, anti-cancer, and leishmanicidal activities [10,16]. In addition to treatments with isolated flavonoids, a previous study evaluated the optimization of the miltefosine treatment. When the drug was associated with the flavonoid apigenin, a reduction in parasitemia in mice was obtained with only half the dose of the drug when compared with the treatment of the drug alone [17]. As observed in the in silico analysis using the SwissADME web tool, naringenin presents physicochemical properties that favor its bioavailability, opening space for further investigation of its leishmanicidal properties in isolation and in combination. We investigated the combinatorial effect of miltefosine with naringenin through using synergism and isobolagram testing to evaluate the interaction between the natural compound and the commercial drug to optimize the treatment of the drug, reducing its toxicity by associating it with a non-toxic natural compound [18]. The MTT assay performed herein showed values of the IC_{50} of the different proportions (Table 2). A reduction in miltefosine IC_{50} values was observed in all proportions; it was possible to assess that in the 1:1 and 2:1 proportions there was a substantial reduction in the IC_{50} dose, and to evaluate this reduction, the DRI calculation was used [19]. The DRI calculation measures how many times the dose of each drug in combination can be reduced due to the level of interaction up to a certain level of effect when compared to separate treatment. A DRI = 1 value indicates that there is no dose reduction; if the DRI > 1, it indicates a favorable dose reduction that leads to toxicity reduction; if the DRI < 1, the dose of the drug is not favorable for reduction. That is, it can be observed that in the proportions of 1:1, 2:1, and 4:1, they provided a reducing dose of miltefosine without reducing its effect, which, on the contrary, had a greater effect at lower doses than in the trial with the drug alone. The calculation of ΣFICI made it possible to construct the isobologram for better visualization of the interaction between the compounds. In Figure 2, it can be seen that the proportions of 1:1, 2:1, and 4:1 were below the indifference line with ΣFICI values of 0.53, 0.57, and 0.96, respectively. The 6:1 ratio presented a ΣFICI value of 1.16, slightly above the indifference line. According to the criteria for evaluating the interaction between compounds described in Section 4.3, it was concluded that the compounds in all proportions showed additive behavior (1 > ΣFICI > 0.5), with the ΣFICI values and the χΣFICI value of 0.803, defining the interaction between the compounds in general as additive. The additive effect between two drugs commonly refers to non-interaction or inertism between the substances being observed when the effect of the combination between different drugs is the sum of the effects of these drugs tested separately [19]. In general, it establishes a demarcation between the synergistic and antagonistic natures in the investigation of the interaction between drugs. Additive interactions have already been observed in several studies with combinations of leishmanicidal compounds [19–21]. The use of drugs with an additive effect in a combination can reduce chances of resistance, bringing the possibility of shortening treatment time [20], making this strategy attractive to mitigate the adverse effects present in the treatment of leishmaniasis. In summary, the combination of naringenin with miltefosine in vitro was able to potentiate the action of the drug, reducing the IC_{50} of the drug by approximately two times and requiring a lower dose of miltefosine to eliminate a considerable percentage of *L. amazonensis*.

4. Materials and Methods

4.1. *In Silico Study*

The structures of naringenin and miltefosine were used to evaluate their theoretical physicochemical properties and the presence of PAIN. The predictions were calculated using the SwissADME web tool [22], considering Lipinski's rule of five (RO5) [23], followed by the additional rule proposed by Veber [24].

4.2. *Growth Curve*

Promastigote forms of the *L. amazonensis* strain (IFLA/BR/67/PH8) were maintained in an M199 medium with Hanks' salts (Sigma-Aldrich Brazil Ltd., São Paulo, Brazil) at 25 °C for inoculum production to be used in our experiments. The culture was maintained by replication every three to four days. The number of cells was measured in a hemocytometer and optical microscope, and the growth curve was performed in triplicate.

4.3. *Antipromastigote Activity In Vitro*

The in vitro antipromastigote activity of miltefosine and naringenin was evaluated in promastigote forms of *L. amazonensis* using the 3-[4,5-dimethyl-thiazol-2-yl]-2,5-diphenyl-tetrazolium bromide (MTT) (Sigma-Aldrich Brazil Ltd., São Paulo, Brazil) assay, with the drug tested alone and combined with naringenin [25] for a 48-h treatment. Commercial naringenin with a purity of 98% (Sigma-Aldrich Brazil Ltd., São Paulo, Brazil) and commercial miltefosine (Cayman Chemical, São Paulo, Brazil) were used, and stock solutions with concentrations of 50 mg/mL and 1 mg/mL were prepared in DMSO (Sigma-Aldrich Brazil Ltd., São Paulo, Brazil). We performed these tests to construct an isobologram to obtain the values of the FICI. The parasites were incubated at 25 °C for 48 h of treatment. After incubation, 50 µL of MTT solution (10 mg/mL) was added to each well. The plates were maintained at 37 °C for 4 h. To solubilize the formazan crystals, 20 µL of 10% sodium dodecyl sulfate (SDS) (Sigma-Aldrich Brazil Ltd., São Paulo, Brazil) and 50 µL of 100% DMSO were added to each well. Plate readings were performed on a microplate reader using a wavelength of 550 nm. All tests were performed in biological triplicate and technical quintuplicate. The results are expressed as the compound concentration capable of inhibiting parasite growth by 50% (IC_{50}). The assay was performed in a 96-well flat-bottom microplate with a final volume of 200 µL. To perform the assay, the concentration of promastigote forms kept in the exponential phase was adjusted to 1×10^6 cells/mL. To calculate the IC_{50} of miltefosine alone, seven dilutions of the initial 200 µM solution of the drug were performed, where each new 2× dilution of the initial dose, the ranges of 100 µM, 50 µM, 25 µM, 12.5 µM, 6.25 µM, 3.125 µM, and 1.5625 µM were obtained in the plate. In addition, an assay was performed with the isolated flavonoid. Following the same dilution strategy used for miltefosine but with different ranges of concentrations that are 1376.4 µM, 688.2 µM, 344.1 µM, 172.05 µM, 86.025 µM, 43.015 µM, 21.50 µM, and 10.75 µM, for these tests, the parasites were first seeded in the plate with M199 medium containing 0.75% DMSO with naringenin. After carrying out tests to evaluate the antipromastigote activity of the compounds in isolation, the next step was to carry out tests combining doses of naringenin and miltefosine in proportions of 1:1, 2:1, 4:1, and 6:1. With the IC_{50} values of the proportions, it was possible to evaluate the interactions of naringenin and miltefosine in the parasite's growth by calculating the fractional inhibitory concentration index (FICI) [26] and the dose reduction index (DRI) to evaluate the possibility of a decrease in the dosage of miltefosine in the combination assay without reducing its effect [19].

The isobologram was plotted with the sum of the FICIs and the averages of the sums of the FICI ratios, with ΣFICI calculated to determine the nature of the interaction between the natural compound and the drug, with $\Sigma FICI \geq 0.5$ indicating a synergistic effect, $0.5 > \Sigma FICI < 4$ additive effect, and $\Sigma FICI > 4$ antagonistic effect [27]. The formulas used to calculate the FICI and DRI are described below:

$$\Sigma FICI = \left[\frac{IC_{50} drug\ A\ combination}{IC_{50} drug\ A\ alone}\right] + \left[\frac{IC_{50} drug\ B\ combination}{IC_{50}\ drug\ B\ alone}\right] \quad (1)$$

$$DRI = \left(\frac{IC_{50} drug\ alone}{IC_{50} drug\ combination}\right) \quad (2)$$

4.4. Statistical Analysis

Statistical analysis and the construction of the isobologram was performed using GraphPad Prism 8.0.1 (GraphPad Software, Inc., San Diego, CA, USA). The results of the IC_{50} assays were transformed into log values and analyzed by a dose–response inhibition curve. A p-value ≤ 0.05 was considered statistically significant. The results were plotted with their means and standard deviations. The experiments were realized in biological triplicates and technical quintuplicates.

5. Conclusions

Although further work is needed, including tests with amastigotes, these results show that the association of naringenin with miltefosine has promising antileishmanial activity in vitro experiments, demonstrating that the flavonoid alone has an antipromastigote effect in *L. amazonensis* and can optimize the treatment of the commercial drug, increasing its efficiency.

Author Contributions: V.L.L.: conceived the presented idea, developed the theory, performed the experiments and formal analyses, conducted the validation tests, and wrote the paper draft and correction. G.G.: supervised the experimenter and conducted the review and correction of the paper draft. B.S.: performed the experimentation, performed the correction of the paper draft, and managed the material of the study. V.C.C.: managed the material of the study, wrote the paper draft, and conducted the review and correction of the paper. R.F.d.C.V.: project administration, supervised the experimenter, responsible for the funding acquisition, and conducted the review and correction of the paper draft. F.B.F.: project administration, supervised the experimenter, conducted the review and correction of the paper draft, and provided the resources for the study. All authors have read and agreed to the published version of the manuscript.

Funding: This study is part of a Ph.D. degree for Vinícius Lessa at the Universidade Federal do Paraná. Vinícius Lessa was sponsored by a fellowship from the Coordenação de Aperfeiçoamento de Pessoal de Nível Superior (CAPES) at the time of this study. FF has a grant from CNPq for productivity in research (309862/2015-9).

Institutional Review Board Statement: Not applicable.

Informed Consent Statement: Not applicable.

Data Availability Statement: The data presented in this study are available upon request from the corresponding author.

Acknowledgments: We would like to thank the researcher Juliano Bordignon of the Molecular Virology Laboratory of the Instituto Carlos Chagas for providing a sample of naringenin to carry out this work.

Conflicts of Interest: The authors declare that they have no conflicts of interest.

References

1. Alvar, J.; Vélez, I.D.; Bern, C.; Herrero, M.; Desjeux, P.; Cano, J.; Jannin, J.; Boer, M.D.; the WHO Leishmaniasis Control Team. Leishmaniasis Worldwide and Global Estimates of Its Incidence. *PLoS ONE* **2012**, *7*, e35671. [CrossRef]
2. Silveira, F.T.; Lainson, R.; Corbett, C.E. Clinical and Immunopathological Spectrum of American Cutaneous Leishmaniasis with Special Reference to the Disease in Amazonian Brazil: A Review. *Mem. Inst. Oswaldo Cruz* **2004**, *99*, 239–251. [CrossRef]
3. Anversa, L.; Tiburcio, M.G.S.; Richini-Pereira, V.B.; Ramirez, L.E. Human Leishmaniasis in Brazil: A General Review. *Rev. Assoc. Med. Bras.* **2018**, *64*, 281–289. [CrossRef]
4. De Oliveira, A.L.L.; Brustoloni, Y.M.; Fernandes, T.D.; Dorval, M.E.C.; Da Cunha, R.V.; Bóia, M.N. Severe Adverse Reactions to Meglumine Antimoniate in the Treatment of Visceral Leishmaniasis: A Report of 13 Cases in the Southwestern Region of Brazil. *Trop. Doct.* **2009**, *39*, 180–182. [CrossRef]
5. Kim, S.; Chen, J.; Cheng, T.; Gindulyte, A.; He, J.; He, S.; Li, Q.; Shoemaker, B.A.; Thiessen, P.A.; Yu, B.; et al. PubChem 2023 Update. *Nucleic Acids Res.* **2023**, *51*, D1373–D1380. [CrossRef]
6. Machado, P.R.; Ampuero, J.; Guimarães, L.H.; Villasboas, L.; Rocha, A.T.; Schriefer, A.; Sousa, R.S.; Talhari, A.; Penna, G.; Carvalho, E.M. Miltefosine in the Treatment of Cutaneous Leishmaniasis Caused by Leishmania Braziliensis in Brazil: A Randomized and Controlled Trial. *PLoS Negl. Trop. Dis.* **2010**, *4*, e912. [CrossRef]
7. Lewin, G.; Cojean, S.; Gupta, S.; Verma, A.; Puri, S.K.; Loiseau, P.M. In Vitro Antileishmanial Properties of New Flavonoids against Leishmania Donovani. *Biomed. Prev. Nutr.* **2011**, *1*, 168–171. [CrossRef]
8. Morel, S.; Helesbeux, J.-J.; Séraphin, D.; Derbré, S.; Gatto, J.; Aumond, M.-C.; Abatuci, Y.; Grellier, P.; Beniddir, M.A.; Le Pape, P.; et al. Anti-AGEs and Antiparasitic Activity of an Original Prenylated Isoflavonoid and Flavanones Isolated from Derris Ferruginea. *Phytochem. Lett.* **2013**, *6*, 498–503. [CrossRef]
9. Lin, C.; Zeng, Z.; Lin, Y.; Wang, P.; Cao, D.; Xie, K.; Luo, Y.; Yang, H.; Yang, J.; Wang, W.; et al. Naringenin Suppresses Epithelial Ovarian Cancer by Inhibiting Proliferation and Modulating Gut Microbiota. *Phytomedicine* **2022**, *106*, 154401. [CrossRef]
10. Kaur, G.; Chauhan, K.; Kaur, S. Immunotherapeutic Potential of Codonopsis Clematidea and Naringenin against Visceral Leishmaniasis. *Biomed. Pharmacother.* **2018**, *108*, 1048–1061. [CrossRef]
11. National Center for Biotechnology Information. Available online: https://www.ncbi.nlm.nih.gov/ (accessed on 7 May 2024).
12. Jean, S.-S.; Hsieh, T.-C.; Hsu, C.-W.; Lee, W.-S.; Bai, K.-J.; Lam, C. Comparison of the Clinical Efficacy between Tigecycline plus Extended-Infusion Imipenem and Sulbactam plus Imipenem against Ventilator-Associated Pneumonia with Pneumonic Extensively Drug-Resistant Acinetobacter Baumannii Bacteremia, and Correlation of Clinical Efficacy with in Vitro Synergy Tests. *J. Microbiol. Immunol. Infect.* **2016**, *49*, 924–933. [CrossRef]
13. Fisusi, F.A.; Akala, E.O. Drug Combinations in Breast Cancer Therapy. *Pharm. Nanotechnol.* **2019**, *7*, 3–23. [CrossRef]
14. Shyr, Z.A.; Cheng, Y.-S.; Lo, D.C.; Zheng, W. Drug Combination Therapy for Emerging Viral Diseases. *Drug Discov. Today* **2021**, *26*, 2367–2376. [CrossRef]
15. van Griensven, J.; Balasegaram, M.; Meheus, F.; Alvar, J.; Lynen, L.; Boelaert, M. Combination Therapy for Visceral Leishmaniasis. *Lancet Infect. Dis.* **2010**, *10*, 184–194. [CrossRef]
16. Gervazoni, L.F.O.; Barcellos, G.B.; Ferreira-Paes, T.; Almeida-Amaral, E.E. Use of Natural Products in Leishmaniasis Chemotherapy: An Overview. *Front. Chem.* **2020**, *8*, 579891. [CrossRef]
17. Emiliano, Y.S.S.; Almeida-Amaral, E.E. Efficacy of Apigenin and Miltefosine Combination Therapy against Experimental Cutaneous Leishmaniasis. *J. Nat. Prod.* **2018**, *81*, 1910–1913. [CrossRef]
18. Foucquier, J.; Guedj, M. Analysis of Drug Combinations: Current Methodological Landscape. *Pharmacol. Res. Perspect.* **2015**, *3*, e00149. [CrossRef]
19. Wang, C.; Wu, P.; Shen, X.-L.; Wei, X.-Y.; Jiang, Z.-H. Synthesis, Cytotoxic Activity and Drug Combination Study of Tertiary Amine Derivatives of 2′,4′-Dihydroxyl-6′-Methoxyl-3′,5′-Dimethylchalcone. *RSC Adv.* **2017**, *7*, 48031–48038. [CrossRef]
20. Gonçalves-Oliveira, L.F.; Souza-Silva, F.; De Castro Côrtes, L.M.; Veloso, L.B.; Santini Pereira, B.A.; Cysne-Finkelstein, L.; Lechuga, G.C.; Bourguignon, S.C.; Almeida-Souza, F.; Da Silva Calabrese, K.; et al. The Combination Therapy of Meglumine Antimoniate and Oxiranes (Epoxy-α-Lapachone and Epoxymethyl-Lawsone) Enhance the Leishmanicidal Effect in Mice Infected by Leishmania (*Leishmania*) Amazonensis. *Int. J. Parasitol. Drugs Drug Resist.* **2019**, *10*, 101–108. [CrossRef]
21. Murphy, M.P.; Bayir, H.; Belousov, V.; Chang, C.J.; Davies, K.J.A.; Davies, M.J.; Dick, T.P.; Finkel, T.; Forman, H.J.; Janssen-Heininger, Y.; et al. Guidelines for Measuring Reactive Oxygen Species and Oxidative Damage in Cells and in Vivo. *Nat. Metab.* **2022**, *4*, 651–662. [CrossRef]
22. Daina, A.; Michielin, O.; Zoete, V. SwissADME: A Free Web Tool to Evaluate Pharmacokinetics, Drug-Likeness and Medicinal Chemistry Friendliness of Small Molecules. *Sci. Rep.* **2017**, *7*, 42717. [CrossRef]
23. Lipinski, C.A. Lead- and Drug-like Compounds: The Rule-of-Five Revolution. *Drug Discov. Today Technol.* **2004**, *1*, 337–341. [CrossRef]
24. Veber, D.F.; Johnson, S.R.; Cheng, H.-Y.; Smith, B.R.; Ward, K.W.; Kopple, K.D. Molecular Properties That Influence the Oral Bioavailability of Drug Candidates. *J. Med. Chem.* **2002**, *45*, 2615–2623. [CrossRef]
25. Fumarola, L.; Spinelli, R.; Brandonisio, O. In Vitro Assays for Evaluation of Drug Activity against *Leishmania* spp. *Res. Microbiol.* **2004**, *155*, 224–230. [CrossRef]

26. Vitale, R.G.; Afeltra, J.; Dannaoui, E. Antifungal Combinations. In *Antifungal Agents*; Humana Press: Totowa, NJ, USA, 2005; Volume 118, pp. 143–152, ISBN 978-1-59259-943-1.
27. Seifert, K.; Croft, S.L. In Vitro and In Vivo Interactions between Miltefosine and Other Antileishmanial Drugs. *Antimicrob. Agents Chemother.* **2006**, *50*, 73–79. [CrossRef]

pharmaceuticals MDPI

Article

Potential of *Aframomum melegueta* and *Xylopia aethiopica* Against *Taenia* spp.: Plant-Based Remedies as Novel Anthelmintics

Fekandine V. Douti [1], Gnatoulma Katawa [1,*], Kathrin Arndts [2,3], Fagdéba D. Bara [1], Essimanam R. Awesso [1], Simplice D. Karou [1], Achim Hoerauf [2,3,4] and Manuel Ritter [2,3,*]

1 Unité de Recherche en Immunologie et Immuno-Modulation (UR2IM), Laboratoire de Microbiologie et de Contrôle de Qualité des Denrées Alimentaires, École Supérieure des Techniques Biologiques et Alimentaires (ESTBA), Université de Lomé, Lomé 01 BP 1515, Togo; doufekandine@gmail.com (F.V.D.); fagdeba.bara@gmail.com (F.D.B.); roseawesso@gmail.com (E.R.A.); simplicekarou@hotmail.com (S.D.K.)
2 Institute for Medical Microbiology, Immunology and Parasitology (IMMIP), University Hospital Bonn (UKB), 53127 Bonn, Germany; kathrin.arndts@ukbonn.de (K.A.); hoerauf@uni-bonn.de (A.H.)
3 German-West African Centre for Global Health and Pandemic Prevention (G-WAC), Partner Site Bonn, 53127 Bonn, Germany
4 German Centre for Infection Research (DZIF), Partner Site Bonn-Cologne, 53127 Bonn, Germany
* Correspondence: mahkatawa@yahoo.fr (G.K.); manuel.ritter@ukbonn.de (M.R.); Tel.: +228-93-04-06-61 (G.K.); +49-228-287-11453 (M.R.)

Abstract: Background/Objectives: Taeniasis, a zoonotic infection, is a common foodborne disease. Niclosamide and praziquantel have proven to be effective in treating it, but the use of the same drugs can lead to resistance, so alternative drugs need to be explored. This study investigated the anthelmintic potential of derived fractions from hydroethanolic extracts (HEs) of *Aframomum melegueta* (AM) and *Xylopia aethiopica* (XA), two medicinal plants known for their diverse bioactive properties. **Methods:** AM-HE fractions (dichloromethane fraction (DCMF), ether fraction (EF), aqueous fraction (AF)) and XA-HE fractions (chloroform fraction (CF), ether fraction (EF), and aqueous fraction (AF)) were used, and in vitro anthelmintic activity was assessed against *Taenia* spp. by using an adult motility assay for the worm's paralysis time determination. The parasiticidal and parasitostatic activity was also tested on *Taenia* spp. adult worms. Cell viability was further evaluated using propidium iodide (PI) staining, with albendazole (20 mg/mL) as the reference drug. **Results:** The three fractions of each plant exhibited significant, dose-dependent anthelmintic activity, with AM-HE and XA-CF showing the greatest effects at 20 mg/mL. AM-EF demonstrated significant activity at 0.4% and 0.8%. Irreversibility tests revealed that most of the treated worms remained paralysis, except those exposed to the AF of both plants. PI staining confirmed the dose-dependent mortality of *Taenia* cells treated with HE, DCMF, and AF of AM. **Conclusions:** These results underscore the potential of AM and XA extracts and fractions as alternative treatments for helminth infections. Further, in vivo studies are warranted to confirm their safety and therapeutic efficacy.

Keywords: *Aframomum melegueta*; *Xylopia aethiopica*; fractions; anthelminthic; *Taenia* spp.

1. Introduction

Taeniasis is an intestinal infection that affects both humans and animals, caused by the adult stages of tapeworms. These parasites belong to the class of *Cestoda*, the family of *Taeniidae*, and the genus *Taenia* [1]. Three species are known to infect humans: *Taenia asiatica*

(Asian tapeworm) [2], *Taenia saginata* (beef tapeworm), and *Taenia solium* (pork tapeworm). While *T. asiatica* is restricted to Asia, *T. saginata* and *T. solium* have a global distribution.

The transmission of taeniasis is influenced by several environmental factors, including the dispersal of parasite eggs in the soil, often due to the inadequate disposal of human and animal waste, and the use of sewage sludge or contaminated water for agricultural irrigation [3]. Intermediate hosts such as cattle and pigs can ingest *Taenia* eggs, leading to cysticercosis, a tissue infection that affects the muscles, skin, eyes, and the nervous system [4].

Humans typically become infected with *Taenia* by eating undercooked or raw beef and pork meat from infected animals. In the human intestine, the larvae develop into adult tapeworms, causing taeniasis, a disease with significant human and veterinary health implications [5,6]. The disease also imposes an economic burden, including treatment costs, lost productivity, and the condemnation of infected meat [1]. Taeniasis is particularly prevalent in low- and middle-income countries in Latin America, Asia, and Africa, where inadequate sanitation, poor meat inspection practices, and limited access to proper cooking facilities are common [6,7]. An estimated 40–60 million people worldwide are affected by the disease [8].

Taeniasis treatment includes antiparasitic drugs such as niclosamide for *Taenia solium* [9] and combined with praziquantel for *Taenia saginata* [10]. The latter would act by opening calcium channels in the tapeworm's membrane, causing an influx of calcium ions, leading to uncontrolled muscle contraction and paralysis [11]. Moreover, praziquantel in combination with corticosteroids is also effective against neurocysticercosis caused by *T. solium* [12]. In addition, fenbendazole and mebendazole have been successfully used for the treatment of cysticercosis in pigs in combination with laxatives such as magnesium sulphate for the expulsion of dead worms [1]. Although the drugs currently used for the treatment of taeniasis and neurocysticercosis are effective, their judicious administration in terms of the dose and duration of treatment is important. Frequent use of the same molecules has been reported as one of the factors contributing to the emergence of helminth resistance to different groups of available anthelmintics [13]. This resistance highlights the urgent need to develop new alternative agents [14].

Traditional medicine, especially herbal remedies, is the first line of treatment [15] for several types of infectious diseases [16] in African communities, especially in Togo [17]. Some herbal medicines have been reported to have hypoglycemic [18], antihypertensive [19], antimalarial [20], and antimicrobial properties [21], as well as others such as antidiabetic, anticancer, anti-inflammatory, and antioxidant activity and hepatoprotective and neuroprotective effects [22].

Numerous studies have demonstrated the anthelmintic potential of many medicinal plants against different worms such as *Haemonchus contortus* [23] and *Heligmosomoides bakeri* [24]. In recent years, the efficacy of plants as anthelmintics has been evaluated in several readily available experimental models such as *Caenorhabditis elegans* [25,26]; *Haemonchus contortus* [27]; *Eisenia fetida* [28]; *Trypanosoma brucei brucei*; and *Leishmania tarentolae* [29]. One study has shown that the essential oil of *Thymus bovei* had a stronger anthelmintic effect on *Pheretima posthuma* than piperazine citrate, the reference drug that was used [30]. In addition, the effectiveness of plants as anthelmintics against *Taenia* species commonly found in domestic animals such as cattle, pigs, goats, and sheep has been investigated in some studies. This is the case of a study which evaluated the anthelmintic properties of *Gongronema latifolium*, *Piper guineense*, and *Ocimum gratissimum* on bovine feces and demonstrated significant efficacy against *Taenia saginata* eggs [31].

In Togo, our previous research has identified *Khaya senegalensis*, *Aframomum melegueta*, and *Xylopia aethiopica* as plants traditionally used to treat helminth infections [32]. In addition, these plants have demonstrated anti-inflammatory activity; they are anti-Th17-Th2 in subjects with hyperreactive onchocerciasis [33]. Our tests also revealed that extracts from *A. melegueta* and *X. aethiopica* exhibit no toxic effects at therapeutic doses, supporting their traditional use and underscoring the need for further scientific validation [34].

This study aimed to investigate the anthelmintic activity of fractions derived from hydroethanolic extracts of *A. melegueta* and *X. aethiopica* against adult *Taenia* worms.

2. Results

2.1. Bio-Guided Extraction and Partitioning

The bio-guided extraction and fractionation of hydroethanolic extracts from *A. melegueta* (AM) and *X. aethiopica* (XA) yielded three fractions for each plant. Both plants produced an aqueous fraction (AF) and an ether fraction (EF). In addition, *A. melegueta* produced a dichloromethane fraction (DCMF), while *X. aethiopica* produced a chloroform fraction (CF).

2.2. Anthelmintic Activity of AM and XA Fractions on Taenia spp. Worms

The anthelmintic activity of hydroethanolic extracts (HEs) and their fractions (DCMF, CF, AF, EF) from AM and XA was evaluated using *Taenia* spp. worms. All of the tested fractions induced a loss of motility in the worms. The time required for worm paralysis after treatment with AM fractions at different concentrations is shown in Figure 1. Among the treatments, 20 mg/mL of AM hydroethanolic extract (Figure 1a) showed the most potent anthelmintic effects. Statistical analysis revealed a significant difference between the hydroethanolic extract of AM (Figure 1a) at a concentration of 20 mg/mL and the negative control, also called medium (RPMI 1640 + 10% FBS). In contrast, no significant differences were observed for the dichloromethane fraction (Figure 1b) and the medium at any concentration. Similarly, a comparison of the medium with different concentrations of the aqueous fraction (Figure 1c) showed no significant differences. However, the ether fraction (Figure 1d) showed significant differences compared to the medium at concentrations of 0.4% and 0.8%. Notably, after a median incubation time of 4 h, all worms in the negative control group (RPMI 1640 + 10% FBS) lost their motility. All fractions were tested in parallel with the same negative control. This experiment was repeated four times.

Figure 2 shows the time taken for *Taenia* worms to lose motility when treated with hydroethanolic extract (HE) and fractions of *X. aethiopica* (XA) at different concentrations. After 4 h of incubation, most of the worms in the treatment groups were paralyzed at all concentrations of HE and fractions, while the worms in the negative control or medium (RPMI 1640 + 10% FBS) group remained motile. The most effective anthelmintic activity was observed at a concentration of 20 mg/mL of the XA chloroform fraction (Figure 2b) with a motility loss time comparable to the reference drug albendazole. Statistical analysis revealed a significant difference when we compared the negative control with the chloroform fraction at concentrations of 20 mg/mL. However, no significant differences were observed between the HE (Figure 2a), AF (Figure 2c), and EF (Figure 2d) of XA.

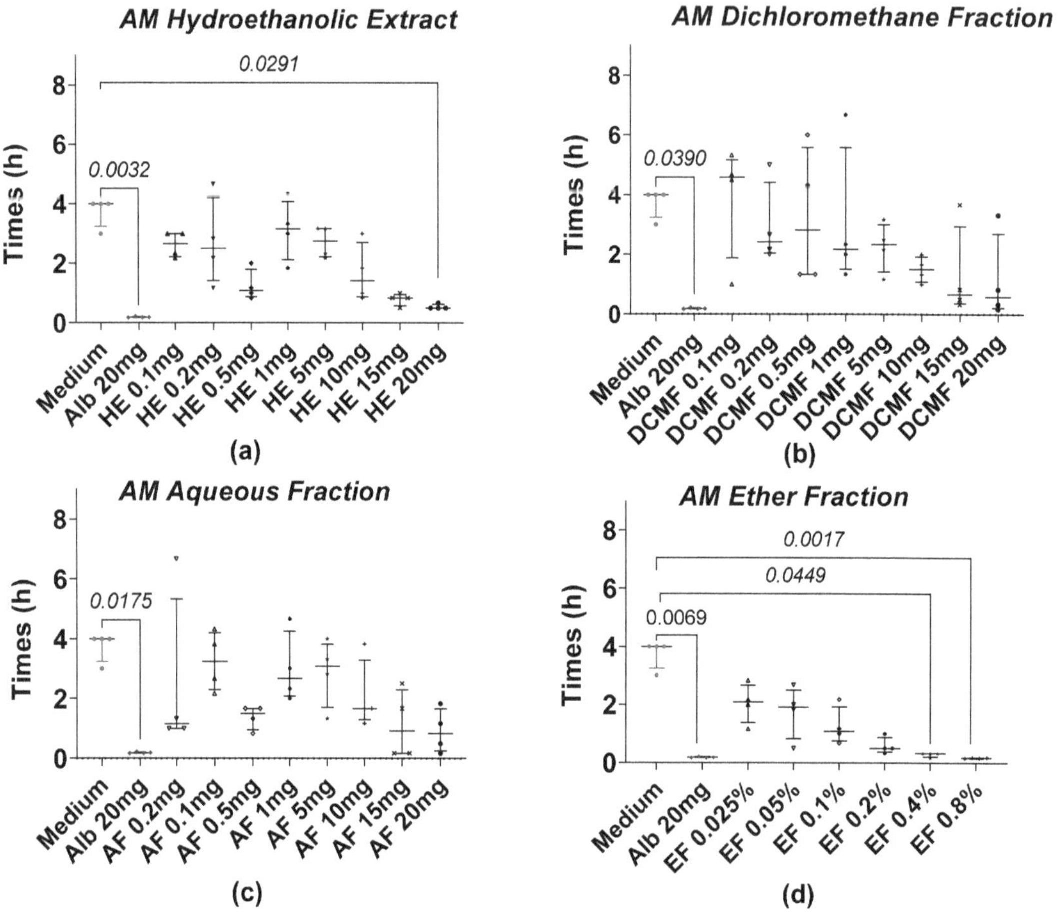

Figure 1. Loss of motility of the tapeworm in the presence of AM extract and fractions. (**a**) The hydroethanolic extract (HE), (**b**) the dichloromethane fraction (DCMF), (**c**) the aqueous fraction (AF), and (**d**) the ether fraction (EF). Alb refers to Albendazole. The green dots represent the negative control (medium), the red dots represent the reference drug (albendazole), and the black dots represent the different concentrations of plant extracts. Data are expressed as the median, and each point represents the mean time of loss of motility from 4 independent experiments with 5 worms per experiment. Statistical analysis was performed using the Kruskal–Wallis and Dunn's post hoc tests.

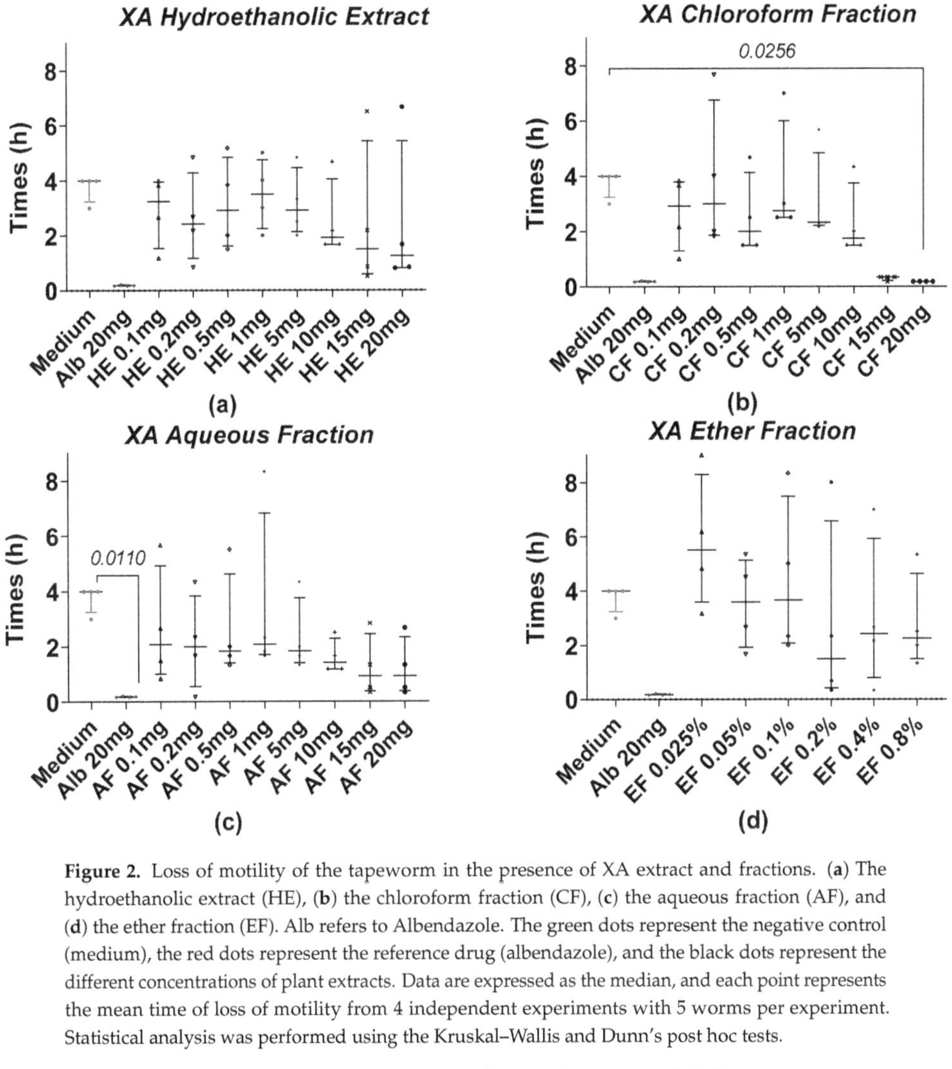

Figure 2. Loss of motility of the tapeworm in the presence of XA extract and fractions. (**a**) The hydroethanolic extract (HE), (**b**) the chloroform fraction (CF), (**c**) the aqueous fraction (AF), and (**d**) the ether fraction (EF). Alb refers to Albendazole. The green dots represent the negative control (medium), the red dots represent the reference drug (albendazole), and the black dots represent the different concentrations of plant extracts. Data are expressed as the median, and each point represents the mean time of loss of motility from 4 independent experiments with 5 worms per experiment. Statistical analysis was performed using the Kruskal–Wallis and Dunn's post hoc tests.

2.3. *Anthelmintic Activity of HE and Fractions of AM and XA on Taenia Cells*

To discover if our plant extracts act in the same way on the cells as on the whole worms, we treated the worms with the plant extract before and after isolating their cells with collagenase to analyze the percentage of dead cells by PI staining.

2.3.1. *Taenia* Worm Cells' Extraction Before Treatment with Extracts and PI Staining

The effects of HE and fractions of AM and XA on *Taenia* cells obtained by enzymatic digestion with collagenase after treatment with plant extract are shown in Figures 3 and 4, respectively. For AM, the mortality of *Taenia* cells under the effect of hydroethanolic extract (Figure 3a), dichloromethane (Figure 3b), and aqueous fractions (Figure 3c) was dose-dependent. Significant differences were observed between the medium and the HE, DCMF, and AF at concentrations of 5, 10, 15, and 20 mg/mL, whereas the EF (Figure 3d) showed significance only at 0.4%. For *XA*, the hydroethanolic extract (Figure 4a), the chloroform fraction (Figure 4b), the aqueous fraction (Figure 4c), and the ether fraction (Figure 4d) showed no significant differences compared to the negative control (medium).

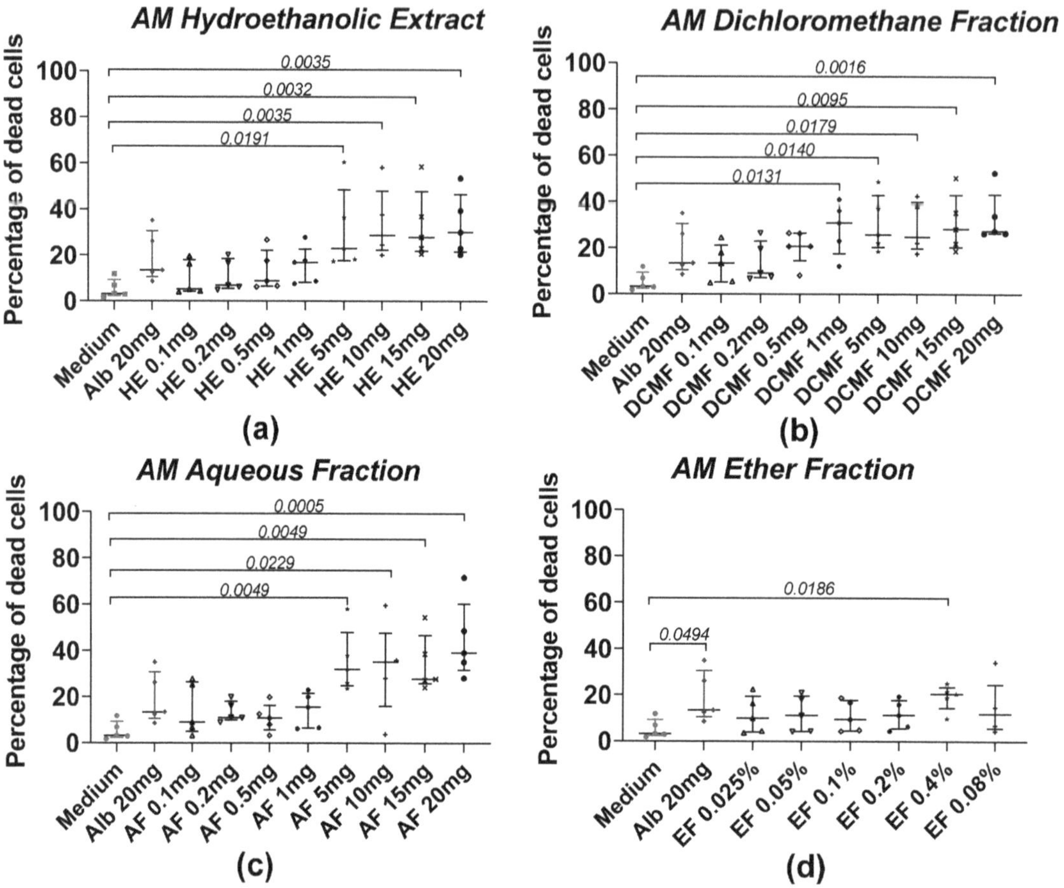

Figure 3. Induction of worm cell death by different fractions of AM. (**a**) The hydroethanolic extract (HE), (**b**) the dichloromethane fraction (DCMF), (**c**) the aqueous fraction (AF), and (**d**) the ether fraction (EF). Alb refers to Albendazole. The green dots represent the negative control (medium), the red dots represent the reference drug (albendazole), and the black dots represent the different concentrations of plant extracts. Data were expressed as the median, and each point represents the percentage of cell death of one worm. The experiment was performed on 5 worms. Statistical analysis was performed using the Kruskal–Wallis and Dunn's multiple comparison post hoc test.

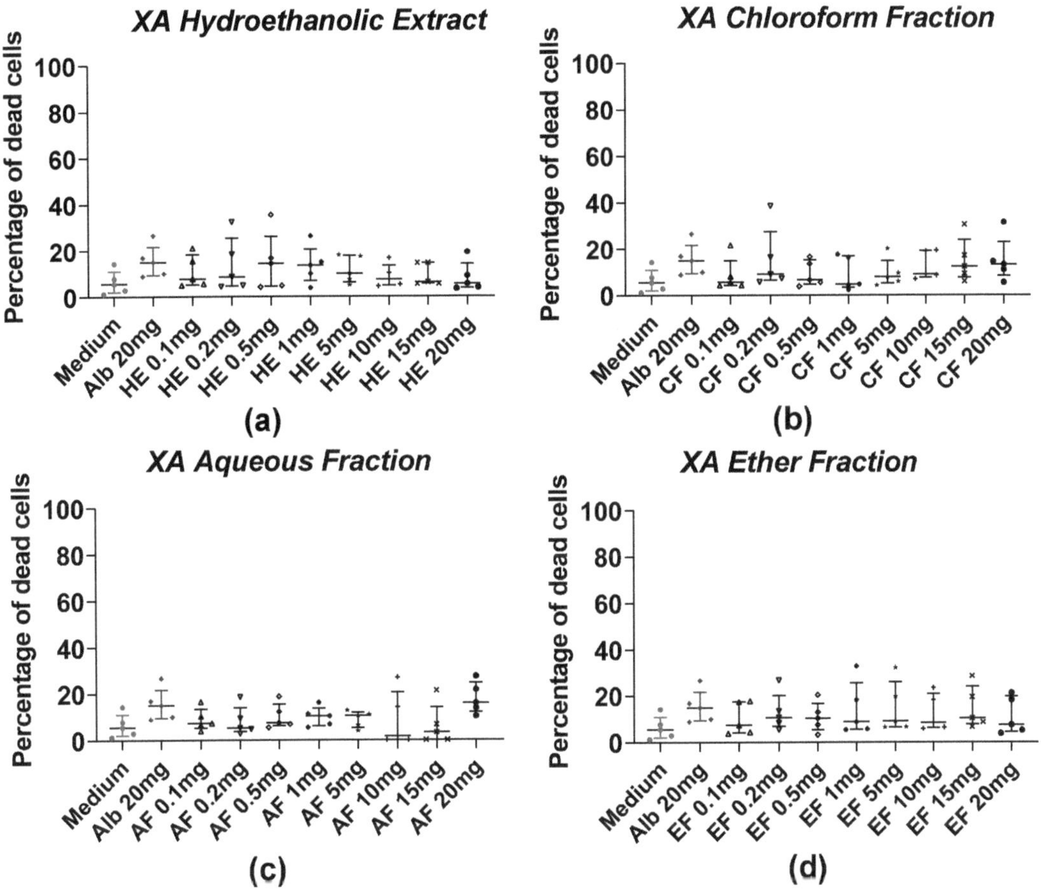

Figure 4. Induction of worm cell death by different fractions of XA. (**a**) The hydroethanolic extract (HE), (**b**) the chloroform fraction (CF), (**c**) the aqueous fraction (AF), and (**d**) the ether fraction (EF). Alb refers to Albendazole. The green dots represent the negative control (medium), the red dots represent the reference drug (albendazole), and the black dots represent the different concentrations of plant extracts. Data were expressed as the median, and each point represents the percentage of cell death of one worm. The experiment was performed on 5 worms. Statistical analysis was performed using the Kruskal–Wallis and Dunn's multiple comparison post hoc test.

2.3.2. Treatment of *Taenia* Worms with Extracts Before Cell Extraction and PI Staining

Figure 5 shows the percentage of dead cells after the loss of motility of worms treated with HE and fractions of AM and XA at a concentration of 20 mg/mL. In general, all of the fractions induce cell death, highlighting that the fractions actually kill the worms and do not just cause starvation, emphasizing that the herbal remedies work and are an option for novel drugs. Furthermore, for AM, the dichloromethane and aqueous fractions showed significant differences compared to the medium (Figure 5a). For XA, only CF showed significant differences when it was compared to the medium (Figure 5b).

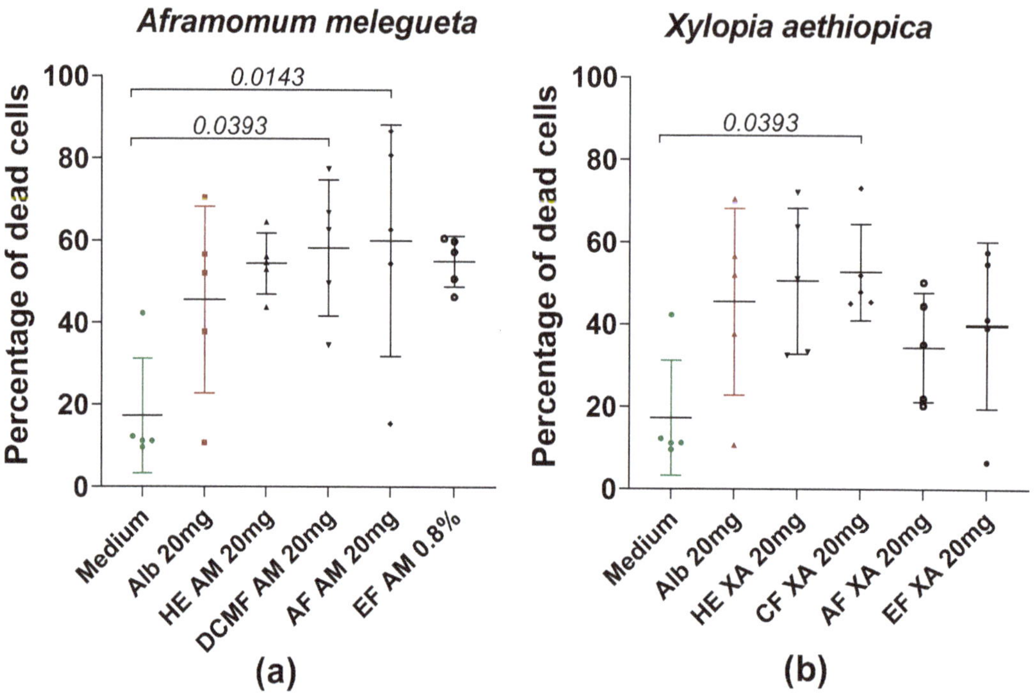

Figure 5. Percentage of dead cells after loss of motility of worms in the presence or absence of hydroethanolic extract (HE) and fractions of AM (**a**) and XA (**b**) at a concentration of 20 mg/mL. Alb refers to Albendazole. The green dots represent the negative control (medium), the red dots represent the reference drug (albendazole), and the black dots represent the different concentrations of plant extracts. Data are expressed as the median, and each point represents the percentage of cell death of one worm. The experiment involved 5 worms. Statistical analysis was conducted using the Kruskal–Wallis and Dunn's multiple comparison.

2.4. Irreversibility of the Effect of AM and XA Fractions on Taenia spp. Worms

To demonstrate the irreversibility of the anthelmintic activity of the AM and XA extracts and fractions, additional tests were performed using the most effective concentrations: 10, 15, and 20 mg/mL for HE, DCMF, CF, and AF, and 0.2%, 0.4%, and 0.8% for EF. Table 1 summarizes the times at which *Taenia* worms remained paralyzed after being exposed to the hydroethanolic extract (HE) and fractions (DCMF, CF, AF, and EF) of AM and XA and then placed in medium. The main goal of this test was to highlight that most of the worms were paralyzed (did not wake up) by our plant extracts and fractions.

Table 1. Time to recovery motility or not of *Taenia* worms in the medium after loss of motility in the HE and fractions (DCMF, CF, AF, and EF) of AM and XA.

Extracts	Concentrations (mg/mL)	Initial Time of Loss of Motility (h)	Transfer in Medium	
			Wake Up Time (h)	Paralysis Time (h)
Medium		4.82	-	-
		A. melegueta		
HE	10	1.16	-	-
	15	1.06	-	-
	20	1	-	-
DCMF	10	1.28	2.11	6
	15	1.44	-	-
	20	0.94	-	-
AF	10	1.78	0.17	0.33
	15	1.72	0.17	0.50
	20	1.67	0.61	1.50
EF	0.2%	0.61	-	-
	0.4%	0.44	-	-
	0.8%	0.28	-	-
		X. aethiopica		
HE	10	2.33	-	-
	15	2.17	-	-
	20	2	0.17	0.21
CF	10	3.22	-	-
	15	2.94	-	-
	20	2.89	0.56	2
AF	10	3.50	0.44	2
	15	3.22	0.5	2
	20	2.94	0.56	2
EF	0.2%	2.17	-	-
	0.4%	3	-	-
	0.8%	1.94	-	-

Abbreviations used: HE—hydroethanolic extract; DCMF—dichloromethane fraction; AF—aqueous fraction; EF—ether fraction; CF—chloroform fraction. Post hoc test.

In AM, when worms that had lost motility in the HE (all concentrations tested) were transferred to the medium (RPMI + 10% FBS), they showed no revival of motility. Similarly, no revival was observed in worms treated with the dichloromethane fraction (15 and 20 mg/mL) and the ether fraction (0.2, 0.4, and 0.8%), and they were transferred to the medium after paralysis. Regarding XA, worms treated at a concentration of 10 and 15 mg/mL of the HE did not recover their motility in the medium. Also, no revival was observed for worms treated with the chloroform fraction (15 and 20 mg/mL). As for the ether fraction, no revival was observed in worms treated with different concentrations and then placed in the medium after paralysis.

3. Discussion

Resistance to anthelmintics is a major public health problem. Several cases of resistance have been reported for helminthiasis caused by hookworm, ascariasis, and schistosomiasis [35,36]. Although the resistance reported for taeniasis is very rare, resistance remains a threat and thus requires the development of alternative treatments [37].

Plants have long been recognized as valuable sources of bioactive molecules to treat various diseases. Since then, numerous studies have investigated their biological activities against parasites, especially helminths [38,39]. Various worm species were used to evaluate the anthelmintic potential of plant extracts, as in a study by Buza et al. that demonstrated the anthelmintic activity of six aqueous medicinal plant extracts against donkey strongyles [40]. In another study, *Lumbricus terretris* worms were used to test the anthelmintic activity of aqueous and ethanolic extracts of *Vernonia amygdalina* and *Alstonia boonei* [41].

The present study is the first to evaluate the anthelmintic activity of two hydroethanolic extracts and six fractions derived from *A. melegueta* (AM) and *X. aethiopica* (XA) against whole worms and cells of *Taenia* spp in vitro. Our results show that all of the extracts and fractions of AM and XA have anthelmintic activity against *Taenia* spp. at both the tissue and cellular levels, with AM having a more pronounced effect on cells than XA.

These results highlight the potential of plant-based remedies as novel anthelmintics [42].

The effectiveness of an anthelmintic drug often varies depending on the developmental stage of the target parasite. Many drugs are effective only against larval stages [43], and those that target larvae may fail to act on adult worms.

For AM, the hydroethanolic extract (HE) and ether fraction (EF) showed significant anthelmintic effects. All worms were immobilized or killed within 9 h, contrasting with the 120 h timeframe reported by Mengome et al. on *Loa loa* microfilariae [22]. This difference likely stems from variations in parasite species, the concentrations used, and experimental conditions. While studies like those of Lakshmi et al. [23] emphasize the influence of methodology on the outcomes, our findings suggest that HE and EF are promising candidates for further studies. In contrast, only the chloroform fraction of XA demonstrated significant activity against *Taenia* spp. This aligns with previous reports of XA's efficacy against parasitic infections [44]. The observed activity of XA may be attributed to its rich phytochemical composition, particularly alkaloids and terpenoids, which have documented anthelmintic effects [45]. These compounds likely disrupt cellular metabolism, leading to parasite death [46].

The better activity of AM compared to XA could be explained by the difference in phytochemical composition and therefore their different mode of action. Our previous study on these plants had shown that the hydroethanolic extracts of AM were more concentrated in polyphenols and flavonoids than XA [34].

Flavonoids, a diverse group of plant-derived polyphenolic compounds, have demonstrated significant anthelmintic activity against several parasitic worms. Their mechanisms of action are diverse, targeting different stages of the parasite life cycle and influencing different physiological processes. Some flavonoids have been shown to affect the neuromuscular system of worms, leading to reduced motility and subsequent paralysis. For example, quercetin and naringenin have been shown to significantly inhibit the motility of liver flukes such as *Opisthorchis felineus*, suggesting interference with neuromuscular function [47]. Flavonoids are thought to act synergistically with other phytochemicals to enhance anthelmintic efficacy. In *Pithecellobium dulce*, the combination of flavonoids such as kaempferol and quercetin with phenolic acids resulted in a potent ovicidal effect against *Haemonchus contortus*, indicating that flavonoids contribute significantly to the overall anthelmintic activity of plant extracts.

Irreversibility tests showed that some extracts were parasiticidal, irreversibly damaging worms, while others showed parasitostatic, temporarily paralyzing them. This dual activity underscores the importance of selecting appropriate fractions for targeted applications. For example, parasiticidal effects that inhibit essential worm metabolism and cause irreversible damage are desirable for achieving complete eradication in therapeutic applications [48,49].

Our cell viability assays using propidium iodide (PI) staining confirmed the dose-dependent anthelmintic activity of AM, with HE inducing higher cell mortality than albendazole. Notably, the hydroethanolic extract showed a synergistic action of its bioactive components, which may enhance its overall efficacy. However, further studies are required to isolate and characterize these components to identify the most active biomolecules.

A key observation was the higher mortality rate of extracted cells after the exposure of worms to the extracts compared to direct application on cells. For example, at 20 mg/mL, HE and AM fractions achieved mortality rates above 50% when acting extracellularly, compared to rates below 45% in direct cellular assays. This suggests that the extracts are more effective on extracellular targets, possibly by disrupting worm membranes and cellular components. These results are consistent with previous studies emphasizing the extracellular activity of flavonoids, a major component of AM. Considering the observed toxicity of the ether fraction (EF) in previous experiments, the evaluation of less toxic solvents should be prioritized in future research.

Hydroethanolic extracts, which have shown significant efficacy with potentially safer profiles, may be more suitable for subsequent animal studies. This approach is consistent with the need to balance efficacy and safety in the development of plant-based anthelmintics. In addition, according to the results obtained for the irreversibility test of the anthelmintic activity of our extracts, the hydroethanolic extracts and the ethereal fractions of AM and XA would contain biomolecules that would irreversibly paralyze *Taenia* worms. Since the main objective of our study was to find bioactive compounds, it would be more appropriate to isolate bioactive molecules directly from hydroethanolic extracts to implement new anthelmintic drugs.

4. Materials and Methods

4.1. Plant Material

The plant material used in this study consisted of the seeds of *A. melegueta* K. Schum. and the fruits of *X. aethiopica* (Dunal) A. Rich. (Figure 6). Both are spices with a rich history of culinary and medicinal use in West Africa and are recognized for their therapeutic properties [50,51].

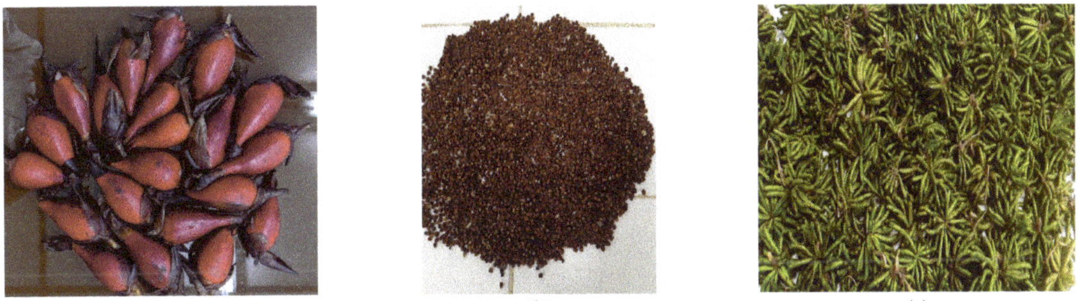

(a) (b) (c)

Figure 6. Plant material used in this study: (**a**) fruits of *Aframomum melegueta* K. Schum.; (**b**) seeds of *Aframomum melegueta* K. Schum.; (**c**) fruits of *Xylopia aethiopica* (Dunal) A. Rich.

The fruits of *A. melegueta* and *X. aethiopica* were collected, and botanical verification was carried out at the Botanical Laboratory of the Faculty of Science at the University of Lomé. The identification process was carried out using the International Plant Names

Index (IPNI) to confirm the taxonomy of the plants. The voucher specimen was deposited at the Herbarium of the University of Lomé. The chemical characterization of the plants was previously described [34].

4.2. Plant Extraction

Fresh *A. melegueta* seeds and *X. aethiopica* fruits were washed and air-dried for two months at room temperature (18–25 °C) under controlled laboratory conditions and then crushed. The extraction of plant materials was performed by percolation. A total of 500 g of dried powdered seeds of *A. melegueta* and fruits of *X. aethiopica* was processed with 2 L of a 70% ethanol–water solution (70:30) for 72 h, with stirring every 24 h. After the first extraction, the filtrate was collected, and another 2 L of the ethanol–water solution was added to the remaining residue to repeat the process. The resulting extract was subsequently filtered through cotton and then through 11 µm Whatman No. 1 paper (Sigma-Aldrich, St. Louis, MO, USA) to ensure purity.

To obtain the hydroethanolic extract, a portion of the filtrate was evaporated to dryness at 50 °C under reduced pressure using a rotary evaporator (Buchi, Flawil, Switzerland). The remaining filtrate was partially evaporated to remove ethanol, leaving an aqueous extract.

4.3. Bio-Guided Partition

Bio-guided partition was carried out on the aqueous extract according to the modified method of Dosso et al. (2017) [52]. In our case, the solvents with increasing polarity used are petroleum ether, dichloromethane (for AM), and chloroform (for XA).

Equal volumes of the aqueous fraction and petroleum ether (Park Scientific Limited, Northampton, UK) (1:1) were mixed, vigorously homogenized, and allowed to decant, resulting in two distinct layers: an organic phase (ether fraction) and an aqueous phase. The aqueous phase was further partitioned with dichloromethane or chloroform (Chemicals & Metals Co, Gyeonggi, Republic of Korea). After mixing and decanting, two layers were obtained: an organic phase (dichloromethane or chloroform fraction) and a final aqueous phase. The aqueous phase was freeze-dried at 50 °C to obtain the aqueous fraction.

4.4. Collection of Worms

Taenia spp. worms, approximately 0.5–2 m long and 0.5–1 cm wide, were collected from the gut of naturally infected cattle and sheep slaughtered at the "Office National des Abattoirs Frigorifiques" (ONAF) in Lomé, Togo.

Isotonic saline water (B. BRAUN, Melsungen, Germany) was used to wash all the worms and to remove all fecal material. The worms were immediately placed in RPMI 1640 medium (Gibco, Paisley, Scotland, UK) to maintain viability during transport to the laboratory. Slaughter of the animals began at 4 a.m. The time taken to wash all the intestines and collect the worms, if present, and then transport them to the laboratory varied between 4 and 6 h. However, once in the laboratory, the viability of worms was assessed by heating them in RPMI 1640 medium (Thermo Fisher Scientific, Waltham, MA, USA) at 45 °C in a water bath (Figure 7). A four-point scoring system ranging from 0 to 3 was used to describe the motility of worms in the different Petri dishes [53]. The vigorous movement of worms was scored at 3, the sluggish shaking of worms was scored at 2, the intermittent shaking of worms was scored at 1, and no movement (immotile) was scored at 0.

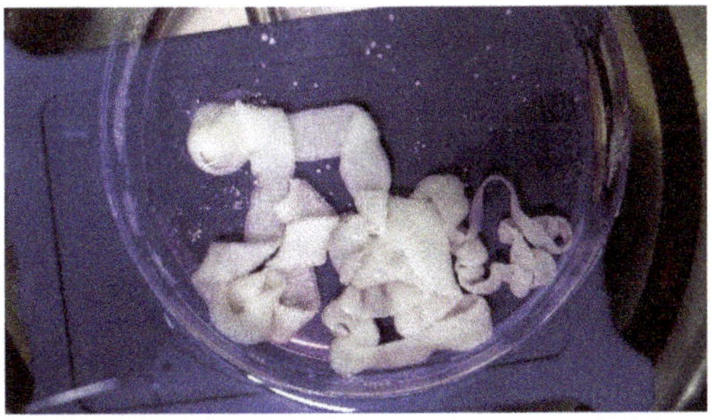

Figure 7. Tapeworm motility test in RPMI 1640 at 45 °C in a water bath.

For the tests, worms that scored 3 were randomly divided into the different treatment groups.

4.5. Anthelmintic Activity on Taenia Worms

The in vitro anthelmintic tests of *A. melegueta* and *X. aethiopica* hydroethanolic-derived fractions on tapeworms were performed by a combination of the methods described by Akter et al. (2014) using five worms [54] and Lalthanpuii et al. (2020) for the motility test at 45 °C [55] with minor modifications. In our case, we modified by using *Taenia* spp. worms isolated on cattle and sheep and the reference drug albendazole at a concentration of 20 mg/mL.

Before treatment, stock solutions of the ether fractions (AM-EF and XA-FE) were obtained by dissolution in DMSO. Six dilutions of 0.025%, 0.05%, 0.1%, 0.2%, 0.4%, and 0.8% of each fraction were then prepared in 15 mL of RPMI medium supplemented with 10% heat-inactivated fetal bovine serum (FBS, PAN Biotech, Aidenbach, Germany). However, stock solutions of hydroethanolic extracts, dichloromethane, chloroform, and aqueous fractions (AM-HE, AM-DCMF, AM-AF, XA-HE, XA-CF, and XA-AF) were prepared in water. Eight dilutions (0.1, 0.2, 0.5, 1, 5, 10, 15 and 20 mg/mL) were made in 15 mL of RPMI medium supplemented with 10% heat-inactivated fetal bovine serum.

An anthelmintic assay was carried out by distributing 5 worms into 60 groups, corresponding to each extract concentration. RPMI medium supplemented with 10% heat-inactivated fetal bovine serum was used as the negative control. The reference drug albendazole (CPA GERERICS, Lomé, Togo) was also prepared in RPMI medium supplemented with 10% heat-inactivated fetal bovine serum at 20 mg/mL and served as the positive control. Petri dishes containing worms and plant extracts or controls were incubated at 37 °C, and motility was checked every 10 min after a brief exposure to 45 °C. The time of worm paralysis was recorded after confirming that the worms did not move when heated or when shaken vigorously. Each experiment was replicated four times.

4.6. Anthelmintic Activity on Taenia Cells

To assess the effect of the extract on *Taenia* cells, we performed a propidium iodide (PI) staining on *Taenia* cells derived from dead worms (loss of motility) and on *Taenia* live cells after exposure to the plant compound. Briefly, adult worms were exposed to the extract, as described, and after loss of motility (12–18 h), the five worms were digested with 100 µL of collagenase (Roche Diagnostics, Mannheim, Germany) at a concentration of 2 mg/mL and incubated at 37 °C with 5% CO_2 for 3–4 h. In addition, five live worms were digested with collagenase, as described, and the obtained cells were co-cultured with the extracts for 12–18 h. Cells from dead worms and the exposed cells were then stained with PI. The rate of cell cytotoxicity in both cases was compared. The gating strategy used is presented in Figure 8.

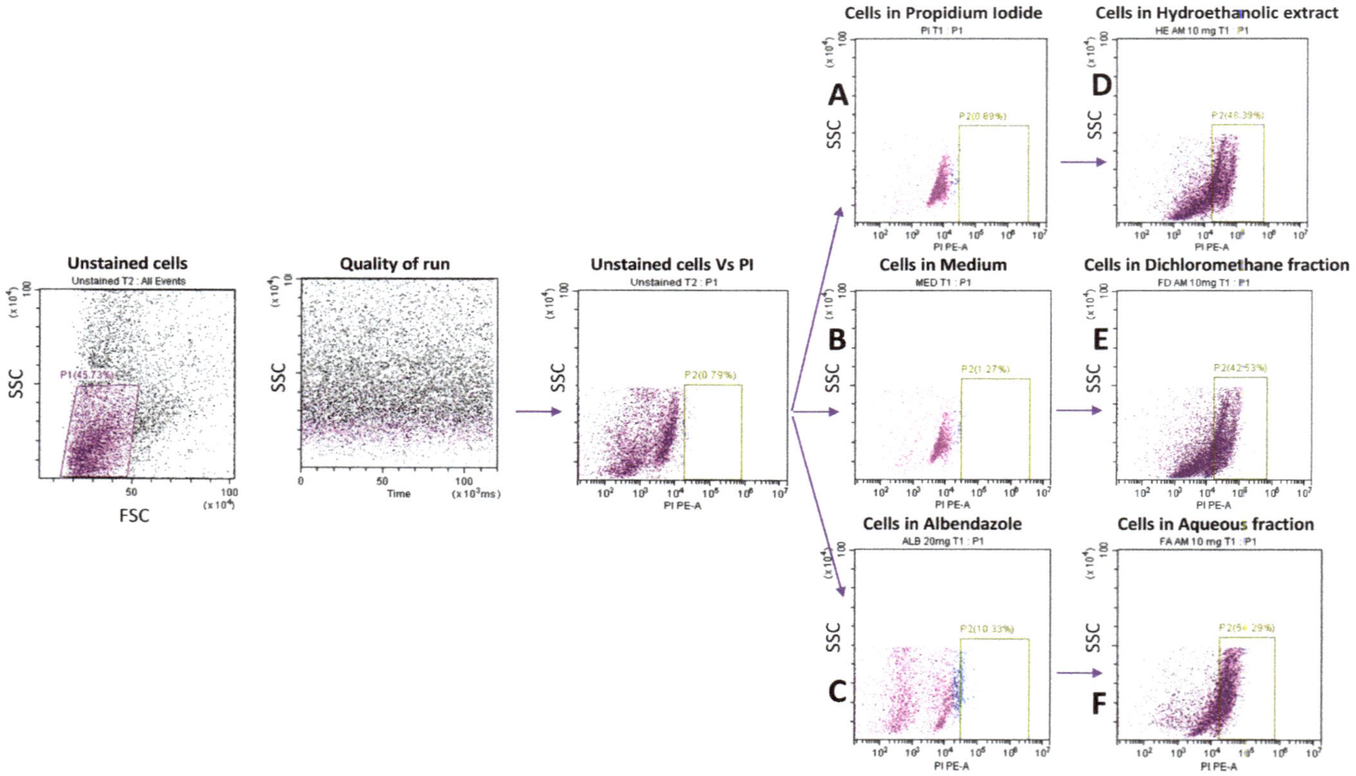

Figure 8. The anthelmintic effect of AM extract and fractions on Taenia cells (1 × 10^4 cells/well) was left alone (Med) or stimulated with 20 mg/mL of ALB and 10 mg/mL of HE, FD, and FA for 12 h. Cells were stained with propidium iodide dye (PI) and acquired by flow cytometry. A: PI cells gate, B, C, D, E, and F are PI+ cells alone, in the presence of medium, albendazole, and 10 mg/mL of HE, FD, and FA, respectively.

4.7. Propidium Iodide Staining of Taenia Cells

After the incubation period, the supernatant was carefully removed from each well, and the remaining cells were stained with propidium iodide (PI) (Avantor, Radnor, PA, USA) for flow cytometry analysis. After removing the supernatant from the wells, 200 µL of FACS buffer (PBS + 2% FBS) was added to each well. Cells were collected in hemolysis tubes and centrifuged at 1500 rpm for 5 min. The supernatant was discarded, and the cells were incubated with 100 µL of PI in the dark. After incubation for 15 min at 4 °C, the cells were washed again with 200 µL of FACS buffer, resuspended in another 100 µL of FACS buffer, and analyzed using a Cytoflex flow cytometer (Beckman Coulter, Brea, CA, USA). Data were processed using CytExpert 2.1 software (Beckman Coulter, Brea, CA, USA). The percentage of cells expressing propidium iodide (PI) was assessed. The gating strategy used is described in Figure 8.

4.8. Assessment of Motility Recovery of Taenia spp. Worms

To determine whether the anthelmintic activity of the AM and XA fractions was irreversible, a separate set of experiments was performed using the most effective concentrations: 10, 15, and 20 mg/mL for HE, DCMF, CF, and AF, and 0.2%, 0.4%, and 0.8% for EF. After complete loss of motility (score 0) upon exposure to these concentrations, they were transferred back to the culture medium (RPMI 1640 + 10% FBS) alone and observed for any recovery of motility (Figure 9). This irreversibility test was performed to distinguish between the reversible and irreversible anthelmintic effects of the plant fractions tested.

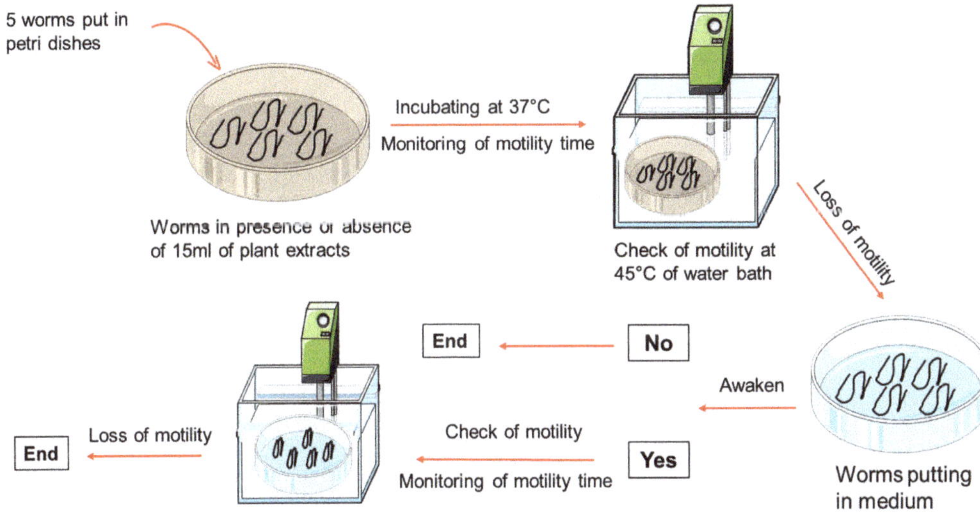

Figure 9. Schematic overview of the experimental design.

4.9. Statistical Analysis

Statistical analysis of the data was performed using the GraphPad PRISM 8.0.2 software (GraphPad Software, Inc., La Jolla, CA, USA). A D'Agostino–Pearson normality test was used to test for the distribution of the values before testing for statistical significance between the groups. Since the variables were nonparametrically distributed, Kruskal–Wallis tests were performed to compare more than two treated groups with the control group. If the Kruskal–Wallis test was significant, Dunn's multiple comparison post-test was performed to further compare the groups. Data were considered significant for *p*-values of 0.05 or less (* $p < 0.05$, ** $p < 0.01$, *** $p < 0.001$).

5. Conclusions

This study revealed that the HEs and fractions (EF and DCMF/CF) of each plant exhibited significant, dose-dependent anthelmintic activity against *Taenia* spp. In particular, AM-HE and XA-CF showed a high effectiveness at 20 mg/mL and AM-EF at 0.4% and 0.8%. These results underscore the potential of AM and XA extracts and fractions as alternative treatments for helminth infections and provide scientific evidence of the efficacy of these plant extracts. While their efficacy is promising, further research is needed to isolate active compounds, refine solvent selection, and evaluate safety profiles in animal models. By focusing on these aspects, future studies may pave the way for the development of effective herbal anthelmintics.

Author Contributions: Conceptualization, F.V.D. and G.K.; methodology, F.V.D. and E.R.A.; software, F.V.D.; validation, G.K., K.A. and M.R.; formal analysis, F.V.D.; investigation, G.K. and M.R.; resources, G.K.; data curation, F.V.D.; writing—original draft preparation, F.V.D.; writing—review and editing, F.D.B., K.A. and M.R.; visualization, A.H.; supervision, G.K. and S.D.K.; project administration, G.K.; funding acquisition, G.K. and M.R. All authors have read and agreed to the published version of the manuscript.

Funding: This research was funded by the German Research Foundation (DFG), grant number LA2746/1-2, within the "German African Cooperation Projects in Infectiology".

Institutional Review Board Statement: This study received approval N° 003/2023/C2EA dated 15 February 2023, from the Comité d'éthique pour l'expérimentation animale (C2EA) of the Laboratoire de Microbiologie et de Contrôle de Qualité des Denrées Alimentaires (LAMICODA), École Supérieure des Techniques Biologiques et Alimentaires (ESTBA), University of Lome'.

Informed Consent Statement: Not applicable.

Data Availability Statement: The original contributions presented in this study are included in the article. Further inquiries can be directed to the corresponding authors.

Acknowledgments: We thank all the workers of the "Office National des Abatoirs et Frigorifiques", especially butchers and veterinarians, for helping us by providing the worms.

Conflicts of Interest: The authors declare that this research was conducted in the absence of any commercial or financial relationships that could be construed as potential conflicts of interest.

Abbreviations

AF	Aqueous fraction
AM	*Aframomum melegueta*
CF	Chloroform fraction
DCMF	Dichloromethane fraction
EF	Ether fraction
FBS	Fetal bovine serum
HE	Hydroethanolic extract
PBS	Phosphate-buffered saline
RPMI	Roswell Park Memorial Institute medium
XA	*Xylopia aethiopica*

References

1. Gebrie, M.; Engdaw, T.A. Review on taeniasis and its zoonotic importance. *Eur. J. Appl. Sci.* **2015**, *7*, 182–191.
2. Ito, A.; Wandra, T.; Yamasaki, H.; Nakao, M.; Sako, Y.; Nakaya, K.; Margono, S.S.; Suroso, T.; Gauci, C.; Lightowlers, M.W.; et al. Cysticercosis/taeniasis in Asia and the Pacific. *Vector-Borne Zoonotic Dis.* **2004**, *4*, 95–107. [CrossRef] [PubMed]
3. Jansen, F.; Dorny, P.; Gabriël, S.; Dermauw, V.; Johansen, M.V.; Trevisan, C. The survival and dispersal of Taenia eggs in the environment: What are the implications for transmission? A systematic review. *Parasit. Vectors* **2021**, *14*, 88. [CrossRef] [PubMed]

4. Galán-Puchades, M.T.; Fuentes, M.V. *Taenia asiatica*: The most neglected human Taenia and the possibility of cysticercosis. *Korean J. Parasitol.* **2013**, *51*, 51–54. [CrossRef]
5. Mlowe, F.; Karimuribo, E.; Mkupasi, E.; Churi, A.; Nyerere, A.D.; Schmidt, V.; Ngowi, H.; Winkler, A.S.; Mlangwa, J. Challenges in the Diagnosis of *Taenia solium* Cysticercosis and Taeniosis in Medical and Veterinary Settings in Selected Regions of Tanzania: A Cross-Sectional Study. *Vet. Med. Int.* **2022**, *2022*, 1–15. [CrossRef]
6. Okello, A.L.; Thomas, L.F.J.R.M.; Policy, H. Human taeniasis: Current insights into prevention and management strategies in endemic countries. *Risk Manag. Healthc. Policy* **2017**, *10*, 107–116. [CrossRef]
7. Edao, A.; Dima, F.G.; Deressa, F.B. Prevalence of bovine cysticercosis and status of human taeniasis in and around Asella town, Tiyoworeda, south east Ethiopia. *Glob. J. Med. Res.* **2016**, *16*, 18–26.
8. Parija, S.C. Taeniasis. In *Textbook of Parasitic Zoonoses*, 1st ed.; Parija, S.C., Chaudhury, A., Eds.; Springer: Singapore, 2022; pp. 337–351.
9. Wardle, M.T.; Allen, S.E.; Gamboa, R.; Vilchez, P.; O'Neal, S.E.; Muro, C.; Lescano, A.G.; Moyano, L.M.; Gonzalvez, G.E.; González, A.E.; et al. Mass chemotherapy with niclosamide for the control of *Taenia solium*: Population-based safety profile and treatment effectiveness. *Lancet Reg. Health Am.* **2024**, *38*, 100876. [CrossRef]
10. Lateef, M.; Zargar, S.A.; Khan, A.R.; Nazir, M.; Shoukat, A. Successful treatment of niclosamide- and praziquantel-resistant beef tapeworm infection with nitazoxanide. *Int. J. Infect. Dis.* **2008**, *12*, 80–82. [CrossRef]
11. Thomas, C.M.; Timson, D.J. The Mechanism of Action of Praziquantel: Can New Drugs Exploit Similar Mechanisms? *Curr. Med. Chem.* **2020**, *27*, 676–696. [CrossRef]
12. World Health Organization. *WHO Guidelines on Management of Taenia solium Neurocysticercosis*, 1st ed.; World Health Organization: Geneva, Switzerland, 2021.
13. Fissiha, W.; Kinde, M.Z. Anthelmintic Resistance and Its Mechanism: A Review. *Infect. Drug Resist.* **2021**, *14*, 5403–5410. [CrossRef] [PubMed]
14. Twumasi, E.B.; Akazue, P.I.; Kyeremeh, K.; Gwira, T.M.; Keiser, J.; Cho-Ngwa, F.; Flint, A.; Anibea, B.; Bonsu, E.Y.; Amewu, R.K.; et al. Antischistosomal, antionchocercal and antitrypanosomal potentials of some Ghanaian traditional medicines and their constituents. *PLoS Negl. Trop. Dis.* **2021**, *14*, 0008919. [CrossRef]
15. Tandon, V.; Yadav, A.; Roy, B.; Das, B. Phytochemicals as cure of worm infections in traditional medicine systems. *Emerg. Trends Zool.* **2011**, *16*, 351–378.
16. Chaughule, R.; Barve, R. Role of herbal medicines in the treatment of infectious diseases. In *Infectious Diseases*; Atta-ur-Rahman, Bian, K., Eds.; Bentham Science: Mumbai, India, 2024; Volume 37, pp. 74–91.
17. Tchacondo, T.; Karou, S.; Batawila, K.; Agban, A.; Ouro-Bang'na, K.; Anani, K.; Gbeassor, M.; De Souza, C. Herbal remedies and their adverse effects in tem tribe traditional medicine in Togo. *Afr. J. Tradit. Complement. Altern. Med.* **2011**, *8*, 45–60. [CrossRef]
18. Ogbonnia, S.; Adekunle, A.; Bosa, M.; Enwuru, V. Evaluation of acute and subacute toxicity of *Alstonia congensis* Engler (Apocynaceae) bark and *Xylopia aethiopica* (Dunal) A. Rich (Annonaceae) fruits mixtures used in the treatment of diabetes. *Afr. J. Biotechnol.* **2008**, *7*, 701–705.
19. Karou, S.D.; Tchacondo, T.; Djikpo Tchibozo, M.A.; Abdoul-Rahaman, S.; Anani, K.; Koudouvo, K.; Batawila, K.; Agbonon, A.; Simpore, J.; de Souza, C. Ethnobotanical study of medicinal plants used in the management of diabetes mellitus and hypertension in the Central Region of Togo. *Pharm. Biol.* **2011**, *49*, 1286–1297. [CrossRef]
20. Akinyele, S.T.; Elusiyan, C.A.; Omisore, N.O.; Adewunmi, C.O. ANTIMALARIAL activities and alkaloids from *Crinum jagus* (Thomps) DANDY. *J. Ethnopharmacol.* **2022**, *296*, 115359. [CrossRef]
21. Chiejina, N.V.; Ukeh, J.A. Antimicrobial properties and phytochemical analysis of methanolic extracts of *Aframomum melegueta* and *Zingiber officinale* on fungal diseases of tomato fruit. *J. Nat. Sci. Res.* **2012**, *2*, 10–16.
22. Alolga, R.N.; Wang, F.; Zhang, X.; Li, J.; Tran, L.P.; Yin, X. Bioactive Compounds from the Zingiberaceae Family with Known Antioxidant Activities for Possible Therapeutic Uses. *Antioxidants* **2022**, *11*, 1281. [CrossRef]
23. Lone, B.A.; Chishti, M.Z.; Bhat, F.A.; Tak, H.; Bandh, S.A. In vitro and in vivo anthelmintic activity of *Euphorbia helioscopia* L. *Vet. Parasitol.* **2012**, *189*, 317–321. [CrossRef]
24. Grzybek, M.; Kukula-Koch, W.; Strachecka, A.; Jaworska, A.; Phiri, A.M.; Paleolog, J.; Tomczuk, K. Evaluation of anthelmintic activity and composition of pumpkin (*Cucurbita pepo* L.) seed extracts—In vitro and in vivo studies. *Int. J. Mol. Sci.* **2016**, *17*, 1456. [CrossRef] [PubMed]
25. Hernando, G.; Turani, O.; Bouzat, C. Caenorhabditis elegans muscle Cys-loop receptors as novel targets of terpenoids with potential anthelmintic activity. *PLoS Negl. Trop. Dis.* **2019**, *13*, e0007895. [CrossRef] [PubMed]
26. Liu, M.; Lu, J.-G.; Yang, M.-R.; Jiang, Z.-H.; Wan, X.; Luyten, W. Bioassay-Guided Isolation of Anthelmintic Components from *Semen pharbitidis*, and the Mechanism of Action of Pharbitin. *Int. J. Mol. Sci.* **2022**, *23*, 15739. [CrossRef] [PubMed]
27. Ahmed, A.H.; Ejo, M.; Feyera, T.; Regassa, D.; Mummed, B.; Huluka, S.A. In vitro anthelmintic activity of crude extracts of *Artemisia herba-alba* and *Punica granatum* against *Haemonchus contortus*. *J. Parasitol. Res.* **2020**, *2020*, 4950196. [CrossRef]

28. Giri, K.; Singh, A.; Palandurkar, K.M.; Banerjee, T.; Chaurasia, S. Evaluation of antihelmintic activity of indigenous plants found in India including *Butea monosperma*, *Origanum majorana*, *Piper longum* and *Embelia ribes* and GC-MS phytochemical analysis of plant extracts. *Pharmacogn. J.* **2021**, *13*, 1464–1471. [CrossRef]
29. Krstin, S.; Sobeh, M.; Braun, M.S.; Wink, M. Anti-Parasitic Activities of *Allium sativum* and *Allium cepa* against *Trypanosoma b. brucei* and *Leishmania tarentolae*. *Medicines* **2018**, *5*, 37. [CrossRef]
30. Jaradat, N.; Adwan, L.; K'Aibni, S.; Shraim, N.; Zaid, A.N. Chemical composition, anthelmintic, antibacterial and antioxidant effects of *Thymus bovei* essential oil. *BMC Complement. Altern. Med.* **2016**, *16*, 418. [CrossRef]
31. Ngozi, U.D.; Ohalete, C.; Ibiam, U.; Okechukwu, R. Medicinal plants effectiveness against helminths of cattle. *J. Appl. Biosci.* **2015**, *86*, 7909–7917. [CrossRef]
32. Ataba, E.; Katawa, G.; Ritter, M.; Ameyapoh, A.H.; Anani, K.; Amessoudji, O.M.; Tchadié, P.E.; Tchacondo, T.; Batawila, K.; Ameyapoh, Y.; et al. Ethnobotanical survey, anthelmintic effects and cytotoxicity of plants used for treatment of helminthiasis in the Central and Kara regions of Togo. *BMC Complement. Med. Ther.* **2020**, *20*, 212. [CrossRef]
33. Katawa, G.; Ataba, E.; Ritter, M.; Amessoudji, O.M.; Awesso, E.R.; Tchadié, P.E.; Bara, F.D.; Douti, F.V.; Arndts, K.; Tchacondo, T.; et al. Anti-Th17 and anti-Th2 responses effects of hydro-ethanolic extracts of *Aframomum melegueta*, *Khaya senegalensis* and *Xylopia aethiopica* in hyperreactive onchocerciasis individuals' peripheral blood mononuclear cells. *PLoS Negl. Trop. Dis.* **2022**, *16*, e0010341. [CrossRef]
34. Ataba, E.; Katawa, G.; Toudji, G.A.; Ritter, M.; Holali Ameyapohh, A.; Edlom Tchadié, P.; Batawila, K.; Tchacondo, T.; Ameyapoh, Y.; Hoerauf, A.; et al. Toxicity, chemical composition, anti-inflammatory and antioxidant activities of plants used for the treatment of helminth infections in the Kara and Central region of Togo. *J. Appl. Biosci.* **2020**, *156*, 16114–16131. [CrossRef]
35. Doenhoff, M.J.; Cioli, D.; Utzinger, J. Praziquantel: Mechanisms of action, resistance and new derivatives for schistosomiasis. *Curr. Opin. Infect. Dis.* **2008**, *21*, 659–667. [CrossRef] [PubMed]
36. Moser, W.; Schindler, C.; Keiser, J. Efficacy of recommended drugs against soil transmitted helminths: Systematic review and network meta-analysis. *BMJ* **2017**, *358*, j4307. [CrossRef] [PubMed]
37. Jato, J.; Orman, E.; Duah Boakye, Y.; Oppong Bekoe, E.; Oppong Bekoe, S.; Asare-Nkansah, S.; Spiegler, V.; Hensel, A.; Liebau, E.; Agyare, C.; et al. Anthelmintic agents from African medicinal plants: Review and prospects. *Evid. Based Complement. Altern. Med.* **2022**, *2022*, 8023866. [CrossRef]
38. Athanasiadou, S.; Githiori, J.; Kyriazakis, I. Medicinal plants for helminth parasite control: Facts and fiction. *Animal* **2007**, *1*, 1392–1400. [CrossRef]
39. Wink, M. Medicinal plants: A source of anti-parasitic secondary metabolites. *Molecules* **2012**, *17*, 12771–12791. [CrossRef]
40. Buza, V.; Cătană, L.; Andrei, S.M.; Ștefănuț, L.C.; Răileanu, Ș.; Matei, M.C.; Vlasiuc, I.; Cernea, M. In vitro anthelmintic activity assessment of six medicinal plant aqueous extracts against donkey strongyles. *J. Helminthol.* **2020**, *94*, e147. [CrossRef]
41. Danquah, C.; Koffuor, G.; Annan, K.; Ketor, E.C. The anthelmintic activity of *Vernonia amygdalina* (asteraceae) and *Alstonia boonei* de wild (apocynaceae). *J. Med. Biomed. Sci.* **2012**, *1*, 21–27.
42. Liu, M.; Panda, S.K.; Luyten, W. Plant-Based Natural Products for the Discovery and Development of Novel Anthelmintics against Nematodes. *Biomolecules* **2020**, *10*, 426. [CrossRef]
43. Sangshetti, J.N.; Shinde, D.B.; Kulkarni, A.; Arote, R. Two decades of antifilarial drug discovery: A review. *RSC Adv.* **2017**, *7*, 20628–20666. [CrossRef]
44. Elufioye, T.O.; Ogunlude, A.T. Nigerian Medicinal Plants with Potential for the Treatment of Neglected Tropical Disease: Onchocerciasis. *Trop. J. Nat. Prod. Res.* **2018**, *2*, 338–348. [CrossRef]
45. Aguoru, C.; Pilla, C.; Olasan, J.O. Phytochemical screening of *Xylopia aethiopica* with emphasis on its medicinally active principles. *J. Med. Plant Res.* **2016**, *10*, 306–309.
46. Bhambhani, S.; Kondhare, K.R.; Giri, A.P. Diversity in Chemical Structures and Biological Properties of Plant Alkaloids. *Molecules* **2021**, *26*, 3374. [CrossRef] [PubMed]
47. Mordvinov, V.A.; Ponomarev, D.V.; Pakharukov, Y.V.; Pakharukova, M.Y. Anthelmintic Activity of Antioxidants: In Vitro Effects on the Liver Fluke *Opisthorchis felineus*. *Pathogens* **2021**, *10*, 284. [CrossRef]
48. Reuter, S.; Beisler, T.; Kern, P. Combined albendazole and amphotericin B against *Echinococcus multilocularis* in vitro. *Acta Trop.* **2010**, *115*, 270–274. [CrossRef]
49. Richter, D.; Richter, J.; Grüner, B.; Kranz, K.; Franz, J.; Kern, P. In vitro efficacy of triclabendazole and clorsulon against the larval stage of *Echinococcus multilocularis*. *Parasitol. Res.* **2013**, *112*, 1655–1660. [CrossRef]
50. Fleischer, T.C.; Mensah, M.L.; Mensah, A.Y.; Komlaga, G.; Gbedema, S.Y.; Skaltsa, H. Antimicrobial activity of essential oils of *Xylopia aethiopica*. *Afr. J. Tradit. Complement. Altern. Med.* **2008**, *5*, 391–393. [CrossRef]
51. Ogwu, M.C.; Dunkwu-Okafor, A.; Omakor, I.A.; Izah, S.C. Medicinal spice, *Aframomum melegueta*: An overview of the phytochemical constituents, nutritional characteristics, and ethnomedicinal values for sustainability. In *Herbal Medicine Phytochemistry*; Izah, S.C., Ogwu, M.C., Akram, M., Eds.; Springer: Cham, Switzerland, 2024; pp. 221–243.

52. Dosso, M.; Soro, D.; Koffi, A.E.; Traore, F.; N'guessan, J.D. Isolement par partition bio guidé du principe actif myostimulant de l'extrait aqueux de *Mareya micrantha* (Benth) Mull. Arg.(Euphorbiaceae). *J. Appl. Biosci.* **2017**, *114*, 11336–11344. [CrossRef]
53. Njouendou, A.J.; Ritter, M.; Kien, C.A.; Esum, M.E.; Ndongmo, W.P.C.; Fombad, F.F.; Gandjui, N.V.T.; Njiokou, F.; Enyong, P.; Pfarr, K.; et al. Dataset on in vitro maintenance of *Mansonella perstans* microfilariae and drug testing. *Data Brief* **2020**, *28*, 104930. [CrossRef]
54. Akter, K.N.; Karmakar, P.; Das, A.; Anonna, S.N.; Shoma, S.A.; Sattar, M.M. Evaluation of antibacterial and anthelmintic activities with total phenolic contents of Piper betel leaves. *Avicenna J. Phytomed.* **2014**, *4*, 320–329.
55. Lalthanpuii, P.B.; Lalchhandama, K. Phytochemical analysis and in vitro anthelmintic activity of *Imperata cylindrica* underground parts. *BMC Complement. Med. Ther.* **2020**, *20*, 332. [CrossRef]

pharmaceuticals

MDPI

Article

Kaempferol Mitigates *Pseudomonas aeruginosa*-Induced Acute Lung Inflammation Through Suppressing GSK3β/JNK/c-Jun Signaling Pathway and NF-κB Activation

Jue Wang [1], Linlin Zhang [2], Lu Fu [3] and Zheng Pang [1,*]

[1] Innovative Institute of Chinese Medicine and Pharmacy, Shandong University of Traditional Chinese Medicine, Jinan 250355, China; wangjue2299@163.com
[2] Institute of Pharmacy, Shandong University of Traditional Chinese Medicine, Jinan 250355, China; linlin66210@outlook.com
[3] School of Medicine, Shandong University of Traditional Chinese Medicine, Jinan 250355, China; 18810550962@163.com
* Correspondence: 60230021@sdutcm.edu.cn; Tel.: +86-531-89628345

Abstract: Background: *Pseudomonas aeruginosa*, one of the common bacterial pathogens causing nosocomial pneumonia, is characterized as highly pathogenic and multidrug-resistant. Kaempferol (KP), a natural flavonoid, has been shown to exhibit effectiveness in treating infection-induced lung injury. **Methods:** We applied network pharmacology to explore the underlying mechanisms of KP in treating *P. aeruginosa* pneumonia and further validated them through a mouse model of acute bacterial lung infection and an in vitro macrophage infection model. **Results:** The in vivo studies demonstrated that treatment with KP suppressed the production of proinflammatory cytokines, including TNF, IL-1β, IL-6, and MIP-2, and attenuated the neutrophil infiltration and lesions in lungs, leading to an increased survival rate of mice. Further studies revealed that KP treatment enhanced the phosphorylation of GSK3β at Ser9 and diminished the phosphorylation of JNK, c-Jun, and NF-κB p65 in lungs in comparison to the mice without drug treatment. Consistently, the in vitro studies showed that pretreatment with KP reduced the activation of GSK3β, JNK, c-Jun, and NF-κB p65 and decreased the levels of the proinflammatory cytokines in macrophages during *P. aeruginosa* infection. **Conclusions:** KP reduced the production of proinflammatory cytokines by inhibiting GSK3β/JNK/c-Jun signaling pathways and NF-κB activation, which effectively mitigated the *P. aeruginosa*-induced acute lung inflammation and injury, and elevated the survival rates of mice.

Keywords: kaempferol; *Pseudomonas aeruginosa*; acute pulmonary inflammation; macrophage; GSK3β; JNK/c-Jun; NF-κB

1. Introduction

Pseudomonas aeruginosa, an opportunistic pathogen, tends to cause serious infections in immunocompromised patients. It has become one of the most predominant pathogens causing hospital-acquired infections globally, accounting for 23% of intensive care unit-acquired infections and 26% of ventilator-associated pneumonia cases [1]. The multiple virulence factors of *P. aeruginosa* facilitate its colonization of the respiratory tract and induce host cells to produce inflammatory mediators, which is accompanied by inflammatory cell infiltration, increased alveolar-capillary permeability, and lung epithelial barrier disruption [2,3]. Furthermore, this bacterium can interfere with intracellular signaling pathways and disrupt cell membrane integrity by injecting virulence effectors into the cells and secreting enzymes and toxins that disrupt cell junctions, leading to apoptosis and necrosis [1]. In addition, the Toll-like receptors (TLRs) of the host immune cells recognize the pathogen-associated molecular patterns (PAMPs) of *P. aeruginosa*, initiating multiple signaling pathways that promote the release of inflammatory mediators, which in turn attract inflammatory cells and further upregulate the inflammation level in lungs [4]. Currently, antibiotic therapy remains the major tool for treating *P. aeruginosa* pneumonia [5,6]. However, the antibiotic resistance of *P. aeruginosa* is a severe issue, and it shows increasing resistance to many commonly used antibiotics [7]. It has been found that *P. aeruginosa* is capable of forming biofilms, which not only physically shield the bacteria from antibiotic penetration but also enable the bacteria to develop resistance mutations in this state, resulting in a major therapeutic challenge [8]. In addition, the efflux pumps of *P. aeruginosa* reduce antibiotic susceptibility by expelling the antibiotics out of bacterial cells, leading to the development of multidrug resistance, and it promotes the formation of biofilm, which makes the bacteria more difficult to eradicate [9]. Antibiotic abuse has resulted in the emergence of multidrug-resistant *P. aeruginosa* strains. Statistically, 23–46% of *P. aeruginosa* infections that cause pneumonia in intensive care units are multidrug-resistant [10]. Consequently, there is an urgent need to find new alternative agents to treat the infections caused by multidrug-resistant *P. aeruginosa* [7]. Natural bioactive compounds have been shown to have excellent pharmacological activities both in preventing the infection of *P. aeruginosa* and modulating the host immune response [11]. Additionally, natural flavonoid compounds have been shown to treat acute lung injury by activating antioxidant pathways and inhibiting inflammatory pathways [12].

Kaempferol (KP), a dietary flavonoid widely distributed in the plant kingdom, exerts anti-inflammatory, antioxidant, antibacterial, anticancer, neuroprotective, and hepatoprotective effects [13–16]. Previous studies have reported that KP can reduce intestinal inflammation [17], airway inflammation [18], and neuroinflammation [19,20]; ameliorate inflammatory bone disease [21]; and protect blood vessels from inflammatory injury [22], demonstrating the broad anti-inflammatory effects of KP. In particular, KP was identified to attenuate the lipopolysaccharide (LPS)- or virus-induced lung injury by inhibiting MAPK and NF-κB signaling pathways [23–25]. Additionally, KP has been found to inhibit a variety of pathogenic bacteria [26,27]. A previous study found that KP reduced the *Staphylococcus aureus*-induced pneumonia by attenuating the production of virulence factors [28]. In addition, many KP-containing herbs have exhibited antimicrobial activity against *P. aeruginosa* [27]. However, the efficacy of KP on *P. aeruginosa*-induced acute pneumonia and the underlying mechanisms have not yet been elucidated.

This research utilized network pharmacology to predict the therapeutic mechanisms of KP in treating P. aeruginosa pneumonia. Glycogen synthase kinase 3 beta (GSK3β) was one of the key targets in the protein–protein interaction (PPI) network, and it has been revealed to exert a crucial function in modulating the activity of inflammation-related proteins [29, 30]. Previous studies have shown that the activity of GSK3β was significantly enhanced in the P. aeruginosa-induced keratitis and the inhibition of its activity could downregulate the corneal inflammation [31]. The alteration of GSK3β activity has been found to act on its downstream targets, JNK, c-Jun, and NF-κB, to regulate inflammatory responses [30,32]. Moreover, JNK, c-Jun, and NF-κB p65 were also the key targets identified in the PPI network, and JNK, c-Jun, and NF-κB were identified to regulate the lung inflammation induced by P. aeruginosa infection [33–35]. In addition, the data of molecular docking suggested that KP exhibited high binding affinities with the protein targets, including GSK3β, JNK1, and NF-κB p65. Therefore, we hypothesized that KP mitigates P. aeruginosa pneumonia by inhibiting GSK3β/JNK/c-Jun and NF-κB signaling pathways. To validate it, we employed a murine model of P. aeruginosa pneumonia. The results indicated that treatment with KP dampened the P. aeruginosa-induced lung damage by reducing the production of

TNF, IL-1β, IL-6, and macrophage inflammatory protein (MIP)-2, and impairing neutrophil infiltration, thus leading to a reduced mortality rate of mice. Moreover, the phosphorylation of GSK3β (Ser9) was increased, whereas the phosphorylation of JNK, c-Jun, and NF-κB p65 was decreased in the lung tissues of the P. aeruginosa-infected mice after KP treatment. Alveolar macrophage is one of the major contributors to the inflammatory cytokine storm in patients with bacterial pneumonia [36]. In addition, macrophages play an important role in host defense against P. aeruginosa infection by recognizing bacterial molecules and activating the inflammatory response [37]. Therefore, we used macrophages to study the in vitro efficacy of KP against P. aeruginosa infection. Similarly, pretreatment with KP resulted in reduced proinflammatory cytokine production; impaired phosphorylation of JNK, c-Jun, and NF-κB p65; and upregulated the phosphorylation of GSK3β at Ser9 in the P. aeruginosa-infected macrophages. Overall, these findings revealed that KP was a potential therapeutic agent for combating acute P. aeruginosa pneumonia, which could alleviate the lung inflammation through suppressing GSK3β/JNK/c-Jun signaling pathway and NF-κB activation.

2. Results

2.1. Network Pharmacology-Based Prediction of the Mechanisms of KP in the Treatment of P. aeruginosa Pneumonia

Seventy-four overlapping targets were identified between KP and *P. aeruginosa* pulmonary infection, which were regarded as the potential targets of KP in treating *P. aeruginosa* pneumonia (Figure 1A). The interactions at the protein level of the potential targets were obtained by the PPI network (Figure 1B). The top 25 targets in Figure 1B were shown in Table 1 with degree values. The larger size and darker coloration of the target signify a higher degree of centrality, indicating a more important role as a core protein in binding to other proteins. Among the core targets, TNF, EGFR, AKT1, MMP9, JUN, PTGS2, PPARG, GSK3B, ICAM1, HMOX1, RELA, and MAPK8 have been found to play essential roles in the *P. aeruginosa*-induced inflammatory response [31,38–44]. Moreover, 461 Gene Ontology (GO) terms, including 331 biological process (BP), 48 cellular component (CC), and 82 molecular function (MF) terms were obtained, and the top 20 items were displayed according to their *p*-values (Figure 1C–E). The size of the bubbles in the graph was correlated with the number of targets involved in each term, and the color was correlated with the *p*-value. The predominant processes of BP included the negative regulation of the apoptotic process, the response to xenobiotic stimulus, protein autophosphorylation, inflammatory response, the negative regulation of gene expression, and the response to hypoxia (Figure 1C). The CC clusters predominantly included the nucleus, plasma membrane, cytosol, membrane raft, extracellular exosome, extracellular space, and perinuclear region of the cytoplasm (Figure 1D). The MF clusters mainly involved functions such as protein binding, enzyme binding, protein serine/threonine/tyrosine kinase activity, and protein kinase activity and binding (Figure 1E). These data suggested that KP might regulate the inflammatory response to *P. aeruginosa* infection by influencing the protein binding and activity in the cell membrane, cytoplasm, and nucleus. Furthermore, 123 Kyoto Encyclopedia of Genes and Genomes (KEGG) terms were identified, and the top 20 terms ranked according to the number of involved targets were shown in Figure 1F. The top 20 KEGG enriched pathways sorted by *p*-value were listed in Table 2. In particular, the IL-17, TNF, MAPK, and PI3K-AKT signaling pathways have been found to promote the *P. aeruginosa*-induced lung inflammation [33–35,44]. These findings suggested that the regulation of the inflammatory response could be the possible mechanism of KP in treating *P. aeruginosa* pneumonia.

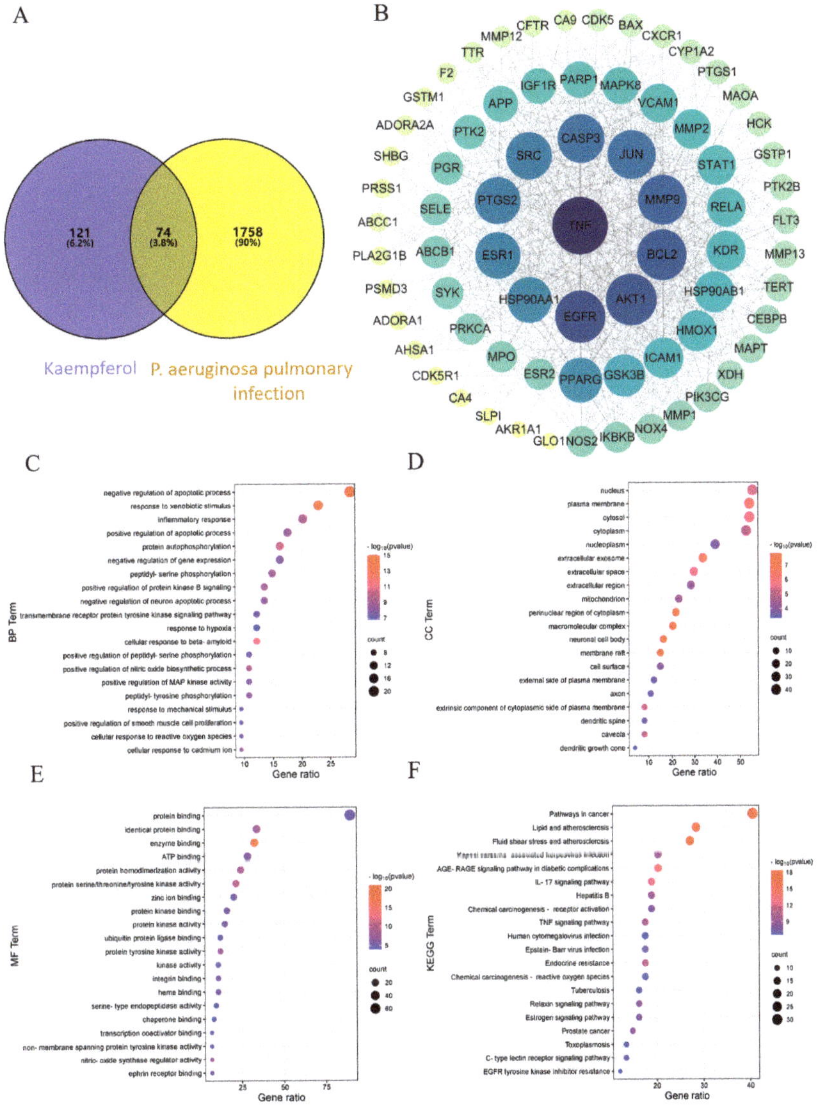

Figure 1. Prediction of the mechanisms of KP in treating *P. aeruginosa* pneumonia by network pharmacology. A total of 121 KP targets and 1758 *P. aeruginosa* pulmonary infection-related targets were collected, and 74 potential targets of KP-*P. aeruginosa* pulmonary infection were obtained by establishing a Venn diagram (**A**). The gray edges in the PPI network represented the potential connections between the targets, while the size and color depth of a node corresponding to the target were positively correlated with the degree of association with other targets (**B**). Gene Ontology (GO) enrichment included biological process (BP) (**C**), cellular component (CC) (**D**), and molecular function (MF) (**E**). Kyoto Encyclopedia of Genes and Genomes (KEGG) enrichment analysis was utilized to obtain the KP-regulated signaling pathways (**F**). Data were displayed as bubble charts. The vertical axis represented the GO or KEGG pathway items, and the horizontal axis represented the number of target genes in each item. The size of the bubble represented the percentage. The colors of the bubbles were correlated with their p-values.

Table 1. The top 25 targets of KP on *P. aeruginosa* pulmonary infection in the PPI network.

Number	UniProt ID	Target Name	Degree
1	P01375	TNF	60
2	P00533	EGFR	52
3	P31749	AKT1	51
4	P10415	BCL2	50
5	P14780	MMP9	49
6	P05412	JUN	47
7	P42574	CASP3	47
8	P12931	SRC	45
9	P35354	PTGS2	45
10	P03372	ESR1	44
11	P07900	HSP90AA1	43
12	P37231	PPARG	42
13	P49841	GSK3B	38
14	P05362	ICAM1	36
15	P09601	HMOX1	36
16	P08238	HSP90AB1	36
17	P35968	KDR	35
18	Q04206	RELA	34
19	P42224	STAT1	34
20	P08253	MMP2	34
21	P19320	VCAM1	33
22	P45983	MAPK8	31
23	P09874	PARP1	30
24	P05067	APP	29
25	P08069	IGF1R	29

Table 2. The top 20 KEGG-enriched pathways sorted by *p*-value.

ID	Description	Gene Ratio	*p*-Value	Count
hsa05200	Pathways in cancer	40.54	4.91×10^{-18}	30
hsa05417	Lipid and atherosclerosis	28.38	9.89×10^{-17}	21
hsa05418	Fluid shear stress and atherosclerosis	27.03	4.22×10^{-19}	20
hsa05022	Pathways of neurodegeneration—multiple diseases	21.62	3.28×10^{-6}	16
hsa04933	AGE-RAGE signaling pathway in diabetic complications	20.27	2.37×10^{-14}	15
hsa05167	Kaposi sarcoma-associated herpesvirus infection	20.27	2.33×10^{-10}	15
hsa04151	PI3K-Akt signaling pathway	20.27	5.04×10^{-7}	15
hsa05010	Alzheimer disease	20.27	1.34×10^{-6}	15
hsa04657	IL-17 signaling pathway	18.92	2.58×10^{-13}	14
hsa05161	Hepatitis B	18.92	2.96×10^{-10}	14
hsa05207	Chemical carcinogenesis—receptor activation	18.92	8.13×10^{-9}	14
hsa01522	Endocrine resistance	17.57	1.03×10^{-11}	13
hsa04668	TNF signaling pathway	17.57	6.37×10^{-11}	13
hsa05169	Epstein–Barr virus infection	17.57	4.67×10^{-8}	13
hsa05208	Chemical carcinogenesis—reactive oxygen species	17.57	1.39×10^{-7}	13
hsa05163	Human cytomegalovirus infection	17.57	1.53×10^{-7}	13
hsa04010	MAPK signaling pathway	17.57	3.53×10^{-6}	13
hsa04926	Relaxin signaling pathway	16.22	4.17×10^{-9}	12
hsa04915	Estrogen signaling pathway	16.22	8.54×10^{-9}	12
hsa05152	Tuberculosis	16.22	1.35×10^{-7}	12

2.2. KP Reduces the Mortality but Has a Limited Effect on Bacterial Clearance in the Lungs of Mice

A survival study was conducted to evaluate the therapeutic effects of KP on *P. aeruginosa*-induced acute pneumonia (Figure 2A). The results showed that the survival rates of the mice of kaempferol low-dose (KPL) (20%) and kaempferol high-dose (KPH) (60%) groups were both higher than that of the mice of the Saline group (10%). Moreover, the survival rate of the mice in the KPH group was higher than that in the dexamethasone (Dex) group (40%), demonstrating a better therapeutic effect of KPH than Dex. Consistently, the disease scores of the mice from the KP-treated groups were lower than those of the mice of the Saline group (Figure 2B). These results indicate that KP ameliorated the disease status of the *P. aeruginosa* lung-infected mice and decreased their mortality, suggesting the therapeutic and protective effects of KP on *P. aeruginosa*-induced acute pneumonia. To further explore the in vivo inhibitory effect of KP on *P. aeruginosa*, the bacterial burden in bronchoalveolar lavage fluid (BALF) and lung tissues was examined (Figure 2C,D). The data revealed that the number of bacteria in the BALF and lungs was reduced in the KP-treated groups in comparison to the Saline group but did not attain statistical significance. This indicated that KP exerted a limited effect on bacterial clearance in vivo, and the increased survival rate of the KP-treated mice might be attributed to the alleviated inflammatory response in the lungs.

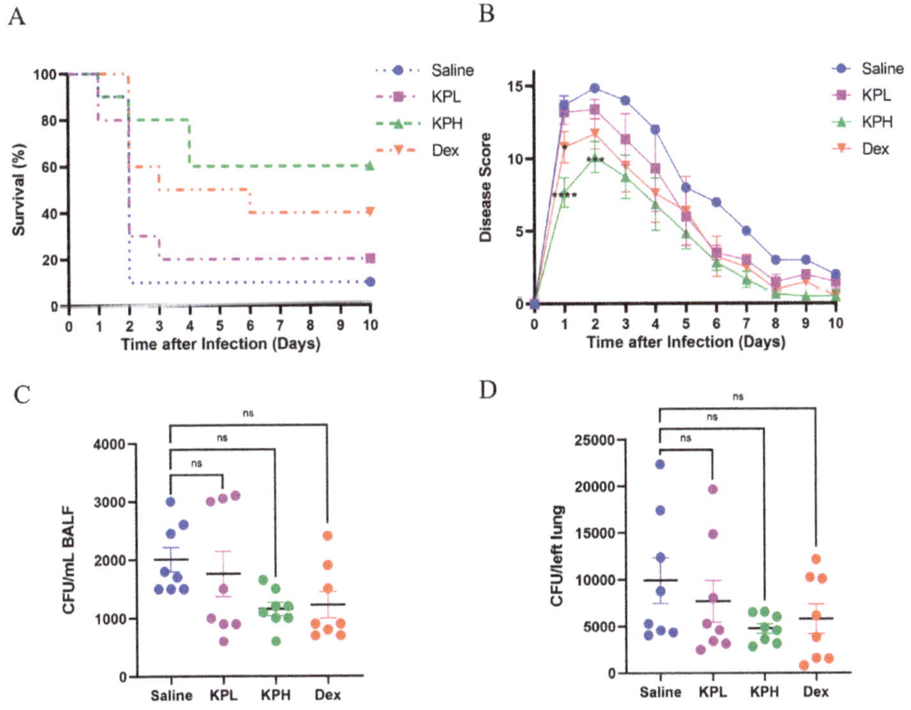

Figure 2. Treatment with KP enhances survival rates but has a limited impact on the bacterial clearance in the lungs during acute *P. aeruginosa* lung infection. The mice from each group were administered 1×10^9 colony-forming unit (CFU)/mouse of PAO1 intranasally for the survival study. The survival rates (**A**) and disease scores (**B**) were recorded daily for 10 days after infection (data are expressed as mean ± standard error of the mean (SEM); $n = 10$; * $p < 0.05$, *** $p < 0.001$, **** $p < 0.0001$). For analyzing bacterial burden, the mice were treated with 5×10^8 CFU of PAO1 per mouse intranasally, and the CFU number in bronchoalveolar lavage fluid (BALF) (**C**) and the lungs (**D**) were analyzed after 24 h of infection (data are expressed as mean ± SEM; $n = 8$; ns: non-significant).

2.3. *KP Dampens the P. aeruginosa-Induced Acute Lung Injury and Impairs Neutrophil Recruitment*

Hematoxylin and eosin (H&E) staining was applied to assess the influence of KP on the *P. aeruginosa*-induced lung injury. The images displayed that the mice in the Saline group had serious lung tissue lesions with obvious alveolar collapse and alveolar septal thickening associated with the infiltration of a large number of inflammatory cells. By contrast, the lesions were significantly attenuated in the KP-treated groups (Figure 3A). Furthermore, the KP-treated group had lower histological scores of lung injury compared with those of the Saline group (Figure 3B). Neutrophil recruitment is one of the important characteristics of acute *P. aeruginosa* pneumonia, and the excessive infiltration of neutrophils can cause severe damage in lung tissue [34]. Myeloperoxidase (MPO), a heme-containing peroxidase predominately produced in neutrophils, is commonly used as a biomarker for quantitatively assessing the number of infiltrated neutrophils. The data showed that the MPO activity was significantly increased in both the lung tissues and BALF of mice upon *P. aeruginosa* lung infection. However, the MPO activity of BALF and lungs was observably decreased in the KP-treated mice in a dose-dependent manner (Figure 3C,D). The excessive inflammatory response in the lungs can lead to a cytokine storm characterized by a significant increase in cytokines, such as TNFα, IL-6, IL-1β, and IFNγ, and increase vascular permeability, which causes blood proteins to leak into the alveoli [45,46]. The total protein concentration of BALF and lung tissues was measured by bicinchoninic acid (BCA) assay, and the results showed that KP treatment was able to dose-dependently reduce the protein concentrations of the BALF and lung tissues in mice after infection (Figure 3E,F). These findings suggested that treatment with KP ameliorated histopathological changes, impaired neutrophil infiltration, and reduced pulmonary vascular permeability during *P. aeruginosa* lung infection.

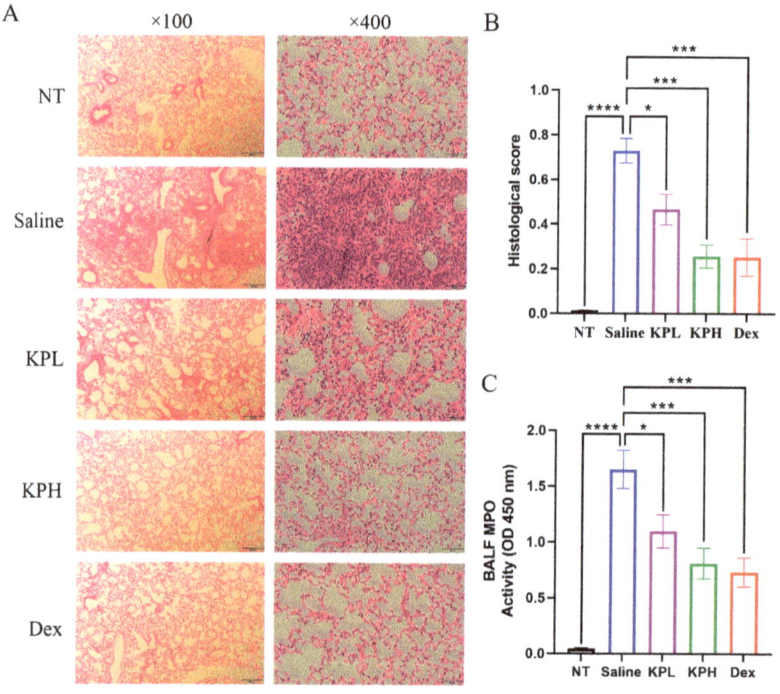

Figure 3. *Cont.*

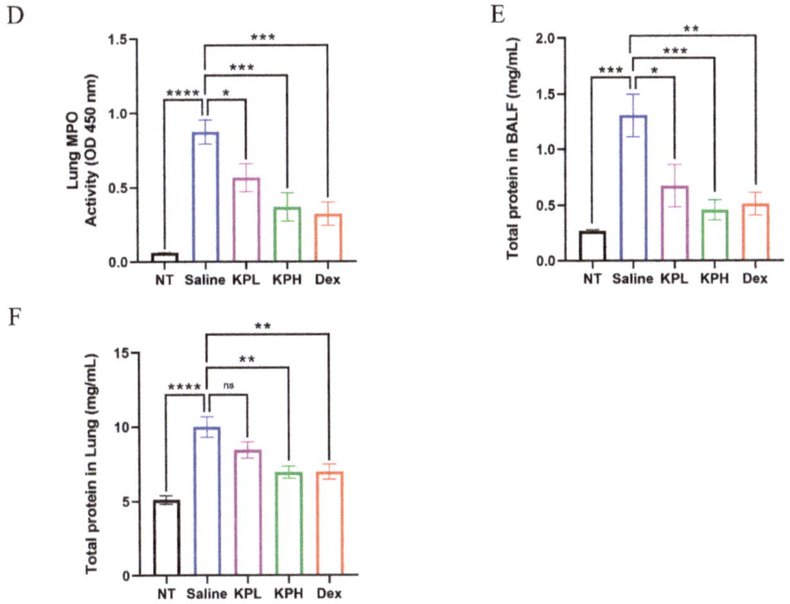

Figure 3. KP ameliorates the *P. aeruginosa*-induced acute lung injury, reduces neutrophil infiltration, and decreases pulmonary vascular permeability. The mice from the Saline, kaempferol low-dose (KPL), kaempferol high-dose (KPH), and dexamethasone (Dex) groups were intranasally administered with 5×10^8 CFU/mouse of PAO1 for 24 h, whereas the mice from the uninfected (NT) group received a mock infection with saline. The post-caval lobes of the lungs were subjected to hematoxylin and eosin (H&E) staining, and imaged at magnifications of 100× and 400× (**A**). The histological score of lung injury was evaluated in each mouse (**B**) (data are expressed as mean ± SEM; $n = 6$; * $p < 0.05$, *** $p < 0.001$, **** $p < 0.0001$). The myeloperoxidase (MPO) activity was examined in the BALF (**C**) and lung (**D**) lysates. The total protein content of BALF (**E**) and left lung (**F**) was detected by bicinchoninic acid (BCA) assay (data are expressed as mean ± SEM; $n = 8$; * $p < 0.05$, ** $p < 0.01$, *** $p < 0.001$, **** $p < 0.0001$, ns: non-significant).

2.4. KP Inhibits the P. aeruginosa-Induced Proinflammatory Cytokine Production in Lungs

In response to infections, the host body produces proinflammatory cytokines to activate and modulate the immune response. However, the overproduction of cytokines leads to excessive inflammation and damage to tissues [45]. The levels of cytokines, TNF, IL-1β and IL-6, and chemokine MIP-2 in lungs were previously reported to be upregulated after *P. aeruginosa* infection [47]. We examined the levels of TNF, IL-1β, IL-6, and MIP-2 in the BALF and lung tissues of mice by enzyme-linked immunosorbent assay (ELISA) (Figure 4). The results showed that the levels of TNF, IL-1β, IL-6, and MIP-2 were significantly elevated in both the BALF and lung tissues of mice after *P. aeruginosa* lung infection, while KP treatment reduced the levels of these cytokines in a dose-dependent manner. To exclude the confounding factors caused by KP, the effects of KP on cytokine production in uninfected mice were examined, and we found that the levels of TNF, IL-1β, IL-6, and MIP-2 in the lungs of KP groups were not significantly different from those of Saline group (Figure S1). Our data showed that KP exhibited an inhibitory effect on the *P. aeruginosa*-induced pneumonia in vivo.

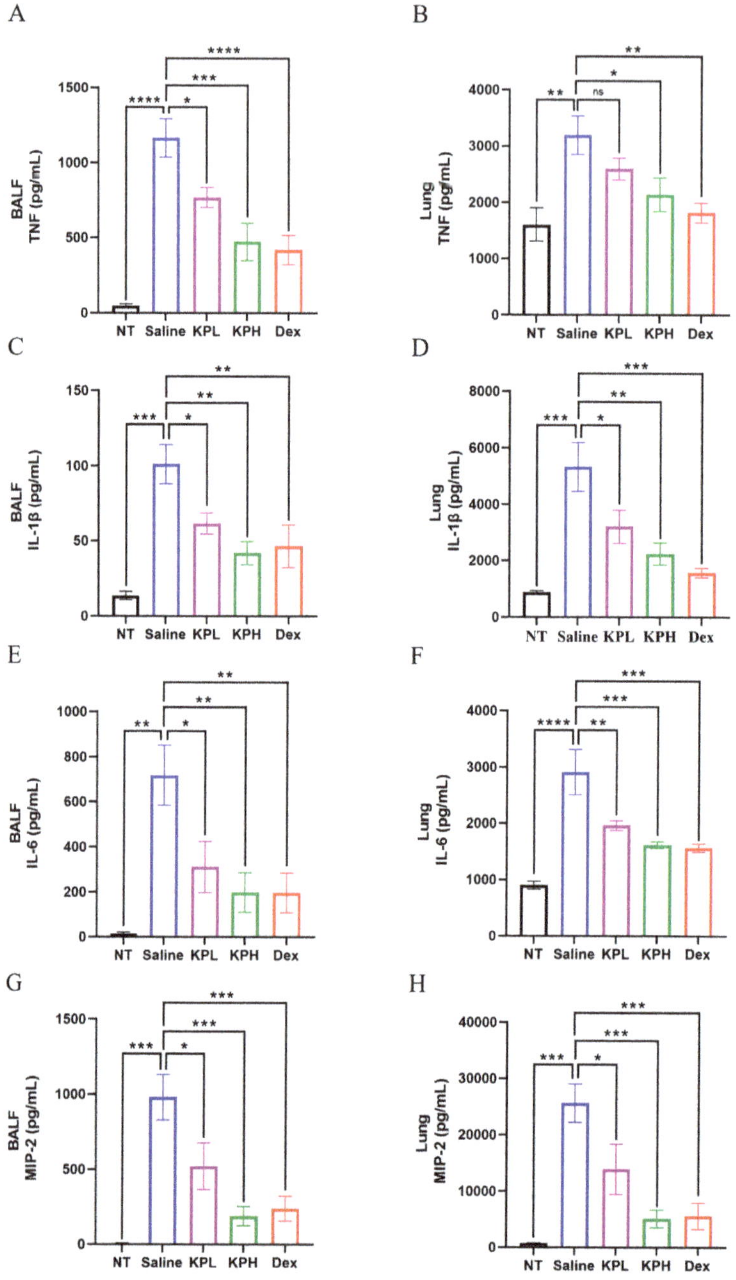

Figure 4. KP inhibits the production of proinflammatory cytokine in the lungs during *P. aeruginosa* acute pulmonary infection. The mice in the Saline, KPL, KPH, and Dex groups were given 5×10^8 CFU of PAO1 per mouse through intranasal infection for 24 h, whereas the mice in the NT group were received a mock infection with saline. The levels of TNF (**A**,**B**), IL-1β (**C**,**D**), IL-6 (**E**,**F**), and macrophage inflammatory protein (MIP)-2 (**G**,**H**) in the BALF and lung tissues of the mice were determined by ELISA (Data are expressed as mean ± SEM; $n = 8$; * $p < 0.05$, ** $p < 0.01$, *** $p < 0.001$, **** $p < 0.0001$, ns: non-significant).

2.5. Binding Activity of KP with GSK3β, JNK1, c-Jun, and NF-κB p65

GSK3β (GSK3B) and its downstream proteins, JNK1 (MAPK8), c-Jun (JUN), and NF-κB p65 (RELA) were identified through network pharmacology screening and molecularly docked with KP to further predict the ability of KP to interact with these targets (Figure 5). Table 3 demonstrated the binding energies of KP to the core target proteins, GSK3β, JNK1, c-Jun, and NF-κB p65. The smaller value of the binding energy indicates that easier intermolecular binding occurs, and it is widely accepted that the high binding affinity between drugs and protein molecules occurs when the binding energy is below −5 kcal/mol [34,35]. The docking results showed a good binding affinity of KP with GSK3β (−5.44 kcal/mol), JNK1 (−5.03 kcal/mol), and NF-κB p65 (−5.56 kcal/mol). This finding implied that KP might regulate the inflammatory response by affecting the binding capacity of these proteins or modulating their activation levels.

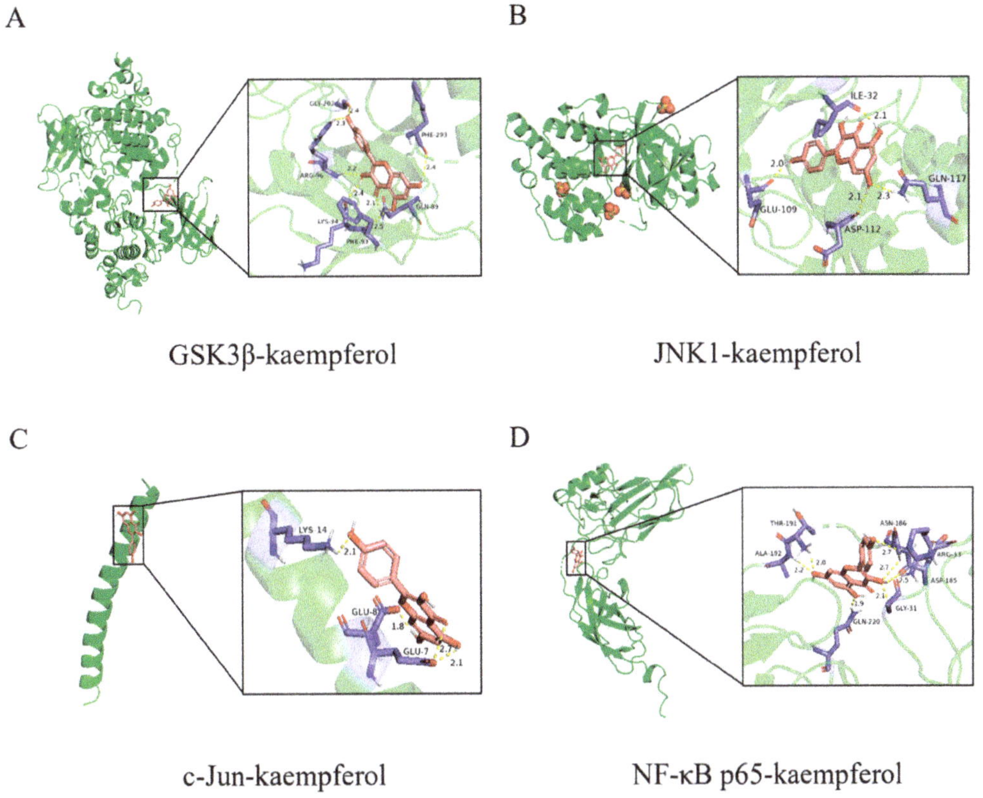

Figure 5. Molecular docking of KP with target proteins. KP was docked with glycogen synthase kinase 3 beta (GSK3β) (**A**), JNK1 (**B**), c-Jun (**C**), and NF-κB p65 (**D**), and the data were visualized using PyMOL 2.4.0.

Table 3. The molecular docking of KP with target proteins.

Target Name	PDB ID	Protein	Binding Energy (kcal/mol)
GSK3B	1Q5K	GSK3β	−5.44
MAPK8	3PZE	JNK1	−5.03
JUN	5FV8	c-Jun	−4.18
RELA	1IKN	NF-κB p65	−5.56

2.6. KP Suppresses GSK3β/JNK/c-Jun Signaling Pathway and NF-κB Activation In Vivo

GSK3β is active under basal conditions and inactivated by phosphorylation at Ser9 [30]. The PAMPs from pathogens are recognized by TLRs and increase the activity of GSK3β [48,49]. Furthermore, the increased activity of GSK3β aggravates inflammatory response, whereas GSK3β inhibition has been proven to alleviate lung injury [29,50,51]. GSK3β activates JNK by phosphorylating MEKK1 [52] and increases IκB degradation and NF-κB activation by regulating IκB kinase [53]. In addition, previous studies showed that GSK3β can also directly phosphorylate NF-κB p65 [54]. To assess the effect of KP on the GSK3β/JNK/c-Jun and NF-κB signaling pathways in vivo, the expression or phosphorylation levels of GSK3β, JNK, c-Jun, and NF-κB p65 in the lungs were examined (Figure 6 and Figure S2). The results showed that neither *P. aeruginosa* infection nor drug treatment significantly affected the mRNA transcription and protein expression of GSK3β, JNK, c-Jun, and NF-κB p65. Upon *P. aeruginosa* lung infection, the phosphorylation levels of JNK, c-Jun and NF-κB p65 were significantly increased, while the phosphorylation of GSK3β at Ser9 was decreased. Furthermore, the phosphorylation of JNK, c-Jun and NF-κB p65 was downregulated, whereas the phosphorylation level of GSK3β at the Ser9 was significantly increased in the KP-treated groups compared with the Saline group. These results suggested that KP inhibited the GSK3β/JNK/c-Jun signaling pathway and NF-κB activation in treating the *P. aeruginosa*-induced acute pneumonia.

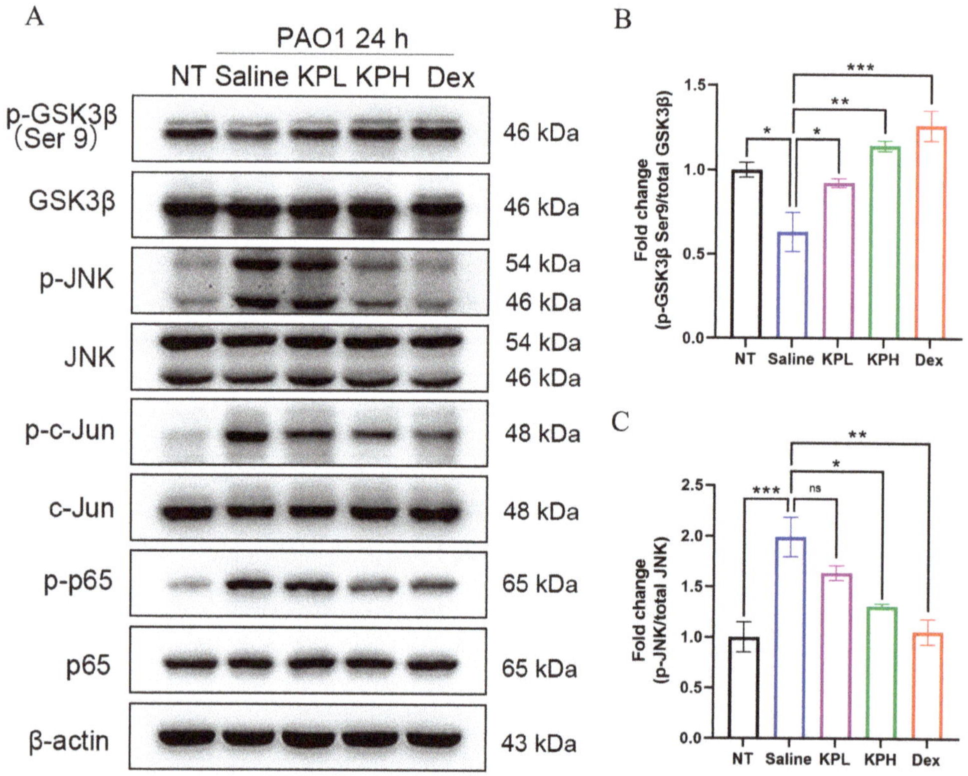

Figure 6. *Cont.*

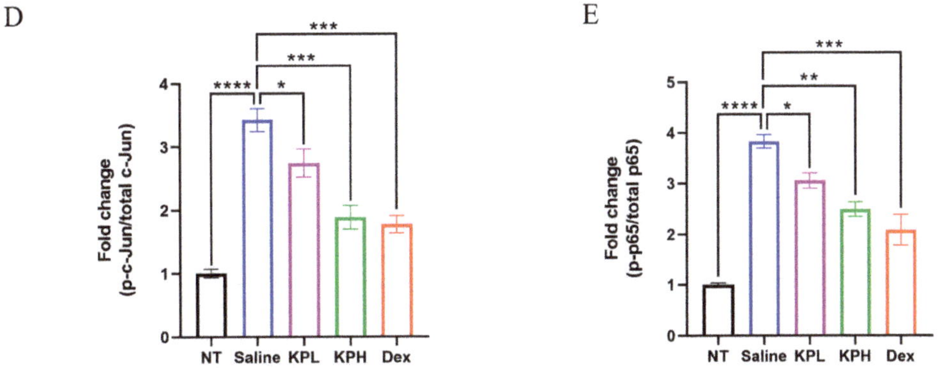

Figure 6. KP inhibits the activation of GSK3β, JNK, c-Jun, and NF-κB p65 in the lungs of mice infected with *P. aeruginosa*. The phosphorylation of GSK3β (Ser9), JNK, c-Jun, and NF-κB p65 in the lung lysates of the mice from the NT, Saline, KPL, KPH, and Dex groups was examined by Western blot analysis (**A**). Densitometry analysis of the phosphorylated GSK3β (Ser9) (**B**), JNK (**C**), c-Jun (**D**), and NF-κB (**E**) was normalized to their total proteins (data are expressed as mean ± SEM; $n = 3$; * $p < 0.05$, ** $p < 0.01$, *** $p < 0.001$, **** $p < 0.0001$, ns: non-significant). β-actin was applied as the loading control.

2.7. KP Reduces the Expression of Proinflammatory Cytokines in Macrophages During P. aeruginosa Infection

Macrophages, the sentinel cells in the lungs, regulate the inflammatory response by recognizing bacteria and secreting inflammatory mediators [37]. Mouse bone marrow-derived macrophages (BMDMs) were used for further in vitro experiments. No significant cytotoxic effect was found across a range of KP concentrations (25, 50, 100, and 120 μM) compared to the blank control group (Figure 7A). The levels of proinflammatory cytokines including TNF, IL-1β, IL-6, and MIP-2 were measured in the cell-free supernatants of the *P. aeruginosa*-infected BMDMs at 3 h post-infection (Figure 7B–E). The results showed that the *P. aeruginosa* significantly induced the production of these cytokines, which were decreased dose-dependently in the cells pretreated with KP at different concentrations (25, 50, and 100 μM). In addition, we conducted a time-course experiment to assess the duration of the effect of KP on cytokine production. The results showed that KP exhibited an inhibitory effect on the production of TNF, IL-1β, IL-6, and MIP-2 in the *P. aeruginosa*-infected BMDMs at 3, 6, and 12 h (Figure 7F–I). It suggested that KP diminished the expression of proinflammatory cytokines in BMDMs during *P. aeruginosa* infection in vitro.

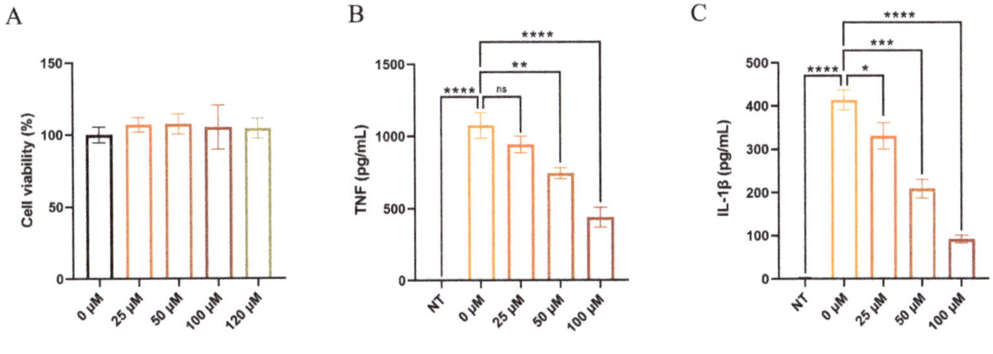

Figure 7. *Cont.*

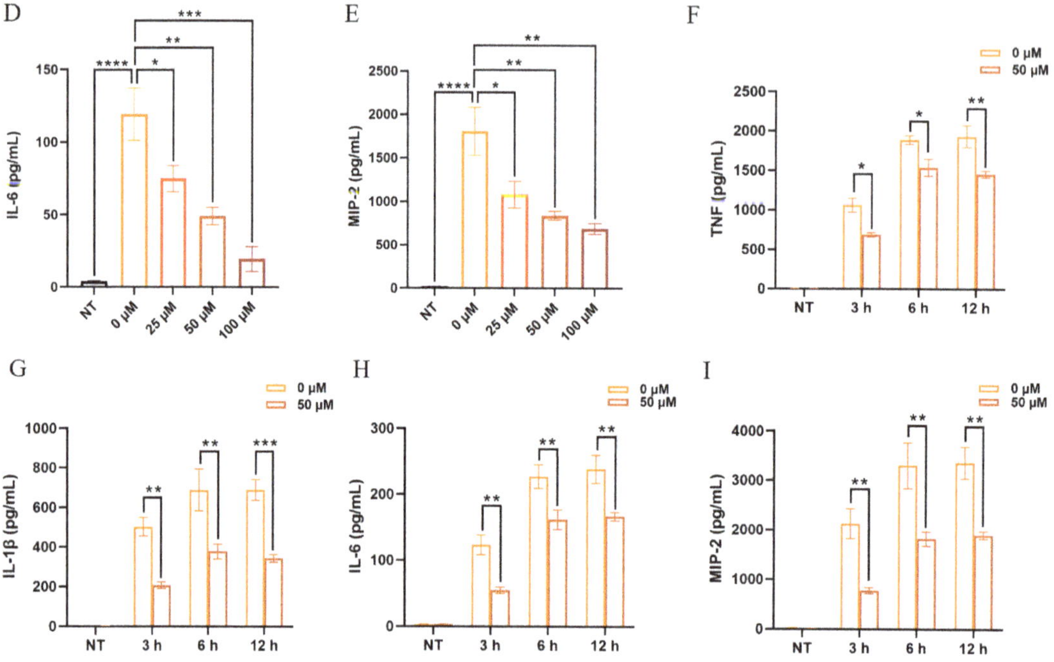

Figure 7. Pretreatment with KP reduces the proinflammatory cytokine production in macrophages upon *P. aeruginosa* infection. The cell viability of KP- (25, 50, 100, and 120 μM) or mock-treated mouse bone-marrow-derived macrophages (BMDMs) was detected with a CCK-8 kit (**A**) (Data are expressed as mean ± SEM; $n = 4$). BMDMs were pretreated with KP (0, 25, 50, and 100 μM) for 1 h and then infected with PAO1 or mock-infected (NT) for 3 h. The levels of TNF (**B**), IL-1β (**C**), IL-6 (**D**), and MIP-2 (**E**) in the cell-free supernatants were determined by enzyme-linked immunosorbent assay (ELISA). For time-course experiments, BMDMs were pretreated with 50 μM KP or PBS (0 μM) for 1 h and then infected with PAO1 for 3 h, 6 h and 12 h. The levels of TNF (**F**), IL-1β (**G**), IL-6 (**H**), and MIP-2 (**I**) were determined in cell-free supernatants. (Data are expressed as mean ± SEM; $n = 3$; * $p < 0.05$, ** $p < 0.01$, *** $p < 0.001$, **** $p < 0.0001$, ns: non-significant).

2.8. KP Inhibits the Activation of GSK3β, JNK, c-Jun, and NF-κB in Macrophages During *P. aeruginosa* Infection

To investigate the impact of KP on GSK3β/JNK/c-Jun and NF-κB signaling pathways in macrophages, the expression and phosphorylation levels of GSK3β, JNK, c-Jun, and NF-κB p65 were analyzed in the KP-pretreated BMDMs upon *P. aeruginosa* infection (Figure 8 and Figure S3). The results showed that *P. aeruginosa* infection did not significantly affect the mRNA transcription and protein expression of GSK3β, JNK, and NF-κB p65 but significantly increased the activation of these proteins. Interestingly, *P. aeruginosa* infection elevated the mRNA and protein expression levels of c-Jun in BMDMs and increased its phosphorylation as well. Furthermore, KP dose-dependently increased the phosphorylation of GSK3β at Ser9 and decreased the phosphorylation of JNK, c-Jun, and NF-κB p65. Those results were consistent with the in vivo results, indicating that KP could attenuate GSK3β/JNK/c-Jun signaling pathway and NF-κB activation in BMDMs during *P. aeruginosa* infection.

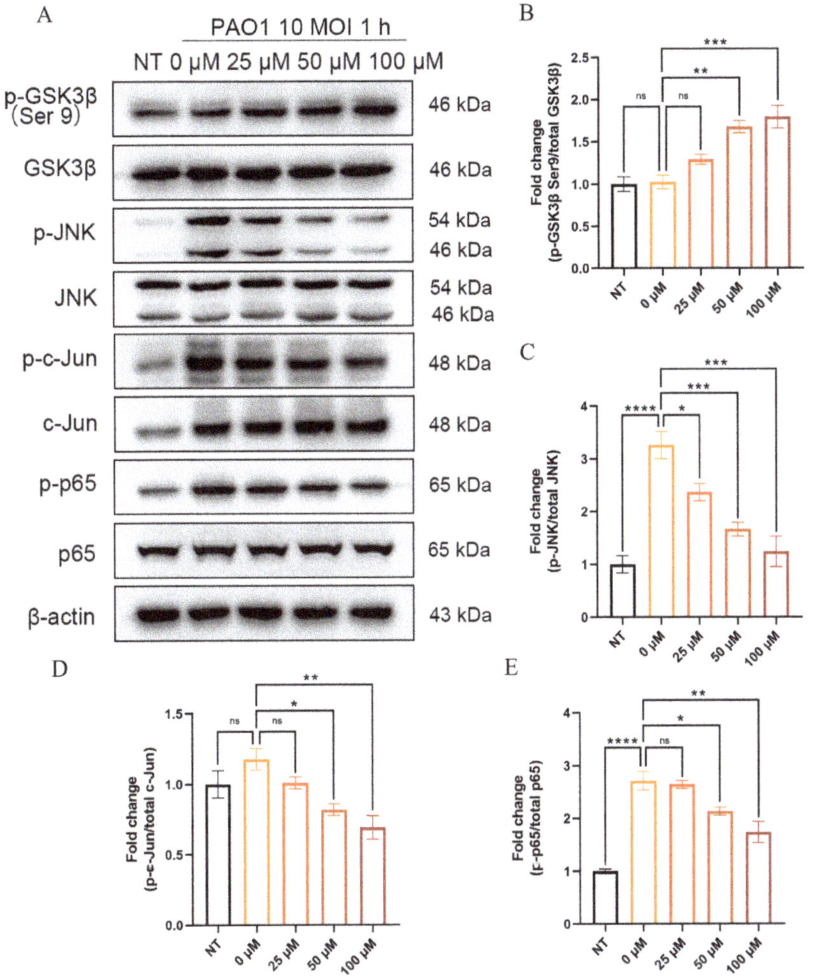

Figure 8. KP diminishes the activation of GSK3β, JNK, c-Jun, and NF-κB p65 in macrophages during *P. aeruginosa* infection. BMDMs were pretreated with KP (0, 25, 50, and 100 μM) for 1 h and then infected with PAO1 or mock-infected (NT) for 1 h. The phosphorylation of GSK3β (Ser9), JNK, c-Jun, and NF-κB p65 in BMDMs was examined by Western blot analysis (**A**). The densitometry analysis of the phosphorylated GSK3β (**B**), JNK (**C**), c-Jun (**D**), and NF-κB p65 (**E**) was normalized to their total proteins (data are expressed as mean ± SEM; $n = 3$; * $p < 0.05$, ** $p < 0.01$, *** $p < 0.001$, **** $p < 0.0001$, ns: non-significant). β-actin was applied as the loading control.

3. Discussion

Pseudomonas aeruginosa commonly causes nosocomial infections, and the mortality of ventilator-associated pneumonia induced by *P. aeruginosa* infection is 32–42.8% [1]. The lung infection caused by this bacterium activates many inflammatory pathways, which can cause severe lung damage [2]. Furthermore, *P. aeruginosa* utilizes endogenous and acquired resistance mechanisms against most antibiotics, which makes the treatment much more difficult [7]. There is an urgent need to develop novel antibiotics and find alternative therapeutic strategies.

Natural bioactive compounds have displayed promising potential in combating *P. aeruginosa* infections and can be used as alternative or complementary drugs to conventional antibiotics [11]. Flavonoids are plant secondary metabolites that have been found to possess antimicrobial and anti-inflammatory activities [55,56]. In addition, some flavonoids have shown considerable efficacy in treating the *P. aeruginosa*-induced lung injury [35,57,58]. For example, quercetin effectively reduced the expression of the *P. aeruginosa*-induced proinflammatory cytokines by repressing NF-κB pathway in H292 cells [58], and it has been demonstrated to mitigate *P. aeruginosa* pneumonia in mice by modulating the PI3K/AKT/NF-κB signaling pathway [35]. Baicalin was identified to alleviate acute pneumonia induced by multidrug-resistant *P. aeruginosa* by inhibiting the TLR4/NF-κB pathway [57]. KP belongs to the flavonoid family and is a safe and effective natural dietary compound with anti-inflammatory and antimicrobial properties [13]. The effects of KP on treating the *P. aeruginosa*-induced acute pneumonia and the underlying mechanisms are unknown.

This research first utilized network pharmacology to study the underlying mechanisms of KP in treating *P. aeruginosa* pneumonia. The results showed that TNF was located in the center of the PPI network, and JUN, GSK3B, RELA, and MAPK8 were listed in the top 25 core targets. KP was previously reported to function as an inhibitor of GSK3β [59], which is regarded as a central regulator of the immune response to bacterial infection and is involved in many bacterial-induced inflammatory diseases by regulating the expression of inflammatory mediators [29,48]. Moreover, GSK3β is inhibited through phosphorylation at Ser9, and the absence or inhibition of this protein has been found to dampen the activation of JNK and NF-κB, leading to decreased expression of proinflammatory cytokines [30,32]. JNK is a member of the MAPK family that can phosphorylate and activate c-Jun, which forms a dimeric transcription factor activating protein-1 (AP-1) with c-Fos and mediates lung inflammatory response [44,60]. GSK3β phosphorylates MEKK1 through physical binding, and the activated MEKK1 further phosphorylates JNKK1 to activate JNK [52]. NF-κB is a master regulator in the host inflammatory response to harmful stimuli, which remains inactive in the cytoplasm by binding to the IκB. After the phosphorylation and degradation of IκB, the NF-κB dimer moves to the nucleus and activates the transcription of proinflammatory cytokines, thus promoting pulmonary inflammation [35,61]. GSK3β has been found to directly phosphorylate NF-κB p65 or indirectly activate NF-κB by affecting the activity of IκB kinase [29,53,54]. The data of molecular docking demonstrated that KP had a high binding activity with GSK3β, JNK1, and NF-κB p65. Therefore, we hypothesized that KP might alleviate the *P. aeruginosa*-induced acute pneumonia by regulating the GSK3β/JNK/c-Jun and NF-κB signaling pathways. A mouse model of acute *P. aeruginosa* pneumonia and an in vitro macrophage infection model were carried out for further validation.

Pseudomonas aeruginosa acute infections induce the overproduction of multiple proinflammatory cytokines in the host, leading to severe tissue lesions [62]. The suppression of cytokine overproduction has become a major strategy for the treatment of pneumonia [45]. KP was previously reported to inhibit the production of several proinflammatory cytokines, including IL-1β, TNF, IL-6, IL-17, IL-18, and MIP-2 [19,63,64]. Among them, TNF is a key proinflammatory cytokine mediating inflammation and could enhance the lung inflammatory response induced by *P. aeruginosa* via the JNK and NF-κB signaling pathways [44]. IL-1β is promptly produced in response to infections, and decreased production of IL-1β was found to alleviate the *P. aeruginosa*-induced lung tissue damage and reduce the mortality of mice [65]. IL-6 is essential in triggering acute inflammation, which promotes the production of a variety of inflammatory mediators [66]. MIP-2 is a potent chemokine for neutrophil recruitment into the inflamed lung [67]. Our study demonstrated that KP could effectively inhibit the *P. aeruginosa*-induced production of TNF, IL-1β, IL-6, and MIP-2 in the lungs of mice and macrophages, thus attenuating the severity of lung tissue damage and reducing the risk of systemic inflammation.

Multiple PAMPs of *P. aeruginosa* can activate TLRs and trigger host innate immune responses [62]. GSK3β is a highly conserved and ubiquitously expressed serine/threonine kinase that is able to regulate the inflammatory response by promoting TLR signaling [49]. The GSK3β inhibitor SB216763 has been found to attenuate the corneal inflammation caused by *P. aeruginosa* and reduce the levels of IL-1β and IL-6 [31]. Moreover, KP was previously reported to effectively inhibit GSK3β activation in the treatment of many diseases, such as myocardial ischemia/reperfusion injury and heart failure [59,68]. Additionally, GSK3β can directly phosphorylate many inflammatory mediators, such as NF-κB, IKK, IκB, MEKK1, JNK, TBK1, and NRF2 [32,48,49,52–54]. The inhibition of GSK3β and its downstream pathways has become an important strategy to mitigate lung injury [50,51]. A previous study showed that the deletion of GSK3β inhibited the degradation of IκB kinase, which led to the reduced activation and nuclear translocation of NF-κB [30]. In addition, GSK3β inhibition has been reported to reduce the activation of JNK, c-Jun, and NF-κB [30,32]. Furthermore, JNK and NF-κB are essential to regulate the expression of the cytokines, including TNF, IL-1β, IL-6, and MIP-2, and their activation levels were positively correlated to the severity of the *P. aeruginosa*-induced lung damage [34,44,47]. Previous studies have shown that KP treatment attenuated neuroinflammation by decreasing the phosphorylation of JNK and the nuclear translocation of NF-κB in microglia [19]. KP was able to significantly inhibit the phosphorylation of JNK and p38, which in turn inhibited the expression of NFATc1 and attenuated the wear particle-induced inflammatory osteolysis [21]. Furthermore, KP was found to inhibit intestinal inflammatory responses by reducing the activation of the TLR4/NF-κB pathway [17]. Further studies revealed that KP dose-dependently increased the levels of the phosphorylation-mediated inactivation of GSK3β in the lungs of mice and macrophages during *P. aeruginosa* infection, leading to the significant suppression of JNK, c-Jun, and NF-κB p65 phosphorylation. Interestingly, in the in vivo experiments, GSK3β in the KPH and Dex groups exhibited a higher level of phosphorylation inactivation than that in uninfected (NT) mice. GSK3 is one of the most substrate-rich protein kinases in cells and was originally found to regulate glucose metabolism and energy homeostasis [69]. GSK3β is a well-studied isoform of GSK3, which has been found to be involved in a wide range of diseases, including metabolic diseases, inflammatory diseases, neurological disorders, cancer, and atherosclerosis [29,48,69–72]. Under normal physiological conditions, GSK3β activity is finely regulated by a variety of signaling pathways, such as the PI3K/AKT and Wnt/β-catenin pathways [29,48,73]. These pathways dynamically regulate the phosphorylation status of GSK3β according to intra- and extracellular signaling changes, maintaining a relative balance between activation and inactivation. We speculated that this balance might be disrupted by the bacterial infection in this study, and the drug treatment decreased GSK3β activation, which led to higher levels of GSK3β phosphorylation. These findings suggested that KP ameliorated the *P. aeruginosa*-induced acute pneumonia through the inhibition of the GSK3β/JNK/c-Jun signaling pathway and NF-κB activation.

This study suggested an alternative strategy for the treatment of acute *P. aeruginosa* lung infection and might also provide a basis for the treatment and management under chronic inflammatory conditions, such as cystic fibrosis, bronchiectasis, and chronic obstructive pulmonary disease. Additionally, although KP has demonstrated inhibitory effects against a wide range of pathogens [27], we did not find significant bacteriostatic effects of KP against *P. aeruginosa* in vivo. The therapeutic effects exerted by KP against *P. aeruginosa* pneumonia were mainly attributed to the suppression of the host inflammatory response. This study also suggested a combination of KP and antibiotics in treating bacterial infections, in which KP might enhance the efficacy of antibiotics by modulating host immune response and reducing the dosage of antibiotics and the risk of the development of drug resistance. Future studies could explore the therapeutic efficacy of KP in combination with antibiotics in bacterial pneumonia.

4. Materials and Methods

4.1. Target Gene Analysis of KP

The KP targets were from the SwissTargetPrediction database (http://swisstargetprediction.ch/ (accessed on 11 February 2025)), the ETCM database (http://www.tcmip.cn/ETCM/ (accessed on 11 February 2025)), and the TCMSP database (https://www.tcmsp-e.com/ (accessed on 11 February 2025)) with the screening criteria of "Homo sapiens" and p-value > 0.1. The names of the target genes were gained from the UniProt database (https://www.uniprot.org/ (accessed on 11 February 2025)). Subsequently, the obtained target names of KP were integrated.

4.2. Target Gene Analysis of P. aeruginosa Pneumonia

The PharmGKB database (https://www.pharmgkb.org/ (accessed on 11 February 2025)), GeneCards database (https://www.genecards.org/ (accessed on 11 February 2025)), and OMIM database (https://www.omim.org/ (accessed on 11 February 2025)) were used to search the target genes of *P. aeruginosa* pneumonia with the keyword "*P. aeruginosa* pulmonary infection". The obtained target genes were integrated.

The targets of KP and *P. aeruginosa* pneumonia were imported into Venny 2.1.0 (https://bioinfogp.cnb.csic.es/tools/venny/ (accessed on 11 February 2025)) to obtain the intersecting targets, which were regarded as the potential targets of KP for treating *P. aeruginosa* pneumonia.

4.3. PPI Network

The intersecting targets were input into the STRING database (https://cn.string-db.org/ (accessed on 11 February 2025)), "Organisms" was limited to "Homo sapiens", "medium confidence (0.400)" was set, and the targets without connection to others were hidden. Finally, the PPI network was exported and visualized via Cytoscape 3.9.1 (Cytoscape Consortium, San Diego, CA, USA).

4.4. GO and KEGG Pathway Enrichment Analysis

To understand the functions of the intersecting targets and potential pathways regulated by KP, the intersecting targets were input into the DAVID database (https://david.ncifcrf.gov/ (accessed on 11 February 2025)) with the restriction of "Homo sapiens". Subsequently, the top 20 items of the KEGG pathway and GO involving BP, CC, and MF were imported into the bioinformatics website (https://www.bioinformatics.com.cn/ (accessed on 11 February 2025)) in descending order of p-value for visualization.

4.5. Molecular Docking

The three-dimensional (3D) structure of KP was optimized for energy-minimized structure by the MM2 functionality of Chem3D 19.0.0.22 (PerkinElmer Informatics, Inc., Wellesley, MA, USA). The 3D structures of the target proteins, GSK3β, JNK1, c-Jun, and NF-κB p65, were acquired from the RCSB Protein Data Bank database (https://www.rcsb.org/ (accessed on 11 February 2025)), and water molecules and ligands were removed using PyMOL 2.4.0 (Schrödinger, Inc., New York, NY, USA). Subsequently, the protein molecules were hydrogen-modified and docked with the KP molecule by AutoDockTools

1.5.6 (Scripps Research Institute, San Diego, CA, USA). Finally, the docking results with the lowest binding energy were visualized by PyMOL 2.4.0.

4.6. Reagents

KP for in vivo and in vitro experiments was supplied by Macklin Biochemical Co., Ltd. (Cat#: K812225; Shanghai, China). The standard of KP was purchased from Shanghai Yuanye Biotechnology (Cat#: B21126; Shanghai, China). Dex was purchased from MedChemExpress (Cat#: HY-14648, Shanghai, China). Enhanced Cell Counting Kit 8 (CCK8) was purchased from Elabscience Biotechnology (Cat#: E-CK-A362; Wuhan, China). The TNF (EK0527), IL-6 (EK0411), IL-1β (EK0394), and MIP-2 (EK0452) ELISA Kits were purchased from Boster Biological Technology (Wuhan, China). The SteadyPure Universal RNA Extraction Kit (AG21017), Evo M-MLV Reverse Transcription Premixed Kit (AG11728), and SYBR Green Pro Taq HS Premixed qPCR Kit (AG11701) were purchased from Accurate Biotechnology (Hunan, China). Antibodies for β-actin (AF0003), BCA Protein Assay Kit (P0011), ECL substrate kit (P0018S), goat anti-rabbit (A0208), and anti-mouse (A0216) IgG were obtained from Beyotime Biotechnology (Shanghai, China). The antibodies for phospho-NF-κB p65 (3033), NF-κB p65 (8242), phospho-GSK3β (Ser9) (5558), GSK3β (12456), phospho- JNK (9251), JNK (9252), phospho-c-Jun (Ser73) (3270), and c-Jun (9165) were supplied by Cell Signaling Technology (Danvers, MA, USA).

4.7. Determination of KP Content

The composition and content of the KP sample were determined by high-performance liquid chromatogram (HPLC). The sample and standard of KP were dissolved in acetonitrile and filtered through a microporous membrane, respectively. Chromatographic conditions: the chromatographic column was SHIMSEN Superb IIC18 (4.6 × 250 mm, 5 μm); the mobile phase was acetonitrile:water = 32:68; the column temperature was 30 °C; the flow rate was 1.00 mL/min; the injection volume was 10 μL; and the detection wavelength of the UV detector (Agilent 1260 liquid chromatography system, Agilent Technologies, Inc., Santa Clara, CA, USA) was 265 nm.

According to the HPLC graph, the KP sample and standard had the same retention time under the same chromatographic conditions (Figure 9). In addition, the integration result displayed that the relative peak area of the KP sample was 97.85%, which indicated a high purity of the KP sample.

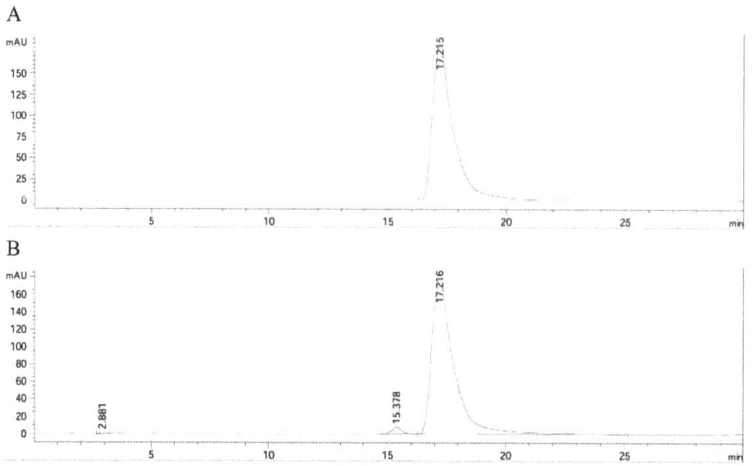

Figure 9. High-performance liquid chromatogram of the KP standard (**A**) and sample (**B**). The pink line indicated the baseline, and the blue line represented the detected signal above the baseline. Peaks were labeled with their respective retention times.

4.8. Bacterial Culture

The *P. aeruginosa* strain PAO1 was utilized in the experiments. Briefly, bacteria were cultured in LB broth with shaking at 37 °C in the early stationary phase. After washing with PBS and centrifuging at 13,000 rpm for 3 min, the bacteria were resuspended for subsequent experiments.

4.9. Animals and Drug Treatment

The male C57BL/6N mice (Charles River Laboratories, Beijing, China) aged 8 weeks with a body weight of 22 ± 2 g were acclimatized in a specific pathogen-free (SPF) facility for one week before the experimental research was conducted. The animal protocol has been approved by the Animal Ethics Committee of Shandong University of Traditional Chinese Medicine (protocol number: SDUTCM20240716002).

The mice were randomly divided into 5 groups, each of which contained 8 mice, including the NT, Saline, KPL (10 mg/kg), KPH (30 mg/kg), and Dex (2.5 mg/kg) groups. All mice were administered with drugs or saline via intraperitoneal injection. The mice in the NT group received an intranasal simulation with saline, whereas the mice from the other groups were intranasally administered with PAO1. Drugs were given 1 h before the infection, and a subsequent dose was administered 8 h after the first dose.

4.10. Lung Infection and Tissue Processing

The mice from the Saline, KPL, KPH, and Dex groups received 5×10^8 colony-forming unit (CFU) of PAO1 per mouse through intranasal infection, while the mice in the NT group were given an equal volume of saline. Subsequently, the mice were euthanized after 24 h of infection, and BALF was obtained by lung lavage with 1 mL PBS. For CFU counting, 10 μL BALF was spread onto an LB agar plate, followed by 24 h incubation at 37 °C. The supernatants for cytokine detection were collected from the remaining BALF after centrifugation at 1200 rpm for 5 min at 4 °C. After erythrocytes were lysed, the BALF cells were lysed with 250 μL of 0.5% cetyltrimethylammonium chloride (CTAC) and then centrifuged to collect the supernatants for MPO assay.

The left lungs were ground in HEPES buffer (50 mM; 4 μL per 1 mg lung) to obtain lung homogenates. For CFU counting, 10 μL homogenates were applied onto an LB agar plate, followed by 24 h incubation at 37 °C. Subsequently, the remaining homogenates were centrifuged at 13,000 rpm for 10 min at 4 °C, and the supernatants were collected for cytokine detection. The pellets were homogenized in 0.5% CTAC (4 μL per 1 mg lung) and centrifuged to obtain extracts for measuring MPO activity.

4.11. Survival Study and Disease Scores

A survival study was applied to explore the therapeutic efficacy of KP and disease progression, which was based on a 21-point scoring system [35]. Briefly, the mice were administered 1×10^9 CFU/mouse of PAO1 intranasally. The drugs or saline were administered on the infection day and day 1 post-infection. Subsequently, the survival rates and disease scores of mice were recorded daily for 10 days after infection. The detailed scoring system was shown in Table 4.

Table 4. The scoring rules of the disease status of mice.

Score	0	1	2	3
Hair feature	Normal	Lack of grooming	Rough	Very obvious rough
Body posture	Normal	Hunched sitting position	A hunched stance with the head lying on the ground	Prone and unable to stay in an upright posture
Activity/Behavior	Normal	Minor changes in behavior	Decreased activity with increased respiratory rate	Only moves when stimulated
Appetite	Normal	Reduced appetite	Not eating food after the last checkpoint	Not eating food for the last two checkpoints
Hydration	Normal	Mild dehydration	Moderate dehydration	Severe dehydration
Change in weight compared with pre-infection	<5.0%	<10.0%	10.0–15.0%	>15.0%
Body temperature (ventral surface temperature)	33–34 °C	28–32.5 °C	25–27.5 °C	<24.5 °C

Total possible score = 21; Endpoint for euthanasia > 15.

4.12. Histological Assessment

The post caval lobes of mouse lung tissues were soaked in 10% formalin for 2 days. Subsequently, the lung tissues were dehydrated with ascending gradients of ethanol, transparently treated with xylene, and embedded in paraffin. The tissues were then sectioned, treated with xylene to remove the paraffin, and rehydrated with descending gradients of ethanol. Finally, the tissue sections were subjected to H&E staining. The images of the lung sections were observed and photographed at 100× or 400× magnification using a microscope (Olympus IX73, Olympus Corporation, Tokyo, Japan).

The score of lung injury was evaluated histologically according to a previously reported scoring criterion [74]. Briefly, at 400× magnification, 20 random non-repeating fields of view were sought and scored according to neutrophils in the alveolar space, neutrophils in the interstitial space, hyaline membranes, proteinaceous debris filling the airspaces, and alveolar septal thickening. Specifically, scoring was based on the following guidelines: (A) the number of neutrophils in the alveolar space (0:none, 1:1–5, 2:>5); (B) the number of neutrophils in the interstitial space (0:none, 1:1–5, 2:>5); (C) the number of hyaline membranes (0:none, 1:1, 2:>1); (D) the extent to the filling of airspace with protein fragments (0: none, 1:1, 2:>1); (E) multiples of alveolar septal thickening (0:<2×, 1:2×–4×, 2:>4×). Scoring formula: score = $[(20 \times A) + (14 \times B) + (7 \times C) + (7 \times D) + (2 \times E)]/(\text{number of fields} \times 100)$. Finally, the histologic score for each sample was calculated by the provided formula.

4.13. Protein Concentration Assay

The total protein concentration of the BALF and lung supernatants of mice was detected by BCA assay. Briefly, 10 μL samples were mixed with 200 μL BCA reagents and incubated at 37 °C for 30 min. Subsequently, the OD was measured at 562 nm, and the total protein concentration of each sample was calculated based on the standard curve and dilution factors.

4.14. MPO Assay

The neutrophil infiltration in the lungs of mice was evaluated by MPO assay [34]. In brief, 75 μL lysates from BALF cells or lung tissues were mixed with 75 μL substrate, a mixture of 2.2 mM H_2O_2, 3 mM TMB dihydrochloride, and 120 μM resorcinol, and the same volume of deionized water mixed with the substrate was used as a blank control. After incubation at room temperature for 2 min, the reaction was terminated with 150 μL H_2SO_4 (2 M), and the OD was measured at 450 nm.

4.15. Macrophage Culture and Infection

The bone marrow cells from the mouse femur and tibia were cultured with DMEM medium containing 1% penicillin–streptomycin, 10 ng/mL macrophage colony-stimulating factor, and 10% FBS. The culture medium was half-replaced every 2–3 days. On day 7, the DMEM medium with only 10% FBS was used for the following experiments. After the pretreatment with KP for 1 h, the cells were infected with PAO1 (MOI: 10) or mock-infected (NT) with PBS. Furthermore, the cell pellets were lysed for Western blot analysis of p-GSK3β at Ser9, GSK3β, p-JNK, JNK, p-c-Jun, c-Jun, p-NF-κB p65, and NF-κB p65 at 1 h after infection, whereas the cell-free supernatants were obtained for cytokine detection at 3 h, 6h, and 12h after infection.

4.16. Cell Viability Assay

Cells were seeded at a density of 1×10^4 per well in a 96-well plate and treated with KP at concentrations of 0, 25, 50, 100, or 120 μM. After incubation at 37 °C for 12 h, 10 μL CCK-8 solution was added to each well, and the incubation was continued for an additional 4 h. The OD was measured at 450 nm.

4.17. Cytokine Analysis

The concentrations of TNF, IL-6, IL-1β, and MIP-2 in the lung tissues, BALF or cell-free supernatants were examined by ELISA, and the experimental processes were conducted according to the manufacturer's instructions.

4.18. Real-Time Quantitative PCR (RT-qPCR)

The mRNA transcription levels of *GSK3β*, *JNK1*, *c-Jun*, and *p65 (RelA)* were examined by RT-qPCR. The total RNA extraction, reverse transcription, and qPCR analyses of lung tissues and cells were performed using SteadyPure Universal RNA Extraction Kit, Evo M-MLV Reverse Transcription Premixed Kit, and SYBR Green Pro Taq HS Premixed qPCR Kit, respectively. The experimental processes were conducted according to the manufacturer's instructions. β-actin served as the endogenous control. Primer sequences were listed in Table 5.

Table 5. Forward and backward primer sequences for RT-qPCR analysis.

Name	Primer Sequence (5′ → 3′)
GSK3β	F: CCCTCCACATGCTCGGATTCA
	R: ATTGGTCTGTCCACGGTCTCC
JNK1	F: AGAAACTGTTCCCCGATGTGC
	R: GCTGGAGAGCTTCATCTACGGA
c-Jun	F: AAACTCCGAGCTGGCATCCAC
	R: GCTGCGTTAGCATGAGTTGGC
p65 (RelA)	F: TCGCCACCGGATTGAAGAGAA
	R: CGGGGTTCAGTTGGTCCATTG
β-actin	F: CATCCGTAAAGACCTCTATGCCAAC
	R: ATGGAGCCACCGATCCACA

4.19. Western Blotting

The phosphorylation levels of GSK3β, JNK, c-Jun, and NF-κB p65 were analyzed. The cells and right lungs of mice were lysed in radioimmunoprecipitation assay (RIPA) buffer for 30 min and then centrifuged to obtain the lysates at 4 °C. The cell or lung lysates were collected to denature at 95 °C for 5 min. The proteins were separated using electrophoresis in 10% SDS polyacrylamide gel and transferred to a 0.45 μm polyvinylidene difluoride (PVDF) membrane. Subsequently, the membrane was blocked with 5% skim milk at room temperature for 1.5 h and incubated overnight with primary antibody. The next day, the washed membrane was probed with a secondary antibody for 2 h. Finally, the ECL substrate was applied onto the membrane, and images were generated with the Vilber Lourmat Fusion FX imaging system (Vilber Lourmat, Marne La Vallée, France).

4.20. Statistical Analysis

Statistical analysis was conducted using GraphPad Prism 9.5.0. Data are expressed as mean ± standard deviation. One-way analysis of variance (ANOVA) with Dunnett's multiple comparisons test was applied for multiple group comparisons. A *p*-value < 0.05 was regarded as statistically significant.

5. Conclusions

Altogether, this research first applied network pharmacology to explore the underlying mechanisms of KP in treating *P. aeruginosa* pneumonia and validated them through in vivo and in vitro studies. The results of network pharmacology suggested that KP might treat *P. aeruginosa* pneumonia by modulating GSK3β/JNK/c-Jun signaling pathway and NF-κB. Further experimental results proved that KP reduced the production of proinflammatory cytokines by inhibiting GSK3β/JNK/c-Jun signaling pathways and NF-κB activation, which effectively mitigated the *P. aeruginosa*-induced acute lung inflammation and injury and elevated the survival rates of mice. In the future, we will focus on evaluating the synergistic therapeutic potential of KP in combination with antibiotics.

Supplementary Materials: The following supporting information can be downloaded at: https://www.mdpi.com/article/10.3390/ph18030322/s1. The results of the effect of KP on proinflammatory cytokine production in the lungs of uninfected mice were shown in Figure S1. The results of the effect of KP on the gene expression of GSK3β, JNK, c-Jun, and NF-κB p65 in the lungs of mice and BMDMs infected with *P. aeruginosa* were shown in Figure S2 and Figure S3, respectively.

Author Contributions: Conceptualization, Z.P.; methodology, Z.P and L.Z.; software, J.W. and L.Z.; validation, J.W., L.Z. and L.F.; formal analysis, J.W.; investigation, J.W.; resources, Z.P.; data curation, Z.P.; writing—original draft preparation, J.W.; writing—review and editing, L.F. and Z.P.; visualization, J.W.; supervision, Z.P.; project administration, Z.P.; funding acquisition, Z.P. All authors have read and agreed to the published version of the manuscript.

Funding: This research was funded by the Natural Science Foundation of Shandong Province (Grant No.: ZR2024QH012), and the National Natural Science Foundation of China (Grant No.: 82002112).

Institutional Review Board Statement: The animal study protocol was approved by the Animal Ethics Committee of Shandong University of Traditional Chinese Medicine, protocol number: SDUTCM20240716002, date: 16 July 2024.

Data Availability Statement: Data will be made available on request.

Conflicts of Interest: The authors have declared that no competing interests exist.

References

1. Qin, S.; Xiao, W.; Zhou, C.; Pu, Q.; Deng, X.; Lan, L.; Liang, H.; Song, X.; Wu, M. *Pseudomonas aeruginosa*: Pathogenesis, virulence factors, antibiotic resistance, interaction with host, technology advances and emerging therapeutics. *Signal Transduct. Target. Ther.* **2022**, *7*, 199. [CrossRef]
2. Deshpande, R.; Zou, C. *Pseudomonas aeruginosa* Induced Cell Death in Acute Lung Injury and Acute Respiratory Distress Syndrome. *Int. J. Mol. Sci.* **2020**, *21*, 5356. [CrossRef] [PubMed]
3. Jurado-Martín, I.; Sainz-Mejías, M.; McClean, S. *Pseudomonas aeruginosa*: An Audacious Pathogen with an Adaptable Arsenal of Virulence Factors. *Int. J. Mol. Sci.* **2021**, *22*, 3128. [CrossRef] [PubMed]
4. Gonçalves-de-Albuquerque, C.F.; Silva, A.R.; Burth, P.; Rocco, P.R.; Castro-Faria, M.V.; Castro-Faria-Neto, H.C. Possible mechanisms of *Pseudomonas aeruginosa*-associated lung disease. *Int. J. Med. Microbiol. IJMM* **2016**, *306*, 20–28. [CrossRef] [PubMed]
5. El Solh, A.A.; Alhajhusain, A. Update on the treatment of *Pseudomonas aeruginosa* pneumonia. *J. Antimicrob. Chemother.* **2009**, *64*, 229–238. [CrossRef]
6. Bassetti, M.; Vena, A.; Russo, A.; Croxatto, A.; Calandra, T.; Guery, B. Rational approach in the management of *Pseudomonas aeruginosa* infections. *Curr. Opin. Infect. Dis.* **2018**, *31*, 578–586. [CrossRef]
7. Pang, Z.; Raudonis, R.; Glick, B.R.; Lin, T.J.; Cheng, Z. Antibiotic resistance in *Pseudomonas aeruginosa*: Mechanisms and alternative therapeutic strategies. *Biotechnol. Adv.* **2019**, *37*, 177–192. [CrossRef] [PubMed]
8. Thi, M.T.T.; Wibowo, D.; Rehm, B.H.A. *Pseudomonas aeruginosa* Biofilms. *Int. J. Mol. Sci.* **2020**, *21*, 8671. [CrossRef] [PubMed]
9. Lorusso, A.B.; Carrara, J.A.; Barroso, C.D.N.; Tuon, F.F.; Faoro, H. Role of Efflux Pumps on Antimicrobial Resistance in *Pseudomonas aeruginosa*. *Int. J. Mol. Sci.* **2022**, *23*, 15779. [CrossRef] [PubMed]
10. Fernández-Barat, L.; Ferrer, M.; De Rosa, F.; Gabarrús, A.; Esperatti, M.; Terraneo, S.; Rinaudo, M.; Li Bassi, G.; Torres, A. Intensive care unit-acquired pneumonia due to *Pseudomonas aeruginosa* with and without multidrug resistance. *J. Infect.* **2017**, *74*, 142–152. [CrossRef]
11. Pang, Z.; Zhu, Q. Traditional Chinese Medicine is an Alternative Therapeutic Option for Treatment of *Pseudomonas aeruginosa* Infections. *Front. Pharmacol.* **2021**, *12*, 737252. [CrossRef] [PubMed]
12. He, Y.Q.; Zhou, C.C.; Yu, L.Y.; Wang, L.; Deng, J.L.; Tao, Y.L.; Zhang, F.; Chen, W.S. Natural product derived phytochemicals in managing acute lung injury by multiple mechanisms. *Pharmacol. Res.* **2021**, *163*, 105224. [CrossRef]
13. Alam, W.; Khan, H.; Shah, M.A.; Cauli, O.; Saso, L. Kaempferol as a Dietary Anti-Inflammatory Agent: Current Therapeutic Standing. *Molecules* **2020**, *25*, 4073. [CrossRef]
14. Ren, J.; Lu, Y.; Qian, Y.; Chen, B.; Wu, T.; Ji, G. Recent progress regarding kaempferol for the treatment of various diseases. *Exp. Ther. Med.* **2019**, *18*, 2759–2776. [CrossRef]
15. Imran, M.; Rauf, A.; Shah, Z.A.; Saeed, F.; Imran, A.; Arshad, M.U.; Ahmad, B.; Bawazeer, S.; Atif, M.; Peters, D.G.; et al. Chemo-preventive and therapeutic effect of the dietary flavonoid kaempferol: A comprehensive review. *Phytother. Res. PTR* **2019**, *33*, 263–275. [CrossRef] [PubMed]
16. Rajendran, P.; Rengarajan, T.; Nandakumar, N.; Palaniswami, R.; Nishigaki, Y.; Nishigaki, I. Kaempferol, a potential cytostatic and cure for inflammatory disorders. *Eur. J. Med. Chem.* **2014**, *86*, 103–112. [CrossRef] [PubMed]
17. Bian, Y.; Lei, J.; Zhong, J.; Wang, B.; Wan, Y.; Li, J.; Liao, C.; He, Y.; Liu, Z.; Ito, K.; et al. Kaempferol reduces obesity, prevents intestinal inflammation, and modulates gut microbiota in high-fat diet mice. *J. Nutr. Biochem.* **2022**, *99*, 108840. [CrossRef] [PubMed]

18. Gong, J.H.; Shin, D.; Han, S.Y.; Kim, J.L.; Kang, Y.H. Kaempferol suppresses eosionphil infiltration and airway inflammation in airway epithelial cells and in mice with allergic asthma. *J. Nutr.* **2012**, *142*, 47–56. [CrossRef]
19. Liu, Z.; Yao, X.; Sun, B.; Jiang, W.; Liao, C.; Dai, X.; Chen, Y.; Chen, J.; Ding, R. Pretreatment with kaempferol attenuates microglia-mediate neuroinflammation by inhibiting MAPKs-NF-κB signaling pathway and pyroptosis after secondary spinal cord injury. *Free. Radic. Biol. Med.* **2021**, *168*, 142–154. [CrossRef]
20. Cheng, X.; Yang, Y.L.; Yang, H.; Wang, Y.H.; Du, G.H. Kaempferol alleviates LPS-induced neuroinflammation and BBB dysfunction in mice via inhibiting HMGB1 release and down-regulating TLR4/MyD88 pathway. *Int. Immunopharmacol.* **2018**, *56*, 29–35. [CrossRef] [PubMed]
21. Yu, X.; Wu, Q.; Ren, Z.; Chen, B.; Wang, D.; Yuan, T.; Ding, H.; Wang, Y.; Yuan, G.; Wang, Y.; et al. Kaempferol attenuates wear particle-induced inflammatory osteolysis via JNK and p38-MAPK signaling pathways. *J. Ethnopharmacol.* **2024**, *318*, 117019. [CrossRef] [PubMed]
22. Yao, H.; Sun, J.; Wei, J.; Zhang, X.; Chen, B.; Lin, Y. Kaempferol Protects Blood Vessels From Damage Induced by Oxidative Stress and Inflammation in Association with the Nrf2/HO-1 Signaling Pathway. *Front. Pharmacol.* **2020**, *11*, 1118. [CrossRef]
23. Qian, J.; Chen, X.; Chen, X.; Sun, C.; Jiang, Y.; Qian, Y.; Zhang, Y.; Khan, Z.; Zhou, J.; Liang, G.; et al. Kaempferol reduces K63-linked polyubiquitination to inhibit nuclear factor-κB and inflammatory responses in acute lung injury in mice. *Toxicol. Lett.* **2019**, *306*, 53–60. [CrossRef]
24. Zhang, R.; Ai, X.; Duan, Y.; Xue, M.; He, W.; Wang, C.; Xu, T.; Xu, M.; Liu, B.; Li, C.; et al. Kaempferol ameliorates H9N2 swine influenza virus-induced acute lung injury by inactivation of TLR4/MyD88-mediated NF-κB and MAPK signaling pathways. *Biomed. Pharmacother. = Biomed. Pharmacother.* **2017**, *89*, 660–672. [CrossRef] [PubMed]
25. Chen, X.; Yang, X.; Liu, T.; Guan, M.; Feng, X.; Dong, W.; Chu, X.; Liu, J.; Tian, X.; Ci, X.; et al. Kaempferol regulates MAPKs and NF-κB signaling pathways to attenuate LPS-induced acute lung injury in mice. *Int. Immunopharmacol.* **2012**, *14*, 209–216. [CrossRef]
26. Xu, L.; Fang, J.; Ou, D.; Xu, J.; Deng, X.; Chi, G.; Feng, H.; Wang, J. Therapeutic potential of kaempferol on *Streptococcus pneumoniae* infection. *Microbes Infect.* **2023**, *25*, 105058. [CrossRef]
27. Periferakis, A.; Periferakis, K.; Badarau, I.A.; Petran, E.M.; Popa, D.C.; Caruntu, A.; Costache, R.S.; Scheau, C.; Caruntu, C.; Costache, D.O. Kaempferol: Antimicrobial Properties, Sources, Clinical, and Traditional Applications. *Int. J. Mol. Sci.* **2022**, *23*, 15054. [CrossRef]
28. Yin, N.; Yang, X.; Wang, L.; Zhang, C.; Guan, J.; Tao, Y.; Guo, X.; Zhao, Y.; Song, W.; Wang, B.; et al. Kaempferol inhibits the expression of α-hemolysin and protects mice from methicillin-resistant *Staphylococcus aureus*-induced lethal pneumonia. *Microb. Pathog.* **2022**, *162*, 105336. [CrossRef] [PubMed]
29. Cortés-Vieyra, R.; Silva-García, O.; Gómez-García, A.; Gutiérrez-Castellanos, S.; Álvarez-Aguilar, C.; Baizabal-Aguirre, V.M. Glycogen Synthase Kinase 3β Modulates the Inflammatory Response Activated by Bacteria, Viruses, and Parasites. *Front. Immunol.* **2021**, *12*, 675751. [CrossRef]
30. Takada, Y.; Fang, X.; Jamaluddin, M.S.; Boyd, D.D.; Aggarwal, B.B. Genetic deletion of glycogen synthase kinase-3beta abrogates activation of IkappaBalpha kinase, JNK, Akt, and p44/p42 MAPK but potentiates apoptosis induced by tumor necrosis factor. *J. Biol. Chem.* **2004**, *279*, 39541–39554. [CrossRef]
31. Chen, K.; Fu, Q.; Ye, C.; Zhan, X.; Lu, J.; Du, M.; Feng, Y.; Liang, P.; Wang, W. The Regulating Role of SB216763 in *Pseudomonas aeruginosa* Keratitis. *Clin. Lab.* **2019**, *65*, 1829–1835. [CrossRef] [PubMed]
32. Kwon, Y.J.; Yoon, C.H.; Lee, S.W.; Park, Y.B.; Lee, S.K.; Park, M.C. Inhibition of glycogen synthase kinase-3β suppresses inflammatory responses in rheumatoid arthritis fibroblast-like synoviocytes and collagen-induced arthritis. *Jt. Bone Spine* **2014**, *81*, 240–246. [CrossRef] [PubMed]
33. Dai, J.; Guan, H.; Zhang, L.; Jiang, H.; Su, W.; Wang, J.; Jia, X.; Pang, Z. Fatty Acids Derived from Royal Jelly Exert Anti-Inflammatory and Antibacterial Activities in the Treatment of *Pseudomonas aeruginosa*-Induced Acute Pneumonia. *J. Med. Food* **2025**, *28*, 44–57. [CrossRef] [PubMed]
34. Gu, M.; Su, W.; Dai, J.; Wang, J.; Jia, X.; Yao, J.; Zhang, G.; Zhu, Q.; Pang, Z. Jingfang granule alleviates *Pseudomonas aeruginosa*-induced acute lung inflammation through suppression of STAT3/IL-17/NF-κB pathway based on network pharmacology analysis and experimental validation. *J. Ethnopharmacol.* **2024**, *318*, 116899. [CrossRef]
35. Jia, X.; Gu, M.; Dai, J.; Wang, J.; Zhang, Y.; Pang, Z. Quercetin attenuates *Pseudomonas aeruginosa*-induced acute lung inflammation by inhibiting PI3K/AKT/NF-κB signaling pathway. *Inflammopharmacology* **2024**, *32*, 1059–1076. [CrossRef] [PubMed]
36. Xiao, K.; Cao, Y.; Han, Z.; Zhang, Y.; Luu, L.D.W.; Chen, L.; Yan, P.; Chen, W.; Wang, J.; Liang, Y.; et al. A pan-immune panorama of bacterial pneumonia revealed by a large-scale single-cell transcriptome atlas. *Signal Transduct. Target. Ther.* **2025**, *10*, 5. [CrossRef] [PubMed]
37. Moser, C.; Jensen, P.; Thomsen, K.; Kolpen, M.; Rybtke, M.; Lauland, A.S.; Trøstrup, H.; Tolker-Nielsen, T. Immune Responses to *Pseudomonas aeruginosa* Biofilm Infections. *Front. Immunol.* **2021**, *12*, 625597. [CrossRef]

38. McClellan, S.A.; Huang, X.; Barrett, R.P.; Lighvani, S.; Zhang, Y.; Richiert, D.; Hazlett, L.D. Matrix metalloproteinase-9 amplifies the immune response to *Pseudomonas aeruginosa* corneal infection. *Investig. Ophthalmol. Vis. Sci.* **2006**, *47*, 256–264. [CrossRef]
39. Abdalla, M.Y.; Hoke, T.; Seravalli, J.; Switzer, B.L.; Bavitz, M.; Fliege, J.D.; Murphy, P.J.; Britigan, B.E. *Pseudomonas* Quinolone Signal Induces Oxidative Stress and Inhibits Heme Oxygenase-1 Expression in Lung Epithelial Cells. *Infect. Immun.* **2017**, *85*, e00176-17. [CrossRef] [PubMed]
40. Hobden, J.A.; Masinick-McClellan, S.; Barrett, R.P.; Bark, K.S.; Hazlett, L.D. *Pseudomonas aeruginosa* keratitis in knockout mice deficient in intercellular adhesion molecule 1. *Infect. Immun.* **1999**, *67*, 972–975. [CrossRef]
41. Ferreira, B.L.; Ramírez-Moral, I.; Otto, N.A.; Salomão, R.; de Vos, A.F.; van der Poll, T. The PPAR-γ agonist pioglitazone exerts proinflammatory effects in bronchial epithelial cells during acute *Pseudomonas aeruginosa* pneumonia. *Clin. Exp. Immunol.* **2022**, *207*, 370–377. [CrossRef] [PubMed]
42. Sadikot, R.T.; Zeng, H.; Azim, A.C.; Joo, M.; Dey, S.K.; Breyer, R.M.; Peebles, R.S.; Blackwell, T.S.; Christman, J.W. Bacterial clearance of *Pseudomonas aeruginosa* is enhanced by the inhibition of COX-2. *Eur. J. Immunol.* **2007**, *37*, 1001–1009. [CrossRef] [PubMed]
43. Xu, Y.; Duan, C.; Kuang, Z.; Hao, Y.; Jeffries, J.L.; Lau, G.W. *Pseudomonas aeruginosa* pyocyanin activates NRF2-ARE-mediated transcriptional response via the ROS-EGFR-PI3K-AKT/MEK-ERK MAP kinase signaling in pulmonary epithelial cells. *PLoS ONE* **2013**, *8*, e72528. [CrossRef] [PubMed]
44. Yang, Y.W.; Jiang, Y.Z.; Hsu, C.M.; Chen, L.W. *Pseudomonas aeruginosa* Ventilator-Associated Pneumonia Induces Lung Injury through TNF-α/c-Jun NH2-Terminal Kinase Pathways. *PLoS ONE* **2017**, *12*, e0169267. [CrossRef] [PubMed]
45. Dukhinova, M.; Kokinos, E.; Kuchur, P.; Komissarov, A.; Shtro, A. Macrophage-derived cytokines in pneumonia: Linking cellular immunology and genetics. *Cytokine Growth Factor Rev.* **2021**, *59*, 46–61. [CrossRef] [PubMed]
46. Wautier, J.L.; Wautier, M.P. Vascular Permeability in Diseases. *Int. J. Mol. Sci.* **2022**, *23*, 3645. [CrossRef] [PubMed]
47. Tsay, T.B.; Jiang, Y.Z.; Hsu, C.M.; Chen, L.W. *Pseudomonas aeruginosa* colonization enhances ventilator-associated pneumonia-induced lung injury. *Respir. Res.* **2016**, *17*, 101. [CrossRef]
48. Wang, H.; Kumar, A.; Lamont, R.J.; Scott, D.A. GSK3β and the control of infectious bacterial diseases. *Trends Microbiol.* **2014**, *22*, 208–217. [CrossRef] [PubMed]
49. Ko, R.; Lee, S.Y. Glycogen synthase kinase 3β in Toll-like receptor signaling. *BMB Rep.* **2016**, *49*, 305–310. [CrossRef]
50. Wang, Y.M.; Gong, F.C.; Qi, X.; Zheng, Y.J.; Zheng, X.T.; Chen, Y.; Yang, Z.T.; Qing, Y.; Mao, E.Q.; Chen, E.Z. Mucin 1 Inhibits Ferroptosis and Sensitizes Vitamin E to Alleviate Sepsis-Induced Acute Lung Injury through GSK3β/Keap1-Nrf2-GPX4 Pathway. *Oxid Med. Cell Longev.* **2022**, *2022*, 2405943. [CrossRef]
51. Becker, E., Jr.; Husain, M.; Bone, N.; Smith, S.; Morris, P.; Zmijewski, J.W. AMPK activation improves recovery from pneumonia-induced lung injury via reduction of er-stress and apoptosis in alveolar epithelial cells. *Respir. Res.* **2023**, *24*, 185. [CrossRef] [PubMed]
52. Kim, J.W.; Lee, J.E.; Kim, M.J.; Cho, E.G.; Cho, S.G.; Choi, E.J. Glycogen synthase kinase 3 beta is a natural activator of mitogen-activated protein kinase/extracellular signal-regulated kinase kinase kinase 1 (MEKK1). *J. Biol. Chem.* **2003**, *278*, 13995–14001. [CrossRef]
53. Wilson, W., 3rd; Baldwin, A.S. Maintenance of constitutive IkappaB kinase activity by glycogen synthase kinase-3alpha/beta in pancreatic cancer. *Cancer Res.* **2008**, *68*, 8156–8163. [CrossRef]
54. Schwabe, R.F.; Brenner, D.A. Role of glycogen synthase kinase-3 in TNF-alpha-induced NF-kappaB activation and apoptosis in hepatocytes. *Am. J. Physiol. Gastrointest Liver Physiol.* **2002**, *283*, G204–G211. [CrossRef] [PubMed]
55. Farhadi, F.; Khameneh, B.; Iranshahi, M.; Iranshahy, M. Antibacterial activity of flavonoids and their structure-activity relationship: An update review. *Phytother. Res. PTR* **2019**, *33*, 13–40. [CrossRef] [PubMed]
56. Al-Khayri, J.M.; Sahana, G.R.; Nagella, P.; Joseph, B.V.; Alessa, F.M.; Al-Mssallem, M.Q. Flavonoids as Potential Anti-Inflammatory Molecules: A Review. *Molecules* **2022**, *27*, 2901. [CrossRef] [PubMed]
57. Li, L.; Cui, H.; Zhang, Y.; Xie, W.; Lin, Y.; Guo, Y.; Huang, T.; Xue, B.; Guo, W.; Huang, Z.; et al. Baicalin ameliorates multidrug-resistant *Pseudomonas aeruginosa* induced pulmonary inflammation in rat via arginine biosynthesis. *Biomed. Pharmacother. = Biomed. Pharmacother.* **2023**, *162*, 114660. [CrossRef] [PubMed]
58. Ahn, H.I.; Jang, H.J.; Kwon, O.K.; Kim, J.H.; Oh, J.H.; Kim, S.H.; Oh, S.R.; Han, S.B.; Ahn, K.S.; Park, J.W. Quercetin Attenuates the Production of Pro-Inflammatory Cytokines in H292 Human Lung Epithelial Cells Infected with *Pseudomonas aeruginosa* by Modulating ExoS Production. *J. Microbiol. Biotechnol.* **2023**, *33*, 430–440. [CrossRef] [PubMed]
59. Zhou, M.; Ren, H.; Han, J.; Wang, W.; Zheng, Q.; Wang, D. Protective Effects of Kaempferol against Myocardial Ischemia/Reperfusion Injury in Isolated Rat Heart via Antioxidant Activity and Inhibition of Glycogen Synthase Kinase-3β. *Oxid Med. Cell Longev.* **2015**, *2015*, 481405. [CrossRef] [PubMed]
60. Karin, M.; Liu, Z.; Zandi, E. AP-1 function and regulation. *Curr. Opin. Cell Biol.* **1997**, *9*, 240–246. [CrossRef]
61. Lawrence, T. The nuclear factor NF-kappaB pathway in inflammation. *Cold Spring Harb Perspect. Biol.* **2009**, *1*, a001651. [CrossRef] [PubMed]

62. Lin, C.K.; Kazmierczak, B.I. Inflammation: A Double-Edged Sword in the Response to *Pseudomonas aeruginosa* Infection. *J. Innate. Immun.* **2017**, *9*, 250–261. [CrossRef] [PubMed]
63. Jia, Y.; Li, C.; Yin, M.; Lin, J.; Zhang, L.; Li, N.; Jiang, N.; Xu, Q.; Wang, Q.; Gu, L.; et al. Kaempferol ameliorate the prognosis of *Aspergillus fumigatus* keratitis by reducing fungal load and inhibiting the Dectin-1 and p38 MAPK pathway. *Exp. Eye Res.* **2022**, *216*, 108960. [CrossRef]
64. Li, N.; Chen, S.; Deng, W.; Gong, Z.; Guo, Y.; Zeng, S.; Xu, Q. Kaempferol Attenuates Gouty Arthritis by Regulating the Balance of Th17/Treg Cells and Secretion of IL-17. *Inflammation* **2023**, *46*, 1901–1916. [CrossRef] [PubMed]
65. Wonnenberg, B.; Bischoff, M.; Beisswenger, C.; Dinh, T.; Bals, R.; Singh, B.; Tschernig, T. The role of IL-1β in *Pseudomonas aeruginosa* in lung infection. *Cell Tissue Res.* **2016**, *364*, 225–229. [CrossRef] [PubMed]
66. Uciechowski, P.; Dempke, W.C.M. Interleukin-6: A Masterplayer in the Cytokine Network. *Oncology* **2020**, *98*, 131–137. [CrossRef] [PubMed]
67. Driscoll, K.E. Macrophage inflammatory proteins: Biology and role in pulmonary inflammation. *Exp. Lung Res.* **1994**, *20*, 473–490. [CrossRef]
68. Zhang, L.; Guo, Z.; Wang, Y.; Geng, J.; Han, S. The protective effect of kaempferol on heart via the regulation of Nrf2, NF-κβ, and PI3K/Akt/GSK-3β signaling pathways in isoproterenol-induced heart failure in diabetic rats. *Drug Dev. Res.* **2019**, *80*, 294–309. [CrossRef] [PubMed]
69. Wang, L.; Li, J.; Di, L.J. Glycogen synthesis and beyond, a comprehensive review of GSK3 as a key regulator of metabolic pathways and a therapeutic target for treating metabolic diseases. *Med. Res. Rev.* **2022**, *42*, 946–982. [CrossRef] [PubMed]
70. Lauretti, E.; Dincer, O.; Praticò, D. Glycogen synthase kinase-3 signaling in Alzheimer's disease. *Biochim. Biophys. Acta. Mol. Cell Res.* **2020**, *1867*, 118664. [CrossRef]
71. Cai, X.; Zhao, Y.; Yang, Y.; Wu, X.; Zhang, L.; Ma, J.A.; Ji, J.; Boström, K.I.; Yao, Y. GSK3β Inhibition Ameliorates Atherosclerotic Calcification. *Int. J. Mol. Sci.* **2023**, *24*, 11638. [CrossRef] [PubMed]
72. Tan, Z.; Boyapati, K.; Tressler, C.M.; Jenkinson, N.M.; Glunde, K. Glutamine transporter SLC38A3 promotes breast cancer metastasis via Gsk3β/β-catenin/EMT pathway. *Cancer Lett.* **2024**, *586*, 216653. [CrossRef] [PubMed]
73. Liao, S.; Wu, J.; Liu, R.; Wang, S.; Luo, J.; Yang, Y.; Qin, Y.; Li, T.; Zheng, X.; Song, J.; et al. A novel compound DBZ ameliorates neuroinflammation in LPS-stimulated microglia and ischemic stroke rats: Role of Akt(Ser473)/GSK3β(Ser9)-mediated Nrf2 activation. *Redox Biol.* **2020**, *36*, 101644. [CrossRef] [PubMed]
74. Matute-Bello, G.; Downey, G.; Moore, B.B.; Groshong, S.D.; Matthay, M.A.; Slutsky, A.S.; Kuebler, W.M. An official American Thoracic Society workshop report: Features and measurements of experimental acute lung injury in animals. *Am. J. Respir. Cell Mol. Biol.* **2011**, *44*, 725–738. [CrossRef] [PubMed]

pharmaceuticals

MDPI

Article

Investigating the Antibacterial, Antioxidant, and Anti-Inflammatory Properties of a Lycopene Selenium Nano-Formulation: An In Vitro and In Vivo Study

Reem Binsuwaidan [1], Thanaa A. El-Masry [2], Maysa M. F. El-Nagar [2,*], Enas I. El Zahaby [3], Mohamed M. S. Gaballa [4] and Maisra M. El-Bouseary [5,*]

[1] Department of Pharmaceutical Sciences, College of Pharmacy, Princess Nourah bint Abdulrahman University, P.O. Box 84428, Riyadh 11671, Saudi Arabia; rabinsuwaidan@pnu.edu.sa
[2] Department of Pharmacology and Toxicology, Faculty of Pharmacy, Tanta University, Tanta 31527, Egypt; thanaa.elmasri@pharm.tanta.edu.eg
[3] Department of Pharmaceutics, Faculty of Pharmacy, Delta University for Science and Technology, Gamasa 35712, Egypt; enas.elzahabi@deltauniv.edu.eg
[4] Department of Pathology, Faculty of Veterinary Medicine, Benha University, Toukh 13736, Egypt; mohamed.gaballah@fvtm.bu.edu.eg
[5] Department of Microbiology and Immunology, Faculty of Pharmacy, Tanta University, Tanta 31527, Egypt
* Correspondence: maysa_elnagar@outlook.com (M.M.F.E.-N.); maysra_mohamed@pharm.tanta.edu.eg (M.M.E.-B.)

Abstract: Background: The potent antioxidant lycopene has attracted a large amount of research attention given its potential health benefits. We aimed to assess the antimicrobial, anti-inflammatory, and antioxidant properties of lycopene (Lyc), selenium nanoparticles (Se-NPs), and lycopene selenium nanoparticles (Lyc-Se-NPs). Methods: FTIR, polydispersity index, and zeta potential evaluations provided a complete characterization of the synthesized Lyc-Se-NPs. The broth dilution method and a crystal violet microtiter plate assay were employed to assess the antibacterial and antibiofilm activity, respectively. The rat wound infection model was performed to study the anti-inflammatory effect. Findings: The Lyc-Se-NPs had a zeta potential range of −16.93 to −31.04 mV and a mean particle size of 126.6 ± 3.12 nm. All peaks' percentage transmittance decreased, according to the FTIR analysis of the Lyc-Se-NPs, with the exception of one peak at 2924.22 cm^{-1}, which is suggestive of C-H stretching. The mean scavenging concentrations for Lyc-Se-NPs in the DPPH and ABTS radical scavenging experiments were 3.85 ± 0.65 and 4.26 ± 0.7 μg/mL, respectively. For *S. aureus*, the Lyc-Se-NPs' MIC values varied from 64 to 1024 μg/mL. CLSM verified that *S. aureus* treated with sub-MICs of Lyc-Se-NPs showed a significant reduction in biofilm formation. Furthermore, the group treated with 50 mg of Lyc-Se-NPs showed the quickest rate of wound healing. They demonstrated a notable elevation of the HO^{-1} content in skin tissues, together with the greatest downregulation of TNF-α, IL-1β, and COX-2. Conclusions: The distinguishing features of Lyc-Se-NPs reveal that this unique compound is a promising antibacterial, antioxidant, and anti-inflammatory agent.

Keywords: lycopene selenium nanoparticles; antibacterial; anti-inflammatory; antioxidant; wound infection

1. Introduction

Plants are the greatest source of a wide range of medications, and approximately 80% of people in more economically developed countries use traditional medicine today [1].

Carotenoids are significant phytoconstituents that are thought to be largely responsible for fruits' and vegetables' health-protective properties [2].

The carotenoid lycopene is the pigment that provides tomatoes, melons, papayas, and red peppers with their distinctive red hue [3]. Tomatoes are one of the main sources of lycopene [4], which makes up 65–98% of the total weight of carotenoids in tomatoes, depending on the variety [4]. Lycopene is a widely used pigment that is well-liked by the food industry for both its nutritional value and culinary addition status [5]. Moreover, lycopene is a potent antioxidant that has attracted a lot of attention for its related health benefits. For instance, it is well-known for its capacity to neutralize oxidative stress and scavenge free radicals, both of which can be related to the treatment of many chronic illnesses, such as cancer, cardiovascular disease, and age-associated degeneration of eyes [6]. Also, lycopene may have antibacterial properties due to its antioxidant activity. Unfortunately, its use as a treatment option has been highly restricted due to its sensitivity to oxidants, light, and heat; its inability to dissolve in water; its minimal solubility in oils at ambient temperatures; its low bioavailability (10–30% of dietary lycopene) [7]; and the fact that it forms crystals during storage due to its high melting point. However, by using lycopene in the form of polymeric nanoparticles (NPs), these disadvantages of the phytochemical can be overcome. It is commonly recognized that polymeric nanoparticles (NPs) improve a formulation's solubility, stability, absorption, and drug-loading capability [8].

Selenium is a key element, forming a structural component of antioxidant enzymes including glutathione peroxidase and thioredoxin reducates [9]. As such, it may assume a vital function in preserving health, meaning selenium has garnered increasing attention in recent years [10]. Thyroid hormone metabolism and other critical metabolic processes, as well as the proper operation of the immune system, depend on selenium. The element also prevents oxidative-stress-induced cell death by integrating with antioxidant enzymes. Moreover, selenoproteins (proteins containing selenium) are important for redox control and the elimination of reactive oxygen species (ROS) [11], as well as important to the antioxidant, antimicrobial, and antitumor systems [12].

Traditional selenium compounds are used sparingly since the safe dose level is low, limiting their applicability, but nanometer-sized materials have properties that differ from those of bulk materials, and some of them have found entirely new applications. Elemental selenium is one of these materials [13], with selenium nanoparticles (Se-NPs) found to be a more effective and safe form of selenium that has high bioavailability and low toxicity [14].

Furthermore, a pioneering study demonstrated Se-NPs' antibacterial activity. The authors found that Se-NPs with a diameter of roughly 100 nm effectively suppress the development of *Staphylococcus aureus* at concentrations as low as 7.8 μg/mL [15]. The majority of their trials also showed significant antibacterial efficiency against *Enterococcus faecalis*, *Streptococcus mutans*, and *Porphyromonas gingivalis*, as well as low toxicity and excellent antioxidant action [15].

Wounds pose a significant worldwide health issue to medical facilities, medical personnel, patients, and their families, with serious social and economic implications [16]. Plants have traditionally been used over the centuries as both preventative and therapeutic measures for the wounded. Many plant concoctions, including the leaves of *Marrubium vulgare* L., *Aloe vera*, and *Elaeis guineensis Jacq*, have been used to treat wounds [17]. When the skin is harmed, the body naturally responds by healing the wound, which involves passing through four predetermined phases—hemostasis, inflammation, proliferation, and remodeling [18]. Since numerous elements are involved, the process of wound healing is complicated. Bacteria and fungi can easily colonize wounds, impeding the healing process. In order to prevent sepsis-causing infections of deeper bodily tissues and blood circulation, physicians advise applying topical antibiotics [19]. However, some topical antibiotics exhibit cytotoxicity, which hinders the healing of wounds. Additionally, wound healing and cleaning may be hampered by antibiotic resistance. As an alternative, given their antibacterial, wound-healing, and biocompatible qualities, medicinal plant formulations can be used with some success [20].

Consequently, this investigation assessed the antibacterial, antioxidant, and anti-inflammatory properties of selenium/lycopene nanoparticles in comparison to the utilization of these two elements independently. To the best of our knowledge, this is the first research to investigate the antibacterial and antibiofilm activity of lycopene and a lycopene-selenium nanoformulation against *S. aureus* clinical isolates.

2. Results

2.1. Characterization of Lycopene, Selenium Nanoparticles, and Selenium/Lycopene Nanoparticles

In this study, the SeNPs were synthesized by a simple wet chemical approach from ascorbic acid with biocompatibility and good reducing characteristics utilizing poloxamer 407 as a stabilizer.

Dynamic Light Scattering (DLS) analysis revealed a single peak with 94.62 ± 0.79% intensity and a mean particle size of 126.6 ± 3.12 nm. The zeta potential ranged from −16.93 to −31.04 mV, with an average of −23.47 ± 7.11 mV. The average value of the PDI was 0.3271 ± 0.023 (Table 1). The average drug content of the colloidal dispersion was 31.85 ± 3.33 µg/mL.

Table 1. Particle size, zeta potential, and polydispersity index (PDI) of lycopene nanoparticles.

Character	Mean ± SD	Range
Particle size (nm)	126.6 ± 3.12	124.6 to 130.2
Zeta potential mV	−23.47 ± 7.11	−16.93 to −31.04
PDI	0.3271 ± 0.023	0.31 to 0.35
Drug content (µg/mL)	31.85 ± 3.33	29.40 to 35.64

The SEM examination of lycopene (magnification power 3000) illustrated irregular flakes, while selenium nanoparticles (magnification 40,000) contained homogenous spherical particles, and lycopene nanoparticles (magnification 40,000) showed almost the same appearance as selenium nanoparticles (Figure 1A(a,b)). A TEM examination of the lycopene nanoparticles also showed the spherical shape of the nanoparticles, with a particle size less than 100 nm (Figure 1A(d)).

FTIR of lycopene showed the characteristic peak at 2925.21 cm^{-1}, which corresponds to C-H stretching. Then, FTIR of selenium/lycopene nanoparticles revealed a decrease in the percentage transmittance of all peaks, except for the peak at 2924.22 cm^{-1}, which corresponds to C-H stretching. The FTIR of selenium nanoparticles did not exhibit the C-H stretching at 2925.21 cm^{-1}. A characteristic peak was observed at 3285.27 cm^{-1} which represents the hydroxyl group and the peak for C=O stretching around 1700 cm^{-1} (Figure 1B) [21].

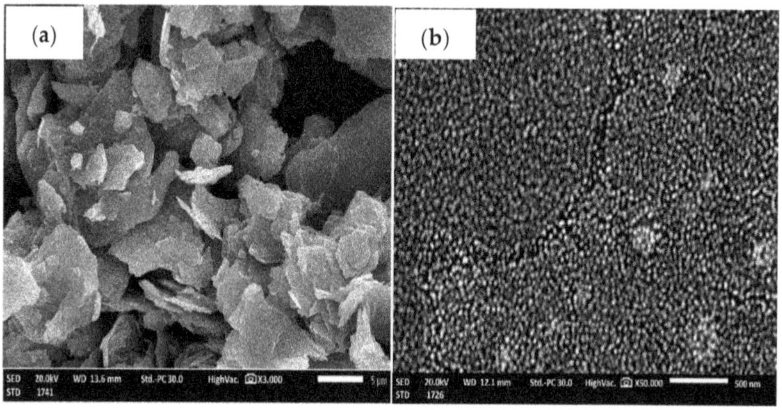

Figure 1. *Cont.*

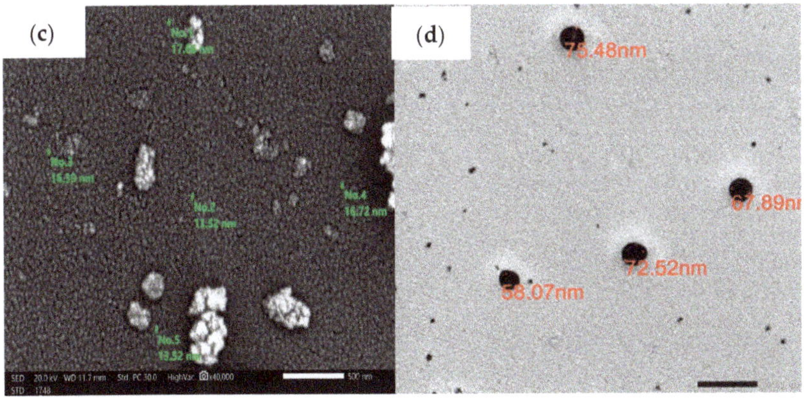

(A)

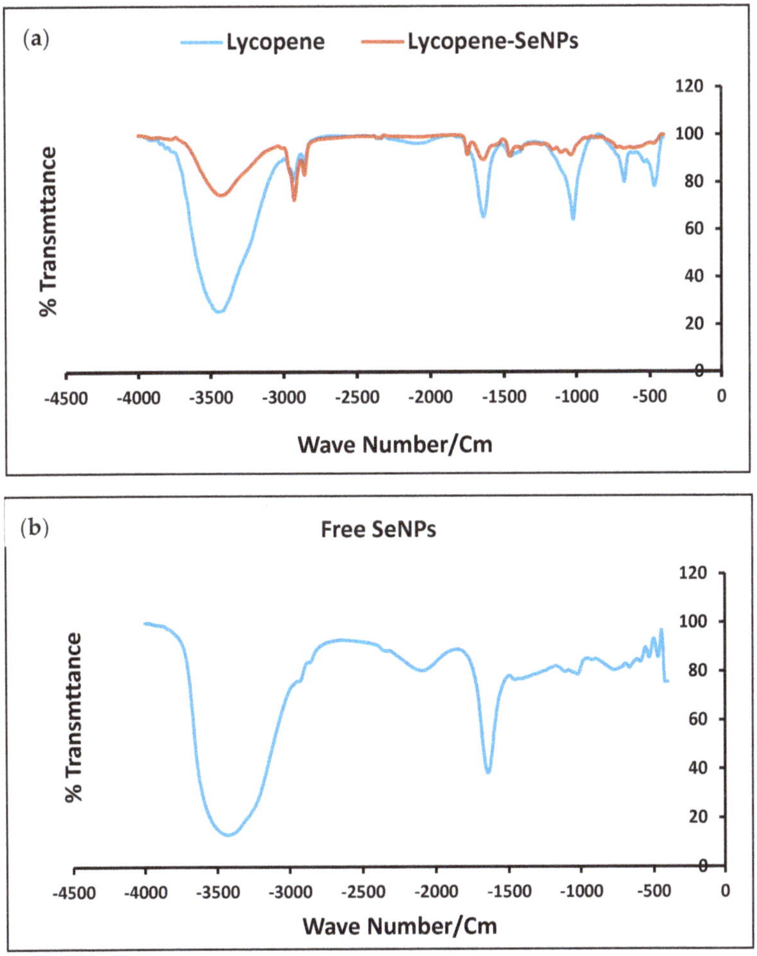

(B)

Figure 1. (**A**) SEM of lycopene (**a**), selenium nanoparticles (**b**), and selenium/lycopene nanoparticles (**c**), and TEM of selenium/lycopene nanoparticles (**d**). (**B**) FTIR of lycopene and selenium/lycopene nanoparticles (**a**), and FTIR of Selenium nanoparticles (**b**).

2.2. *Antioxidant Activity Assay*

2.2.1. DPPH Radical Scavenging Assay

To assess the antioxidant activity, the DPPH radical scavenging activity was quantified (Figure 2A). Treatments with free Se-NPs, lycopene, and Lyc-Se-NPs were found to generate concentration-dependent DPPH radical scavenging activity (Figure 2A). Lyc-Se-NPs showed superior activity over free Se-NPs and lycopene. The mean scavenging concentrations (IC_{50}, expressing 50% of scavenging) were 7.73 ± 1.4, 6.48 ± 0.95, and 3.85 ± 0.65 μg/mL for free Se-NPs, lycopene, and lycopene-Se-NPs, respectively, while the IC_{50} of ascorbic acid as a positive control was 2.53 μg/mL (Figure 2A).

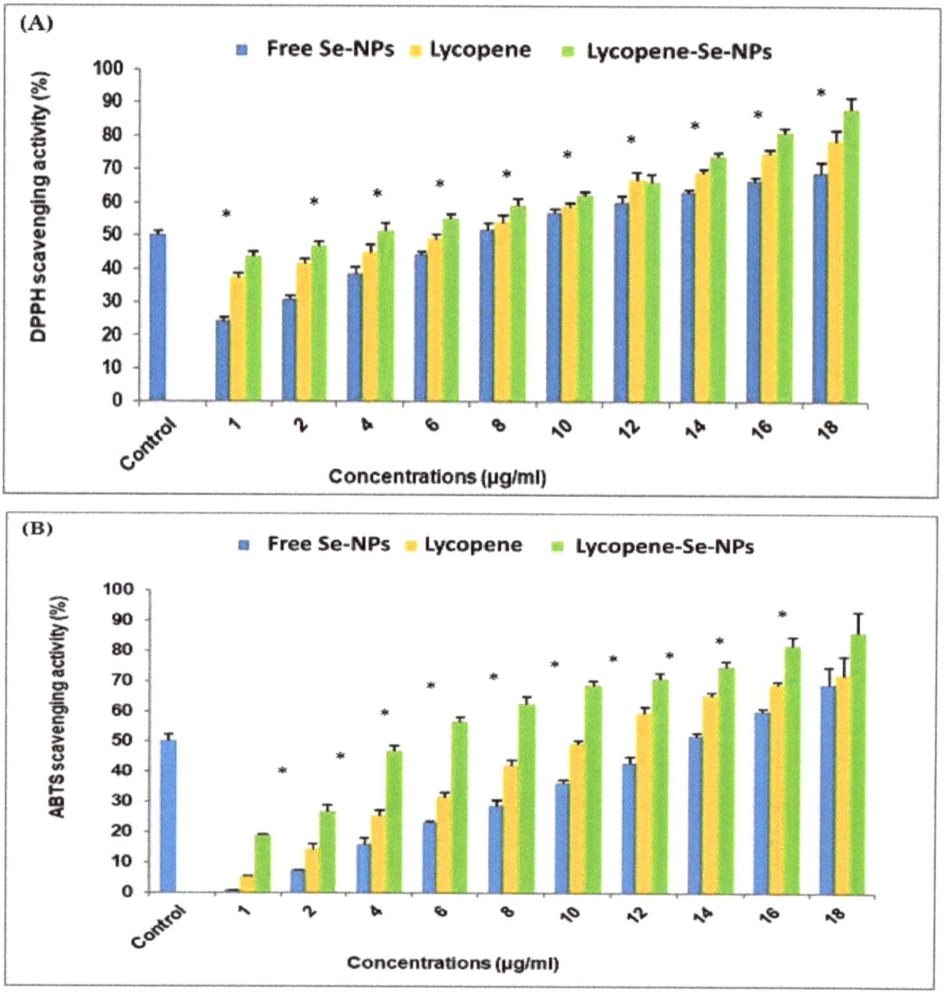

Figure 2. The antioxidant activity of free Se-NPs, lycopene, and Lyc-Se-NPs, evaluated by a DPPH radical scavenging assay (**A**) and ABTS radical scavenging assay (**B**). Results are expressed as the mean ± SD (n = 3). Control: ascorbic acid, Se-NPs: selenium nanoparticles. * Significant vs. control group (ascorbic acid) per each concentration ($p < 0.05$).

2.2.2. ABTS Radical Scavenging Assay

The DPPH and ABTS assay findings were similar, with the Lyc-Se-NP antioxidant efficacy exceeding that of free Se-NPs and Lyc (Figure 2B). The IC_{50} values of the ABTS scavenging assay were established to be 13.42 ± 1.09, 10.14 ± 2.6, and 4.26 ± 0.7 µg/mL for free Se-NPs, lycopene, and lycopene-Se-NPs, respectively, while the IC_{50} of gallic acid as a positive control was 2.55 µg/mL (Figure 2B).

2.3. In Vitro Antibacterial Activity

Lycopene (Lyc) and lycopene selenium nanoparticles (Lyc-Se-NPs) displayed antibacterial activity against the *S. aureus* reference strain, as determined via the agar-well diffusion method (Table 2).

Table 2. Inhibition zone diameters of the tested compounds against different bacterial strains.

Bacterial Reference Strain	Inhibition Zone Diameter (mm)				
	Lyc	Selenium	Lyc-Se-NPs	Gentamicin	DMSO
S. aureus (ATCC 25923)	11.3 ± 0.58 [#a]	12 ± 0.00 [*#a]	17.3 ± 0.58 *	18 ± 1.00 *	10 ± 0.00
E. coli (ATCC 25922)	11 ± 0.00 #	11 ± 1.00 #	12 ± 0.00 *#	20.67 ± 0.58 *	10 ± 0.00
P. aeruginosa (ATCC 27853)	11 ± 0.00 #	11 ± 0.00 #	12 ± 1.00 *#	20 ± 1.00 *	10 ± 0.00
P. mirabilis (ATCC 35659)	10 ± 0.00 #	10 ± 0.00 #	10.67 ± 0.58 #	16.67 ± 0.58 *	10 ± 0.00
K. pneumoniae (ATCC 700603)	11 ± 1.00 #	10 ± 0.00 #	11 ± 0.00 #	20 ± 2.00 *	10 ± 0.00

Data were recorded as the mean ± SD (n = 3). * Significant vs. DMSO, # significant vs. gentamicin, [a] significant vs. Lyc-Se-NPs. Se-NPs: selenium nanoparticles. Each group differed significantly from the others at $p \leq 0.05$.

A broth microdilution assay was employed to determine the MIC values of Lyc, selenium, and Lyc-Se-NPs against *S. aureus* isolates (n = 20) (see Supplementary Table S1), which ranged from 256 to 1024 µg/mL and from 64 to 1024 µg/mL for Lyc and Lyc-Se-NPs, respectively (Table 3).

Table 3. MIC values of Lyc, selenium, and Lyc-Se-NPs against the tested *S. aureus* clinical isolates (n = 20).

MIC (µg/mL)	Number of Isolates (%)			
	Lyc	Selenium	Lyc-Se-NPs	Gentamicin
16	0 (0)	0 (0)	0 (0)	3 (15)
32	0 (0)	0 (0)	0 (0)	5 (25)
64	0 (0)	0 (0)	8 (40)	5 (25)
128	0 (0)	0 (0)	4 (20)	4 (20)
256	3 (15)	0 (0)	5 (25)	2 (10)
512	7 (35)	1 (5)	2 (10)	1 (5)
1024	4 (20)	2 (10)	1 (5)	0 (0)
>1024	6 (30)	17 (85)	0 (0)	0 (0)

2.4. Growth Curves of S. aureus Clinical Isolates

The impacts of 1/2, 1/4, and 1/8 MICs of the tested compounds on the bacterial growth curve were tested to determine the best concentrations, that is, those that did not affect the growth of bacteria, to be employed in further investigations (see Supplementary Figure S1). Our findings showed that1/4 and 1/8 MICs had no significant effect on the growth of *S. aureus* clinical isolates (Figure 3).

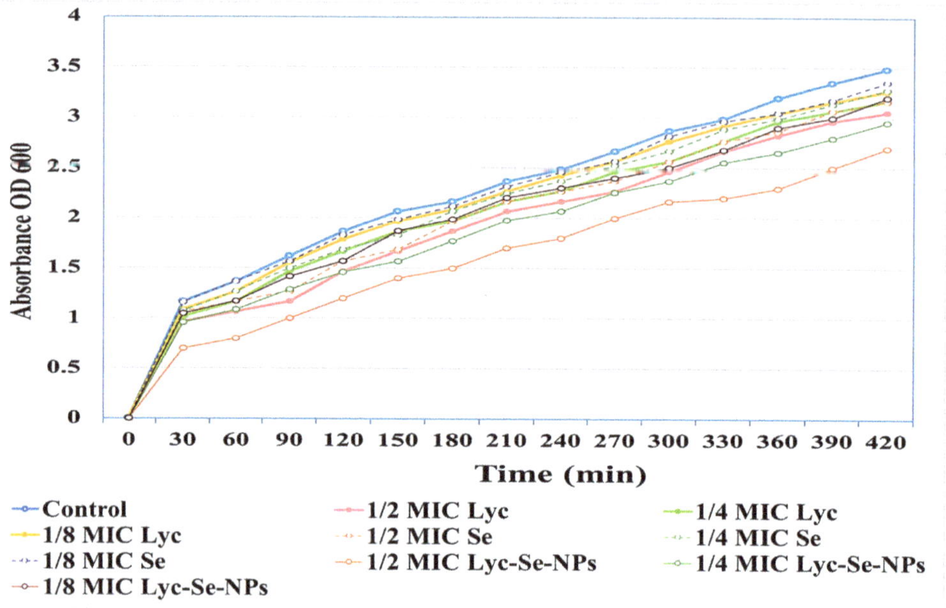

Figure 3. Growth curve of *S. aureus* (S16) clinical isolate cultured in the absence and presence of 1/2, 1/4, and 1/8 MICs of tested compounds at different time intervals.

2.5. In Vitro Antibiofilm Activity

The total number of biofilm-producing *S. aureus* isolates was reduced from 19 to 11, 16, and 18 following treatments with 1/2, 1/4, and 1/8 MICs of Lyc-Se-NPs, respectively (see Supplementary Table S1). Moreover, these treatments reduced the percentage of strong biofilm-forming isolates from 25% to 5%, 10%, and 15%, respectively (Table 4).

Table 4. Effect of the treatment by the tested compounds at sub-MICs on the biofilm formation.

Categories of Biofilm Production	Number of Isolates (%)									
	Pre-Treatment	Post-Treatment								
		Lyc			Selenium			Lyc-Se-NPs		
		1/8 MIC	1/4 MIC	1/2 MIC	1/8 MIC	1/4 MIC	1/2 MIC	1/8 MIC	1/4 MIC	1/2 MIC
None	1 (5)	2 (10)	2 (10)	4 (20)	1 (5)	1 (5)	2 (10)	2 (10)	4 (20)	9 (45)
Weak	4 (20)	8 (40)	8 (40)	8 (40)	6 (30)	6 (30)	5 (25)	9 (45)	8 (40)	6 (30)
Moderate	10 (50)	6 (30)	6 (30)	5 (25)	8 (40)	8 (40)	8 (40)	6 (30)	6 (30)	4 (20)
Strong	5 (25)	4 (20)	4 (20)	3 (15)	5 (25)	5 (25)	5 (25)	3 (15)	2 (10)	1 (5)
Total producers	19 (95)	18 (90)	18 (90)	16 (80)	19 (95)	19 (95)	18 (90)	18 (90)	16 (80)	11 (55)

2.6. Confocal Laser Scanning Microscopy (CLSM)

The impact of 1/4 MICs of the tested compounds on *S. aureus* biofilm formation was confirmed using CLSM with the double-staining technique (Figure 4). The percentages of reduction after exposure to 1/4 MICs of Lyc, selenium, and Lyc-Se-NPs were 33.3, 11, and 66.7%, respectively (Figure 5).

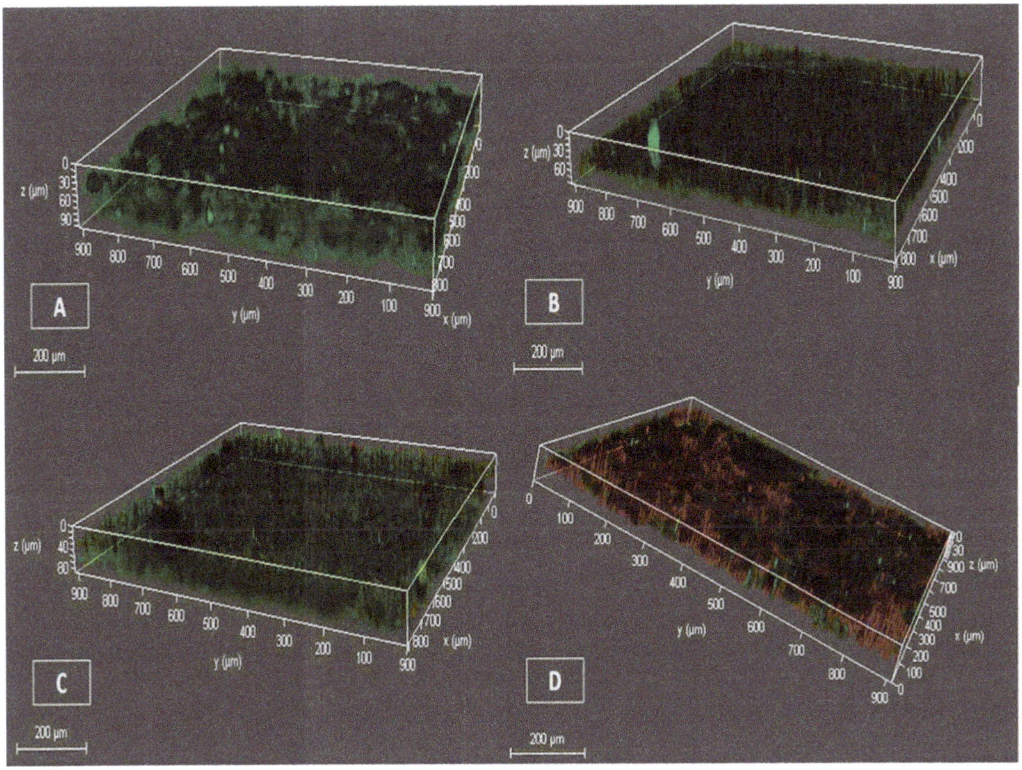

Figure 4. CLSM of *S. aureus* (S16) clinical isolate to detect biofilm thickness pre- and post-treatment with 1/4 MIC of the tested compounds. (**A**) Untreated *S. aureus* biofilm. (**B**) Lyc-treated biofilm. (**C**) Selenium-treated biofilm. (**D**) Lyc-Se-NP-treated biofilm.

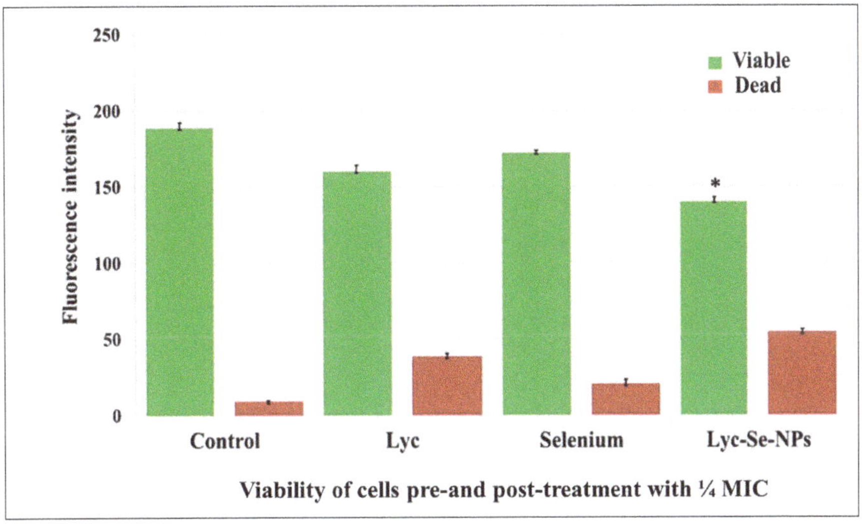

Figure 5. Change in fluorescence intensity with change in viability pre- and post-treatment with 1/4 MIC of the tested compounds. * Significant vs. untreated group ($p < 0.05$).

2.7. In Vivo Study

2.7.1. Wound Healing

On day two, the wound areas across all groups remained relatively similar, with minimal signs of healing. The untreated (Figure 6(A2)) group exhibited the largest wound areas, showing no notable signs of contraction or healing. In contrast, slight wound contraction was observed in the combination groups, specifically the gentamicin (Figure 6(B2)), Lyc-Se-NP (25 mg) (Figure 6(E2)), and Lyc-Se-NP (50 mg) (Figure 6(F2)) treatment groups. These groups demonstrated early signs of wound healing, albeit marginal, compared to the other groups. The lycopene-only (Figure 6(C2)) and free Se-NP (Figure 6(D2)) groups showed negligible changes in wound size in comparison to the untreated group.

In the same context, on day four, each group showed varying degrees of healing. The wound areas of the gentamicin (Figure 6(B4)), lycopene-only (Figure 6(C4)), free Se-NP (Figure 6(D4)), Lyc-Se-NP (25 mg) (Figure 6(E4)), and Lyc-Se-NP (50 mg) (Figure 6(F4)) treatment groups were notably smaller in comparison to those of the untreated (Figure 6(A4)) group. The Lyc-Se-NP group (50 mg) (Figure 6(F4)) exhibited the most significant reduction in wound size, indicating an accelerated healing process.

As time progressed, on day seven, the wound areas of each group decreased gradually. At this stage, each group displayed varying degrees of wound contraction and scabbing. The lycopene-only (Figure 6(C7)) and free Se-NP (Figure 6(D7)) groups showed significant healing, resulting in smaller wound areas compared to the untreated (Figure 6(A7)) group, but less than the gentamicin (Figure 6(B7)) group. The Lyc-Se-NP (25 mg) (Figure 6(E7)) and Lyc-Se-NP (50 mg) (Figure 6(F7)) groups demonstrated marked reductions in wound size compared to both the untreated (Figure 6(A7)) and gentamicin (Figure 6(B7)) groups, with the Lyc-Se-NP group (50 mg) (Figure 6(F7)) displaying the most advanced healing signs. Over time, all treatment groups showed a reduction in wound areas, with varying degrees of contraction and scabbing. The groups are arranged in order of healing efficacy as follows: Lyc-Se-NPs (50 mg) > Lyc-Se-NPs (25 mg) > gentamicin > lycopene only > free Se-NPs.

The Lyc-Se-NP (50 mg) treated group exhibited the fastest wound healing process, achieving near-complete healing within six days post-wounding in comparison to the control group. The wound regions in the Lyc-Se-NP group (50 mg) were nearly covered with epidermis, and the wound areas were almost completely closed. The average wound closure rate (WCR) is displayed in Table 5.

Table 5. Average wound closure rates (WCRs).

Groups	Day 2 (%)	Day 4 (%)	Day 7 (%)
Untreated	8.22 ± 0.23	12.58 ± 0.48	20.23 ± 0.43
Gentamicin	17.65 ± 0.19 *	34.05 ± 0.33 *	50.10 ± 0.45 *
Lycopene only	13.05 ± 0.22 *#	24.58 ± 0.23 *#	36.17 ± 0.62 *#
Free Se-NPs	12.15 ± 0.18 *#	23.15 ± 0.25 *#	35.67 ± 0.15 *#
Lyc-Se-NPs (25 mg)	21.17 ± 0.16 *#ab	40.08 ± 0.4 *#ab	60.35 ± 0.48 *#ab
Lyc-Se-NPs (50 mg)	25.13 ± 0.23 *#abc	45.22 ± 0.35 *#abc	70.23 ± 0.52 *#abc

Data were recorded as the mean ± SD (n = 6). * Significant vs. untreated group, # significant vs. gentamicin group, [a] significant vs. lycopene-only group, [b] significant vs. free Se-NP group, and [c] Lyc-Se-NPs (25 mg). Se-NPs: selenium nanoparticles. Each group differed significantly from the others at $p \leq 0.05$.

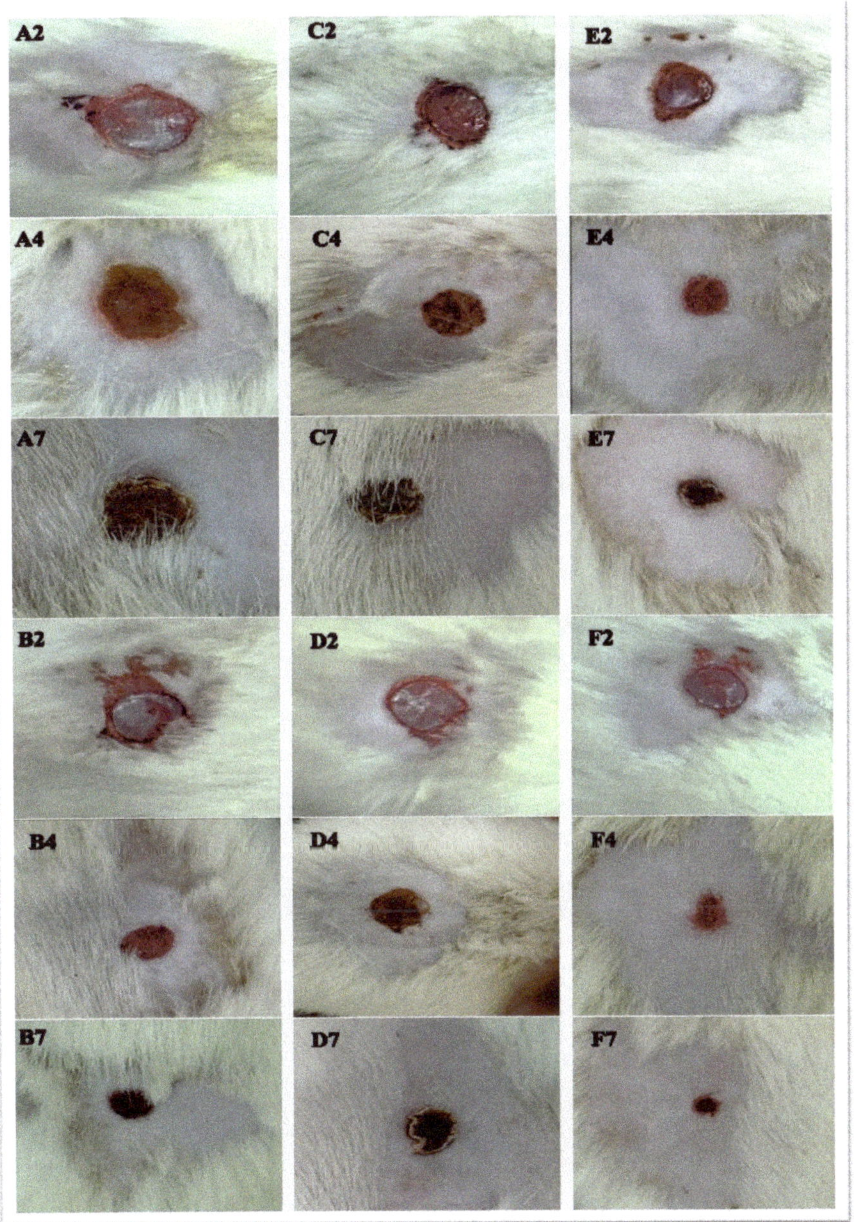

Figure 6. Experimental study of a rat wound-healing model untreated or after treatment with the standard, lycopene only, free Se-NPs, Lyc-Se-NPs (25 mg), or Lyc-Se-NPs (50 mg). The untreated group (**A2**,**A4**,**A7**) exhibited larger wound areas compared to the gentamicin (**B2**,**B4**,**B7**), lycopene-only (**C2**,**C4**,**C7**), free Se-NP (**D2**,**D4**,**D7**), Lyc-Se-NP (25 mg) (**E2**,**E4**,**E7**), and Lyc-Se-NP (50 mg) (**F2**,**F4**,**F7**) groups.

2.7.2. Impacts of Different Treatments on Inflammatory Markers (TNF-α, IL-1β, and COX-2) Contents in Skin Tissues

The results showed that the contents of inflammatory markers (TNF-α, IL-1β, and COX-2) declined in all treatment groups, but to varying degrees (Figure 7A–C). The Lyc-Se-NP (50 mg) treatment demonstrated the most pronounced downregulating effects (Figure 7A–C).

Lyc-Se-NPs (50 mg) and Lyc-Se-NPs (25 mg) induced a significant reduction in the levels of inflammatory markers TNF-α (76.34 and 71.81%, respectively), IL-1β (892.04 and 82.31%, respectively), and COX-2 (94.35 and 79.42%, respectively) in comparison with the untreated control group. In addition, the gentamicin-treated group displayed notable anti-inflammatory activity, as revealed by a marked decrease in TNF-α, IL-1β, and COX-2 levels (58.84%, 53.75%, and 25%, respectively) compared to the untreated group (Figure 7A–C).

Furthermore, Lyc-Se-NPs (50 mg) and Lyc-Se-NPs (25 mg) brought about a significant reduction in the levels of inflammatory markers TNF-α, IL-1β, and COX-2 compared to the lycopene-only and free Se-NP groups (Figure 7A–C).

2.7.3. Impacts of Different Treatments on the Anti-Inflammatory Marker (HO-1) Content in Skin Tissues

According to the results, all treatment groups showed an increase in anti-inflammatory marker (HO-1) content, but to varying degrees (Figure 8). Lyc-Se-NP (50 mg) treatment produced the most notable downregulating effects. Figure 8 shows that treatments with gentamicin, lycopene only, free Se-NPs, Lyc-Se-NPs (25 mg), and Lyc-Se-NPs (50 mg) produced remarkable amplification of 4.67, 3.74, 3.38, 5.54, and 7.67-fold, respectively, in HO-1 content compared to the untreated group (Figure 8). In addition, treatment with Lyc-Se-NPs (50 mg) produced substantial increases of 82.94%, 97.69%, and 32.61% in HO-1 content compared to lycopene only, free Se-NPs, and Lyc-Se-NPs (25 mg), respectively (Figure 8).

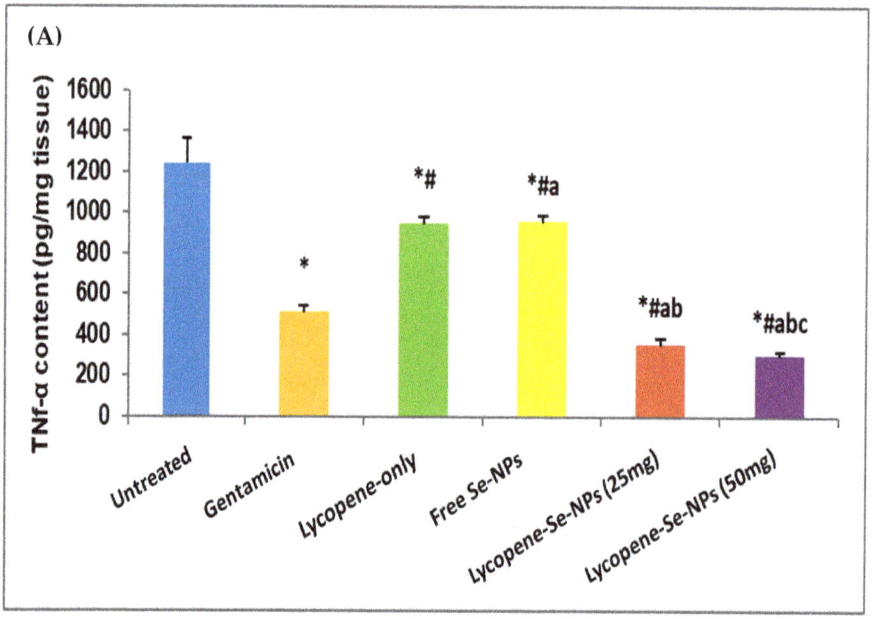

Figure 7. *Cont.*

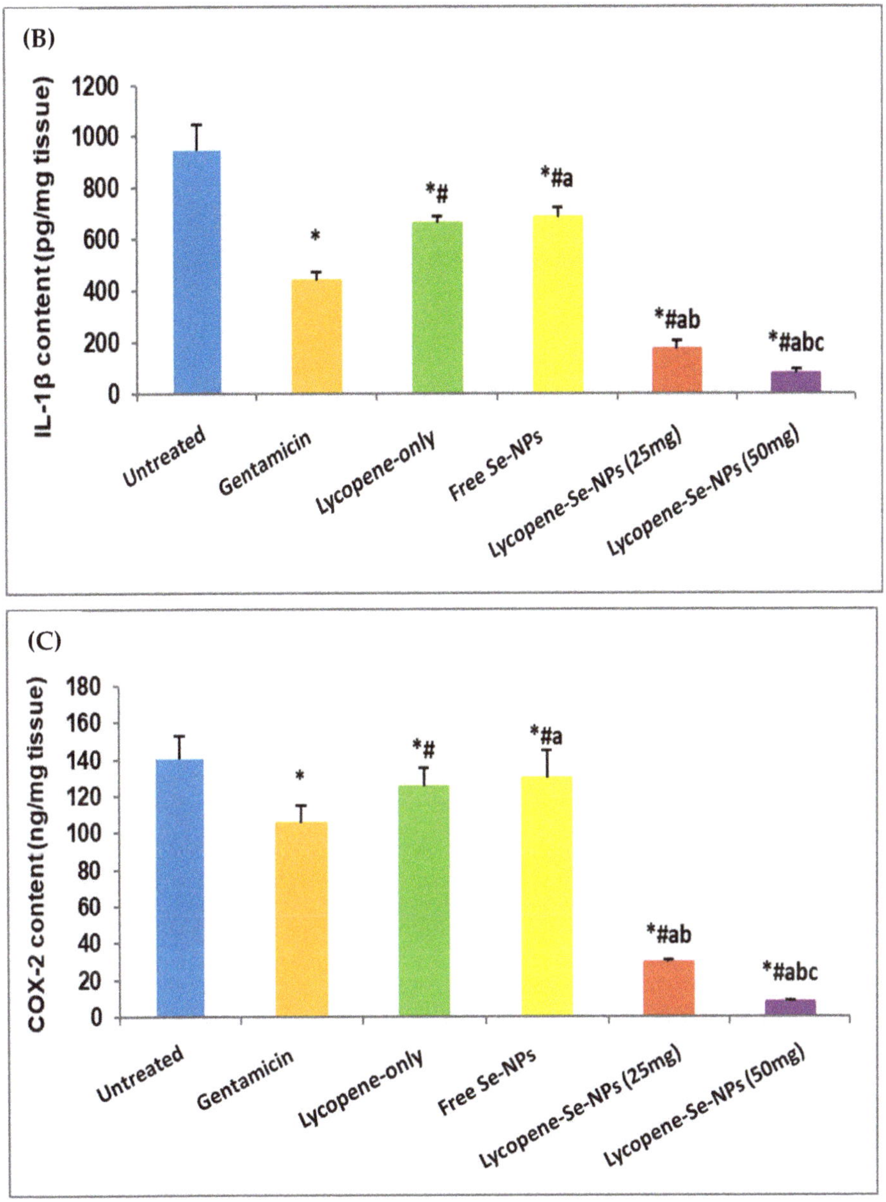

Figure 7. Impacts of different treatments on contents of inflammatory markers TNF-α (**A**), IL-1β (**B**), and COX-2 (**C**) in skin tissues. Data were recorded as mean ± SD (n = 6). * Significant vs. untreated group, [#] significant vs. gentamicin group, [a] significant vs. lycopene-only group, [b] significant vs. free Se-NP group, and [c] Lyc-Se-NPs (25 mg). Se-NPs: selenium nanoparticles. Each group differed significantly from the others at $p < 0.05$.

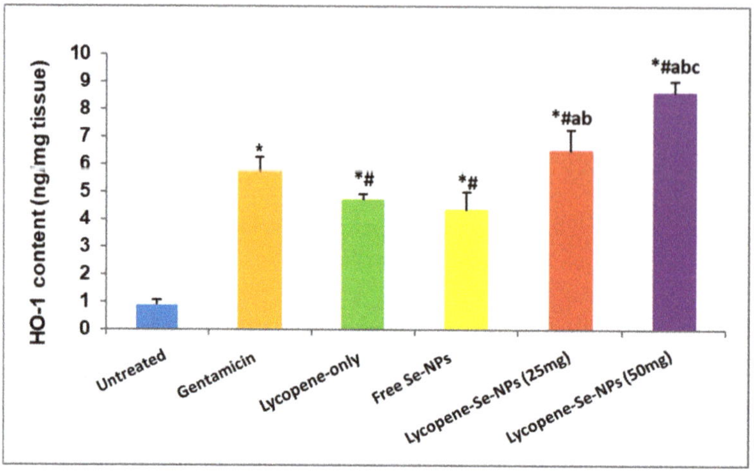

Figure 8. Impacts of different treatments on anti-inflammatory marker (HO-1) content in skin tissues. Data were recorded as mean ± SD ($n = 6$). * Significant vs. untreated group, # significant vs. gentamicin group, [a] significant vs. lycopene-only group, [b] significant vs. free Se-NP group, and [c] Lyc-Se-NPs (25 mg). Se-NPs: selenium nanoparticles. Each group differed significantly from the others at $p < 0.05$.

2.7.4. Histopathological Evaluation of Skin

The skin section in the untreated group demonstrated delayed healing with persistent fibrin deposition, no granulation tissue, ulceration, scab formation, tissue debris, and inflammatory cell infiltration. The epidermis exhibited necrotic areas and a loss of epithelial integrity (Figure 9(A1)). The dermis had a severe inflammatory infiltrate featuring neutrophils and macrophages (Figure 9(A2)).

In contrast, in the gentamicin group, there was evidence of a more advanced healing process at the wound site, including the initial formation of granulation tissue and early collagen deposition, indicating improved wound healing. The epidermis showed moderate re-epithelialization, with a few layers of epithelial epidermal cells formed under the scab (Figure 9(B1)). The dermis exhibited an insignificant inflammatory response with fewer neutrophils (Figure 9(B2)).

In the lycopene-only group, the epidermis exhibited mild preservation of its architecture, with fewer necrotic areas. The dermis showed a mild to moderate inflammatory response, with a reduced presence of neutrophils and macrophages (Figure 9(C1)). The wound site showed enhanced granulation tissue formation and improved collagen organization, indicating accelerated wound closure (Figure 9(C2)).

Similarly to the lycopene-only group, in the free Se-NP group, the epidermis displayed preserved layers, with one to two layers of degenerated epithelial epidermal cells formed under the scab. The dermis showed a mild inflammatory infiltrate, predominantly lymphocytic (Figure 9(D1)). The wound site exhibited enhanced vascularization and increased collagen synthesis, promoting early tissue repair (Figure 9(D2)).

With Lyc-Se-NP (25 mg) treatment, the epidermis maintained an intact barrier with minimal signs of necrosis and more healthy epidermal layers (Figure 9(E1)). The dermis had a mild inflammatory response, with a balanced presence of neutrophils and macrophages (Figure 9(E2)). The wound site exhibited robust granulation tissue formation and collagen remodeling, indicating the synergistic effects of Lyc and selenium.

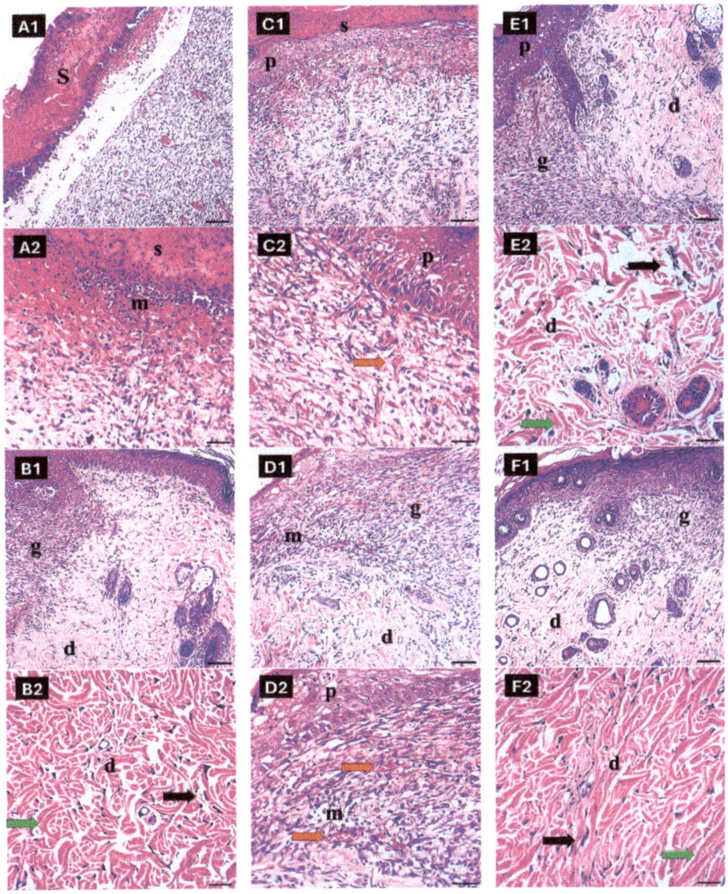

Figure 9. Histopathological examination of wound healing and tissue integrity across different study groups. In the untreated group (**A1**,**A2**), delayed wound healing is evident, characterized by persistent fibrin deposition, absence of granulation tissue, and extensive inflammatory cell infiltration. The epidermis shows necrotic areas and disrupted epithelial integrity, while the dermis exhibits severe inflammatory infiltration with neutrophils and macrophages. The gentamicin group (**B1**,**B2**) demonstrates advanced healing with initial granulation tissue formation and early collagen deposition. The epidermis displays moderate re-epithelialization, and the dermis shows a significantly reduced inflammatory response. In the lycopene-only group (**C1**,**C2**), mild preservation of epidermal architecture and reduced necrosis can be observed. Enhanced granulation tissue formation and improved collagen organization indicate accelerated wound closure. The free Se-NP group (**D1**,**D2**) similarly shows preserved epidermal layers, mild inflammatory infiltrate (predominantly lymphocytic), and increased vascularization and collagen synthesis at the wound site, suggesting improved early tissue repair. The Lyc-Se-NP (25 mg) group (**E1**,**E2**) exhibits intact epidermal layers, minimal necrosis, and a balanced inflammatory response with robust granulation tissue and collagen remodeling, reflecting the synergistic effects of the treatment. In the Lyc-Se-NP (50 mg) group (**F1**,**F2**), the skin structure is well organized with complete preservation of epidermal layers and advanced wound closure. Dense collagen bundles and mature vascular networks are prominent, indicating the optimal therapeutic efficacy of the high-dose combination. Scab (S), granulation tissue (g), dermis (d), epidermis (p), inflammatory cells (m), and arrow mark for neovascularization (red arrow), fibroblast infiltration (black arrow), and fibrous tissue (green arrow).

Moreover, when treated with Lyc-Se-NPs (50 mg), the skin had a well-organized architecture, with the three main layers (epidermis, dermis, and hypodermis) distinguishable. Plenty of sebaceous glands and hair follicles were in various stages of maturation. The epidermis showed complete preservation of its layers, with no signs of necrosis. The normal keratinization process over the entire wound confirmed the full differentiation of keratinocytes (Figure 9(F1)). The wound site showed advanced closure, with dense collagen bundles and mature vascular networks (Figure 9(F2)), indicating the optimal therapeutic efficacy of Lyc-Se-NPs (50 mg). The semiquantitative scoring of wound healing parameters is presented in Table 6.

Table 6. Semi-quantitative scoring of wound healing parameters.

Parameter	Untreated	Gentamicin	Lycopene	Free Se-NPs	Lyc-Se-NPs (25 mg)	Lyc-Se-NPs (50 mg)
Necrosis	++++	++	+++	+++	+	ND
Inflammation	++++	+	++	++	+	ND
Granulation tissue	ND	++	++	++	+++	++++
Vascularization	+	+++	++	++	++	++++
Epithelization	ND	+++	+	+	+++	++++

In the scoring system, ND stands for "not detectable", + indicates a "mild score", ++ represents a "moderate score", +++ denotes a "moderate to high score", and ++++ signifies a "high score".

2.7.5. Masson's Trichrome Examination for Dermal Collagen (%) in Skin Sections

In the untreated group, the skin's outer layer (epidermis) showed a disrupted structure with a significant loss of epithelial integrity (Figure 10(A1)). The layer underneath (dermis) displayed insufficient collagen deposition and was mostly made up of fibrin with a lack of organized granulation tissue. The collagen fibers were poorly oriented and disorganized (Figure 10(A2)). In contrast, the gentamycin group showed partial preservation of epidermal architecture, with early re-epithelialization evident. Wound sites displayed the onset of collagen deposition (Figure 10(B1)). They improved connective tissue organization, with more orderly granulation tissue beginning to form, indicative of enhanced wound healing compared to the negative control (Figure 10(B2)).

The epidermis in the lycopene-only group exhibited better preservation with minimal necrosis (Figure 10(C1)). Enhanced collagen organization and granulation tissue formation at the wound site suggested accelerated wound closure and tissue repair (Figure 10(C2)). Similarly, the free Se-NP group displayed an intact epidermal barrier (Figure 10(D1)), with minimal necrosis and improved collagen synthesis and maturation, contributing to early tissue repair and wound closure (Figure 10(D2)).

The Lyc-Se-NP (25 mg) group showed a fully preserved epidermis with no necrotic areas (Figure 10(E1)), robust granulation tissue formation, and dense collagen bundles (Figure 10(E2)). This indicates a synergistic effect of lycopene and selenium in promoting wound healing. Similarly, the Lyc-Se-NP (50 mg) group maintained an intact epidermis with no necrotic areas (Figure 10(F1)), and the dermis showed advanced closure with dense collagen deposition and well-developed vascular networks (Figure 10(F2)), highlighting the optimal therapeutic effectiveness of Lyc-Se-NPs (50 mg). The results of our dermal collagen (%) evaluation are presented in Figure 11.

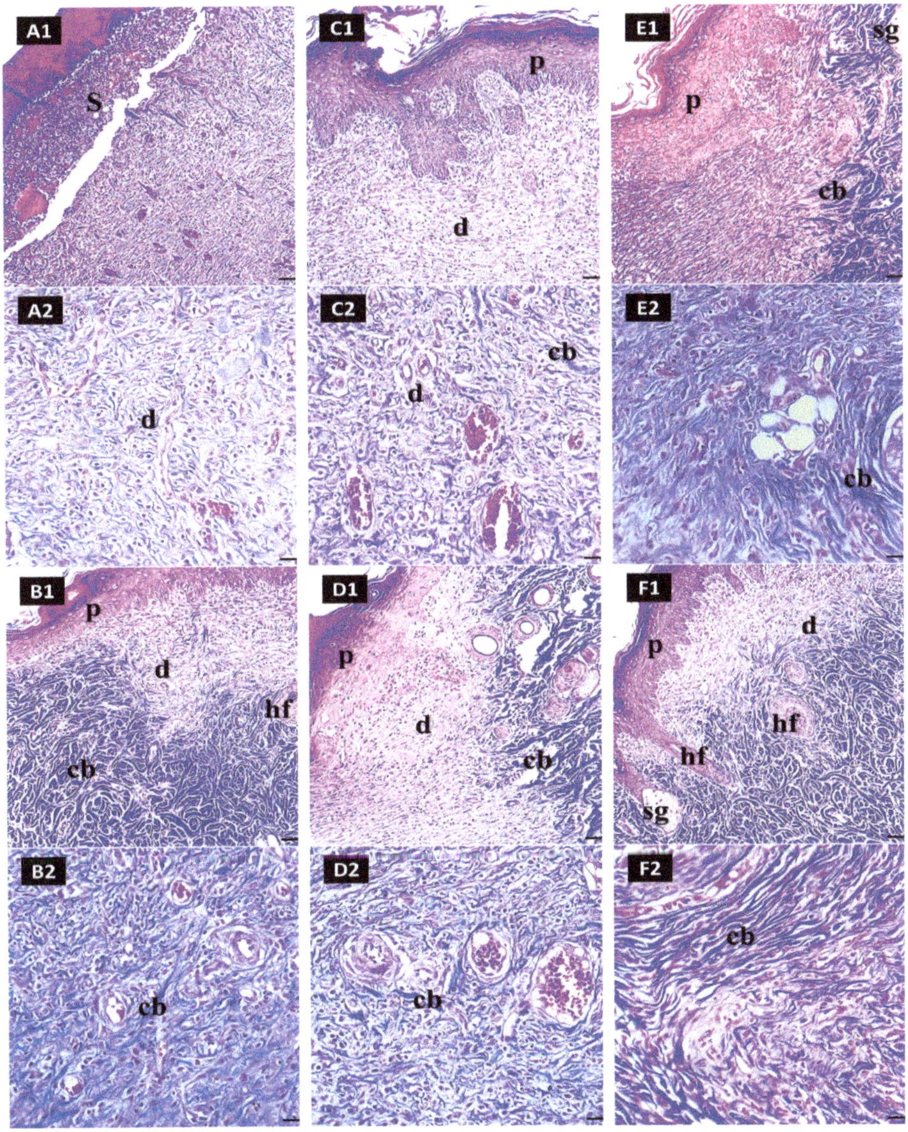

Figure 10. Histopathological assessment of wound healing across different treatments. The untreated group (**A1**,**A2**) exhibits a disrupted epidermal structure, poor collagen deposition, and disorganized fibers, reflecting inadequate wound repair. The gentamicin (**B1**,**B2**) group shows partial preservation of the epidermis, initial collagen deposition, and improved granulation tissue organization, indicating better healing. The lycopene-only group (**C1**,**C2**) has enhanced epidermal preservation and improved collagen organization, suggesting accelerated wound repair. The free Se-NP group (**D1**,**D2**) demonstrates an intact epidermis, minimal necrosis, and improved collagen synthesis. The Lyc-Se-NP (25 mg) group (**E1**,**E2**) shows complete epidermal preservation, robust granulation, and dense collagen bundles, indicating a synergistic effect of the treatments. The Lyc-Se-NP (50 mg) group (**F1**,**F2**) exhibits optimal healing with a well-preserved epidermis, advanced collagen deposition, and mature vascular networks, underscoring the efficacy of the high-dose combination. (p) epidermis, (d) dermis, (hf) hair follicles, (sg) sebaceous gland, (cb) collagen bundles, (S) scab.

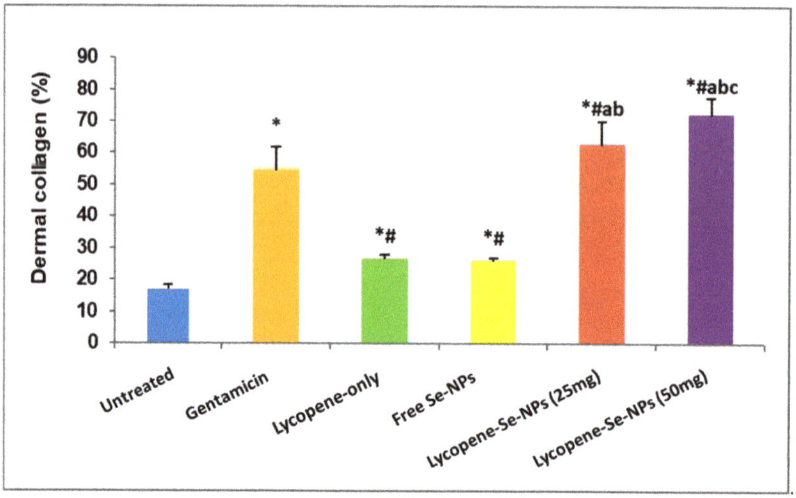

Figure 11. Dermal collagen (%) of skin sections. Data were recorded as mean ± SD (n = 6). * Significant vs. untreated group, # significant vs. gentamicin group, [a] significant vs., lycopene-only group, [b] significant vs. free Se-NP group, and [c] Lyc-Se-NPs (25 mg). Se-NPs: selenium nanoparticles. Each group differed significantly from the others at $p < 0.05$.

2.7.6. Immunohistochemical Staining of NF-κB-p65 in Skin Sections

Distinct variations in NF-κB-p65 activation across different treatment groups were observed when analyzing NF-κB-p65 staining as well as expression in the epidermis. The untreated group (Figure 12(A1,A2)) demonstrated a marked activation of NF-κB-p65, characterized by the highest staining and expression scores, indicating robust NF-κB-p65 activity. The gentamicin group (Figure 12(B1,B2)) showed mild NF-κB-p65 activation, with minor staining and expression levels reflecting a partial response. In contrast, treatments with lycopene only (Figure 12(C1,C2)) or free Se-NPs (Figure 12(D1,D2)) resulted in moderate NF-κB-p65 activation, as evidenced by lower staining and expression scores. In the Lyc-Se-NP (25 mg) group (Figure 12(E1,E2)), NF-κB-p65 activation was reduced further, but not as significantly as it was with the high-dose treatment. Notably, the Lyc-Se-NP (50 mg) group (Figure 12(F1,F2)) exhibited the lowest NF-κB-p65 activation, with minimal staining and expression levels, suggesting an effective suppression of NF-κB-p65 activity. The average scores and classification of NF-κB-p65 are presented in Table 7.

Table 7. Average scores and classification.

Group	Average Staining Score	Average Expression Score	Average Final Score	Classification
Untreated	2.6 ± 0.3	3.5 ± 0.42	10.5 ± 1.7	++++
Gentamicin	1.6 ± 0.52 *	2.1 ± 0.23 *	4.4 ± 1.6	++
Lycopene only	1.4 ± 0.12 *#	2.6 ± 0.21 *#	5.0 ± 1.8	+++
Free Se-NPs	1.5 ± 0.06 *#	2.5 ± 0.19 *#	7.3 ± 1.0	+++
Lyc-Se-NPs (25 mg)	1.3 ± 0.07 *#	1.5 ± 0.04 *#	3.0 ± 0.9	++
Lyc-Se-NPs (50 mg)	0.6 ± 0.08 *#abc	1.4 ± 0.02 *#abc	0.6 ± 0.5	+

Data were recorded as mean ± SD (n = 6). * Significant vs. untreated group, # significant vs. gentamicin group, [a] significant vs. lycopene-only group, [b] significant vs. free Se-NP group, and [c] Lyc-Se-NPs (25 mg). Se-NPs: selenium nanoparticles. Each group differed significantly from the others at $p < 0.05$. ++++: severe, +++ moderate, ++ mild, and + minimal.

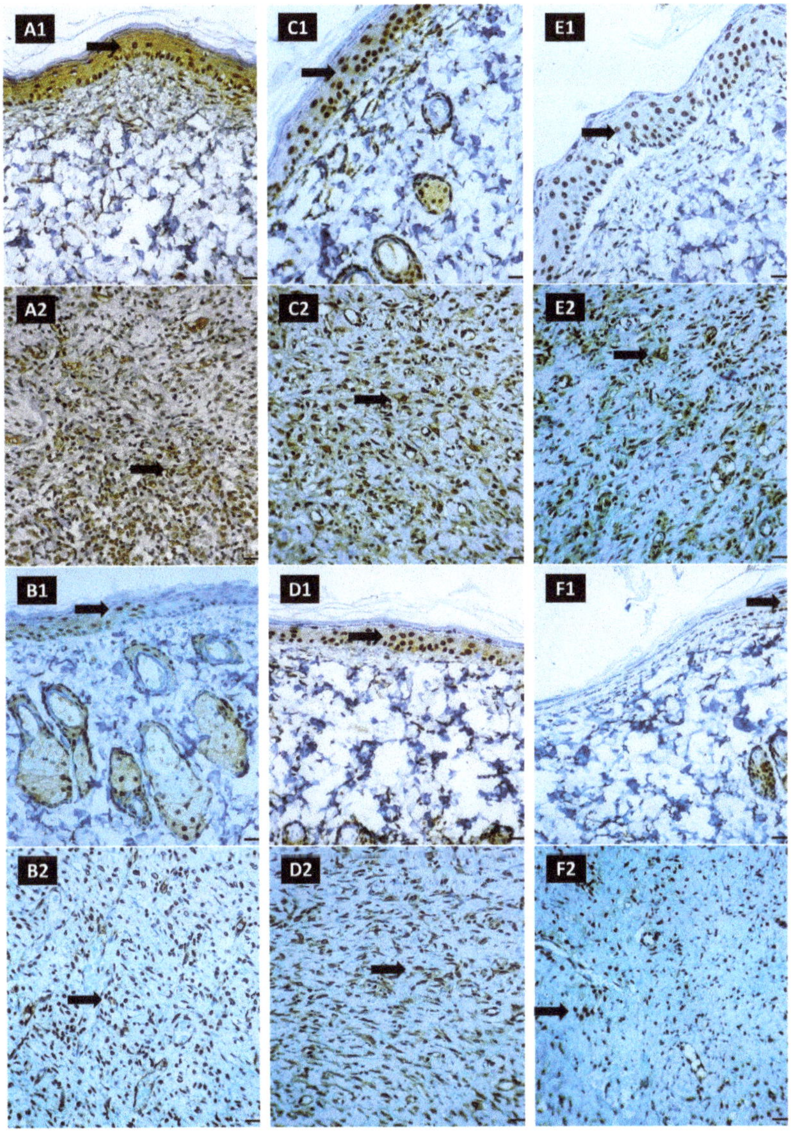

Figure 12. Analysis of NF-κB-p65 activation across different treatment groups. (**A1**,**A2**) show the untreated group with marked NF-κB-p65 activation, characterized by the highest staining and expression scores, indicating robust NF-κB activity. (**B1**,**B2**) depict the gentamicin group with mild NF-κB-p65 activation, evidenced by lower staining and expression levels, reflecting a partial response. (**C1**,**C2**) illustrate the effect of lycopene only, while (**D1**,**D2**) showed the effect of free Se-NPs, both resulting in moderate NF-κB-p65 activation with reduced staining and expression scores. (**E1**,**E2**) present the Lyc-Se-NP (25 mg) group, which further reduced NF-κB-p65 activation but not as effectively as the Lyc-Se-NP (50 mg) group. Finally, (**F1**,**F2**) demonstrate the Lyc-Se-NP (50 mg) group, with the lowest NF-κB-p65 activation, characterized by minimal staining and expression levels, indicating effective suppression of NF-κB-p65 activity. Black arrows indicate positive immunohistochemical expression.

3. Discussion

One of the several tetraterpene compounds included in tomatoes and tomato-based products is lycopene, a member of the carotenoids. It is widely acknowledged to be a strong antioxidant and a carotenoid that is not pro-vitamin A [22]. An investigation of a population in the United States found that lycopene is the predominant carotenoid in plasma and tissues [23]. Lycopene is beneficial in the management of inflammatory events, oxidative-stress-associated illness, diabetes mellitus, cardiovascular problems, and hepatic, neurological, reproductive, and skeletal disorders [23]. However, its application as a therapeutic agent has been severely limited due to its sensitivity to oxidizing agents, light, and temperature; difficulties dissolving in water; low solubility in oil at ambient temperature; and insufficient bioavailability [23].

The results demonstrated relatively small nanoparticles with an average hydrodynamic diameter of 126.6 $\pm$ 3.12 nm, which was confirmed by TEM, showing a smooth spherical particle (90 nm in diameter). Furthermore, the nanoparticles were adequately monodispersed, as indicated by the PDI value (0.3271 $\pm$ 0.023), and they had acceptable stabilities, as illustrated by the zeta potential (-23.47 ± 7.11 mV). Furthermore, FTIR illustrated the interaction between poloxamer 407 and lycopene with the appearance of a peak at 2924.22 cm^{-1}, which could be explained by carbon–hydrogen SP3 bending. As such, FTIR provided great evidence of the formation of metal nanoparticles, as illustrated by the decreases in the percentages of transmittance of almost all functional groups [24].

The results of this study showed that the Lyc-Se-NPs antioxidant, antibacterial, and anti-inflammatory efficacy exceeded those of free Se-NPs and lycopene.

Selenium supplements offer several health advantages, including protection against cancer, heart disease, diabetes, inflammation-related disorders, and the antioxidant system [25,26]. Regarding different selenium forms, reducing selenium to the nanoparticle form may lessen its toxicity. According to a prior study using a mouse model, selenium nanoforms are less harmful than their inorganic and organic counterparts, as demonstrated by the findings that animals treated with Se-NPs experienced less hepatic damage, fewer bone marrow cell deaths, and less DNA damage [27,28]. Moreover, it has been found that the selenium nanoform exhibits a greater antioxidant capacity than the elemental form.

Meanwhile, the most powerful antioxidant is lycopene. It is a crucial reactive oxygen species (ROS) deactivator. As an example, it can eliminate singlet oxygen two and ten times more efficiently than alpha-tocopherol and beta-carotene, respectively [29]. The health advantages of lycopene have garnered significant attention in recent times. Not only is it a strong antioxidant, but several published reviews and meta-analyses have also assessed and authorized its therapeutic efficacy in preventing and treating a broad range of disorders [30]. Moreover, previous research demonstrated that the presence of active ingredients like lycopene is responsible for tomato extract's antibacterial action against a variety of bacteria [27].

Concerning the antibacterial activity of the tested compounds, Lyc and Lyc-Se-NPs showed potential activity against *S. aureus*, with MIC values ranging from 256 to 1024 and 64 to 1024 µg/mL, respectively. Moreover, *S. aureus* treated with sub-MICs of Lyc and Lyc-Se-NPs showed significant antibiofilm action.

It is widely recognized that there are three main stages to the healing of a wound following hemostasis. In the initial stage, inflammation takes place, leading to the accumulation of neutrophils and macrophages at the site of the lesion. The proliferation stage comes next, during which re-epithelization, angiogenesis, granulation tissue development, and fibroplasia occur [28]. Ultimately, the remodeling phase is characterized by neovascularization and the onset of neocollagenesis. In this last stage, the wound heals more slowly. Reducing the healing time and avoiding negative side effects like scarring are the two main objectives of wound-healing interventions [28].

According to reports, sepsis brought on by a secondary bacterial infection, possibly by *P. aeruginosa* or *S. aureus*, can make wound healing extremely difficult. Furthermore, through the activation of inflammatory cytokines, inflammation plays a critical role in wound healing [31]. Pro-inflammatory cytokines have a crucial role in initiating inflammation, drawing out neutrophils, eliminating contaminants and pathogens from the site of the injury, and promoting the formation of metalloproteinases (MMPs). These MMPs are involved in the healing process by destroying damaged extracellular matrices (ECMs) to facilitate tissue restoration [32].

Conversely, prolonged inflammation may exacerbate tissue devastation, leading to chronic wounds, as the produced proteinases and cytokines may magnify tissue destruction [33]. Furthermore, inflammation severely devastates the surrounding tissues, and the injury may develop into a pathological condition that deserves more intensive care [33]. Therefore, anti-inflammatory medications are of great importance in helping treat wounds.

In addition to scavenging singlet ROS, lycopene also inhibits lipid peroxidation. It was demonstrated that HO-1 mRNA was increased by lycopene at 50 and 100 μM, but lycopene was unable to control the expression of COX-2 or NOS2 mRNA. Nevertheless, these doses inhibited the production of the LPS-stimulated COX-2, NOS2, and TNF-α genes in RAW264.7 cells [34]. Furthermore, lycopene protects against inflammation caused by β-amyloid. β-amyloid boosted the expression levels of TLR4, NF-κB p65 mRNA, and IL-6β, and the serum levels of IL-1β, TNF-α, and protein at the choroid plexus. Supplementation with lycopene reduced the levels of inflammatory cytokines, reversed the expression of Aβ1-42, and upregulated TLR4, NF-κB p65 mRNA, and protein at the choroid plexus [35].

In carrageenan-induced inflammation, lycopene supplementation (12.5 mg/kg BW) significantly reduced edema in Swiss mice, as determined by immunostaining for NF-κB, iNOS, and COX-2, and using different phlogistic chemicals. Additionally, it reduced the MPO concentration and leukocyte motility in paw tissue and the peritoneal cavity while raising GSH levels [34].

Additionally, studies have investigated lycopene at various levels (i.e., 0.5, 1.0, 2.0, 4.0, 8.0, 10.0, and 25 μM) for its potential to prevent inflammation brought on by cigarette smoking. Increases in TNF-α, interleukin-10, and interferon-γ concentrations were all reduced by lycopene [36]. In a recent study, Sprague Dawley rats were given a single 200 μg injection of LPS to elicit endotoxin-induced uveitis. Treatment with 10 mg/kg of lycopene intraperitoneally significantly reduced the raised total protein concentration, infiltrating cell number, NO, TNF-α, and IL-6 caused by LPS [37].

4. Materials and Methods

4.1. Drugs and Chemicals

Lycopene capsules (40 mg) were obtained from Puritan's Pride Inc., Ronkonkoma, NY, USA. Poloxamer 407 USP/NF was sourced from BASF Corporation, Florham Park, NJ, USA. We obtained sodium selenite from Lanxess, Netherlands. L-ascorbic acid was sourced from Research-Lab FINE Chem Industries, Mumbai, India. n-hexane and acetone were obtained from El-Nasr Pharmaceutical Chemicals Co., Cairo, Egypt. Gentamicin was sourced from Sigma-Aldrich, Saint Louis, MO, USA. The highest analytical-grade chemicals were used in this study.

4.2. In Vitro Study

4.2.1. Preparation of Selenium Nanoparticles

Lyc-Se-NPs were synthesized by the chemical reduction method utilizing ascorbic acid as a reducing agent and poloxamer 407 as a stabilizer. In brief, the equivalent weight of 40 mg lycopene was dissolved in 3 mL acetone.

Poloxamer 407 (40 mg) was dissolved in 10 mL cold water (4 °C) and was added to 5 mL of sodium selenite (8 mg/mL) mixed with a magnetic stirrer (Stuart, Caliber Scientific, Holland, OH, USA) at 200 rpm for 5 min. Lycopene solution was gradually dropped manually with the aid of a 3 mL plastic syringe, with continuous stirring for an additional 10 min. The solution was then incubated in an ice bath and allowed to equilibrate for 10 min (4 °C). Ascorbic acid (80 mg) was dissolved in 5 mL of distilled water. Using a 5 mL plastic syringe, ascorbic acid was introduced stepwise with continuous stirring until the appearance of a reddish color. The solution was allowed to equilibrate for 2 h, and then the solution was subjected to a probe sonicator (Sonic Vibra Cell, Newtown, CT, USA) for a further 5 min (10 s pulse and 3 s pause) at 69% of its power (130 W), (the solution was incubated in an ice bath).

The colloid dispersion was lyophilized for further investigation. The drug-free nanoparticles were formulated by this same method, except that the addition of lycopene solution was replaced with 3 mL of acetone.

4.2.2. Drug Content

The weight equivalent to 10 mg lycopene was transferred to a 10 mL volumetric flask complete to volume with n-hexane. The UV spectrophotometric scanning was performed utilizing n-hexane as a blank. Lycopene has three peaks of absorbance: 444, 471, and 503 nm [38]. The absorbance of lycopene was investigated at 471 nm, and serial dilution was performed to prepare a standard curve (0.3 to 1.6 µg/mL). The drug content was studied by determining the lycopene absorbance utilizing the UV-VIS spectrophotometric method at 471 nm.

4.2.3. Characterization of Selenium Nanoparticles

Average Particle Size, Zeta Potential Evaluation, Polydispersity Index (PDI), SEM and TEM

Particle size and zeta potential are crucial for nanoformulation efficiency, with PDI indicating distribution uniformity [39]. Furthermore, nanoparticles' cellular uptake, which influences cell and tissue binding, is controlled by their form, dimensions, and zeta potential. Higher zeta potentials result in stronger membrane bonds and increased cellular absorption [40]. The Zeta Sizer Nano (Malvern Panalytical Ltd., Malvern, UK) was used to assess the particle size and zeta potential.

The surface properties and structure of lycopene, drug-free selenium nanoparticles, and Lyc-Se-NPs were verified using the SEM method [41]. One drop of alcoholic solution was then applied to a glass slide. The sample was coated with gold for one minute, and then a 10 kV electron acceleration voltage field emission scanning electron microscope (JEOL, JSM-6510LV, Tokyo, Japan) was used. The size and shape of the Lyc-Se-NPs were evaluated using a transmission electron microscopy (TEM, JEM-2100F, electron microscope, JEOL Ltd., Tokyo, Japan) [41].

Fourier Transform Infrared Spectroscopy Analysis (FTIR)

The system's stability was studied through FTIR analysis, which was carried out to evaluate the interactions or compatibility of the formulations. IR spectra in the range of 4000–400 cm^{-1} were acquired at room temperature using a Perkin–Elmer Fourier transform spectrometer [42] (Bruker, Billerica, MA, USA), and we used FTIR spectra of the lycopene powder, Selenium nanoparticles, and the lycopene-Se-NPs were examined.

4.3. Antioxidant Activity Assay

4.3.1. DPPH Radical Scavenging Assay

The DPPH assay was employed for lycopene, free Se-NPs, and Lyc-Se-NPs at different concentrations (1, 2, 4, 6, 8, 10, 12, 14, 16, and 18 µg/mL) using the method described by [43]. A spectrophotometer (Biosystem 310 plus) was employed to measure the absorbance at 517 nm. The reference chemical was ascorbic acid. By utilizing the log dosage inhibition curve (n = 3), the IC50 value was determined.

The percentage of DPPH scavenging effect was determined as follows:

$$\% \text{ Inhibition} = \frac{A0 - A1}{A0} \times 100$$

where A_0 denotes the absorbance of the control response, and A_1 represents the absorbance in the presence of a test or standard sample.

4.3.2. ABTS Radical Scavenging Assay

ABTS radical scavenging activity was determined for lycopene, free Se-NPs, and Lyc-Se-NPs at different concentrations (1, 2, 4, 6, 8, 10, 12, 14, 16, and 18 μg/mL), following [43] with minor modifications. After incubating for six minutes, the absorbance at 734 nm was measured using a spectrophotometer. The antioxidant activity was assessed as follows:

$$\% \text{ Inhibition} = \frac{\text{A control} - \text{A sample}}{\text{Acontrol}} \times 100$$

where A control represents the absorption of the negative control with solution preparation, and A sample represents the sample absorbance after 6 min.

The chemical utilized as the reference was gallic acid. The IC_{50} value was determined using a graph that displayed the sample concentration needed to scavenge 50% of the ABTS free radicals (n = 3).

4.4. Screening the In Vitro Antibacterial Activity of Lycopene (Lyc) and Lycopene Selenium Nanoparticles (Lyc-Se-NPs)

4.4.1. Microorganisms

The bacterial reference strains were *Escherichia coli* (ATCC 25922), *Staphylococcus aureus* (ATCC 25923), *Proteus mirabilis* (ATCC 35659), *Klebsiella pneumoniae* (ATCC 700603), and *Pseudomonas aeruginosa* (ATCC 27853). A total of 20 *Staphylococcus aureus* clinical isolates were obtained from the culture collection of the Microbiology and Immunology Department, Faculty of Pharmacy, Tanta University.

4.4.2. Agar-Well Diffusion Technique

In the present study, bacterial reference strains were employed to demonstrate the antibacterial activity of lycopene (Lyc), selenium, and lycopene selenium nanoparticles (Lyc-Se-NPs). The screening of the antibacterial activity of Lyc, selenium, and Lyc-Se-NPs proceeded with us establishing cups in Muller–Hinton agar using the agar-well diffusion technique. Bacterial suspensions were prepared to 0.5 McFarland standard in 0.85% saline. Each bacterial reference strain was streaked on a plate with five cups to test the effects of Lyc, selenium, and Lyc-Se-NPs at concentrations of 1000 μg/mL, whereas the other two cups contained gentamicin and DMSO [44].

Antibiotic susceptibility determinations for bacterial isolates were performed according to the Clinical Laboratory Standards Institute (CLSI, 2015 [45]) with the quality control reference strain *Staphylococcus aureus* ATCC 25923. All experiments were conducted in triplicate, and the data are presented as the mean ± standard deviation (SD).

4.4.3. Broth Microdilution Assay

The minimum inhibitory concentration (MIC) values (μg/mL) of Lyc, selenium, and Lyc-Se-NPs against the tested bacterial isolates were determined using the broth microdilution method in a 96-well microtitration plate [46]. The quality control reference strain *Staphylococcus aureus* ATCC 29213 was used. All experiments were conducted in triplicate.

4.4.4. Growth Curves of *S. aureus* Clinical Isolates (Before and After the Treatment with Tested Compounds)

Staphylococcus aureus clinical isolates (n = 20) were cultivated in LB broth at 37 °C with and without 1/2, 1/4, and 1/8 MICs of Lyc, selenium, and Lyc-Se-NPs. The OD value for treated and untreated isolates was kept at 0.3, and the absorbance of samples collected every 30 min from each culture was measured at 600 nm [41].

4.5. In Vitro Antibiofilm Activity

4.5.1. Crystal Violet (CV) Microtiter Plate Assay

The effects of either Lyc, selenium, or Lyc-Se-NPs on *S. aureus* clinical isolates' biofilm were investigated, as described by [41]. In summary, the isolates were cultivated in TSB containing 1% glucose for 24 h at 37 °C with and without sub-MICs (1/2, 1/4, and 1/8 MICs) of either Lyc, selenium, or Lyc-Se-NPs using a 96-well microtiter plate. The formed biofilm was fixed with absolute methanol for 20 min, followed by drying. After that, the staining of biofilm was performed using 200 µL of 0.1% CV for 15 min and then rinsing with water, and the plate was left to dry. The stained biofilms were dissolved with 200 µL glacial acetic acid (33% (*v*/*v*)). Each experiment was executed in triplicate.

The absorbance was evaluated using a microplate reader (Sunrise TM, TECAN, Switzerland) at 595 nm to determine the optical density (OD). If OD $\leq$ ODc, the isolate was recorded as a non-producer; ODc < OD $\leq 2 \times$ ODc as a weak producer; $2 \times$ ODc < OD $\leq 4 \times$ ODc as a moderate producer; and $4 \times$ ODc < OD as a strong producer [41]. The percentage reduction in biofilm formation was determined as follows:

$$\text{Percentage reduction in biofilm formation} = \frac{\text{Control OD595 nm} - \text{Treated OD595 nm}}{\text{Control OD595 nm}} \times 100$$

4.5.2. Testing Biofilm Thickness and Bacterial Viability Using CLSM

The effects of Lyc, selenium, or Lyc-Se-NPs on the formation of bacterial biofilms were identified using confocal laser scanning microscopy (CLSM). Glass slides were submerged in the *S. aureus* inoculated TSB media without and with 1/4 MICs of Lyc, Se, or Lyc-Se-NPs in 6-well plates with a flat bottom. The microplates were incubated at 37 °C for 18 hrs. Afterward, they were treated twice with PBS and stained with 5 µL of acridine orange (AO) and propidium iodide (PI). When living cells were stained, green fluorescence was created, which was visible for 15 min in the absence of light. Red fluorescence was produced when staining dead cells. Finally, we investigated the thickness of the biofilm with CLSM (DMi8, Leica Microsystem, Deerfield, USA) [41].

4.6. In Vivo Study

4.6.1. Animals

A national research center in Egypt provided adult male Wister albino rats weighing 200–220 g. The animals were given regular food and unlimited access to water. This study complied with ethical standards for animal care as well as institutional norms. The University of Tanta's Faculty of Pharmacy research ethics committee, which followed the ARRIVE 2.0 criteria (Code of Protocol: TP/RE/6/23 p-0070), accepted the study protocol.

4.6.2. Wound Model and Experimental Groups

A total of thirty-six rats were randomly assigned to six different groups consisting of six rats each:

(1) Untreated group (infected wound only);
(2) Gentamicin group (infected wound + standard drug gentamycin treatment);
(3) Lycopene-only group (infected wound + lycopene treatment);
(4) Free Se-NP group (infected wound + free Se-NP treatment);
(5) Lyc-Se-NP group (25 mg) (infected wound + Lyc-Se-NP (25 mg) treatment);
(6) Lyc-Se-NP group (50 mg) (infected wound + Lyc-Se-NP (50 mg) treatment).

After isoflurane anesthesia was administered, a small section of each rat's back was meticulously shaved. The dorsal skin was injured via full-thickness excisional skin cuts according to a technique previously described [47]. Different treatments were applied topically to the surface of the wound for seven days.

4.6.3. Assessment of Wound Closure Rates (WCRs)

Animals were placed on a white plastic platform, and pictures of their wounds were taken. Morphometric software (Version 1.5) was used to examine the photos (Image J®,

National Institute of Health, Bethesda, MD, USA), to measure the wound areas on days 0, 2, 4, and 7. The WCR was determined as follows:

$$WCR = (iWA - fWA/iWA) \times 100$$

where WCR is the wound closure rate, iWA is the initial wounded area (day 0), and fWA is the final wounded area (days 2, 4, and 7). This methodology follows the approach detailed by Santos et al. (2021) [48].

4.6.4. Skin Tissue Sample Collection

Rats were given isoflurane anesthesia. Skin wound tissue samples were collected from each group for histopathological and immunohistochemical examination. The remaining tissues were stored at −80 °C for further analysis.

4.6.5. Determination of Inflammatory Marker (TNF-α, IL-1β, and COX-2) and Anti-Inflammatory Marker (HO-1) Contents in Skin Tissues

The contents of inflammatory markers TNF-α, IL-1β, and COX-2 and anti-inflammatory marker HO-1 in skin tissues were evaluated using various commercial ELISA kits purchased from CUSABIO. Co., Houston, TX, USA (Cat. No. CSB-E11987r, CSB-E08055r, CSB-E13399r, and CSB-E08267r, respectively). The assay procedures were achieved according to the manufacturer's instructions.

4.6.6. Histopathological Evaluation and Masson's Trichrome Examination for Dermal Collagen (%) in Skin Sections

Dissected skin wound tissue samples were fixed in 10% neutral buffered formalin. The specimens were sectioned to a thickness of 4 μm after undergoing tissue processing using a standard paraffin embedding technique. The samples were then stained with hematoxylin and eosin (H&E) for light microscopy observation.

Histopathological assessments were conducted using a semiquantitative scoring system to evaluate various aspects of tissue repair, including necrosis, inflammation, fibrin deposition, granulation tissue formation, collagen remodeling, vascularization, and epithelialization. The inflammation scores were based on the presence of neutrophils, monocytes, and plasma cells. The scoring system used ranged from ND (not detectable) to ++++ (high), with intermediate scores indicating + (mild), ++ (moderate), and +++ (moderate to high). This scoring methodology for necrosis, inflammation, fibrin deposition, granulation tissue formation, collagen remodeling, epithelialization, and vascularization was adapted from [49].

The mean area percentage of collagen fiber deposition was assessed through Masson's trichrome staining, with the collagen content analyzed semiquantitatively using ImageJ software 1.54, as outlined by [50].

4.6.7. Immunohistochemical Staining of NF-κB-p65 of Skin Sections

The procedure for applying the immunohistochemical staining approach was as stated in [51]. Dewaxed sections were soaked in a 0.05 M, pH 6.8 citric acid buffer solution to extract antigens. Following that, protein blocks were applied to the sections and H_2O_2 at 0.3%. The samples were then treated with NF-κB-p65 antibody (Santa Cruz, CA, USA, Cat No. sc-166416, 1:100 dilution). After that, half an hour was spent at 37 °C using the secondary antibody coupled with horseradish peroxidase.

The sections were exposed for three minutes to the 3,3′-diaminobenzidine tetrahydrochloride reagent. Finally, Mayer's hematoxylin was used to counterstain the slides. DPX mounting and a wash with distilled water came next. The slides were examined using an Olympus CX21 microscope (Tokyo, Japan).

The immunohistochemical grading was performed semiquantitatively as described by [52] with the average scores used for analysis. The scoring system was defined as follows: 0 = no staining, 1 = light brown–yellow, 2 = brown, and 3 = dark brown staining. Ten fields were evaluated on each slide at 400x magnification. The average positive expression on each slide was scored as follows: 1 = <25%, 2 = 25 to <50%, 3 = 50 to <75%, and 4 = >75%. The final score for each slide was determined by the product of the positive expression percentage and the degree of staining score, resulting in the following classifications: 0 to 1 point was negative (−), 2 to 3 points were weakly positive (+), 4 to 6 points were moderately positive (++), and >6 points were strongly positive (+++).

4.7. Statistical Analysis

The results were shown as the mean ± standard deviation (SD). To compare different groups, a one-way analysis of variance (ANOVA) was employed, and Tukey–Kramer post hoc testing. A significance threshold of $p < 0.05$ was used. GraphPad Prism 5 Software, Inc., San Diego, CA, USA, was employed in order to use to perform the statistical analysis.

5. Conclusions

The present study describes, for the first time, the antibacterial and antibiofilm activity of lycopene and lycopene-selenium nanoformulation on *S. aureus*. Our findings demonstrate that Lyc and Lyc-Se-NPs have powerful antioxidant activity which was confirmed with the findings of both DPPH and ABTS radical scavenging experiments. Moreover, they demonstrated significant anti-inflammatory properties, which were evident by the downregulation of TNF-α, IL-1β, and COX-2. Given the unique characteristics of Lyc-Se-NPs, we propose that this formula should be subject to further research in the field of inflammation management.

Supplementary Materials: The following supporting information can be downloaded at: https://www.mdpi.com/article/10.3390/ph17121600/s1, Table S1. MIC values of tested compounds against *S. aureus* clinical isolates and the effect of the treatment by the tested compounds at sub-MICs on biofilm formation (S; strong producer, M; moderate producer, W; weak producer, N; non-producer); Figure S1. Growth curves of *S. aureus* clinical isolates grown in the absence and presence of 1/2, 1/4, and 1/8 MICs of the tested compounds at different time intervals.

Author Contributions: Conceptualization, T.A.E.-M., M.M.F.E.-N., M.M.E.-B.; data curation, T.A.E.-M., E.I.E.Z., M.M.S.G., M.M.F.E.-N., M.M.E.-B.; investigation, T.A.E.-M., R.B., E.I.E.Z., M.M.F.E.-N., M.M.S.G., M.M.E.-B.; methodology E.I.E.Z., M.M.S.G., M.M.F.E.-N., M.M.E.-B.; project administration, T.A.E.-M.; supervision, T.A.E.-M., R.B.; writing—original draft, M.M.F.E.-N., M.M.E.-B.; writing—review and editing, M.M.F.E.-N., M.M.E.-B. All authors have read and agreed to the published version of the manuscript.

Funding: This research was funded by Princess Nourah bint Abdulrahman University Researchers Supporting Project number (PNURSP2024R304), Princess Nourah bint Abdulrahman University, Riyadh, Saudi Arabia.

Institutional Review Board Statement: All animal procedures were performed according to the institutional guidelines for the care and use of laboratory animals. After informed written consent was obtained from the participant, this study was conducted following the Declaration of Helsinki and as approved by the Research Ethics Committee of the Faculty of Pharmacy, Tanta University (TP/RE/6/23 p-0070).

Informed Consent Statement: Not applicable.

Data Availability Statement: All data generated or analyzed during this study are included in this article.

Acknowledgments: This research was funded by Princess Nourah bint Abdulrahman University Researchers Supporting Project number (PNURSP2024R304), Princess Nourah bint Abdulrahman University, Riyadh, Saudi Arabia.

Conflicts of Interest: The authors declare no conflicts of interest.

References

1. Oyebode, O.; Kandala, N.B.; Chilton, P.J.; Lilford, R.J. Use of Traditional Medicine in Middle-Income Countries: A WHO-SAGE Study. *Health Policy Plan.* **2016**, *31*, 984–991. [CrossRef] [PubMed]
2. Crupi, P.; Faienza, M.F.; Naeem, M.Y.; Corbo, F.; Clodoveo, M.L.; Muraglia, M. Overview of the Potential Beneficial Effects of Carotenoids on Consumer Health and Well-Being. *Antioxidants* **2023**, *12*, 1069. [CrossRef] [PubMed]
3. Ilahy, R.; Tlili, I.; Siddiqui, M.W.; Hdider, C.; Lenucci, M.S. Inside and beyond Color: Comparative Overview of Functional Quality of Tomato and Watermelon Fruits. *Front. Plant Sci.* **2019**, *10*, 769. [CrossRef] [PubMed]
4. Martí, R.; Roselló, S.; Cebolla-Cornejo, J. Tomato as a Source of Carotenoids and Polyphenols Targeted to Cancer Prevention. *Cancers* **2016**, *8*, 58. [CrossRef] [PubMed]
5. Khan, U.M.; Sevindik, M.; Zarrabi, A.; Nami, M.; Ozdemir, B.; Kaplan, D.N.; Selamoglu, Z.; Hasan, M.; Kumar, M.; Alshehri, M.M.; et al. Lycopene: Food Sources, Biological Activities, and Human Health Benefits. *Oxidative Med. Cell. Longev.* **2021**, *2021*, 2713511. [CrossRef] [PubMed]
6. Górecka, D.; Wawrzyniak, A.; Jędrusek-Golińska, A.; Dziedzic, K.; Hamułka, J.; Kowalczewski, P.Ł.; Walkowiak, J. Lycopene in Tomatoes and Tomato Products. *Open Chem.* **2020**, *18*, 752–756. [CrossRef]
7. Rao, A.V.; Rao, L.G. Carotenoids and Human Health. *Pharmacol. Res.* **2007**, *55*, 207–216. [CrossRef]
8. Singh, G.; Pai, R.S. Atazanavir-Loaded Eudragit RL 100 Nanoparticles to Improve Oral Bioavailability: Optimization and in Vitro/in Vivo Appraisal. *Drug Deliv.* **2016**, *23*, 532–539. [CrossRef]
9. Liu, L.; Liu, C.; Hou, L.; Lv, J.; Wu, F.; Yang, X.; Ren, S.; Ji, W.; Wang, M.; Chen, L. Protection against Ischemia/Reperfusion-Induced Renal Injury by Co-Treatment with Erythropoietin and Sodium Selenite. *Mol. Med. Rep.* **2015**, *12*, 7933–7940. [CrossRef]
10. Rayman, M.P. Selenium Intake, Status, and Health: A Complex Relationship. *Hormones* **2020**, *19*, 9–14. [CrossRef]
11. Dagnell, M.; Schmidt, E.E.; Arnér, E.S.J. The A to Z of Modulated Cell Patterning by Mammalian Thioredoxin Reductases. *Free Radic. Biol. Med.* **2018**, *115*, 484–496. [CrossRef] [PubMed]
12. Puri, A.; Mohite, P.; Patil, S.; Chidrawar, V.R.; Ushir, Y.V.; Dodiya, R.; Singh, S. Facile green synthesis and characterization of Terminalia arjuna bark phenolic-selenium nanogel: A biocompatible and green nano-biomaterial for multifaceted biological applications. *Front. Chem.* **2023**, *11*, 1273360. [CrossRef] [PubMed]
13. Filipović, N.; Ušjak, D.; Milenković, M.T.; Zheng, K.; Liverani, L.; Boccaccini, A.R.; Stevanović, M.M. Comparative Study of the Antimicrobial Activity of Selenium Nanoparticles With Different Surface Chemistry and Structure. *Front. Bioeng. Biotechnol.* **2021**, *8*, 624621. [CrossRef] [PubMed]
14. AlBasher, G.; Alfarraj, S.; Alarifi, S.; Alkhtani, S.; Almeer, R.; Alsultan, N.; Alharthi, M.; Alotibi, N.; Al-bass, A.; Abdel Moneim, A.E. Nephroprotective Role of Selenium Nanoparticles Against Glycerol-Induced Acute Kidney Injury in Rats. *Biol. Trace Elem. Res.* **2020**, *194*, 444–454. [CrossRef] [PubMed]
15. Sans-Serramitjana, E.; Obreque, M.; Muñoz, F.; Zaror, C.; Mora, M.d.L.L.; Viñas, M.; Betancourt, P. Antimicrobial Activity of Selenium Nanoparticles (SeNPs) against Potentially Pathogenic Oral Microorganisms: A Scoping Review. *Pharmaceutics* **2023**, *15*, 2253. [CrossRef]
16. Benbow, M. Wound Care: Ensuring a Holistic and Collaborative Assessment. *Br. J. Community Nurs.* **2011**, *16*, S6–S16. [CrossRef]
17. Amri, B.; Martino, E.; Vitulo, F.; Corana, F.; Ben-Kaâb, L.B.; Rui, M.; Rossi, D.; Mori, M.; Rossi, S.; Collina, S. *Marrubium vulgare* l. Leave Extract: Phytochemical Composition, Antioxidant, and Wound Healing Properties. *Molecules* **2017**, *22*, 1851. [CrossRef]
18. Aytekin, A.A.; Tuncay Tanrıverdi, S.; Aydın Köse, F.; Kart, D.; Eroğlu, İ.; Özer, Ö. Propolis Loaded Liposomes: Evaluation of Antimicrobial and Antioxidant Activities. *J. Liposome Res.* **2020**, *30*, 107–116. [CrossRef]
19. Siafaka, P.I.; Zisi, A.P.; Exindari, M.K.; Karantas, I.D.; Bikiaris, D.N. Porous Dressings of Modified Chitosan with Poly(2-Hydroxyethyl Acrylate) for Topical Wound Delivery of Levofloxacin. *Carbohydr. Polym.* **2016**, *143*, 90–99. [CrossRef]
20. Puca, V.; Marulli, R.Z.; Grande, R.; Vitale, I.; Niro, A.; Molinaro, G.; Prezioso, S.; Muraro, R.; Di Giovanni, P. Microbial Species Isolated from Infected Wounds and Antimicrobial Resistance Analysis: Data Emerging from a Three-Years Retrospective Study. *Antibiotics* **2021**, *10*, 1162. [CrossRef]
21. Manaa, H.M.; Hamza, E.M.; Sorour, N.M. Post-Harvest Biocontrol of Fusarium Infection in Tomato Fruits Using Bio-Mediated Selenium Nanoparticles. *AMB Express* **2023**, *13*, 119. [CrossRef] [PubMed]
22. Imran, M.; Ghorat, F.; Ul-haq, I.; Ur-rehman, H.; Aslam, F.; Heydari, M.; Shariati, M.A.; Okuskhanova, E.; Yessimbekov, Z.; Thiruvengadam, M.; et al. Lycopene as a Natural Antioxidant Used to Prevent Human Health Disorders. *Antioxidants* **2020**, *9*, 706. [CrossRef] [PubMed]
23. Forootanfar, H.; Adeli-Sardou, M.; Nikkhoo, M.; Mehrabani, M.; Amir-Heidari, B.; Shahverdi, A.R.; Shakibaie, M. Antioxidant and Cytotoxic Effect of Biologically Synthesized Selenium Nanoparticles in Comparison to Selenium Dioxide. *J. Trace Elem. Med. Biol.* **2014**, *28*, 75–79. [CrossRef] [PubMed]
24. Al-Brakati, A.; Alsharif, K.F.; Alzahrani, K.J.; Kabrah, S.; Al-Amer, O.; Oyouni, A.A.; Habotta, O.A.; Lokman, M.S.; Bauomy, A.A.; Kassab, R.B.; et al. Using Green Biosynthesized Lycopene-Coated Selenium Nanoparticles to Rescue Renal Damage in Glycerol-Induced Acute Kidney Injury in Rats. *Int. J. Nanomed.* **2021**, *16*, 4335–4349. [CrossRef] [PubMed]
25. Hosnedlova, B.; Kepinska, M.; Skalickova, S.; Fernandez, C.; Ruttkay-Nedecky, B.; Peng, Q.; Baron, M.; Melcova, M.; Opatrilova, R.; Zidkova, J.; et al. Nano-Selenium and Its Nanomedicine Applications: A Critical Review. *Int. J. Nanomed.* **2018**, *13*, 2107–2128. [CrossRef]
26. Rayman, M.P. Selenium and Human Health. *Lancet* **2012**, *379*, 1256–1268. [CrossRef]

27. Divyadharsini, V.; Uma Maheswari, T.; Rajeshkumar, S. Assessment of Antimicrobial Activity of Lycopene, Vitamin E, and Lycopene-Vitamin E Combination against *Staphylococcus aureus*, *Streptococcus mutans*, *Enterococcus faecalis*, and *Candida albicans*: An In Vitro Study. *Cureus* **2023**, *15*, e42419. [CrossRef]
28. Okur, M.E.; Karantas, I.D.; Şenyiğit, Z.; Üstündağ Okur, N.; Siafaka, P.I. Recent Trends on Wound Management: New Therapeutic Choices Based on Polymeric Carriers. *Asian J. Pharm. Sci.* **2020**, *15*, 661–684. [CrossRef]
29. Przybylska, S. Lycopene—A Bioactive Carotenoid Offering Multiple Health Benefits: A Review. *Int. J. Food Sci. Technol.* **2020**, *55*, 11–32. [CrossRef]
30. Joshi, B.; Kar, S.K.; Yadav, P.K.; Yadav, S.; Shrestha, L.; Bera, T.K. Therapeutic and Medicinal Uses of Lycopene: A Systematic Review. *Int. J. Res. Med. Sci.* **2020**, *8*, 1195. [CrossRef]
31. Okur, M.E.; Karadağ, A.E.; Okur, N.Ü.; Özhan, Y.; Sipahi, H.; Ayla, Ş.; Daylan, B.; Demirci, B.; Demirci, F. In Vivo Wound Healing and In Vitro Anti-Inflammatory Activity Evaluation of *Phlomis russeliana* Extract Gel Formulations. *Molecules* **2020**, *25*, 2695. [CrossRef] [PubMed]
32. Alsenani, F.; Ashour, A.M.; Alzubaidi, M.A.; Azmy, A.F.; Hetta, M.H.; Abu-Baih, D.H.; Elrehany, M.A.; Zayed, A.; Sayed, A.M.; Abdelmohsen, U.R.; et al. Wound Healing Metabolites from Peters' Elephant-Nose Fish Oil: An In Vivo Investigation Supported by In Vitro and In Silico Studies. *Mar. Drugs* **2021**, *19*, 605. [CrossRef] [PubMed]
33. Schilrreff, P.; Alexiev, U. Chronic Inflammation in Non-Healing Skin Wounds and Promising Natural Bioactive Compounds Treatment. *Int. J. Mol. Sci.* **2022**, *23*, 4928. [CrossRef] [PubMed]
34. Vasconcelos, A.G.; das GN Amorim, A.; dos Santos, R.C.; Souza, J.M.T.; de Souza, L.K.M.; Araújo, T.d.S.L.; Nicolau, L.A.D.; de Lima Carvalho, L.; de Aquino, P.E.A.; da Silva Martins, C.; et al. Lycopene Rich Extract from Red Guava (*Psidium guajava* L.) Displays Anti-Inflammatory and Antioxidant Profile by Reducing Suggestive Hallmarks of Acute Inflammatory Response in Mice. *Food Res. Int.* **2017**, *99*, 959–968. [CrossRef] [PubMed]
35. Liu, C.B.; Wang, R.; Yi, Y.F.; Gao, Z.; Chen, Y.Z. Lycopene Mitigates β-Amyloid Induced Inflammatory Response and Inhibits NF-KB Signaling at the Choroid Plexus in Early Stages of Alzheimer's Disease Rats. *J. Nutr. Biochem.* **2018**, *53*, 66–71. [CrossRef]
36. Campos, K.K.D.; Araújo, G.R.; Martins, T.L.; Bandeira, A.C.B.; de Paula Costa, G.; Talvani, A.; Garcia, C.C.M.; Oliveira, L.A.M.; Costa, D.C.; Bezerra, F.S. The Antioxidant and Anti-Inflammatory Properties of Lycopene in Mice Lungs Exposed to Cigarette Smoke. *J. Nutr. Biochem.* **2017**, *48*, 9–20. [CrossRef]
37. Goncu, T.; Oğuz, E.; Sezen, H.; Koçarslan, S.; Oğuz, H.; Akal, A.; Adibelli, F.M.; Çakmak, S.; Aksoy, N. Anti-Inflammatory Effect of Lycopene on Endotoxin-Induced Uveitis in Rats. *Arq. Bras. Oftalmol.* **2016**, *79*, 357–362. [CrossRef]
38. Cámara, M.; De Cortes Sánchez-Mata, M.; Fernández-Ruiz, V.; Cámara, R.M.; Manzoor, S.; Caceres, J.O. Lycopene: A Review of Chemical and Biological Activity Related to Beneficial Health Effects. In *Studies in Natural Products Chemistry*; Elsevier: Amsterdam, The Netherlands, 2013; Volume 40, ISBN 9780444596031.
39. Mahbubul, I.M. Introduction to Nanofluid. In *Preparation, Characterization, Properties and Application of Nanofluid*; William Andrew: Norwich, NY, USA, 2019; pp. 1–13. [CrossRef]
40. Németh, Z.; Csóka, I.; Semnani Jazani, R.; Sipos, B.; Haspel, H.; Kozma, G.; Kónya, Z.; Dobó, D.G. Quality by Design-Driven Zeta Potential Optimisation Study of Liposomes with Charge Imparting Membrane Additives. *Pharmaceutics* **2022**, *14*, 1798. [CrossRef]
41. Omar, A.; El-Banna, T.E.; Sonbol, F.I.; El-Bouseary, M.M. Potential Antivirulence and Antibiofilm Activities of Sub-MIC of Oxacillin against MDR S. Aureus Isolates: An In-Vitro and In-Vivo Study. *BMC Microbiol.* **2024**, *24*, 295. [CrossRef]
42. Theivandran, G.; Ibrahim, S.M.; Murugan, M. Fourier Transform Infrared (Ft-Ir) Spectroscopic Analysis of *Spirulina fusiformis*. *J. Med. Plants Stud.* **2015**, *3*, 30–32.
43. González-Palma, I.; Escalona-Buendía, H.B.; Ponce-Alquicira, E.; Téllez-Téllez, M.; Gupta, V.K.; Díaz-Godínez, G.; Soriano-Santos, J. Evaluation of the Antioxidant Activity of Aqueous and Methanol Extracts of *Pleurotus ostreatus* in Different Growth Stages. *Front. Microbiol.* **2016**, *7*, 1099. [CrossRef] [PubMed]
44. Alotaibi, B.; Elekhnawy, E.; El-Masry, T.A.; Saleh, A.; El-Bouseary, M.M.; Alosaimi, M.E.; Alotaibi, K.N.; Abdelkader, D.H.; Negm, W.A. Green Synthetized Cu-Oxide Nanoparticles: Properties and Applications for Enhancing Healing of Wounds Infected with *Staphylococcus aureus*. *Int. J. Pharm.* **2023**, *645*, 123415. [CrossRef] [PubMed]
45. *M07-A10*; Methods for Dilution Antimicrobial Susceptibility Tests for Bacteria That Grow Aerobically. Approved Standard Seventh Edition; CLSI—Clinical and Laboratory Standards Institute: Wayne, PA, USA, 2015; pp. 1–64.
46. Elbouseary, M.; El-Said El-Banna, T.; Ibrahim Sonbol, F.; El-Bouseary, M.M.; El-Banna, T.E.; Sonbol, F.I. Prevalence of MRSA among *Staphylococcus aureus* Isolates Recovered From Patients with Otitis Media. *Nat. Sci.* **2018**, *16*, 48–55. [CrossRef]
47. Tramontina, V.A.; Machado, M.A.N.; Nogueira Filho, G.d.R.; Kim, S.H.; Vizzioli, M.R.; Toledo, S.d. Effect of Bismuth Subgallate (Local Hemostatic Agent) on Wound Healing in Rats. Histological and Histometric Findings. *Braz. Dent. J.* **2002**, *13*, 11–16. [PubMed]
48. Santos, T.S.; Dos Santos, I.D.D.; Pereira-Filho, R.N.; Gomes, S.V.F.; Lima-Verde, I.B.; Marques, M.N.; Cardoso, J.C.; Severino, P.; Souto, E.B.; de Albuquerque-Júnior, R.L.C. Histological Evidence of Wound Healing Improvement in Rats Treated with Oral Administration of Hydroalcoholic Extract of Vitis Labrusca. *Curr. Issues Mol. Biol.* **2021**, *43*, 335–352. [CrossRef]
49. Gad, S.B.; Hafez, M.H.; El-Sayed, Y.S. Platelet-Rich Plasma and/or Sildenafil Topical Applications Accelerate and Better Repair Wound Healing in Rats through Regulation of Proinflammatory Cytokines and Collagen/TGF-B1 Pathway. *Environ. Sci. Pollut. Res.* **2020**, *27*, 40757–40768. [CrossRef]

50. Cheng, K.Y.; Lin, Z.H.; Cheng, Y.P.; Chiu, H.Y.; Yeh, N.L.; Wu, T.K.; Wu, J.S. Wound Healing in Streptozotocin-Induced Diabetic Rats Using Atmospheric-Pressure Argon Plasma Jet. *Sci. Rep.* **2018**, *8*, 12214. [CrossRef]
51. Alasmari, A.F.; Ali, N.; Alharbi, M.; Alqahtani, F.; Alasmari, F.; Almoqbel, D.; Alswayyed, M.; Alshammari, A.; Alanazi, M.M.; Alhoshani, A.; et al. Geraniol Ameliorates Doxorubicin-Mediated Kidney Injury through Alteration of Antioxidant Status, Inflammation, and Apoptosis: Potential Roles of NF-κB and Nrf2/Ho-1. *Nutrients* **2022**, *14*, 1620. [CrossRef]
52. Weng, H.; Deng, Y.; Xie, Y.; Liu, H.; Gong, F. Expression and Significance of HMGB1, TLR4 and NF-κB P65 in Human Epidermal Tumors. *BMC Cancer* **2013**, *13*, 311. [CrossRef]

pharmaceuticals

MDPI

Article

Ethanolic Extracts of Cupressaceae Species Conifers Provide Rapid Protection against Barium Chloride-Induced Cardiac Arrhythmia

Meng-Ting Zeng [1,†], Li-Yue Huang [1,†], Xiao-Hui Zheng [1], Yan-Qi Fu [1] and Ching-Feng Weng [1,2,3,*]

1 Functional Physiology Section, Department of Basic Medical Science, Xiamen Medical College, Xiamen 361023, China; 18859868050@163.com (M.-T.Z.); hly0915@163.com (L.-Y.H.); 201500010365@xmmc.edu.cn (X.-H.Z.); xmepb1@163.com (Y.-Q.F.)

2 Institute of Respiratory Disease, Department of Basic Medical Science, Xiamen Medical College, Xiamen 361023, China

3 LEADTEK Research, Inc., New Taipei City 235603, Taiwan

* Correspondence: cfwengcf@gmail.com; Tel.: +86-0592-6270028

† The authors equally contributed this work.

Abstract: Sudden cardiac death (SCD) is responsible for a high percentage of cardiovascular fatalities, with ventricular arrhythmias being the most common cause. Despite numerous clinically available antiarrhythmic drugs (AADs), AADs retain some undesirable arrhythmic effects, and their inappropriate use can lead to severe adverse reactions. The exploration of new therapeutic options against arrhythmias with fewer unreceptive effects is of utmost importance. The ethanolic extracts of seven Cupressaceae species, namely, *Chamaecyparis obtusa*, *Juniperus chinensis* (L.) Ant., *Sabina chinensis* (L.) Ant. cv. Kaizuca, *Platycladus orientalis* (L.) Franco, *Juniperus sabina* L., *Fokienia hodginsii*, and *Juniperus chinensis* 'Pyramidalis' were investigated for their pharmacological effects on barium chloride ($BaCl_2$)-induced arrhythmia using normal II lead electrocardiogram (ECG) measurements in a mouse model. According to the ECG profiles, pretreatment with *C. obtusa*, *P. orientalis*, and *J. sabina* extracts provoked dose-dependent protection against $BaCl_2$-induced arrhythmia, while pretreatment with the other four species and amiodarone did not exert cardioprotective effects. The treatment effects were confirmed using a rat model. The therapeutic effects of *C. obtusa*, *P. orientalis*, and *J. sabina* extracts on the M2 and M3 receptors but not the M1 receptor were mediated by the inhibition of the M2 receptor blocker (methoctramine tetrahydrochloride), M3 antagonist (4-DAMP), or M1 receptor blocker (pirenzepine dihydrochloride). This first-line evidence illustrates that certain Cupressaceae species possess active antiarrhythmic components. The first line of key findings revealed that active components of certain Cupressaceae species have cardioprotective effects, suggesting that these innovative phytochemicals have promising potential for preventing the occurrence of cardiac arrhythmia and reducing sudden cardiac death.

Keywords: Cupressaceae; antiarrhythmia; cardioprotection; herbal medicine; phytochemicals

1. Introduction

Cardiovascular diseases (CVDs) are major causes of health problems and death, representing prominent causes of morbidity and mortality worldwide and a total health and economic burden. Numerous lines of evidence suggest that CVDs include complex remodeling responses, such as hypertension, myocardial ischemia, and valve disease, which lead to poor clinical outcomes, including arrhythmia, heart failure (HF), and sudden cardiac death (SCD). These deleterious effects not only aggravate intrinsic heart disease and influence the eminence of life of patients but also induce SCD, which is life-threatening [1]. As the utmost populous country worldwide, China has ≈290 million patients with CVDs, and thus, CVDs represent the leading cause of death in the Chinese population [2]. In most cases, SCD leads to a sudden and unpredictable death due to an alteration in heart rhythm (sudden cardiac arrest). It estimates about 300,000 to 400,000 deaths annually in the United States and approximately 600,000 deaths annually in China [3,4].

Notably, the pathogenesis of arrhythmia is complicated and unpredictable. Intervention alternatives for arrhythmias include medications, radiofrequency ablation, cardiac resynchronization, implantable cardioverter-defibrillators, artificial pacemakers, and heart transplants [5–9]. Notwithstanding technological advances in catheter ablation therapy, antiarrhythmic drugs (AADs) are a basis for the management of cardiac arrhythmias. Experimental and translational data have demonstrated that regularly used AADs exert numerous effects on the heart, and the manifestation of these effects intensely depends on the specific experimental or clinical settings [10]. In the clinic, the treatment of arrhythmia is mainly based on Western medicine, i.e., propafenone (calcium channel blocker) and propranolol (β receptor blocker), but medical research has shown that AADs also have undesirable arrhythmic effects and that their improper usage can frequently cause more severe adverse reactions. Amiodarone [2-butyl-3-(3′,5′-diiodo-4′α-diethylaminoethoxybenzoyl)-benzofuran] (AMD), a class III antiarrhythmic drug that is an antagonism of Na^+, Ca^{2+}, and K^+ channels, and the β-adrenergic receptors as well, is a highly efficient AAD with potentially serious side effects in humans, such as idiosyncratic hepatotoxic reactions [11] and severe pulmonary toxicity (interstitial pneumonia and lung fibrosis) [12]. Despite numerous clinical options for AADs, pharmacotherapy is still ineffectual for the majority of patients. Additionally, all antiarrhythmic agents that act via diverse ion channels retain life-threatening proarrhythmic potential. Though the long-term consumption of these drugs can release symptoms, they can lead to an inadequate prognosis and may even upsurge mortality; hence, there is an urgent necessity to discover new antiarrhythmic treatment strategies involving natural products [13,14].

New phytoconstituent drugs and their physicochemical properties can be used for the treatment of various diseases because the secondary metabolites of plants include important bioactive compounds that are selected and propagated naturally for application as remedies against various human diseases and health disorders [15]. Remarkably, *Juniperus sabina* L. and *Sonchus oleraceus* (L.) L. are broadly utilized as traditional medicinal plants in China, and their aqueous extracts have been taken as a folk medicine to treat infections, inflammatory diseases, and tumors [16]. Several studies have shown that *J. sabina* L. significantly improves hepato-protective activity, antioxidant activity, antidiabetic activity, and antitumor effects [17–19]. *J. chinensis* has demonstrated noteworthy improvements in anti-proliferative and antifungal activities [20–22]. In addition, *J. formosana Hayata* has been shown to have an inhibitory effect on the progression of kidney disease, urinary disorders, gynecological diseases, and lung cancer [23–25]. The fruit and leaves of junipers are usually used as tea, and minced fruits are applied to lower blood sugar contents in Anatolia [19]. *Chamaecyparis obtusa* was found to be effective in preventing bleeding, possessing antibacterial activity, and exerting antitussive effects [26]. Whether Cupressaceae plants possess antiarrhythmia activity remains to be investigated.

In this study, we attempted to evaluate the efficacy of pretreatment with Cupressaceae in a murine model of barium chloride ($BaCl_2$)-induced arrhythmia. To achieve this goal, seven Cupressaceae species, including *Chamaecyparis obtusa*, *Juniperus chinensis* (L.) Ant., *Sabina chinensis* (L.) Ant. cv. Kaizuca, *Platycladus orientalis* (L.) Franco, *Juniperus sabina* L., *Fokienia hodginsii*, and *Juniperus chinensis* 'Pyramidalis', were collected and extracted with ethanol. The biological function (protection) of the ethanolic extracts against $BaCl_2$-induced arrhythmia was examined using normal II lead electrocardiogram (ECG) measurements in mouse models.

2. Results

2.1. A Survey of the Medicinal Value of Various Conifer Plants

The literature search of electronic databases, including PubMed, MEDLINE, ScienceDirect, Google Scholar, the Cochrane Library, and Web of Science, was performed to identify articles published from inception until May 2023, illustrating that various conifer plant extracts composed of a variety of active components have great medicinal value (Supplemental Table S1 in Supplementary File). For example, *F. hodginsii*, a rich source of structurally diverse diterpenoids, has been used for the treatment of stomach aches, nausea, vomiting, and anti-proliferative activity [27–30], which are dependent on various components. One report shows that the volatile oil (100 mg/kg body weight, p.o.) of *Cupressus funebris* Endl can significantly enhance its anti-inflammatory activity [31]. The volatile oil of *J. chinensis 'Pyramidalis'* has significant antitumor and antibacterial effects [32]. In addition to its blood circulation, diuretic activity, and antibacterial activity, *S. chinensis* L. exerts antidiabetic effects via its α-amylase inhibitory activity [33]. The compounds β-phellandrene, terpinen-4-ol, and bornyl acetate are major constituents of essential oils in *S. chinensis* and have been found to possess effective antifungal activity [22,34]. Three phenolic compounds, cosmosiin, caffeic acid, and p-coumaric acid, were firstly isolated from the leaves of *Cupressus sempervirens* L.; together with cupressuflavone, amentoflavone, rutin, quercitrin, quercetin, and myricitrin, these compounds have been found to have high antioxidant activity, and quercetin, rutin, caffeic acid, and p-coumaric acid are further used for hepatoprotective activity [35]. The previous study affords a promising complementary alternative for the proper use of a selection of essential oil combinations for use in the respiratory tract [36]. In total, 33, 37, and 37 compounds were found in the oils from the leaves of *S chinensis* (L.) Ant, *C. lusitanica* 'Zhongshan' Mill, and *S. chinensis* (L.) Ant. Cv. Kaizuca, respectively. Fourteen compounds were commonly identified, such as thujene, alpha-pinene, camphene, sabinene, beta-myrcene, alpha-terpinene, gamma-terpinene, alpha-terpinolene, bornyl acetate, beta-elemene, alpha-amorphene, germacrene D, delta-cadinene, and elemol. Moreover, each species contained its own particular compounds. Remarkably, the main components are sabinene (20.99%), limonene (19.78%), and bornyl acetate (11.68%) for *S. chinensis* (L.) Ant; alpha-pinene (10.39%), sabinene (11.19%), and delta-3-carene (8.88%) for *C. lusitanica* 'Zhongshan' Mill; and limonene (24.56%) and beta-myrcene (8.04%) for *S. chinensis* (L.) Ant. Cv. Kaizuca [37]. Because of the various associated phytochemicals with numerous medicinal properties, diverse conifer plants might represent a new source of materials with pharmacological properties involved in protection against cardiac arrhythmia that is worth investigating.

2.2. Screening of Various Conifer Plant Extracts in Mice

To investigate the antiarrhythmic effects on conifer plants, mice were gavaged with the crude extracts of *F. hodginsii*, *C. obtusa*, *J. chinensis* (L.) Ant., *S. chinensis* (L.) Ant. cv. Kaizuca, *P. orientalis* (L.) Franco, *J. sabina* L., or *J. chinensis* (0.1 mL/10 g Bwt) for 10 min and injected (i.p.) with 0.8% $BaCl_2$ solution (0.1 mL/10 g Bwt). First, mice were orally administered olive oil alone for 5 or 10 min before $BaCl_2$ injection, and the mice with an ECG of $BaCl_2$-induced arrhythmia failed to show any effect of the addition of olive oil (Figure 1A,C). Olive oil was used to dissolve all the extracts in subsequent experiments. Next, to evaluate time points after administration of the extracts, mice were orally administered the *C. obtusa*, *P. orientalis*, and *J. sabina* extracts for 5 or 10 min followed by a subsequent $BaCl_2$ injection. The results revealed no protective effect at 5 min after administration (Figure 1B), while 10 min prior to $BaCl_2$ injection was found to have a protective effect (Figure 1D). To investigate the protective effect of amiodarone (clinical medicine as a reference), mice were i.p. injected with 0.6% amiodarone (15 mg/kg Bwt) for 10 min before $BaCl_2$ injection, and the ECG signals of the mice appeared normal (Figure 1E). The results further illustrated that $BaCl_2$-induced arrhythmia in mice is remediable via clinical drugs. Subsequently, considering the intestinal absorption of the extracts, the conifer plant extract was intragastrically administered for 10 min, followed by an injection of the $BaCl_2$ solution. After seven conifer plants were screened, *F. hodginsii*, *J. chinensis* (L.) Ant., *S. chinensis* (L.) Ant. cv. Kaizuca, and *J. chinensis* showed no protective effects against $BaCl_2$-induced arrhythmia in mice. Surprisingly, the ECG data revealed protective effects of *C. obtusa*, *P. orientalis*, and *J. sabina* against $BaCl_2$-induced arrhythmia in mice (Figures 2–4).

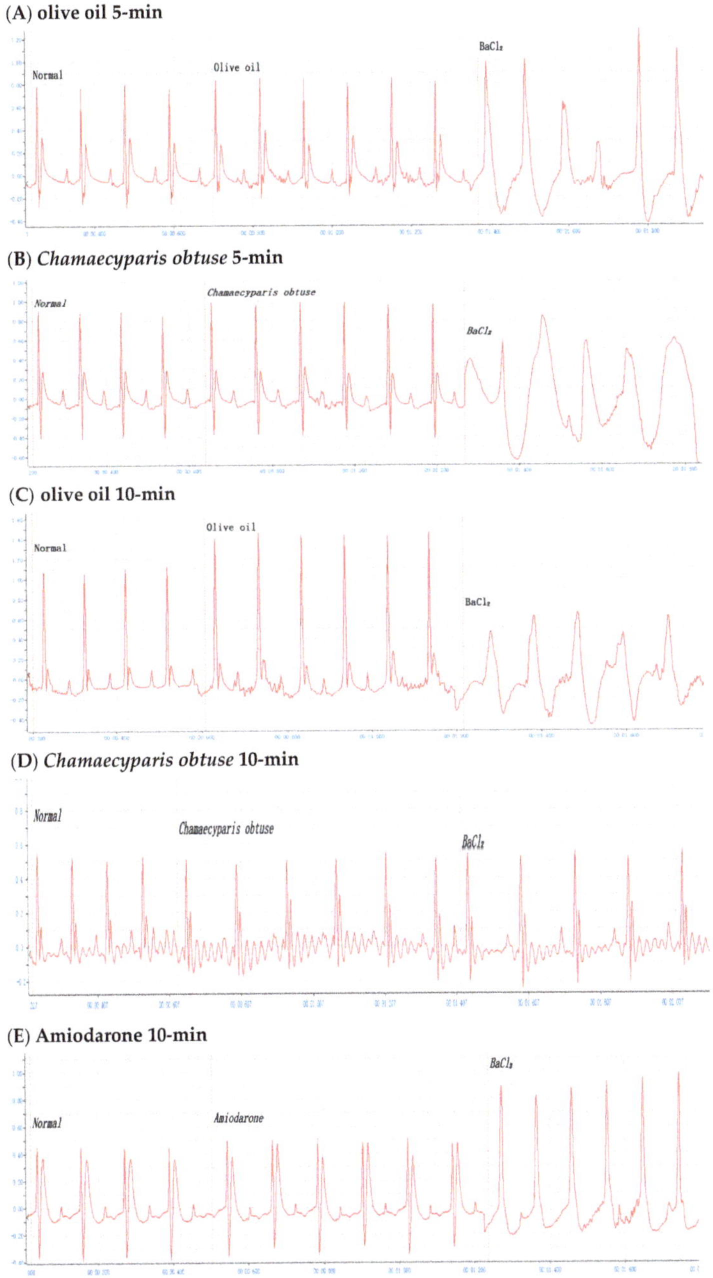

Figure 1. The protective effect of olive oil and *Chamaecyparis obtusa* (0.1 mL/10 g Bwt) at 5-min or 10-min after administration in mice before $BaCl_2$-induced arrhythmia. (**A**) Olive oil for 5-min, (**B**) olive oil for 10-min, (**C**) *Chamaecyparis obtusa* for 5-min, (**D**) *Chamaecyparis obtusa* for 10-min, and (**E**) 0.6% amiodarone (15 mg/kg Bwt) for 10-min.

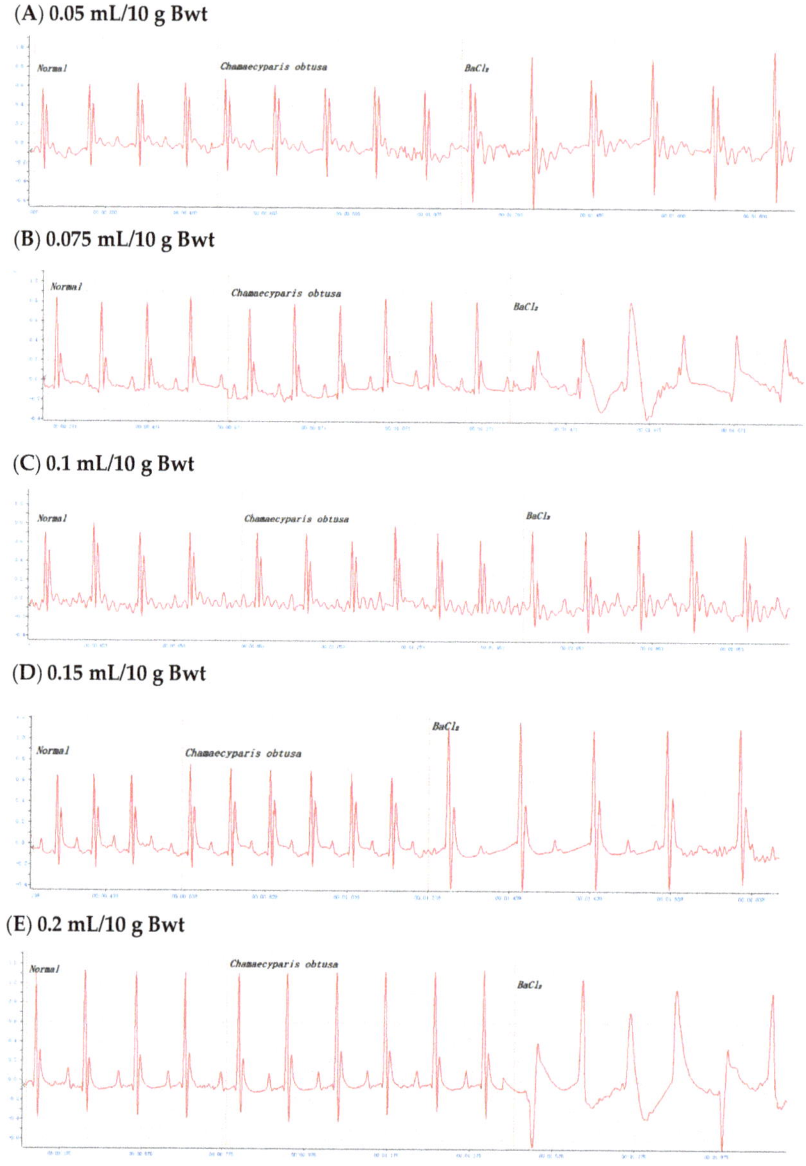

Figure 2. The protective effect of various concentrations of *Chamaecyparis obtusa* in mice after $BaCl_2$-induced arrhythmia: (**A**) 0.05 mL/10 g Bwt, (**B**) 0.075 mL/10 g Bwt, (**C**) 0.1 mL/10 g Bwt, (**D**) 0.15 mL/10 g Bwt, and (**E**) 0.2 mL/10 g Bwt.

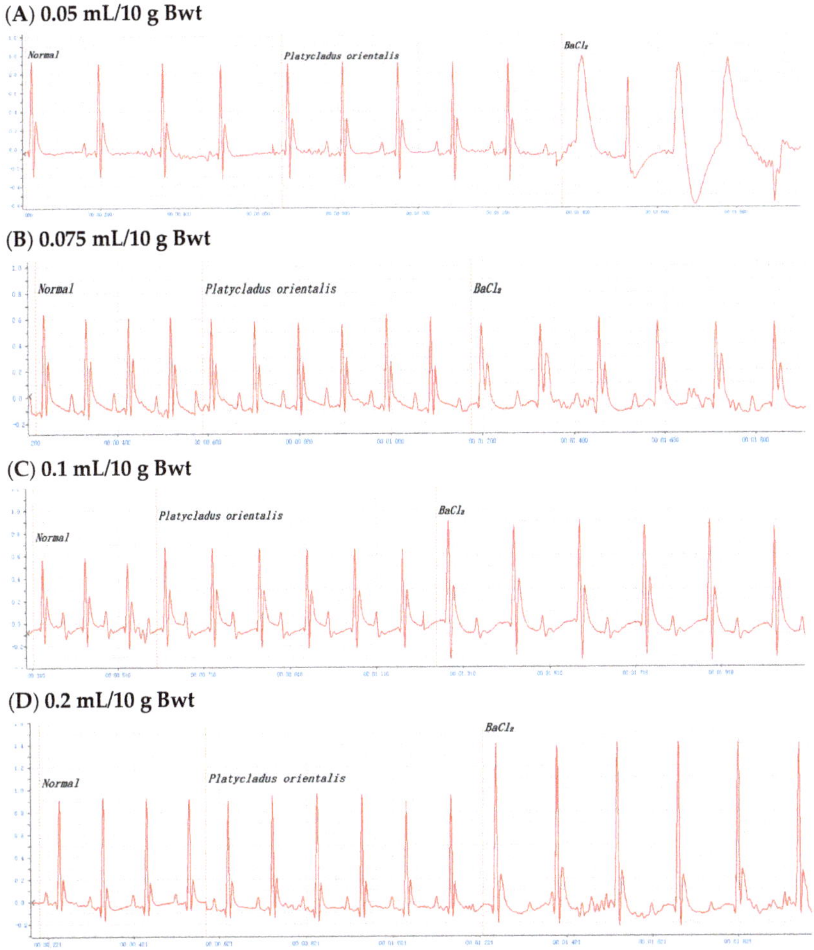

Figure 3. The protective effect of various concentrations of *Platycladus orientalis* in mice after $BaCl_2$-induced arrhythmia: (**A**) 0.05 mL/10 g Bwt, (**B**) 0.075 mL/10 g Bwt, (**C**) 0.1 mL/10 g Bwt, and (**D**) 0.2 mL/10 g Bwt.

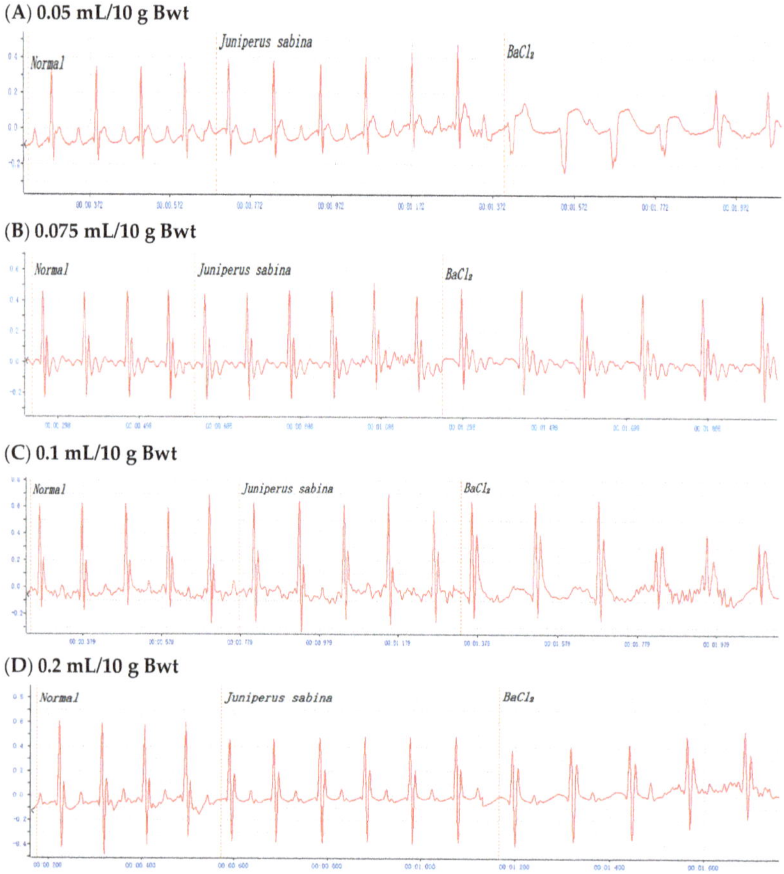

Figure 4. The protective effect of various concentrations of *Juniperus sabina* in mice after $BaCl_2$-induced arrhythmia: (**A**) 0.05 mL/10 g Bwt, (**B**) 0.075 mL/10 g Bwt, (**C**) 0.1 mL/10 g Bwt, and (**D**) 0.2 mL/10 g Bwt.

2.3. Dose-Dependent Protective Effects of *C. obtusa*, *P. orientalis*, and *J. sabina* Extracts on $BaCl_2$-Induced Arrhythmia in Mice

To determine the antiarrhythmic effects of *C. obtusa*, *P. orientalis*, and *J. sabina* on $BaCl_2$-induced arrhythmia in mice, various doses of *C. obtusa*, *P. orientalis*, *and J. sabina* extracts were tested. The data revealed dose-dependent protective effects of the *C. obtusa*, *P. orientalis*, and *J. sabina* extracts, ranging from 0.075 mL/10 g Bwt to 0.15 mL/10 g Bwt or 0.2 mL/10 g Bwt, while 0.05 mL/10 g Bwt had no significant effect (Figures 2–4).

2.4. Efficacy of *C. obtusa*, *P. orientalis*, and *J. sabina* Extracts in Protection against $BaCl_2$-Induced Arrhythmia in Mice

To investigate the protective potential (duration) of $BaCl_2$-induced cardiac arrhythmia, mice were orally administered various doses of *C. obtusa*, *P. orientalis*, and *J. sabina* extracts for 10 min, followed by an injection of the $BaCl_2$ solution. The results showed that with increasing doses of *P. orientalis*, and *J. sabina* extracts, the duration of protection increased with increasing dosage. However, due to the toxicity of *C. obtusa*, the duration of protection increased to 0.15 mL/10 g Bwt (Table 1). These results revealed that *C. obtusa*, *P. orientalis*, and *J. sabina* extracts contain antiarrhythmic characters.

Table 1. The protection duration (min) of barium chloride-induced cardiac arrhythmia pretreated with the ethanol extracts of *Chamaecyparis obtusa, Platycladus orientalis*, and *Juniperus sabina* leaves.

Species	0.05 mL/10 g Bwt	0.075 mL/10 g Bwt	0.10 mL/10 g Bwt	0.15/0.20 mL/10 g Bwt
Chamaecyparis obtusa	0.5 ± 0.2 min	4.0 ± 1.1 min **	5.0 ± 1.1 min **	15.0 ± 2.9 min *** (0.15 mL/10 g)
Platycladus orientalis	1.0 ± 0.4 min	5.0 ± 1.4 min **	5.0 ± 1.7 min **	9.0 ± 2.1 min **
Juniperus sabina	0.5 ± 0.3 min	4.5 ± 1.9 min **	5.0 ± 1.5 min **	10.0 ± 2.3 min ***

Mice was orally pretreated with various concentrations of ethanol extracts of *C. obtusa, P. orientalis*, or *J. sabina* leaves (each dose $n = 6$) for 10 min followed by a 0.8% barium chloride (0.1 mL/10 g Bwt) injection (i.p.). ** $p < 0.01$ and *** $p < 0.005$ compared with 0.05 mL/10 g Bwt.

2.5. Treated Efficacy of *C. obtusa, P. orientalis*, and *J. sabina* Extracts in $BaCl_2$-Induced Arrhythmia in Rats

One report indicated that the ethanol extract of *Sophora flavescens* Ait. has been shown to have antiarrhythmic activity via investigations of cardiac arrhythmias induced by aconitine infusion in mice and by coronary artery ligation in rats [38]. To confirm the potential of $BaCl_2$-induced cardiac arrhythmia treatment with *C. obtusa, P. orientalis*, and *J. sabina* extracts, rats were orally injected with 0.4 mL/100 g Bwt of *C. obtusa, P. orientalis*, and *J. sabina* extracts, respectively, of the $BaCl_2$ solution. The results revealed the antiarrhythmic effects of *C. obtusa, P. orientalis*, and *J. sabina* extracts against $BaCl_2$-induced cardiac arrhythmia in rats (Figure 5). These results were consistent with the results obtained in mice, illustrating that *C. obtusa, P. orientalis*, and *J. sabina* extracts possessed antiarrhythmic effects.

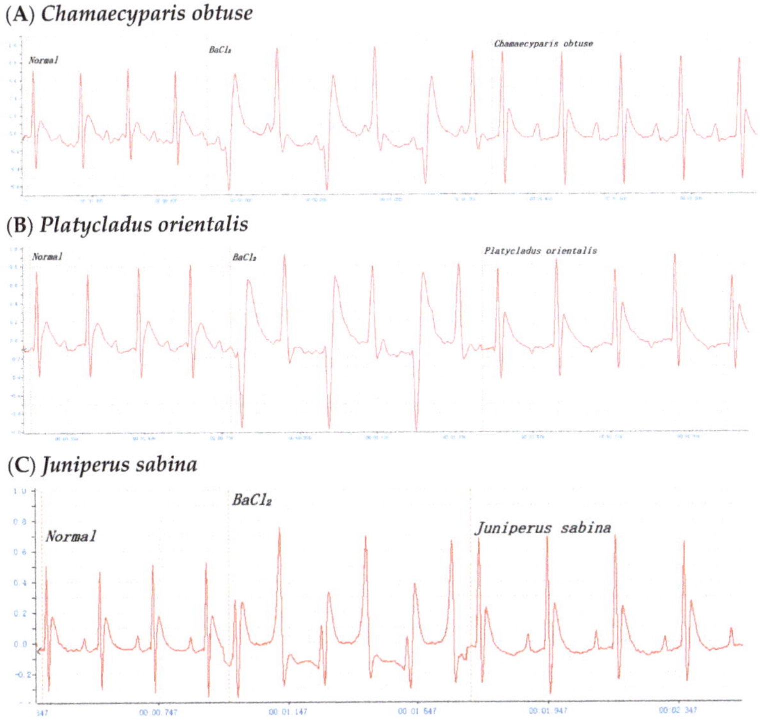

Figure 5. Treatment with 0.4 mL/100 g Bwt of (**A**) *Chamaecyparis obtusa*, (**B**) *Platycladus orientalis*, and (**C**) *Juniperus sabina* in rats after $BaCl_2$-induced arrhythmia.

2.6. The Involvement of the M Receptor in the Antiarrhythmic Effects of C. obtusa, P. orientalis, and J. sabina Extracts Compared with That of Amiodarone in Mice

To further understand which M-receptor type was involved in the antiarrhythmic effects of the *C. obtusa*, *P. orientalis*, or *J. sabina* extracts compared with the reference drug amiodarone, mice were first administered $BaCl_2$; once arrhythmia developed, the mice received pirenzepine dihydrochloride (M1 antagonist, 0.3 mg/kg Bwt), methoctramine tetrahydrochloride (M2 antagonist, 0.3 mg/kg Bwt), or 4-DAMP (M3 antagonist, 1 mg/kg Bwt) for 2 min and then amiodarone, *C. obtusa*, *P. orientalis*, or *J. sabina* extracts (0.1 mL/10 g Bwt) to monitor alterations in the ECG. The results demonstrated that the antiarrhythmic effects of the *C. obtusa*, *P. orientalis*, and *J. sabina* extracts could occur through the M2 (Figure 6) and M3 receptors (Figure 7) but not the M1 receptor (Figure 8).

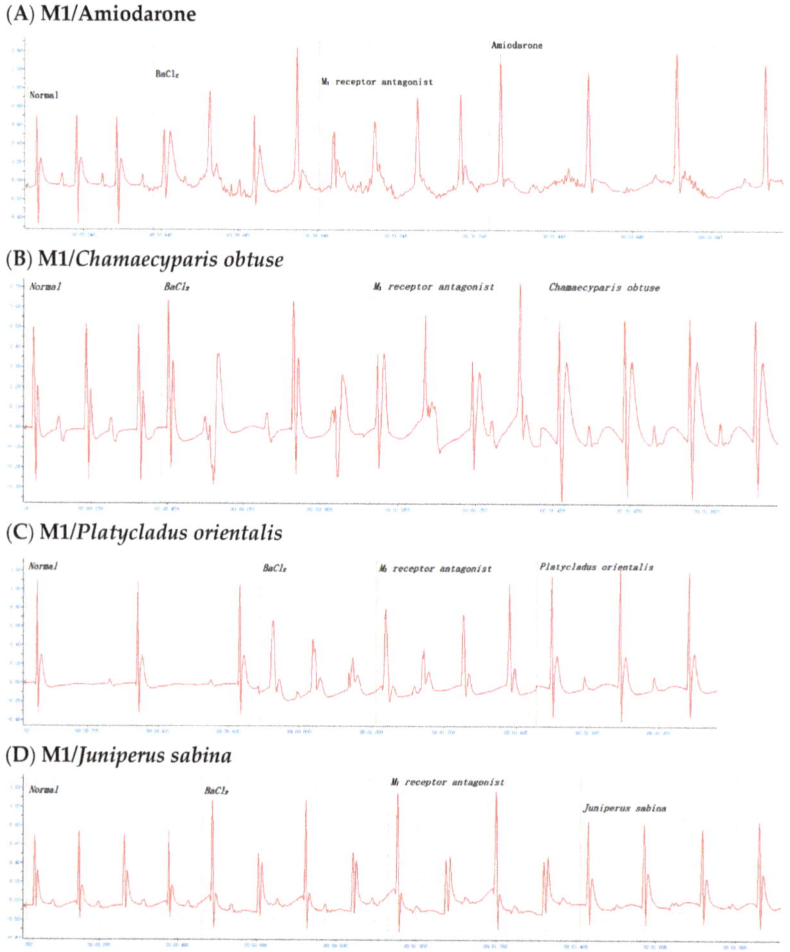

Figure 6. The addition of pirenzepine dihydrochloride (muscarinic receptor M1 antagonist, 0.3 mg/kg) to (**A**) amiodarone or the ethanolic extract (0.1 mL/10 g Bwt) of (**B**) *C. obtusa*, (**C**) *P. orientalis*, and (**D**) *J. sabina* leaves in mice after $BaCl_2$-induced arrhythmia.

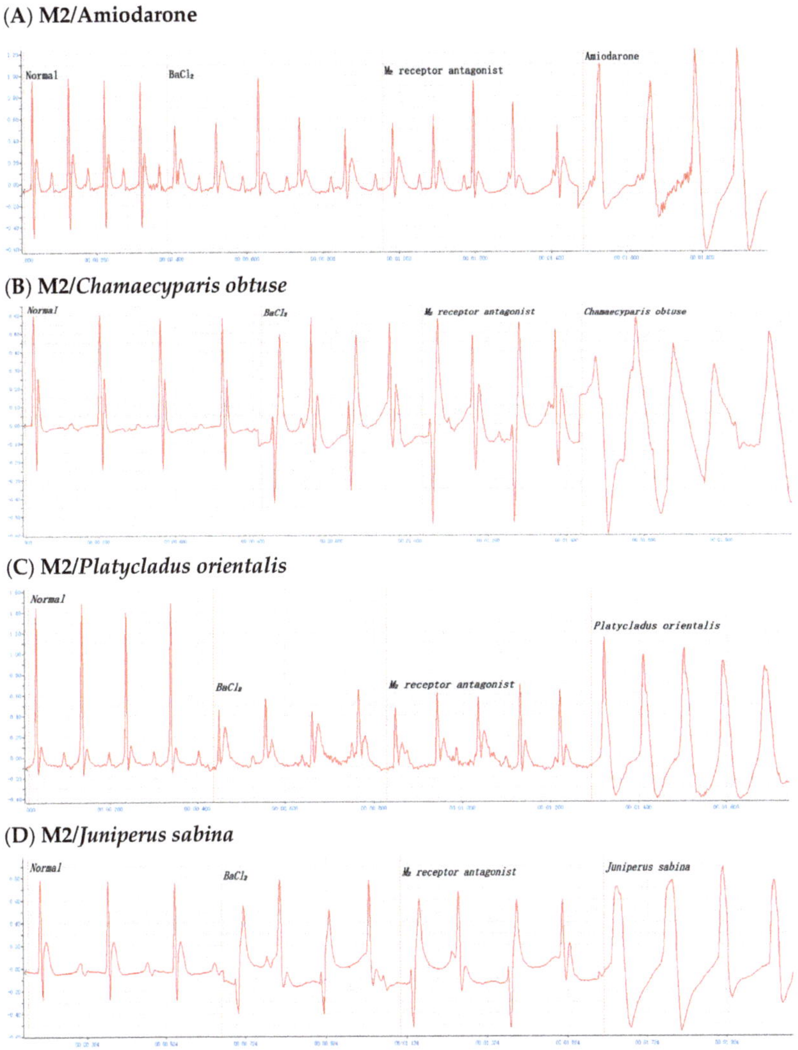

Figure 7. The addition of methoctramine tetrahydrochloride (M2 antagonist, 0.3 mg/kg) with (**A**) amiodarone or ethanolic extract (0.1 mL/10 g Bwt) to (**B**) *C. obtusa*, (**C**) *P. orientalis*, and (**D**) *J. sabina* leaves in mice after $BaCl_2$-induced arrhythmia.

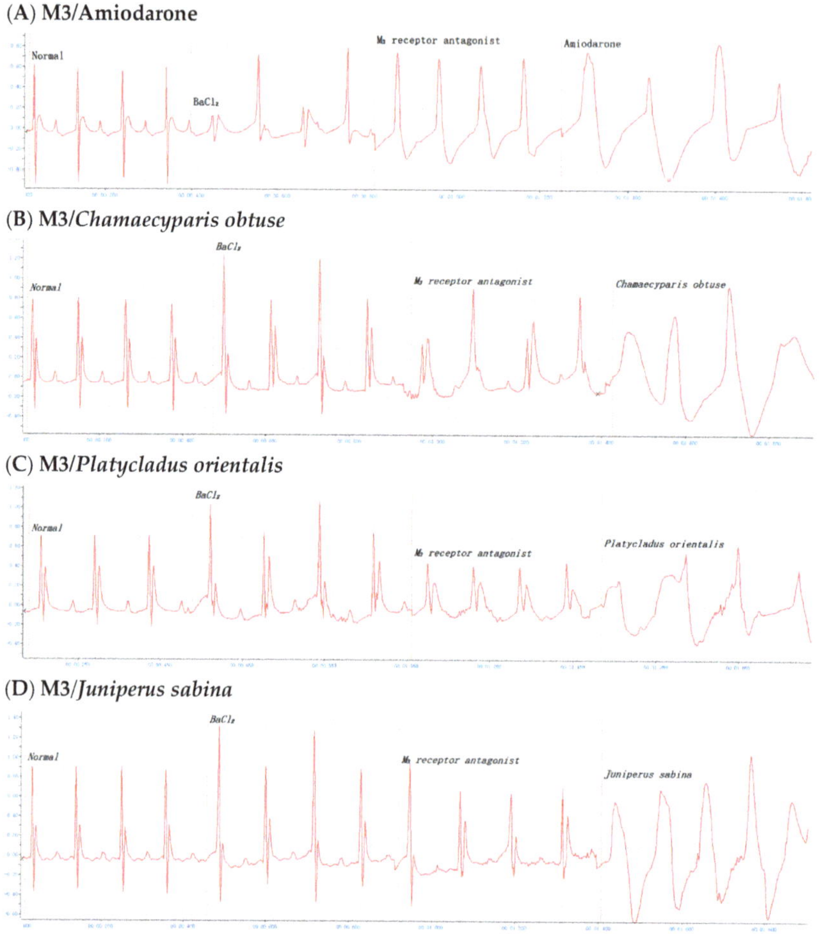

Figure 8. The addition of 4-DAMP (1,1-dimethyl-4-diphenylacetoxypiperidinium iodide, an M3 antagonist, 0.2 mg/kg) to (**A**) amiodarone or the ethanolic extracts (0.1 mL/10 g Bwt) of (**B**) *C. obtusa*, (**C**) *P. orientalis*, and (**D**) *J. sabina* leaves after $BaCl_2$-induced arrhythmia in mice.

3. Discussion

In the present study, we first demonstrated the pharmacological effects of *C. obtusa*, *P. orientalis*, and *J. sabina* extracts in a concentration-dependent manner as the cardioprotective agents against $BaCl_2$-induced arrhythmia. As we know, traditional Chinese medicine (TCM) has played a critical role in ameliorating symptoms, thwarting disease recurrence, reducing toxic side effects, and improving the quality of life. The use of Western medicine for the management of AF is limited, and several studies have revealed that traditional herbs comprise a variety of pharmacologically active constituents that have great efficacy and prospective for the hindrance and treatment of cardiac arrhythmia [39–42] with distinctive advantages, such as few side and adverse effects, low toxicity, a long effect duration, and high compliance. In terms of clinical usage, TCMs with alkaloids, flavonoids, and saponins as the leading effective constituents have a positive effect on the treatment of CVDs such as angina pectoris, arrhythmia, myocardial ischemia, and myocardial infarction (MI) [43]. Another report revealed that Fuzi, *Aconiti lateralis Radix Praeparata*, has been broadly used for 2000 years in TCM for the treatment of acute HF. Notably, the results revealed that the long-term use of Fuzi has a main benefit in averting cardiovascular problems [44]. Calycosin and its derivatives, the major bioactive flavonoids in *Astragalus membranaceus*, have promising potential for the cardiovascular protection of cardiac myocytes and vascular endothelial cells [43]. Wenxin Keli (WXKL), a typical Chinese patent medicine with apparent effectiveness and promising safety, has played a prominent role in the treatment of CVD patients. Accumulating evidence from various cell and animal studies has shown that WXKL plays cardioprotective roles by impeding inflammation, diminishing oxidative stress, mediating vasomotor disorders, decreasing cellular apoptosis, and protecting against endothelial injury, myocardial ischemia, cardiac fibrosis, and cardiac hypertrophy [45]. Furthermore, the action of WXKL may reduce the QT interval and dawdle the heart rate by downregulating sodium channel protein type 5 subunit alpha (SCN5A) and the beta-2 adrenergic receptor (ADRB2) and upregulating muscarinic acetylcholine receptor M2 (CHRM2) during myocardial ischemia. These findings afford novel insight into the molecular mechanisms by which WXKL reduces the prevalence of ventricular arrhythmia [46].

The results of this study disclose that the pharmacological effects of *C. obtusa*, *P. orientalis*, and *J. sabina* extracts exert cardioprotection against $BaCl_2$-induced (inhibiting IK1) arrhythmia. Basal and acetylcholine-gated inward-rectifier K^+-currents (IK1 and IKACh, respectively) play vital roles in cardiac excitability by mediating heart rate variability and susceptibility to atrial arrhythmias and AF. Recent studies have indicated the coexistence of multiple muscarinic acetylcholine receptor (mAChR) subtypes that regulate several distinct K^+ currents in the heart, namely, the inward rectifier K^+ current (IKACh) by M2 and two delayed rectifier K^+ currents, IKM3 and IK4AP, by the M3 and M4 receptors, respectively. Gi-protein-coupled muscarinic receptor M2 is considered the predominant receptor that activates IKACh [47]. Calcium/calmodulin-dependent protein kinase II (CaMKII) is a vital ion channel mediator that participates in excitation–contraction coupling to regulate its electrophysiological function. These effects can be largely abolished by the co-application of the IK1 blocker $BaCl_2$. IK1-dependent suppression of CaMKII activity is a crucial cardiac salvage signaling pathway during Ca^{2+} dyshomeostasis and oxidative stress (reactive oxygen species, ROS). IK1 might be a unique target for the pharmacological conditioning of reperfusion arrhythmia, especially during intervention after unpredictable ischemia [48].

Cardiac autonomic nerve dysfunctions, such as the excitement of the Vagal nerve and inhibition of sympathetic nerves, have been exposed by molecular biology studies [49,50]. Accordingly, arrhythmia can be triggered by the abnormal structure and function of ion channels [51]. Accumulating studies have demonstrated a role for α1-adrenolytics in the management of arrhythmias. The stimulation of α1-adrenoceptor facilitates inositol trisphosphate (IP_3) production and subsequent Ca^{2+} release from the sarcoplasmic reticulum (SR) [52]. Therefore, the blockade of α1-adrenoceptors may result in the stabilization of Ca^{2+} levels, generating antiarrhythmic effects in catecholamine-induced arrhythmias, e.g., catecholaminergic polymorphic ventricular tachycardia. One study has reported that prazosin not only reduced the norepinephrine-induced elongation of AF in mice but also mitigated norepinephrine-induced SR Ca^{2+} leakage and spontaneous SR Ca^{2+} release in cultured atrial cardiomyocytes. These findings confirm that α1-adrenoceptors may have a role in preventing cardiac arrhythmias [53] and have been confirmed in numerous animal studies, thus validating the antiarrhythmic properties of α1-adrenolytics [54–56]. In earlier experiments, 2-methoxyphenylpiperazine derivatives were shown to have a high affinity for α1-adrenoceptors [57], and the activities of these compounds were compared with those of carvedilol, which is a β1- and α1-adrenoceptor blocker with antioxidant properties [58]. Nevertheless, the mechanism by which *C. obtusa*, *P. orientalis*, and *J. sabina* extracts protect against $BaCl_2$-induced arrhythmia requires verification.

The experiments also depict the involvement of the M receptor in the antiarrhythmic effects of *C. obtusa*, *P. orientalis*, and *J. sabina* extracts compared with that of amiodarone in mice. In primary tissues, at least four pharmacological M receptors (M1, M2, M3, M4) are defined, and five muscarinic receptors have been cloned (m1, m2, m3, m4, m5). There are few selective agonists for M-receptor subtypes, and all classical agonists (acetylcholine, carbachol, etc.) are evidently nonselective. Several selective antagonists for M1 (pirenzepine) and M2 receptors (AF-DX 116) have been critically studied [59]. A comparative study of the ability of selective M-cholinoblockers to prevent arrhythmias induced by phosphacol and potassium cyanide showed that the activity of the M1 antagonist pirenzepine is greater than that of the M2 antagonist AF-DX-116; simultaneously, both drugs revealed the equivalent activity with regard to arrhythmias induced by aconitine, calcium chloride, and carbachol [60]. The present results demonstrated that the antiarrhythmia effects of *C. obtusa*, *P. orientalis*, and *J. sabina* extracts could occur through the M2 (Figure 7) and M3 receptors (Figure 8) but not the M1 receptor (Figure 6). One study has reported that (1) the stimulation of the M1 mAChR subtype on sympathetic postganglionic cells results in catecholamine-mediated cardiac stimulation, (2) M1 mAChR is not expressed in the mouse heart, and (3) the administration of ACh to mice induces arrhythmia [61]. The IKACh plays a vital role in cardiac excitability by mediating heart rate variability and vulnerability to atrial arrhythmias. Both inward rectification mechanisms are extrinsic to the KACh channel; from our understanding, this is the first depiction of an extrinsic inward rectification of ionic current attributable to an intrinsic voltage-sensitive property of the G protein-coupled receptor M2 [62]. Recent studies have indicated the presence of multiple mAChR subtypes that regulate several distinct K+ currents in the heart, namely, the IKACh by M2 and the two delayed rectifier K+ currents IKM3 and IK4AP by the M3 and M4 receptors, respectively [63]. This is the first report to demonstrate the downregulation of three types of mAChR-coupled K^+ currents (IKM2, IKM3, and IKM4) and of M2, M3, and M4 mAChR subtype proteins in a canine model of atrial tachycardia (AT)-induced remodeling [64]. Both D,L-sotalol and MS-551 interact with cardiac M2 and peripheral M3 receptors, and they exert anticholinergic activity in cardiac and peripheral tissues at high concentrations [65]. Activation of M3 has been previously shown to promote short-term cardioprotection against ischemic injury with the M3 agonist choline, the antagonist 4-DAMP, or the M2-mAChR antagonist methoctramine followed by the administration of choline. M3-mAChRs denote a promising target for interpreting cardiomyocytes tolerant to ischemic injury [66]. The prevention of ischemia-induced changes in Gi-mediated signal transduction and/or (with certain limitations discussed below) the selective activation of cardiac muscarinic M2 receptors could hence be an alternative pharmacological treatment for acute myocardial ischemia [67]. Atrial G protein-gated inwardly rectifying K+ (GIRK) channels are critical mediators of parasympathetic effects on cardiac physiology. The mouse ventricular GIRK channel is a GIRK channel subunit (GIRK1, GIRK4), a GIRK1/GIRK4 heteromer, and although it contributes to the cholinergic suppression of ventricular myocyte excitability, this impact does not substantively influence cardiac physiology or ventricular arrhythmogenesis in mice [68]. Accumulating evidence indicates the presence of functional M3-mAChRs, in addition to the well-recognized M2-mAChRs, in the hearts of various species comprising humans. Choline improves cardiac function and moderates ischemic myocardial injury by stimulating cardiac M3-mAChRs, which in turn results in changes in the multiple signaling pathways, leading to cytoprotection. These findings suggest that M3-mAChR is a new target for improving cardiac function and preventing cardiac injury during ischemia/reperfusion [69].

Remarkably, bioactive compounds such as phenolics, flavonoids, terpenoids, glycosidic derivatives, alkaloids, iridoids, and saponins from various parts of plants including *Terminalia arjuna* [70] and *Emblica officinalis* fruit [71] have gained important applications in exerting significantly cardioprotective effects. Furthermore, many lines of medicinal values have been discovered from *Cupressus sempervirens* L. (Cupressaceae) including headache, toothaches [72], sneeze bronchitis, obesity, and laryngitis along with biological properties such as anti-inflammatory, anti-microbial, and insecticidal actions [73]. In addition, nineteen various polyphenolic molecules comprising gallic acid, chlorogenic acid, catechin, methyl gallate, coffeic acid, syringic acid, pyrocatechol, rutin, ellagic acid, coumaric acid, vanillin, ferulic acid, naringenin, rosmarinic acid, daidzein, quercetin, cinnamic acid, kaempferol, and hesperetin upon extraction of *C. sempervirens* using supercritical fluid extraction have recently been identified and further been investigated for their antibacterial and anti-biofilm activities [74,75]. To the best of our knowledge, this study is the first investigation to explore the potential benefit of Cupressaceae in the treatment of arrhythmia, making our findings particularly valuable. In the future, we will be treating large animal arrhythmia with the extracts to confirm the efficacy of ethanolic extracts. And the extracts are isolated and purified to obtain the active components via HPLC and NMR. The experiments will further be conducted to investigate the purified components in in vivo and in vitro assays in the treatment of animal arrhythmia to validate the efficacy, acting mechanisms, and toxicity for the completion of preclinical tests.

4. Materials and Methods

4.1. Plant Source and Reagents

Conifer plants (*F. hodginsii* and *C. obtusa*) were collected from Xiamen (Fujian, China), and others (*J. chinensis* (L.) Ant., *S. chinensis* (L.) Ant. cv. Kaizuca, *P. orientalis* (L.) Franco, *J. sabina* L., and *J. chinensis* 'Pyramidalis') were obtained from Jiangsu (China). The experimental plant samples, including the collected plant material, complied with relevant institutional, national, and international guidelines. Leaves of cypress varieties were cleaned thoroughly with water and rinsed with distilled water. The plant materials were dried under shade at room temperature (RT). All chemicals were purchased from Sigma–Aldrich (St. Louis, MO, USA). Pirenzepine dihydrochloride (muscarinic receptor M1 antagonist), methoctramine tetrahydrochloride (M2 antagonist), and 4-DAMP (1,1-dimethyl-4-diphenylacetoxypiperidinium iodide, M3 antagonist) were obtained from MedChemExpress (Shanghai, China).

4.2. Extraction of Cypress Leaves

First, all the dried cypress leaves were cut into small pieces. Second, all the cut leaves were soaked in 75% ethanol (1:10, *w*/*v*) in an ultrasonic bath (KQ-5200 type DE, Kun Shan Ultrasonic Instruments Co., Ltd., Kunshan, Jiangsu, China) to obtain the extraction solutions. Finally, the extraction solutions were dried in an evaporator (DHG-9070A, Shanghai Heheng Instruments and Equipment Co., Ltd., Shanghai, China) at 42 °C to obtain the products as dark green solids. The extracts were then dissolved in olive oil for subsequent experiments. The yield of crude extract was 8.6 ± 1.2%. The experimental concentration was 40 mg/mL.

4.3. Animal Care

All experimental procedures were executed according to the guidelines outlined in the "Guide for the Care and Use of Laboratory Animals, 8th edition" published by the National Institutes of Health, and they fulfilled the ARRIVE guidelines. The animal experiments were approved by the Animal Ethics Committee of Medical College according to the "Guide for the Care and Use of Laboratory Animals" of Xiamen Medical College (approved protocol ID SYXK 2018-0010). Evaluations of experimental animal care were periodically performed in accordance with the Laboratory Animal Guidelines for Ethical Review of Animal Welfare (GB/T 35892-2018, China).

Eighty male ICR mice (6 weeks old, 22 ± 3 g Bwt) and male Sprague Dawley rats (150 ± 30 g Bwt) were obtained from Hangzhou Medical College (Zhejiang, China) and kept at RT (22 ± 2 °C) and a specific humidity (50 ± 10%). A 12/12 h light/dark (6 a.m.–6 p.m.) cycle was maintained throughout the entire study. The mice had free access to a standard laboratory diet (Rodent Feed 1022, Beijing HFK Bioscience Co., Ltd., Beijing, China) and tap water ad libitum. Sprague Dawley rats and ICR mice were anesthetized with 5% isoflurane gas in an inhalation chamber with a vaporizer (R583S rodent gas anesthesia machine, RWD Life Science Co., Ltd., Shenzhen, China), and 2% isoflurane was administered during the entire experimental procedure. The mice were anesthetized according to the protocol supplied in the McGill Standard Operating Procedure (SOP) (#110 for mice and #111 for rats), which describes methods used for mouse and rat anesthesia.

4.4. Antiarrhythmic Activity of the Extract in a Mouse Model of $BaCl_2$-Induced Arrhythmia Prior to (Protection) $BaCl_2$ Induction

Mice were randomly divided into 9 groups: an NS group, a positive control group (amiodarone), and 7 test groups of Cupressaceae leaves. First, the mice were generally anesthetized with 5% inhaled isoflurane in a rodent gas anesthesia machine (RWD Life Science Co., Ltd. Shenzhen, China) and fixed on a plank. Second, acupuncture needles were subcutaneously inserted into the limbs of the mice to monitor and record normal II lead electrocardiograms (ECGs) via the BL-420I biological function experiment system (Techman Inc., Chengdu, Sichuan, China) under 2% isoflurane anesthesia. Then, the anesthetized mice were orally administered different treatments at the test dose. Ten minutes later, a 0.8% barium chloride solution was i.p. injected into each mouse (0.1 mL/10 g Bwt) to induce arrhythmia. ECG signals were individually monitored and recorded during the experiments. The number of mice that maintained a normal rhythm and the duration (5, 10, and 30 min) of normal rhythm mice were recorded to calculate the efficacy of the tested samples in each group. At the end of the experiments, all rats were sacrificed by CO_2 euthanasia. Additional experiments were performed to explore the effect of the muscarinic acetylcholine receptor type on the antiarrhythmic effects of the *C. obtusa*, *P. orientalis*, and *J. sabina* extracts (5 mg/mL of olive oil). Mice were treated with pirenzepine dihydrochloride (an M1 antagonist, 0.3 mg/kg Bwt), methoctramine tetrahydrochloride (an M2 antagonist, 0.3 mg/kg Bwt), or 4-DAMP (an M3 antagonist, 1 mg/kg Bwt) for 2 min and administered amiodarone, *C. obtusa*, *P. orientalis*, or *J. sabina* extracts (0.1 mL/10 g Bwt) to detect alterations in the ECG profile.

4.5. Statistical Analysis

The in vivo data are expressed as means ± SEMs. The results were carried out by using a one-way analysis of variance (ANOVA) for statistical comparisons among treatments. The means within each column followed by different letters are significantly different at $p < 0.05$ according to the post hoc Tukey's test.

5. Conclusions

CVDs are the leading cause of global mortality and impose a considerable economic burden on both governments and individuals. Ethanolic extracts of seven species of Cupressaceae, namely, *Chamaecyparis obtusa*, *Juniperus chinensis* (L.) Ant., *Sabina chinensis* (L.) Ant. cv. Kaizuca, *Platycladus orientalis* (L.) Franco, *Juniperus sabina* L., *Fokienia hodginsii*, and *Juniperus chinensis* 'Pyramidalis' were screened for their cardioprotective effects against $BaCl_2$-induced arrhythmia in a mouse model, and the results of the ECG profiles revealed that pretreatment with *C. obtusa*, *P. orientalis*, and *J. sabina* extracts exerted dose-dependent cardioprotective effects. The cardioprotection of the *C. obtusa*, *P. orientalis*, and *J. sabina* extracts was exerted through the M2- and M3-mAChRs. These treatment effects were also confirmed in a rat model. These first-line key findings reveal that certain Cupressaceae species possess active antiarrhythmic components, suggesting that these innovative phytocompounds might have promising potential for preventing the occurrence of cardiac arrhythmia and reducing SCD. The identification of active phytochemicals and their antiarrhythmic implications in the clinic requires further study.

Supplementary Materials: The following supporting information can be downloaded at: https://www.mdpi.com/article/10.3390/ph17081003/s1, Table S1: The chemo-information and biological functions of Cupressaceae species.

Author Contributions: L.-Y.H. and M.-T.Z. executed the experiment design and carried out the manuscript draft preparation. Y.-Q.F. and X.-H.Z. participated in data analysis. And C.-F.W. critically reviewed and edited the manuscript. All authors have read and agreed to the published version of the manuscript.

Funding: This study received financial support from the Xiamen Medical College Research Grant (Xiamen Medical College: K2019-01 for Ching-Feng Weng; K2020-07 for Xiao-Hui Zheng) by Xiamen Medical College, Xiamen, China.

Institutional Review Board Statement: This study has been reviewed by the Animal Ethics Committee of Medical College (approved protocol ID SYXK 2018-0010).

Informed Consent Statement: Not applicable.

Data Availability Statement: Data are contained within the article and Supplementary Materials.

Acknowledgments: The authors sincerely thank May-Jywan Tsai and Wei-Hao Weng for their technique help. The authors also thank Jun-Xiong Yang and Hao-Wei Zhao for collecting information and Xiamen Medical College for its full support.

Conflicts of Interest: Author Weng, Ching-Feng was employed by the company LEADTEK Research, Inc. The remaining authors declare that the research was conducted in the absence of any commercial or financial relationships that could be construed as a potential conflict of interest.

Abbreviations

AADs (antiarrhythmic drugs); ADRB2 (beta-2 adrenergic receptor); AT (atrial tachycardia); $BaCl_2$ (barium chloride); CaMKII (calcium/calmodulin-dependent protein kinase II); CHRM2 (muscarinic acetylcholine receptor M2); *C. obtuse (Chamaecyparis obtusa);* CVDs (cardiovascular diseases); DAMP (1,1-dimethyl-4-diphenylacetoxypiperidinium iodide); ECG (electrocardiogram); GIRK (Atrial G protein-gated inwardly rectifying K^+); HF (heart failure); IKACh (acetylcholine (ACh)-gated inwardly rectifying K+ current); IP_3 (inositol trisphosphate); *J. sabina* (*Juniperus sabina*); mAChRs (muscarinic acetylcholine receptor subtypes); MI (myocardial infarction); *P. orientalis (Platycladus orientalis*); ROS (reactive oxygen species); SCD (sudden cardiac death); SCN5A (5 subunit alpha); SOP (standard operating procedure); SR (sarcoplasmic reticulum); TCM (traditional Chinese medicine); WXKL (Wenxin Keli).

References

1. Krittayaphong, R.; Rangsin, R.; Thinkhamrop, B.; Hurst, C.; Rattanamongkolgul, S.; Sripaiboonkij, N.; Yindeengam, A. Prevalence and associating factors of atrial fibrillation in patients with hypertension: A nation-wide study. *BMC Cardiovasc. Disord.* **2016**, *16*, 57. [CrossRef] [PubMed]
2. Bei, Y.; Shi, C.; Zhang, Z.; Xiao, J. Advance for Cardiovascular Health in China. *J. Cardiovasc. Transl. Res.* **2019**, *12*, 165–170. [CrossRef] [PubMed]
3. Kusumoto, F.M.; Bailey, K.R.; Chaouki, A.S.; Deshmukh, A.J.; Gautam, S.; Kim, R.J.; Kramer, D.B.; Lambrakos, L.K.; Nasser, N.H.; Sorajja, D. Systematic review for the 2017 AHA/ACC/HRS guideline for management of patients with ventricular arrhythmias and the prevention of sudden cardiac death: A Report of the American College of Cardiology/American Heart Association Task Force on Clinical Practice Guidelines and the Heart Rhythm Society. *Heart Rhythm.* **2018**, *15*, e253–e274. [CrossRef] [PubMed]
4. Wang, W.; Cadrin-Tourigny, J.; Bhonsale, A.; Tichnell, C.; Murray, B.; Monfredi, O.; Chrispin, J.; Crosson, J.; Tandri, H.; James, C.A.; et al. Arrhythmic outcome of arrhythmogenic right ventricular cardiomyopathy patients without implantable defibrillators. *J. Cardiovasc. Electrophysiol.* **2018**, *29*, 1396–1402. [CrossRef] [PubMed]
5. Habibi, M.; Berger, R.D.; Calkins, H. Radiofrequency ablation: Technological trends, challenges, and opportunities. *Europace* **2021**, *23*, 511–519. [CrossRef] [PubMed]
6. Sandhu, A.; Levy, A.; Varosy, P.D.; Matlock, D. Implantable cardioverter defibrillators and cardiac resynchronization therapy in older adults with heart failure. *J. Am. Geriatr. Soc.* **2019**, *67*, 2193–2199. [CrossRef] [PubMed]
7. Al-Khatib, S.M.; Kusumoto, F.M. Implantable cardioverter-defibrillators have stood the test of time! *Circulation* **2019**, *140*, 1540–1542. [CrossRef] [PubMed]
8. Honarbakhsh, S.; Hunter, L.; Chow, A.; Hunter, R.J. Bradyarrhythmias and pacemakers. *BMJ* **2018**, *360*, k642. [CrossRef] [PubMed]
9. Fuchs, M.; Schibilsky, D.; Zeh, W.; Berchtold-Herz, M.; Beyersdorf, F.; Siepe, M. Does the heart transplant have a future? *Eur. J. Cardio-Thorac. Surg.* **2019**, *55*, I38–I48. [CrossRef]
10. Sutanto, H.; Laudy, L.; Clerx, M.; Dobrev, D.; Crijns, H.J.G.M.; Heijman, J. Maastricht antiarrhythmic drug evaluator (MANTA): A computational tool for better understanding of antiarrhythmic drugs. *Pharmacol. Res.* **2019**, *148*, 104444. [CrossRef]

11. Lu, J.; Jones, A.D.; Harkema, J.R.; Roth, R.A.; Ganey, P.E. Amiodarone exposure during modest inflammation induces idiosyncrasy-like liver injury in rats: Role of tumor necrosis factor-alpha. *Toxicol. Sci.* **2012**, *125*, 126–133. [CrossRef] [PubMed]
12. Mahavadi, P.; Henneke, I.; Ruppert, C.; Knudsen, L.; Venkatesan, S.; Liebisch, G.; Chambers, R.C.; Ochs, M.; Schmitz, G.; Vancheri, C.; et al. Altered surfactant homeostasis and alveolar epithelial cell stress in amiodarone-induced lung fibrosis. *Toxicol. Sci.* **2014**, *142*, 285–297. [CrossRef] [PubMed]
13. Brugada, J.; Katritsis, D.G.; Arbelo, E.; Arribas, F.; Bax, J.J.; Blomström-Lundqvist, C.; Calkins, H.; Corrado, D.; Deftereos, S.G.; Diller, G.P.; et al. 2019 ESC Guidelines for the management of patients with supraventricular tachycardia. The Task Force for the management of patients with supraventricular tachycardia of the European Society of Cardiology (ESC). *Eur. Heart J.* **2020**, *41*, 655–720. [CrossRef] [PubMed]
14. Yang, N.J.; Liu, Y.R.; Tang, Z.S.; Duan, J.A.; Yan, Y.F.; Song, Z.X.; Wang, M.G.; Zhang, Y.R.; Chang, B.J.; Zhao, M.L.; et al. Poria cum Radix Pini Rescues Barium Chloride-Induced Arrhythmia by Regulating the cGMP-PKG Signalling Pathway Involving ADORA1 in Zebrafish. *Front. Pharmacol.* **2021**, *12*, 688746. [CrossRef] [PubMed]
15. Wink, M. Modes of Action of Herbal Medicines and Plant Secondary Metabolites. *Medicines* **2015**, *2*, 251–286. [CrossRef] [PubMed]
16. Huyan, T.; Li, Q.; Wang, Y.L.; Li, J.; Zhang, J.Y.; Liu, Y.X.; Shahid, M.R.; Yang, H.; Li, H.Q. Anti-tumor effect of hot aqueous extracts from *Sonchus oleraceus* (L.) L. and *Juniperus sabina L*—Two traditional medicinal plants in China. *J. Ethnopharmacol.* **2016**, *185*, 289–299. [CrossRef] [PubMed]
17. Abdel-Kader, M.S.; Soliman, G.A.; Alqarni, M.H.; Hamad, A.M.; Foudah, A.I.; Alqasoumi, S.I. Chemical composition and protective effect of *Juniperus sabina,* L. essential oil against CCl4 induced hepatotoxicity. *Saudi Pharm. J.* **2019**, *27*, 945–951. [CrossRef] [PubMed]
18. Xu, S.; Li, X.; Liu, S.; Tian, P.; Li, D. *Juniperus sabina,* L. as a Source of Podophyllotoxins: Extraction Optimization and Anti-cholinesterase Activities. *Int. J. Mol. Sci.* **2022**, *23*, 10205. [CrossRef]
19. Orhan, N.; Deliorman Orhan, D.; Gökbulut, A.; Aslan, M.; Ergun, F. Comparative Analysis of Chemical Profile, Antioxidant, In-vitro and In-vivo Antidiabetic Activities of *Juniperus foetidissima* Willd. and *Juniperus sabina* L. *Iran. J. Pharm. Res.* **2017**, *16*, 64–74.
20. Shi, R.; Li, J. Study on the mechanism of *Sabina przewalskii* on chronic obstructive pulmonary disease based on network pharmacology. *J. Qinghai Norm. Univ.* **2022**, *38*, 44–52.
21. Park, S.A.; Jegal, J.; Chung, K.W.; Jung, H.J.; Noh, S.G.; Chung, H.Y.; Ahn, J.; Kim, J.; Yang, M.H. Isolation of tyrosinase and melanogenesis inhibitory flavonoids from *Juniperus chinensis* fruits. *Biosci. Biotechnol. Biochem.* **2018**, *82*, 2041–2048. [CrossRef] [PubMed]
22. Cui, Y.; Nan, P.; Lin, M. Main Volatile Components in the Leaves of *Sabina chinensis* L. Ant. and *Sabina chinensis* L. Ant. Cv. Kaizuca and Their Effects on Bacteria. *J. Environ. Health* **2006**, *1*, 63–65. [CrossRef]
23. Andersen, F.A. Final report on the safety assessment of *Juniperus communis* Extract, *Juniperus oxycedrus* Extract, *Juniperus oxycedrus* Tar, *Juniperus phoenicea* Extract, and *Juniperus virginiana* Extract. *Int. J. Toxicol.* **2001**, *20* (Suppl. S2), 41–56. [CrossRef]
24. Li, R.L.; Wu, P.L.; Li, C.R. Study on the chemical constituents of the branches and leaves of *Juniperus formosana*. *West China J. Pharm.* **2019**, *34*, 5–9.
25. Wu, S.; Lin, Y. Advances in Chinese Juniper leaves. *Chin. J. Ethn. Med.* **2014**, *20*, 55–58.
26. Jiang, J.H.; Li, X.C.; Gao, T.H.; He, D.N.; Chen, F.M.; Zhang, Y.P.; Huang, L.B. Volatile Constituents from the Cupressaceae Plants and Their Antitumor Activities. *J. Fujian For. Sci. Technol.* **2006**, *2*, 52–57. [CrossRef]
27. Wu, X.D.; He, J.; Li, X.Y.; Dong, L.B.; Gong, X.; Song, L.D.; Li, Y.; Peng, L.Y.; Zhao, Q.S. Diterpenoids from the twigs and leaves of *Fokienia hodginsii*. *J. Nat. Prod.* **2013**, *76*, 1032–1038. [CrossRef] [PubMed]
28. Wu, X.D.; Zhong, W.W.; Ding, L.F.; Tu, W.C.; Yang, H.; Gong, X.; Peng, L.Y.; Li, Y.; Xu, Z.Z.; Zhao, Q.S. Sesquiterpenoids from the twigs and leaves of *Fokienia hodginsii*. *J. Asian Nat. Prod. Res.* **2017**, *19*, 666–672. [CrossRef]
29. Hau, D.V.; Sa, N.H.; Tam, N.T.; Diep, N.T.; Hoang Anh, N.T.; Thuy Linh, N.T.; Ngoc Ni, H.T.; Adorisio, S.; Delfino, D.V.; Thuy, T.T. Pro-apoptoticeffect of diterpenoids from *Fokienia hodginsii* on acute myeloid leukemia cells. *Nat. Prod. Res.* **2021**, *35*, 4685–4689. [CrossRef]
30. Zhang, Y.; Yang, S.; Cao, Q.; Zhang, W.; Chen, F. Study on the Chemical Constituents and Biological Activities of Volatile Oil from *Fokienia hodgisii*. *Anhui Agric. Sci.* **2008**, *17*, 7290–7291, 7298.
31. Manimaran, S.; Kumar, B.S.; Khan, S.; Patel, D.; Suresh, B. Anti inflammatory activity of cone vola tile oil of *Cupressus funebris* endl. *Anc. Sci. Life.* **2005**, *25*, 1–3. [PubMed]
32. Liu, Y.X. Analysis of Chemical Constituents of Essential Oil Extracted from Leaves and Seeds of *Sabina chinensis* L. *J. Hubei Univ. Natl.* **2013**, *31*, 414–418, 441.
33. Gu, D.; Fang, C.; Yang, J.; Li, M.; Liu, H.; Yang, Y. Chemical composition and α-amylase inhibitory activity of the essential oil from *Sabina chinensis* cv. *Kaizuca leaves. Nat. Prod. Res.* **2018**, *32*, 711–713. [CrossRef] [PubMed]
34. Zhang, J.; Zhao, Z.; Liang, W.; Bi, J.; Zheng, Y.; Gu, X.; Fang, H. Essential oil from *Sabina chinensis* leaves: A promising green control agent against Fusarium sp. *Front. Plant Sci.* **2022**, *13*, 1006303. [CrossRef] [PubMed]
35. Ibrahim, N.A.; El-Seedi, H.R.; Mohammed, M.M. Phytochemical investigation and hepatoprotective activity of *Cupressus sempervirens,* L. leaves growing in Egypt. *Nat. Prod. Res.* **2007**, *21*, 857–866. [CrossRef] [PubMed]
36. Leigh-de Rapper, S.; Viljoen, A.; van Vuuren, S. Essential Oil Blends: The Potential of Combined Use for Respiratory Tract Infections. *Antibiotics* **2021**, *10*, 1517. [CrossRef] [PubMed]

37. Hao, D.; Zhang, Y.; Dai, H.; Wang, Y. Analysis of volatile constituents in leaves of three cypress species by gas chromatography/mass spectrometry. *Se Pu = Chin. J. Chromatogr.* **2006**, *24*, 185–187. (In Chinese)
38. Dai, S.; Chan, M.Y.; Lee, S.S.; Ogle, C.W. The antiarrhythmic effects of *Sophora flavescens* Ait. in rats and mice. *Am. J. Chin. Med.* **1986**, *14*, 119–123. [CrossRef] [PubMed]
39. He, H.; Han, G.; Li, X.; Lan, H.; Li, Y.; Dou, X.; Guo, Y.; Zhang, M.; Liu, H. Efficacy and Safety of Chinese Medicine in Treating Arrhythmia: Meta-Analysis of Randomized Controlled Trials. *Evid. Based Complement. Alternat Med.* **2021**, *2021*, 9960471. [CrossRef]
40. Yang, Y.; Ge, F.L.; Huang, Q.; Zeng, R.; Zhang, X.Y.; Liu, P.; Luo, G.; Yang, S.J.; Sun, Q. Randomized Controlled Trials of Zhigancao Decoction Combined with Metoprolol in the Treatment of Arrhythmia: A Systematic Review and Meta-Analysis. *Front. Cardiovasc. Med.* **2022**, *9*, 795903. [CrossRef]
41. Yuan, H.; Ma, Q.; Ye, L.; Piao, G. The Traditional Medicine and Modern Medicine from Natural Products. *Molecules* **2016**, *21*, 559. [CrossRef] [PubMed]
42. Bryzgalov, A.O.; Tolstikova, T.G.; Shults, E.E.; Petrova, K.O. Natural Products as a Source of Antiarrhythmic Drugs. *Mini Rev. Med. Chem.* **2018**, *18*, 345–362. [CrossRef]
43. Pan, L.; Zhang, X.F.; Wei, W.S.; Zhang, J.; Li, Z.Z. The cardiovascular protective effect and mechanism of calycosin and its derivatives. *Chin. J. Nat. Med.* **2020**, *18*, 907–915. [CrossRef] [PubMed]
44. Tai, C.J.; El-Shazly, M.; Yang, Y.H.; Tsai, Y.H.; Csupor, D.; Hohmann, J.; Wu, Y.C.; Tseng, T.G.; Chang, F.R.; Wang, H.C. The effectiveness of Fuzi in combination with routine heart failure treatment on chronic heart failure patients. *J. Ethnopharmacol.* **2022**, *289*, 115040. [CrossRef] [PubMed]
45. Tian, G.; Sun, Y.; Liu, S.; Li, C.; Chen, S.; Qiu, R.; Zhang, X.; Li, Y.; Li, M.; Shang, H. Therapeutic Effects of Wenxin Keli in Cardiovascular Diseases: An Experimental and Mechanism Overview. *Front. Pharmacol.* **2018**, *9*, 1005. [CrossRef] [PubMed]
46. Yao, Y.; Liu, Y.; Zeng, Z.; Zhao, Y.; Li, T.; Chen, R.; Zhang, R. Identification of Target Genes of Antiarrhythmic Traditional Chinese Medicine Wenxin Keli. *Cardiovasc. Ther.* **2020**, *2020*, 3480276. [CrossRef] [PubMed]
47. Heijman, J.; Kirchner, D.; Kunze, F.; Chrétien, E.M.; Michel-Reher, M.B.; Voigt, N.; Knaut, M.; Michel, M.C.; Ravens, U.; Dobrev, D. Muscarinic type-1 receptors contribute to IKACh in human atrial cardiomyocytes and are upregulated in patients with chronic atrial fibrillation. *Int. J. Cardiol.* **2018**, *255*, 61–68. [CrossRef] [PubMed]
48. Liu, Q.; Sun, J.; Zhang, L.; Xu, Y.; Wu, B.; Cao, J. The Agonist of Inward Rectifier Potassium Channel (IK1) Attenuates Rat Reperfusion Arrhythmias Linked to CaMKII Signaling. *Int. Heart J.* **2021**, *62*, 1348–1357. [CrossRef]
49. de Araújo, R.B.; Azevedo, B.M.S.; Andrade, T.S.; Abalem, M.F.; Monteiro, M.L.R.; Carricondo, P.C. Subconjunctival 0.1% epinephrine versus placebo in maintenance of mydriasis during vitrectomy: A randomized controlled trial. *Int. J. Retin. Vitr.* **2018**, *4*, 38. [CrossRef]
50. Janssens, U.; Michels, G. Adrenalin bei Patienten mit prähospitalem Herz-Kreislauf-Stillstand: PARAMEDIC2-Studie Adrenaline in patients with out-of-hospital cardiac arrest: PARAMEDIC2 trial. *Med. Klin. Intensivmed. Notfmed.* **2019**, *114*, 63–67. [CrossRef]
51. Torrente, A.G.; Mesirca, P.; Bidaud, I.; Mangoni, M.E. Channelopathies of voltage-gated L-type Cav1.3/α1D and T-type Cav3.1/α1G Ca2+ channels in dysfunction of heart automaticity. *Pflugers Arch.* **2020**, *472*, 817–830. [CrossRef] [PubMed]
52. Escobar, G.J.; LaGuardia, J.C.; Turk, B.J.; Ragins, A.; Kipnis, P.; Draper, D. Early detection of impending physiologic deterioration among patients who are not in intensive care: Development of predictive models using data from an automated electronic medical record. *J. Hosp. Med.* **2012**, *7*, 388–395. [CrossRef] [PubMed]
53. Suita, K.; Fujita, T.; Hasegawa, N.; Cai, W.; Jin, H.; Hidaka, Y.; Prajapati, R.; Umemura, M.; Yokoyama, U.; Sato, M.; et al. Norepinephrine-Induced Adrenergic Activation Strikingly Increased the Atrial Fibrillation Duration through β1- and α1-Adrenergic Receptor-Mediated Signaling in Mice. *PLoS ONE.* **2015**, *10*, e0133664. [CrossRef] [PubMed]
54. Sapa, J.; Kubacka, M. The possible mechanism of hypotensive activity of some pyrrolidin-2-one derivatives with antagonist properties at alpha1-adrenoceptors. *Eur. J. Pharmacol.* **2011**, *673*, 40–48. [CrossRef] [PubMed]
55. Kubacka, M.; Mogilski, S.; Filipek, B.; Marona, H. The hypotensive activity and alpha1-adrenoceptor antagonistic properties of some aroxyalkyl derivatives of 2-methoxyphenylpiperazine. *Eur. J. Pharmacol.* **2013**, *698*, 335–344. [CrossRef] [PubMed]
56. Rapacz, A.; Sapa, J.; Nowiński, L.; Mogilski, S.; Pytka, K.; Filipek, B.; Siwek, A.; Szkaradek, N.; Marona, H. Biofunctional studies of new 2-methoxyphenylpiperazine xanthone derivatives with α_1-adrenolytic properties. *Pharmacol. Rep.* **2015**, *67*, 267–274. [CrossRef]
57. Pytka, K.; Rapacz, A.; Zygmunt, M.; Olczyk, A.; Waszkielewicz, A.; Sapa, J.; Filipek, B. Antidepressant-like activity of a new piperazine derivative of xanthone in the forced swim test in mice: The involvement of serotonergic system. *Pharmacol. Rep.* **2015**, *67*, 160–165. [CrossRef] [PubMed]
58. Pytka, K.; Lustyk, K.; Żmudzka, E.; Kotańska, M.; Siwek, A.; Zygmunt, M.; Dziedziczak, A.; Śniecikowska, J.; Olczyk, A.; Gałuszka, A.; et al. Chemically Homogenous Compounds with Antagonistic Properties at All α1-Adrenoceptor Subtypes but not β1-Adrenoceptor Attenuate Adrenaline-Induced Arrhythmia in Rats. *Front. Pharmacol.* **2016**, *7*, 229. [CrossRef]
59. van Zwieten, P.A.; Doods, H.N. Muscarinic receptors and drugs in cardiovascular medicine. *Cardiovasc. Drugs Ther.* **1995**, *9*, 159–167. [CrossRef]
60. Kosmachev, A.B.; Fil'ko, O.A.; Petrov, V.V. Izuchenie roli otdel'nykh podtipov M-kholinoretseptorov v narushenii serdechnogo ritma razlichnoĭ étiologii the role of M-cholinoreceptor subtypes in heart rhythm disturbances of various etiology. *Eksp. Klin. Farmakol.* **2002**, *65*, 34–36. (In Russian)

61. Hardouin, S.N.; Richmond, K.N.; Zimmerman, A.; Hamilton, S.E.; Feigl, E.O.; Nathanson, N.M. Altered cardiovascular responses in mice lacking the M(1) muscarinic acetylcholine receptor. *J. Pharmacol. Exp. Ther.* **2002**, *301*, 129–137. [CrossRef] [PubMed]
62. Salazar-Fajardo, P.D.; Aréchiga-Figueroa, I.A.; López-Serrano, A.L.; Rodriguez-Elias, J.C.; Alamilla, J.; Sánchez-Chapula, J.A.; Tristani-Firouzi, M.; Navarro-Polanco, R.A.; Moreno-Galindo, E.G. The voltage-sensitive cardiac M2 muscarinic receptor modulates the inward rectification of the G protein-coupled, ACh-gated K+ current. *Pflugers Arch.* **2018**, *470*, 1765–1776. [CrossRef] [PubMed]
63. Shi, H.; Wang, H.; Li, D.; Nattel, S.; Wang, Z. Differential alterations of receptor densities of three muscarinic acetylcholine receptor subtypes and current densities of the corresponding K+ channels in canine atria with atrial fibrillation induced by experimental congestive heart failure. *Cell Physiol. Biochem.* **2004**, *14*, 31–40. [CrossRef] [PubMed]
64. James, A.F.; Hancox, J.C. More types than one: Multiple muscarinic receptor coupled K+ currents undergo remodelling in an experimental model of atrial fibrillation. *Br. J. Pharmacol.* **2007**, *152*, 981–983. [CrossRef] [PubMed]
65. Uemura, H.; Hara, Y.; Endou, M.; Mori, K.; Nakaya, H. Interaction of class III antiarrhythmic drugs with muscarinic M2 and M3 receptors: Radioligand binding and functional studies. *Naunyn Schmiedebergs Arch. Pharmacol.* **1995**, *353*, 73–79. [CrossRef] [PubMed]
66. Zhao, J.; Su, Y.; Zhang, Y.; Pan, Z.; Yang, L.; Chen, X.; Liu, Y.; Lu, Y.; Du, Z.; Yang, B. Activation of cardiac muscarinic M3 receptors induces delayed cardioprotection by preserving phosphorylated connexin43 and up-regulating cyclooxygenase-2 expression. *Br. J. Pharmacol.* **2010**, *159*, 1217–1225. [CrossRef] [PubMed]
67. Rauch, B.; Niroomand, F. Specific M2-receptor activation: An alternative to treatment with beta-receptor blockers? *Eur. Heart J.* **1991**, *12* (Suppl. F), 76–82. [CrossRef]
68. Anderson, A.; Kulkarni, K.; Marron Fernandez de Velasco, E.; Carlblom, N.; Xia, Z.; Nakano, A.; Martemyanov, K.A.; Tolkacheva, E.G.; Wickman, K. Expression and relevance of the G protein-gated K+ channel in the mouse ventricle. *Sci. Rep.* **2018**, *8*, 1192. [CrossRef]
69. Yang, B.; Lin, H.; Xu, C.; Liu, Y.; Wang, H.; Han, H.; Wang, Z. Choline produces cytoprotective effects against ischemic myocardial injuries: Evidence for the role of cardiac m3 subtype muscarinic acetylcholine receptors. *Cell Physiol. Biochem.* **2005**, *16*, 163–174. [CrossRef]
70. Ramesh, P.; Palaniappan, A. Terminalia arjuna, a Cardioprotective Herbal Medicine–Relevancy in the Modern Era of Pharmaceuticals and Green Nanomedicine—A Review. *Pharmaceuticals* **2023**, *16*, 126. [CrossRef]
71. Hashem-Dabaghian, F.; Ziaee, M.; Ghaffari, S.; Nabati, F.; Kianbakht, S. A systematic review on the cardiovascular pharmacology of *Emblica officinalis* Gaertn. *J. Cardiovasc. Thorac. Res.* **2018**, *10*, 118–128. [CrossRef] [PubMed]
72. Nehdi, I.A. Cupressus sempervirens var. horizentalis seed oil: Chemical composition, physicochemical characteristics, and utilizations. *Ind. Crops Prod.* **2013**, *41*, 381–385. [CrossRef]
73. Hasaballah, A.; Shehata, A.; Fouda, M.; Hassan, M.; Gad, M. The biological activity of *Cupressus sempervirens* extracts against *Musca domestica*. *Asian J. Biol.* **2018**, *5*, 1–12. [CrossRef]
74. Mohamed, A. Biological applications of *Cupressus sempervirens* biomass extracted at various levels of pressure using different critical fluid extraction protocol. *Biomass Conv. Bioref.* **2024**. [CrossRef]
75. Zhao, J.; Gu, Z.; Liu, T.; Xu, F.; You, S.; Li, C. Anti-arthritic effects of total flavonoids from Juniperus sabina on complete freund's adjuvant induced arthritis in rats. *Pharmacogn. Mag.* **2016**, *12*, 178–183. [CrossRef]

pharmaceuticals

MDPI

Article

Thymol Protects against 5-Fluorouracil-Induced Hepatotoxicity via the Regulation of the Akt/GSK-3β Pathway in In Vivo and In Silico Experimental Models

Yasmen F. Mahran [1,†], Amira M. Badr [2,*,†], Layla A. Al-Kharashi [2], Hanaa N. Alajami [3], Nouf T. Aldamry [2], Nervana Moustafa Bayoumy [4], Elshaymaa I. Elmongy [5] and Sahar Soliman [6]

[1] Department of Pharmacology and Toxicology, Faculty of Pharmacy, Ain Shams University, Cairo 11566, Egypt; jassie_81@hotmail.com

[2] Department of Pharmacology and Toxicology, College of Pharmacy, King Saud University, Riyadh 11211, Saudi Arabia; lalkharashi@ksu.edu.sa (L.A.A.-K.); naldamri@ksu.edu.sa (N.T.A.)

[3] College of Pharmacy, King Saud University, Riyadh 11211, Saudi Arabia; hanaalajmi16@gmail.com

[4] Department of Physiology, College of Medicine, King Saud University, Riyadh 11211, Saudi Arabia; nbayoumy@ksu.edu.sa

[5] Department of Pharmaceutical Chemistry, Faculty of Pharmacy, Helwan University, Ain Helwan, Cairo 11795, Egypt; shaymaa.taha@pharm.helwan.edu.eg

[6] Department of Physiology and Pharmacology, College of Osteopathic Medicine, Sam Houston State University, Conroe, TX 77304, USA; sahar.soliman@shsu.edu

* Correspondence: amibadr@ksu.edu.sa

† The two authors contributed equally to this work (co-first authors).

Abstract: Background: 5-fluorouracil (5-FU) is a widely used, highly effective chemotherapeutic agent. However, its therapeutic efficacy is often limited by associated adverse effects, with hepatotoxicity being frequently reported with 5-FU therapy. Thymol is a monoterpene found in thyme (*Thymus vulgaris* L., Lamiaceae) and is known for its antioxidant, anti-apoptotic, and anticancer activities. This study aimed to explore the hepatoprotective activity of thymol against 5-FU-induced liver injury. Methods: Rats received two intraperitoneal doses of 5-FU (150 mg/kg) either alone or in combination with thymol at doses of 60 mg/kg or 120 mg/kg. Liver enzymes, oxidative stress, and apoptotic markers, in addition to histopathological changes, were assessed. Results: 5-FU induced marked liver injuries as evidenced by elevated liver enzymes and histopathological changes, in addition to abnormalities of oxidative and apoptotic markers. The administration of thymol ameliorated the 5-FU-induced oxidative damage through increasing hepatic antioxidants and lowering lipid peroxidation. Apoptotic response markers such as Bax, Bcl-2, Bax/Bcl-2 ratio, and PARP were also improved. Furthermore, Western blotting analysis showed that thymol modulated the 5-FU-induced changes in the expression of Akt/GSK-3β and p44/42 MAPK (ERK1/2) signaling pathways. Conclusions: Our research is the first to shed light on thymol's potential protective effect against 5-FU- induced hepatotoxicity by inhibiting oxidative and apoptotic pathways and modulating the Akt/ GSK-3β as well as p44/42 MAPK (ERK1/2) signaling pathways.

Keywords: thymol; 5-flourouracil; hepatotoxicity; apoptosis; GSK-3β signaling; p44/42 MAPK(ERK1/2) signaling

1. Introduction

Chemotherapy is a standard cancer treatment; however, its use can be limited by chemotherapy-induced hepatotoxicity. Efficient antineoplastic agents' therapeutic outcomes are constrained because of the negative clinical side effects that necessitate dose reduction or a discontinuation of the therapy [1]. A fluorinated pyrimidine analog known as 5-fluorouracil (5-FU) is an antimetabolite chemotherapeutic agent extensively used for a variety of cancers, including breast and colorectal cancers [2]. 5-FU works by substituting the reduced thymidine triphosphate in DNA with the deoxyuridine triphosphate and fluorodeoxyuridine triphosphate, leading to DNA strand breaks [3].

Clinically, 5-FU treatment causes substantial systemic toxicities, including hepatotoxicity. Al-Asmari et al. (2016) reported the main mechanisms of 5-FU-induced cytotoxicity, including the overproduction of reactive oxygen species (ROS) and the generation of inflammatory mediators [4]. The use of 5-FU has occasionally been associated with the elevation of hepatic enzymes, such as alanine aminotransferase (ALT), aspartate aminotransferase (AST), and alkaline phosphatase (ALP). Moreover, 5-FU-generated oxidative stress in the liver causes lipid peroxidation and antioxidants depletion, leading to hepatocyte structural and functional abnormalities [5,6]. Thus, the use of antioxidants has been suggested to attenuate 5-FU-induced toxicity [7,8]. Finding approaches to reduce 5-FU-associated hepatotoxicity is crucial, as it may prove beneficial not only for minimizing liver damage but also for maintaining the optimal dosing required for effective chemotherapy, thereby improving the overall clinical outcomes of 5-FU [1].

As the search for effective ways to mitigate 5-FU-associated hepatotoxicity continues, the potential of natural substances, including essential oils from aromatic herbs, is being explored. These oils are known for their distinctive aromas, as well as their diverse therapeutic properties such as insecticidal, antibacterial, and antifungal activities [9]. Thymol, the primary component of the *Thymus vulgaris* component, is frequently used in foods to enhance flavor and taste due to its safety and acceptance [10,11]. In various experimental models, thymol is well known for its chemoprotective activity through antioxidant [12] and anti-inflammatory [13–16] mechanisms, due to its natural monoterpene phenolic composition [17], and has a favorable safety profile [18]. Thymol is also known to improve intestinal barrier integrity and fight off dangerous microbes, both of which contribute to its ability to support the immune system [19]. With regards to thymol's hepatoprotective effect, thymol prevented the hepatic damage mediated by lipopolysaccharides via reducing inflammation and hepatocellular apoptosis [20]. Furthermore, thymol was used to ameliorate the ethanol- and nano titanium dioxide-induced liver injury through its antioxidant qualities [10,21]. However, the hepatoprotective mechanisms of thymol remain poorly understood. Understanding the different protective mechanisms is essential to identify the possible practical applications of thymol [20].

Glycogen synthase kinase-3 (GSK-3) is a ubiquitously expressed serine/threonine kinase with diverse functions in various cell types [22]. It is involved in a variety of cellular functions and regulates various transcription factors that define cell destiny. The role of the Akt/GSK-3β signaling pathway in acetaminophen-induced hepatotoxicity has been documented. Therefore, a detailed exploration of the GSK-3β signaling pathway in disease pathogenesis is warranted [23]. Several studies reported that thymol offered protective effects through the modulation of Akt/GSK-3β signaling in different experimental models [24,25]. Thus, we hypothesized that thymol can protect against 5-FU-induced liver injury by modulating oxidative and apoptotic-signaling molecules. Consequently, this study sought to investigate the potential hepatoprotective effect of thymol against 5-FU-induced liver injury, as well as the underlying protective mechanisms.

2. Results

2.1. Protective Effect of Thymol against 5-FU-Induced Histopathological Changes in Liver Tissues

The histopathological changes in the examined hepatic sections are shown in Figure 1. The control group revealed almost intact histological structures of hepatic parenchyma, with apparent normal hepatocytes showing large vesicular nuclei and intact vasculature. (Figure 1A,B). On the other hand, the administration of 5-FU demonstrated a moderate dilation of hepatic blood vessels (star) and sinusoids accompanied with periportal mononuclear inflammatory cells infiltrations (yellow arrow), scattered throughout the samples. Additionally, alternating intact or degenerated pyknotic hepatocytes in hepatic plates (arrow) were observed (Figure 1C,D).

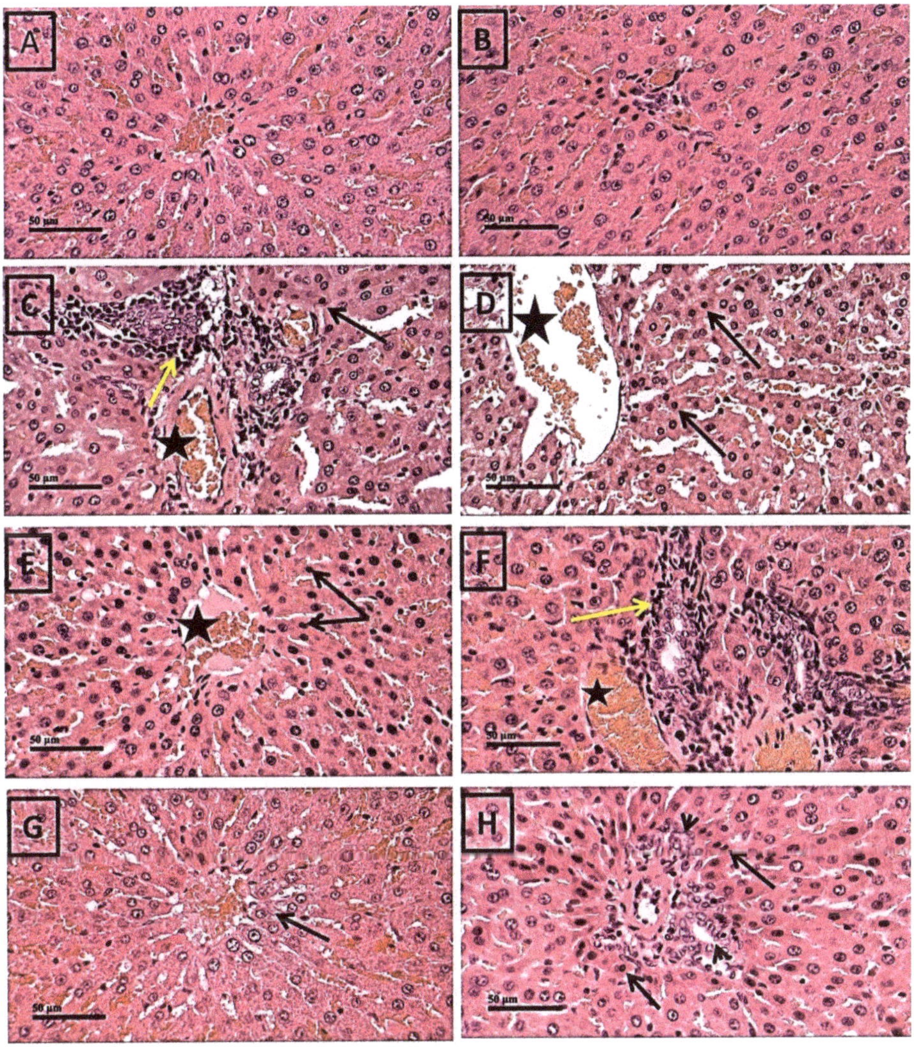

Figure 1. Histological photomicrographs of the liver tissue stained with hematoxylin and eosin staining. (**A**,**B**) Sections of liver tissues from the control rats received only the vehicle orally show normal histological features of hepatic parenchyma with normal hepatocytes. (**C**,**D**) Sections of liver tissues from the 5-FU treated rats that received the vehicle and two doses of 5-FU (150 mg/kg) show a dilatation of hepatic blood vessels (star) in both (**C**,**D**), periportal mononuclear inflammatory cell infiltrations (yellow arrow) in (**C**), and degenerated pyknotic hepatocytes in hepatic plats (arrow) in both (**C**,**D**). (**E**,**F**) Sections of liver tissues from the FU+ Thymol (60 mg) treated group that received thymol (60 mg/kg orally) and two doses of 5-FU (150 mg/kg) show more or less the same records as the 5-FU group with the same annotations. (**G**,**H**) Sections of liver tissues from the FU+ Thymol (120 mg) treated group that received thymol (120 mg/kg orally) and two doses of 5-FU (150 mg/kg) show intact hepatocytes with mild vacuolar changes in pericentral zones (arrow) as shown in (**G**). (**H**) shows few karyopyknotic changes in periportal areas (arrow) and minimal records of inflammatory cell infiltrates in periportal areas (arrowhead). X: 200 bar 200 µm, X: 400 bar 50 µm. FU: 5-fluorouracil.

Concurrent treatment with 60 mg/kg thymol demonstrated a moderate protective effect against 5-FU-induced histopathological liver changes, yielding results comparable to those observed in the 5-FU group (Figure 1E,F). On the other hand, thymol administration (120 mg/kg) attenuated 5-FU-induced pathological changes, showing many apparent intact hepatocytes with mild vacuolar changes in pericentral zones (arrow) or few karyopyknotic changes in periportal areas (arrow). Minimal records of inflammatory cells infiltrating the periportal areas with mild hyperplasia of bile ducts (arrowhead) were observed (Figure 1G,H).

2.2. Effects of Thymol and 5-FU on Liver Enzymes and Oxidative Stress Markers in Liver Tissues

As shown in Table 1, the activities of liver enzymes AST, ALT, ALP, and LDH were markedly increased in the 5-FU treated group to about 142%, 188%, 238%, and 198%, respectively, compared to the control group. However, treatment with thymol (60 mg/kg) decreased serum levels of AST, ALT, ALP, and LDH by 15%, 46%, 61%, and 13%, respectively, compared to the 5-FU group, reflecting the protective effect of thymol. Furthermore, a significant reduction in liver enzymes was observed with thymol at a dose of 120 mg/kg by 35%, 65%, 70%, and 45%, respectively, when compared to the 5-FU group. The protective effect of thymol is dose-dependent, as shown in Table 1.

Table 1. Changes in liver enzymes and oxidative stress markers levels in 5-FU-induced hepatotoxicity in rats treated with thymol at two doses (60 and 120 mg/kg).

Groups	Liver Enzymes				Oxidative Stress Markers		
	AST (U/L)	ALT (U/L)	ALP (U/L)	LDH (U/L)	Glutathione (µg/mg Protein)	TBARSs (nmol/mg Protein)	SOD (U/mg Protein)
Control	92.49 ± 2.02	47.58 ± 3.91	15.89 ±1.32	166.80 ± 1.92	1.70 ± 0.03	0.37 ± 0.02	3.93 ± 0.12
5-FU	131.20 ± 4.39 ^{x}	89.21 ± 1.16 ^{x}	37.80 ± 1.66 ^{x}	330.60 ± 11.58 ^{x}	0.63 ± 0.04 ^{x}	2.60 ± 0.07 ^{x}	0.95 ± 0.049 ^{x}
5-FU + Thymol (60 mg/kg)	112.00 ± 6.88 ^{x,y}	48.25 ± 2.73 ^{y}	15.03 ± 0.85 ^{y}	288.00 ± 11.58 ^{x,y}	1.11 ± 0.04 ^{x,y}	1.68 ± 0.03 ^{x,y}	2.35 ± 0.08 ^{x,y}
5-FU + Thymol (120 mg/kg)	84.58 ± 2.29 ^{y,z}	31.60 ± 4.30 ^{x,y,z}	11.35 ± 0.59 ^{y}	182.00 ± 2.55 ^{y,z}	1.55 ± 0.07 ^{y,z}	0.67 ± 0.05 ^{x,y,z}	3.52 ± 0.08 ^{x,y,z}

Data are presented as mean ± S.D. (n = 6). x, y, or z: The 5-fluorouracil and Fu+ thymol (60 mg/kg) groups, are significantly different from the control at $p < 0.05$.

An increment in oxidative stress was evidenced in the 5-FU-treated group. The levels of SOD and GSH were reduced by 37% and 25%, respectively, compared to the control group. Additionally, the level of TBARSs was significantly elevated by approximately sevenfold in the 5-FU rats, reflecting increased lipid peroxidation. Conversely, the antioxidant effect of thymol was demonstrated by the increase in the level of GSH and SOD, reaching about 76% and 147%, respectively, and decreased the level of TBARSs by 35% at a dose of 60 mg/kg.

On the other hand, the higher thymol dose (120 mg/kg) significantly increased the levels of SOD and GSH to about 270% and 144%, respectively, and the level of TBARSs was almost normalized compared to the control group.

Control; 5-FU rats; 5-FU + Thymol (60 mg/kg): 5-FU rats treated with thymol (60 mg/kg/day, orally); 5-FU + Thymol (120 mg/kg): 5-FU rats treated with thymol (120 mg/kg/day, orally).

x, y, or z: The 5-fluorouracil and 5-FU + thymol (60 mg/kg) groups are significantly different from the control at $p < 0.05$, using ANOVA followed by Tukey–Kramer as a post-hoc test. 5-FU: 5-fluorouracil; AST: aspartate aminotransferase; ALT: alanine aminotransferase; ALP: alkaline phosphatase; LDH: lactate dehydrogenase; SOD: superoxide dismutase; TBARSs: thiobarbituric acid reactive substances.

2.3. Effect of Thymol and 5-Fluorouracil on Apoptotic Marker Expression in Liver Tissues

To investigate the potential anti-apoptotic effects of thymol against 5-FU-induced hepatocellular death, the hepatic expression of caspase-3, the pro-apoptotic protein (Bax), and the anti-apoptotic protein (Bcl-2) were examined across the different groups. In addition, an assessment of the cleaved PARP (89 kDa) and p44/42 MAPK (ERK1/2) hepatic protein expression was also carried out. First, Figure 2 shows microscopic photos of caspase-3 expression in all experimental groups by immunohistochemical staining, where the control showed minimal caspase-3 expression while the FU-treated group showed an intense expression of caspase-3. However, thymol-treated groups show a moderate expression of caspase-3. A statistical analysis of area % of caspase-3 immunostaining revealed a significant induction of caspase-3 expression to about eight-fold in rats treated with 5-FU when compared to the control group. On the other hand, either dose of thymol (60 mg or 120 mg) significantly decreased caspase-3 expression to about 0.75- and 0.5-fold, respectively, compared with the 5-FU group, as shown in Figure 2. Moreover, the immunoblotting analysis showed that 5-FU increased Bax and decreased the Bcl-2 protein level by about 1- and 0.5-fold, respectively, relative to the control group (Figure 3a,b). Thus, the Bax/Bcl-2 ratio in the 5-FU group was significantly elevated to about 1.75 folds when compared to the control group. Nevertheless, treatment with thymol at a dose of 60 mg/kg significantly decreased the Bax/Bcl-2 ratio to a level comparable to that in the control group. Interestingly, the administration of thymol 120 mg/kg was able to decrease the Bax/Bcl-2 ratio to 0.4-fold compared to the control and the thymol 60 mg/kg group (Figure 3c).

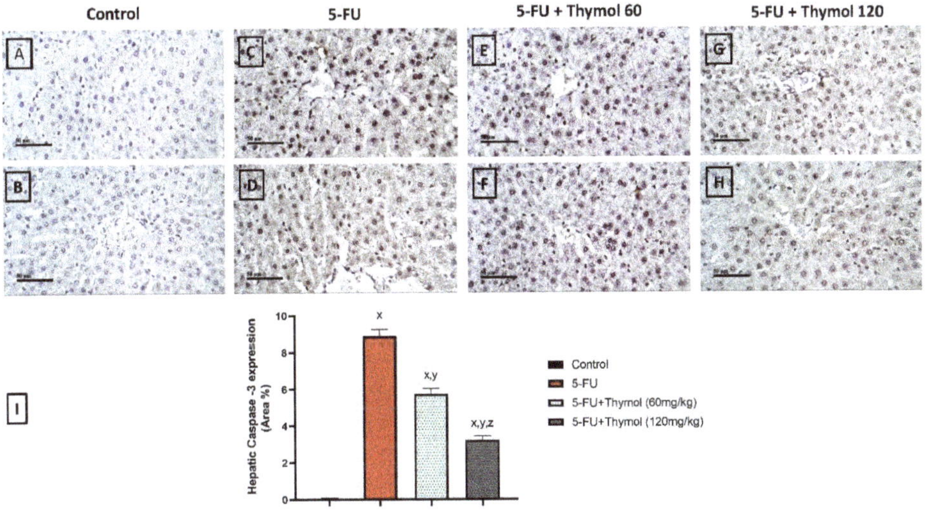

Figure 2. Effect of 5-fluorouracil with or without thymol on caspase-3 expression in liver tissues. (**A–H**) Immunohistochemical images of caspase-3 hepatic expression. (**A**,**B**) Control: normal rats that received only the vehicle orally show minimal caspase-3 expression. (**C**,**D**) FU rats: 5-FU treated rats that received the vehicle and two doses of 5-FU (150 mg/kg) show intense expression of caspase-3. (**E**,**F**) FU+Thymol 60: the FU+ Thymol (60 mg) treated group that received thymol (60 mg/kg orally) and two doses of 5-FU (150 mg/kg) show moderate caspase-3 expression. (**G**,**H**) FU+Thymol 120: the FU+ Thymol (120 mg) treated group that received thymol (120 mg/kg orally) and two doses of 5-FU (150 mg/kg) show moderate caspase-3 expression. (**I**) Statistical analysis of quantitative hepatic expression of caspase-3 as area % of immune-positive staining in all groups. Values are mean ± SEM (n = 5). x, y, or z: The 5-fluorouracil and Fu+ thymol (60 mg/kg) groups, are significantly different from the control at $p < 0.05$. $p \leq 0.05$, as evaluated using ANOVA followed by Tukey–Kramer as a post-hoc test. Scale bar = 50 μm. 5-FU: 5-fluorouracil.

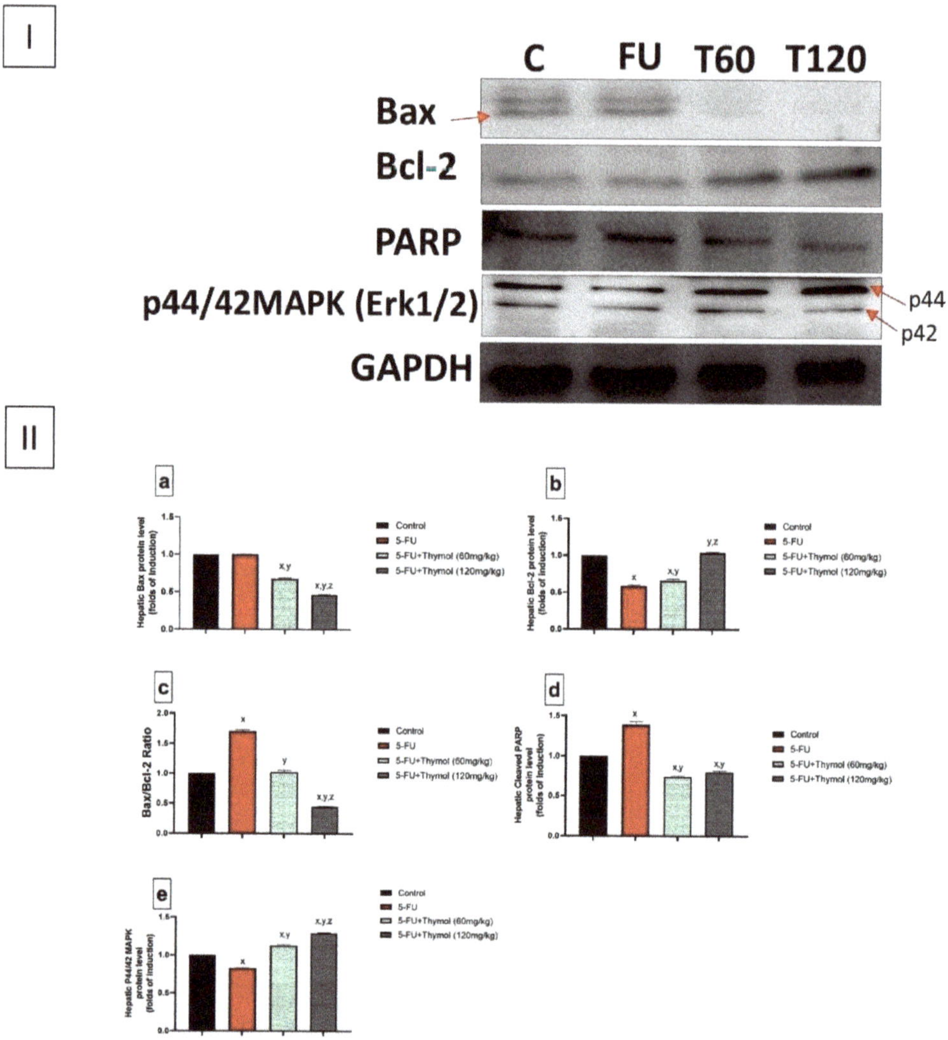

Figure 3. Effects of 5-fluorouracil with or without thymol on the hepatic protein expressions of the apoptotic markers Bax, Bcl-2, PARP, and p44/42 MAPK (ERK1/2) in rats. (**I**) Representative immunoblot of protein levels of Bax (lower band), Bcl-2, PARP, and p44/42 MAPK (ERK1/2) marked for p44 and p42 in liver tissues. (**II**) Quantitative results of the immunoblot of (**a**) Bax, (**b**) Bcl-2, (**c**) Bax/Bcl-2 ratio, (**d**) PARP, and (**e**) p44/42 MAPK (ERK1/2) protein levels are expressed as the ratio of expressed protein /GAPDH. The densities of immunoblots were quantified using analysis software. The relative quantities were normalized to the control and expressed as a fold of induction. Values are mean ± SEM (n = 3). x, y, or z: 5-Fluorouracil and 5-FU+ thymol (60 mg/kg) groups, are significantly different from the control at $p < 0.05$. $p \leq 0.05$ was evaluated using ANOVA followed by Tukey–Kramer as a post-hoc test. 5-FU: 5-fluorouracil. p44/42 MAPK: p44/42 mitogen activated protein kinase.

Next, we checked the effect on cleaved PARP and p44/42 MAPK (ERK1/2) hepatic protein expression. 5-FU strongly induced the expression of hepatic cleaved PARP (89 kDa) protein level by about 1.75-fold as compared to the control. Thymol (60 and 120 mg/kg) significantly decreased the hepatic cleaved PARP protein level below the level of the control group, reaching about 0.75-fold of the 5-FU group (Figure 3d). This shows that thymol might suppress 5-FU-induced liver damage through an inhibition of the apoptotic pathway. In addition, Figure 3e shows that 5-FU administration caused a 0.8-fold downregulation of the hepatic expression of p44/42 MAPK (ERK1/2) when compared to the control group, while thymol co-administration generated a significant p44/42 MAPK (ERK1/2) upregulation in a dose-dependent manner by 1.1-fold for thymol (60 mg/kg) and 1.3-fold for thymol (120 mg/kg), compared to both the control and the 5-FU values (Figure 3e).

2.4. Effect of Thymol and 5-Fluorouracil on Akt1/GSK-3α/β Signaling Pathway Protein Expression in Liver Tissues

To further explore mechanisms of 5-FU-induced liver injury, we investigated the fundamental role of the AKT1/GSK-3α/β signaling pathway in the hepatic tissues. Results showed that 5-FU slightly upregulated the phosphorylation of both Akt1 and GSK-3α/β, which was evidenced by an increase in the ratio of p-Akt1/Akt1 and p-GSK-3α/β/GSK-3α/β by 1.2 and 1.3-folds, respectively, compared with the control group (Figure 4a,b). In this context, we found that the GSK-3α protein was less expressed in the hepatic tissue specimens among all different groups. Thus, the discussion will mainly take the GSK-3β isoform into consideration. However, the co-treatment of 5-FU-injected rats with thymol, either 60 or 120 mg/kg, modulated the Akt/GSK-3α/β signaling via an upregulation of the Akt1 phosphorylation downregulation of GSK-3α/β phosphorylation, compared to the 5-FU treated group, as shown in Figure 4a,b where the ratio of p-Akt1/Akt1 was increased about three-fold and the phosphorylation of GSK-3α/β/ decreased by about 40%.

2.5. Docking Studies of Thymol

This study investigates the protective effect of thymol against 5-FU-induced hepatotoxicity, oxidative stress, and apoptosis. The counteraction of thymol to the aforementioned 5-FU-induced toxicities was also investigated computationally in addition to pharmacologic investigations on the docking of the markers' downloaded proteins where pdbID:7JL7 represented the caspase-3 substrate, pdb ID:1Q5K represented the GSK-3β protein, and PDBID: 4S0P represented the BAX protein. As shown in Figure 5, thymol interaction with caspase-3 target protein involved PHE 250 and ASN 208 as amino acid residues in H-bond and hydrophobic interactions, respectively, and as ASP was not involved in the interactions, this might imply a decrease in caspase-3 levels, which are known to be aspartate specific [26].

Docking on GSK-3β was performed based on reported inhibitors that showed activity against many diseases, such as cancer, Alzheimer's disease, and chronic inflammatory diseases [27–30]. Results recorded a binding energy of −5.283 kcal/mol and were shown totally inside the binding site with a perfect fit of 1.082 Å and an interaction with VAL 135 by a hydrogen bond between the phenolic hydroxy group of thymol and the amino group of valine as shown in Figure 2. These results are consistent with those of the co-crystallized inhibitor "TMU901", which interacts by a hydrogen bond with VAL 135 (Figure 6).

Upon docking in the BAX (pdb: 4S0P) binding pocket, thymol recorded a binding energy of −4.595 kcal/mol and was totally in the site of interaction with a fitting at 1.487 Å but did not show any significant interaction, which is consistent with the biological results of reduced BAX level (Figure 7).

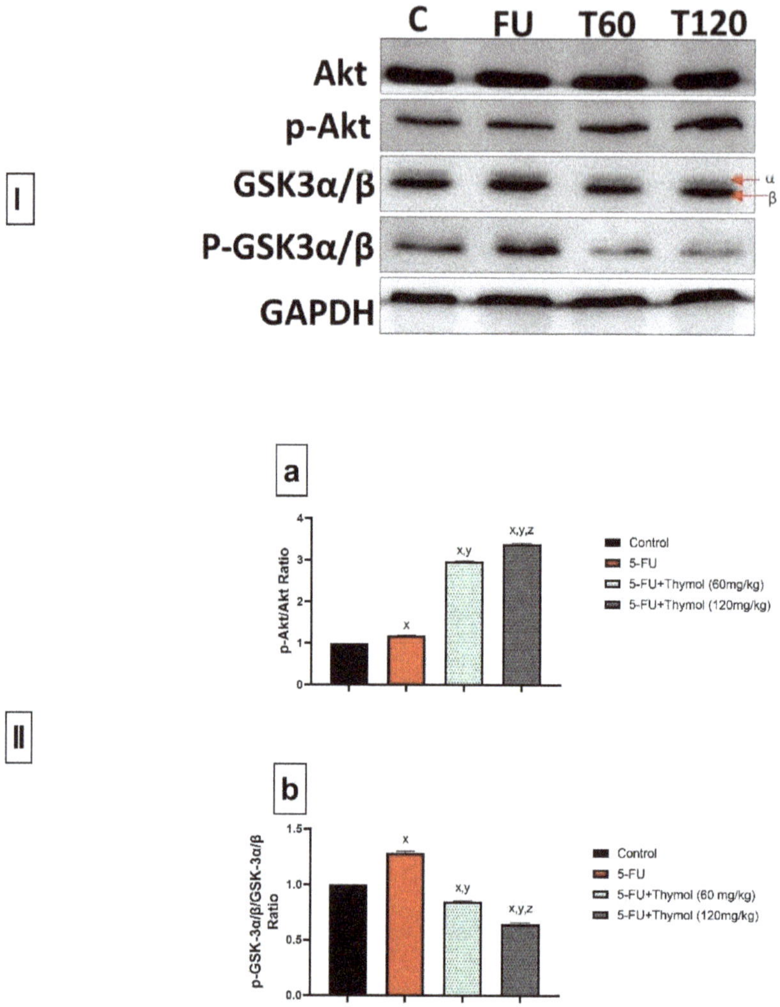

Figure 4. Effects of 5-fluorouracil with or without thymol on the p-AKT/p-GSK3α,3β signaling pathway in liver tissue of rats. (**I**) Representative immunoblot of protein levels of AKT, p-AKT, GSK3α,3β, and p-GSK3α,3β (the upper band for α and the lower band for β) in liver tissues. Proteins were immunoblotted with Akt antibody in "the first upper panel," p-Akt antibody in "the second panel," GSK3α,3β antibody in "the third panel," p-GSK3α,3β antibody in "the fourth panel," and after stripping with GAPDH antibody as a loading control in the "lower panel." (**II**) Quantitative results for the immunoblot, showing (**a**) the ratio of p-Akt/Akt and (**b**) the ratio of p-GSK3α,3β/GSK3α,3β protein levels expressed, and the relative quantities were normalized to the control and expressed as a fold of induction. The densities of immunoblots were quantified using analysis software. Values are mean ± SEM (n = 3). x, y, or z: The 5-fluorouracil and Fu+ thymol (60 mg/kg) groups are significantly different at $p < 0.05$. $p \leq 0.05$ was evaluated using ANOVA followed by Tukey–Kramer as a post-hoc test. 5-FU: 5-fluorouracil; Akt: protein Kinase B; p-Akt: phosphorylated Akt, GSK3α,3β: glycogen synthase kinase 3 α and 3β; p-GSK3α,3β: phosphorylated glycogen synthase kinase 3 α and 3β.

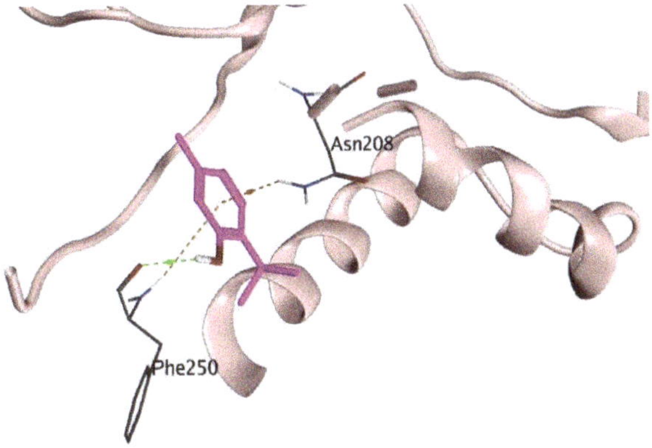

Figure 5. Thymol (in pink) interacting at the caspase-3 site of action with an H-bond as a green dotted line and pi-interactions as brown dotted lines.

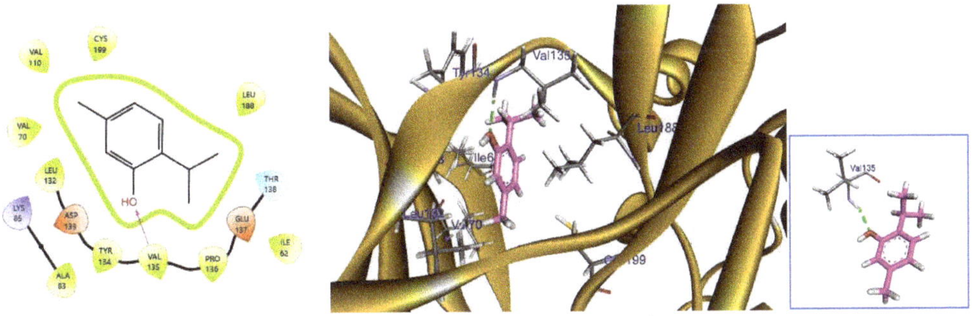

(a) (b)

Figure 6. Thymol in GSK 3β: (**a**) 2D representation of thymol with a perfect fitting inside the active site and (**b**) 3D representation of thymol (in pink) interacting with valine 135 with a hydrogen bond (in green dotted line).

Table 2 presents the docking results for thymol with all of the downloaded proteins, detailing the types of chemical bonding, the amino acids involved in the interaction, and the recorded values for binding affinity and root mean square deviation (RMSD).

Table 2. Binding affinities and type of interactions of thymol with target proteins.

Protein	pdb ID	Binding Energy Kcal/mol	RMSD (Å)	Amino Acid Residues of Interaction	Types of Bonds
Caspase-3	3kjf	−4.16	1.48	PHE 250 ASN 208 PHE 250	H-donor pi-H pi-H
Gsk-3β	1Q5K	−5.28	1.08	VAL 135	H-donor
Bax	4S0P	−4.6	1.49	-	-

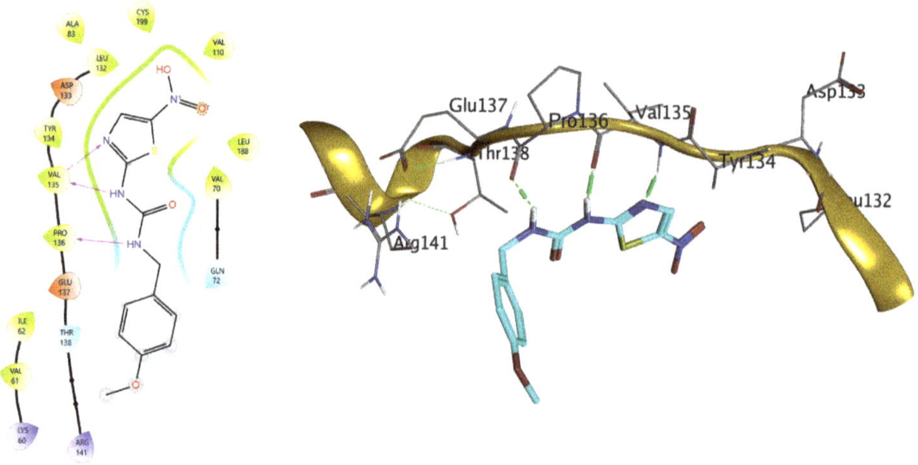

(**a**) (**b**)

Figure 7. Co-crystalized ligand of GSK (displayed in blue colored sticks) in the binding site of GSK target protein (golden ribbon): (**a**) 2D presentation and (**b**) 3D visualization (site view) where hydrogen bonds are represented as dotted green lines.

3. Discussion

It is undeniable that antineoplastic agents have been one of the major therapeutic modalities widely used for the eradication of cancer. However, severe and undesirable adverse effects remain the main complications of cancer therapy that might limit its therapeutic outcomes [31,32]. 5-FU is an effective antineoplastic agent used in the management of several solid tumors. Since 5-FU is mainly metabolized in the liver, dose-related hepatotoxicity has been associated with 5-FU therapy and may be attributed to the production of toxic metabolites [33,34]. The toxic metabolites produced by 5-FU have been blamed as being responsible for hepatic injury resulting in severe hepatotoxicity [35]. Despite the recognized risk, there are few reports examining the liver toxicity caused by 5-FU, and the underlying mechanisms remain poorly understood. Identifying these mechanisms is a critical first step in mitigating 5-FU-induced hepatic injury and developing effective hepatoprotective strategies [34,35].

Furthermore, much attention has been given to the inhibition of oxidative stress- and inflammatory-mediated apoptosis to mitigate liver injury induced by different toxicants [36–38]. It has been documented that thymol offers chemopreventive activity through its antioxidant [15], anti-inflammatory [13], and immunomodulatory mechanisms [14,39]. Therefore, the present study aimed to investigate the possible hepatoprotective effect of thymol against 5-FU-induced liver injury as well as the mechanisms of protection that might underlie it, particularly the oxidative- and inflammatory-mediated apoptosis.

Hepatotoxicity is becoming a serious cause of morbidity and mortality. To induce hepatotoxicity in our model, two doses of 5-FU were injected consecutively and hepatotoxicity was manifested by a moderate significant elevation in liver enzymes, including AST, ALT, ALP, and LDH, compared with the control group. In addition, this elevation was found to be accompanied by marked inflammatory cell infiltration along with pyknotic degeneration in hepatocytes. This elevation in AST and ALT was probably due to the damage of liver biological membranes and endothelial linings resulting from the accumulation of oxidation products and ROS in the liver tissue. Another key hepatic marker enzyme is ALP, which is associated with membrane lipids in canalicular ducts. An elevation of ALP activity in the serum occurs when ALT and AST infiltrate the hepatocytes, thus confirming the occurrence of liver damage and indicating a biliary flow disturbance [40]. In general, these liver enzymes are considered the most significant biological markers of cellular damage and toxicity [2,41], and up to 65% of patients treated with 5-FU were known to have clinically higher levels of these liver enzymes [2,42]. Our results confirmed the previous studies, which reported that 5-FU caused elevated liver enzymes and histopathological changes in liver tissues [1,5,43]. On the other hand, thymol treatment rescued the hepatocellular damage as evidenced by the improvement in serum liver enzymes, which was associated with the considerable recovery of liver histological changes in rats who received thymol in a dose of 120 mg/kg. However, liver damage remained after thymol (60 mg/kg) treatment, including the congestion of hepatic sinusoids together with alternating intact or degenerated pyknotic hepatocytes, and was consistent with a previous study. Moreover, the dose of 120 mg/kg showed considerable improvements in the histopathological examination compared with the 5-FU group.

It is well established that oxidative stress plays a significant role in 5-FU-induced toxicity, primarily through the involvement of reactive oxygen species (ROS) [4,44]. A study by Zeng and coworkers reported that 5-FU produces an excessive amount of ROS by damaging mitochondria morphology, resulting in hepatic dysfunction. These ROS caused lipid peroxidation and a perturbation of antioxidant balance, resulting in cell dysfunction and cell apoptosis [36]. Our findings suggest that 5-FU aggravated the oxidative stress in the liver specimens through a massive production of ROS that was confirmed by a significant increase in lipid peroxidation and depletion of enzymatic antioxidant, such as SOD activity, and non-enzymatic antioxidants, such as GSH content content in the liver. Additionally, dramatic biochemical and histological alterations in liver function and structure were associated with a marked elevation of liver lipid peroxidation and a significant decrease in antioxidants (GSH and SOD). Several previous studies demonstrated the same findings that affirmed the possible mechanism of antioxidants in mitigating 5-FU-induced liver injury [4,36]. Furthermore, thymol in either dose significantly decreased the formation of lipid peroxides, possibly by boosting the antioxidant machinery such as GSH and SOD, preserving them to normal tissue levels. This effect of thymol has been previously demonstrated against doxorubicin-mediated hepatotoxicity via the modulation of oxidative stress because of the thymol phenolic hydroxyl structure that confers the inherent antioxidant activity [18,45]. Thyme oil and thymol act as scavengers for ROS, providing substantial defense against ROS [46].

Another pathway that contributes to the 5-FU cytotoxicity is apoptosis, mediated by oxidative damage. Apoptosis is closely related to oxidative stress and mitigating the oxidative stress can alleviate apoptosis [36]. ROS overproduction results in potential damage to various macromolecules, and when there is insufficient protection from high ROS, cells may not survive, and the induction of apoptosis becomes inevitable [47–50]. Studies have demonstrated that 5-FU administration would cause portal apoptosis through the induction of endoplasmic reticulum stress-related genes and atrophic mitochondria [36,51]. In our experiment, we also observed that following 5-FU treatment, the hepatic expression of the apoptotic enzyme, caspase-3, significantly increased, and the anti-apoptotic protein, Bcl-2, expression was dramatically downregulated together with increased hepatic Bax protein expression, which explains the upregulation of the Bax/Bcl2 ratio in the 5-FU group compared with the control group. However, both Bax and Bcl2 proteins help suppress apoptosis in carcinogenesis rather than stimulate cell proliferation [52]. Our findings were confirmed before by the previously mentioned study [36] and were coincident with the 5-FU-induced reduction in the enzyme activity of SOD and GSH, which are essential indicators to assess the capacity to resist oxidation [50]. Accordingly, we suggested that 5-FU increased ROS production, leading to lipid peroxidation and the reduction of antioxidant enzymes, which might lead to DNA damage and promote cell death. Furthermore, our study also demonstrated that thymol significantly counteracted the 5-FU-induced hepatocyte cell apoptosis by the upregulation of Bcl2 protein expression and corrected both the Bax/Bcl2 ratio and hepatic caspase-3 expression compared with the 5-FU group. Consistently, thymol was known to reduce apoptosis by increasing Bcl-2 expression and decreasing Bax expression in different experimental models, including hepatotoxicity [24,53].

Besides Bax and Bcl-2 hepatic expression, Poly (ADP-ribose) polymerase (PARP) is a key marker involved in liver cell death. PARPs are nuclear enzymes involved in multiple biological processes, including the regulation of oxidative stress, mitochondrial function, inflammatory responses, and DNA repair processes. PARP activity increases after DNA damage induced by ROS to transfer the ADP-ribose moiety of NAD+ to form the poly(ADP ribose) polymers. This step might make changes in the function of many enzymes and structural proteins and initiate caspase-independent cell death [54–56]. During apoptosis, PARP is cleaved into fragments of 89 and 24 kDa. This caspase-mediated cleavage has become a useful hallmark of apoptosis [57]. Recently, PARP activation was demonstrated in the livers of subjects with hepatitis B-mediated cirrhosis or excessive alcohol consumption, and studies reported that the inhibition of PARP has exerted a significant hepatoprotective effect via improving the inflammatory and oxidative stress-related changes induced by alcohol consumption [56,58].

Therefore, in our study, we investigated the cleaved PARP (89 kDa) hepatic expression in all groups, and we found a marked elevation of cleaved PARP protein expression following 5-FU administration, confirming the hepatocellular cell death. However, thymol treatment in either dose decreased the cleaved PARP protein expression, and this finding was previously reported for thymol in experimental models of lipopolysaccharides-induced nephrotoxicity [59]. We suggested that thymol might have an antiapoptotic effect driven by its inhibition of PARP signaling-mediated apoptosis.

Furthermore, mitogen-activated protein (MAP) kinases have been implicated in both cell survival and cell death. The alteration of the extracellular signal-regulated kinases (ERK1/2) pathway, which influences cell proliferation, survival, and homeostasis, has been associated with various disorders, including alcoholic liver disease [60,61]. The activation of p44/42 MAP kinase has been shown to protect against cell death [62,63]. For instance, neurotrophins exerted neuroprotection through the activation of p44/42 MAP kinase in hippocampal neuronal cells [64,65]. Our current study found that 5-FU downregulated the p44/42 MAP kinase phosphorylation, which was coincident with others reporting that ethanol-induced abnormal hepatic methionine metabolism is specifically associated with the inhibition of ERK1/2; the protective agent, betaine, improved this insult by alleviating the ERK1/2 inhibition [66].

In this context, one of the signaling pathways incorporated in inflammation, oxidative stress, and apoptosis is the Akt/GSK-3β signaling pathway [67]. It is known that the Akt/GSK-3β signaling pathway can be activated by Akt phosphorylation upstream and is closely linked to the PI3K/Akt pathway. In addition, a study suggested that sulforaphane inhibits neuroinflammation by modulating the PI3K/Akt/GSK-3β pathway in the rat hippocampus [68,69]. Moreover, it was documented that 5-FU inhibited cell growth and induced apoptosis by targeting Akt/GSK-3β signaling [70]. Therefore, we decided to assess the critical Akt/GSK-3β signaling pathway to further elucidate thymol's protective effects in our experimental model of 5-FU-induced liver damage. The current study found that 5-FU elicited the activation of Akt/GSK-3β phosphorylation, as shown by the significant upregulation of the protein expression of hepatic p-AKT and p-GSK-3β. The phosphorylated Akt protein regulates a diversity of cell death pathways and cell-cycle transitions [71]. In this regard, 5-FU was known to induce drug resistance by activating p-Akt and decreasing chemotherapy sensitivity [72,73].

A study demonstrated that the activation of Akt usually involves phosphorylation at the site of threonine 308, known to phosphorylate GSK-3β on the site of serine 9 [74]. Reviewing the literature, we found that GSK-3β is constitutively active in the cytoplasm, and its activity is induced by being phosphorylated at tyrosine 216 and inhibited by phosphorylation at serine 9 [75]. Shinohara and coworkers suggested that increasing the phosphorylation of both the active and inhibited forms of GSK-3β in acetaminophen-induced hepatotoxicity resulted in an overall increase in GSK-3β activity. This previous study also suggested that GSK-3β, once further activated, is translocated to mitochondria [76]. Nevertheless, the dual and sometimes contradictory roles of GSK-3β in promoting both cell survival and apoptosis in different diseases have not been fully elucidated [23]. In the current study, we demonstrated that thymol treatment modulated Akt/ GSK-3β pathway signaling as shown by the upregulation of Akt phosphorylation and downregulation of GSK-3β phosphorylation. This effect coincided with thymol, which is a proven antioxidant and anti-apoptotic effect in our treated groups. In harmony with our findings, others have demonstrated that thymol reduced the GSK-3β protein expression in an experimental model of monosodium glutamate-induced attention deficit hyperactivity disorder [24]. Furthermore, a study by Wang et al. [25] demonstrated that thymol protected rats from glycerol-induced nephrotoxicity by increasing the phosphorylation of Akt signaling. Based on this study, it is suggested that the anti-inflammatory and anti-oxidative effects of thymol are potentially dependent on the activation of the PI3K/Akt pathway, but the exact mechanism needs further exploration.

4. Materials and Methods

4.1. Materials

4.1.1. Drugs and Chemicals

Thymol was obtained from extrasynthese (Z.I Lyon Nord, Lyon, France). We obtained the 5-FU (Fluorouracil Injection 50 mg/mL Amp) from EBEWE Pharma (Unterach am Attersee, Österreich). Primary and secondary antibodies were products of Abcam (Cambridge, MA, USA). Bax (ab6671), Bcl-2 (ab215715), cleaved PARP (46D11) Rabbit mAb, Akt 1 [(Ser473) (D9E) XP® Rabbit mAb #4060.Cell sig.], phosphorylated-Akt1 (p-AKT1) [(Ser473) (D9E) XP® Rabbit mAb #4060.Cell sig.], GSK-3α/β [(D75D3) Rabbit mAb], phosphorylated-GSK-3α/β (p-GSK-3α/β) [(Ser21/9) (D17D2) Rabbit mAb], and phosphorylated-44/42 MAP kinases [(Erk1/2) (137F5) Rabbit mAb #4695] and anti-glyceraldehydes-3-phosphate dehydrogenase (GAPDH) (ab8245) were used. Other chemicals were of the highest grade and were obtained from Sigma (St. Louis, MO, USA) and Abcam (Cambridge, MA, USA).

4.1.2. Animals

The study was carried out after approval was obtained from the ethical committee at the College of Pharmacy, King Saud University, Riyadh, Saudi Arabia (IRB number: KSU-SE-24-6). Forty male Wistar Rats (7 weeks old, 150–200 g) were supplied by the experimental Animal House, Faculty of Pharmacy, King Saud University, Saudi Arabia. The rats were housed in clean cages for a week before the experiment for acclimatization and kept under standard conditions, 25 °C and 60% humidity, and a 12 h light–dark cycle. In addition, rats were provided free access to a standard diet and water. According to the standard guidelines, standard diet pellets contain not less than 20% protein, 5% fiber, 3.5% fat, 6.5% ash, and a vitamin mixture.

4.2. Methods

4.2.1. Experiment Design

Rats were randomly organized into four different groups and treated for 11 days, as described in Table 3.

Table 3. The experimental groups and their description.

	Description
Control	Normal rats received the vehicle (0.5% DMSO in normal saline) once daily by oral gavage.
5-FU	Rats serving as the positive control group were given the vehicle orally (0.5% DMSO in normal saline) once daily and two doses of 5-FU (150 mg/kg, intraperitoneally (ip)) on days 6 and 7 to induce hepatic toxicity [15,77].

Table 3. *Cont.*

	Description
5-FU + Thymol 60	Rats were given thymol daily (60 mg/kg in 0.5% DMSO in normal saline, orally) and 5-FU (150 mg/kg, ip) on days 6 and 7 [15,78].
5-FU + Thymol 120	Rats were given thymol daily (120 mg/kg in 0.5% DMSO in normal saline, orally) and 5-FU (150 mg/kg, ip) on days 6 and 7 [15,24]

Animals' weights were recorded on the 1st, 6th, and last day of the experiment.

4.2.2. Blood and Liver Sample Collection

Four days after the last 5-FU dose (on the 11th day), animals were anesthetized using carbon dioxide and decapitated, and blood samples were collected from the trunk. The collected blood was centrifuged at 1000 rpm at 4 °C for 30 min, and sera were collected and stored at −80 °C. Lastly, the livers were dissected and rinsed with ice-cold phosphate-buffered saline [79].

A part of the liver was cut and kept in 4% formaldehyde for histopathological and immunohistochemical studies. The other part of the liver was snap frozen in liquid nitrogen and stored at −80 °C for Western blotting. The remaining part was homogenized, kept at −80 °C, and used for other biochemical assays.

4.2.3. Histopathological Examination

Liver specimens were fixed in buffered formalin, processed, and stained with hematoxylin and eosin (H&E), as described previously [80]. Sections were then examined using a light microscope.

4.2.4. Assessment of Serum Liver Enzymes and Oxidative Stress Markers in Liver Tissues

Reduced glutathione (GSH) [81], thiobarbituric acid reactive substances (TBARSs) [82], glutathione peroxidase (GPx), and superoxide dismutase (SOD) [83] were analyzed in liver homogenates using commercially available kits (Biodiagnostic, Cairo, Egypt), in compliance with the instructions of the manufacturer.

Liver enzymes, ALT, AST, ALP, and lactate dehydrogenase (LDH), were measured in sera using standard kits (United Diagnostics Industry, Dammam, Saudi Arabia).

4.2.5. Assessment of Apoptotic Markers in Liver Tissues

The expression of caspase-3 in liver tissues was assessed using the immunohistochemistry technique. In addition, Bax and Bcl-2 protein expressions in liver specimens were evaluated by Western blot analysis. The immunohistochemistry was conducted following the standard protocol used in our lab [16] using the primary antibody against caspase-3 (ab32351; Abcam, Cambridge, UK). The scores for caspase-3 were calculated as the area % of the hepatic immunopositive expression of caspase-3, for which six random fields/section were used.

4.2.6. Western Blot Analysis

The expression of Bax, Bcl2, cleaved PARP, Akt1, GSK-3α/β, and phosphorylated-44/42 MAP kinase proteins in liver tissues was carried out using Western blot analysis as previously described [84].

4.2.7. Assessing the Binding Affinities Using In Silico Modeling

Three proteins were selected for each selected target. Selected targets were caspase-3, GSK-3β, and BAX. Proteins were downloaded from the protein data bank with pdb codes pdb ID:7JL7 representing caspase-3, pdb ID:1Q5K representing GSK-3β, and pdb ID: 4S0P representing BAX target proteins. Ligand and protein structural optimizations were applied by Autodock4 with the aid of UCSF-chimera-1.17.3. Protein preparation, including calculating partial charges, 3D protonation, and strands correction, was performed, and then the protein was saved in pdbqt format. The ligand was optimized by UCSF-chimera and saved in a pdbqt format. A grid box was generated using autogrid 4 allocated at the macromolecule center. Docking was performed using AutoDock4. Results were then visualized using Maestro-2023-4 and Biovia-DS V21.1.0.20298.

4.3. Statistics

Data are represented as means ± standard deviation (SD). Multiple group analyses were performed using one-way ANOVA and then by the Tukey–Kramer post-hoc test. The significance level was accepted at $p < 0.05$. Statistical analyses and graphical representations were performed using GraphPad Prism software version 5 (ISI® software, USA).

5. Conclusions

Collectively, our study elucidated the hepatoprotective mechanisms of thymol against 5-FU-induced hepatocellular injury in rat models. Thymol ameliorated liver damage via its antioxidant and anti-apoptotic effects. Additionally, the present study suggested that the modulation of the Akt/GSK-3β pathway signaling is potentially implicated in the cytoprotecting effect of thymol against 5-FU-induced hepatocellular death. Thus, our study might illustrate a new clinical benefit of thymol as a promising natural chemo-preventive agent in chemotherapy-based therapy for cancer patients.

Author Contributions: Y.F.M.: Conceptualization, Investigation, Methodology, Formal Analysis, Writing—Original Draft, Writing—Review and Editing. A.M.B.: Conceptualization, Investigation, Methodology, Formal Analysis, Writing—Review and Editing, and Project Administration. L.A.A.-K.: Conceptualization, Investigation, Methodology, Formal Analysis, Writing—Original Draft. S.S.: Writing—Review and Editing. H.N.A.: Investigation, Visualization. N.M.B.: Investigation. N.T.A.: Writing–Original Draft. E.I.E.: Investigation, Writing–Original Draft. All authors have read and agreed to the published version of the manuscript.

Funding: This research project was supported by a grant from the Researchers Supporting Project, King Saud University, Riyadh, Saudi Arabia.

Institutional Review Board Statement: The study was carried out after the approval obtained by the ethical committee at the College of Pharmacy, King Saud University, Riyadh, Saudi Arabia (IRB number: KSU-SE-24-6).

Data Availability Statement: Data generated or analyzed during this study are included in this published article.

Acknowledgments: The authors extend their appreciation to the Researchers Supporting Project number (RSPD2024R575), King Saud University, Riyadh, Saudi Arabia for funding this project.

Conflicts of Interest: The authors declare that they have no competing interests.

References

1. Pujari, R.R.; Bandawane, D.D. Hepatoprotective Activity of Gentisic Acid on 5-Fluorouracil-Induced Hepatotoxicity in Wistar Rats. *Turk. J. Pharm. Sci.* **2021**, *18*, 332–338. [CrossRef] [PubMed]
2. Gelen, V.; Şengül, E.; Yıldırım, S.; Atila, G. The Protective Effects of Naringin against 5-Fluorouracil-Induced Hepatotoxicity and Nephrotoxicity in Rats. *Iran. J. Basic Med. Sci.* **2018**, *21*, 404–410. [CrossRef]
3. Ghoshal, K.; Jacob, S.T. An Alternative Molecular Mechanism of Action of 5-Fluorouracil, a Potent Anticancer Drug. *Biochem. Pharmacol.* **1997**, *53*, 1569–1575. [CrossRef]
4. Al-Asmari, A.; Khan, A.; Al-Masri, N. Mitigation of 5-Fluorouracil–Induced Liver Damage in Rats by Vitamin C via Targeting Redox–Sensitive Transcription Factors. *Hum. Exp. Toxicol.* **2016**, *35*, 1203–1213. [CrossRef]
5. Fukuno, S.; Nagai, K.; Yoshida, S.; Suzuki, H.; Konishi, H. Taurine as a Protective Agent for 5-Fluorouracil-Induced Hepatic Damage Related to Oxidative Stress. *Die Pharm. Int. J. Pharm. Sci.* **2016**, *71*, 530–532. [CrossRef]
6. Mansoori, R.; Kazemi, S.; Almasi, D.; Hosseini, S.M.; Karim, B.; Nabipour, M.; Moghadamnia, A.A. Therapeutic Benefit of Melatonin in 5-Fluorouracil-Induced Renal and Hepatic Injury. *Basic Clin. Pharmacol. Toxicol.* **2024**, *134*, 397–411. [CrossRef]
7. Diba, M.; Seghatoleslam, A.; Namavari, M.; Assadi, S.; Vakili, S.N.; Babaei, Z.; Akmali, M. Potential Protective Role of Cyrtopodion Scabrum in Antioxidant Parameters in Serum and Liver of Rats with 5-FU-Induced Oxidative Damage. *Arch. Razi Inst.* **2021**, *76*, 95–105. [CrossRef] [PubMed]

8. Khalaf, H.M.; Hafez, S.M.N.A.; Abdalla, A.M.; Welson, N.N.; Abdelzaher, W.Y.; Abdelbaky, F.A.F. Role of Platelet-Activating Factor and HO-1 in Mediating the Protective Effect of Rupatadine against 5-Fluorouracil-Induced Hepatotoxicity in Rats. *Environ. Sci. Pollut. Res.* **2022**, *29*, 40190–40203. [CrossRef]
9. Saleh, D.O.; Mahmoud, S.S.; Hassan, A.; Sanad, E.F. Doxorubicin-Induced Hepatic Toxicity in Rats: Mechanistic Protective Role of Omega-3 Fatty Acids through Nrf2/HO-1 Activation and PI3K/Akt/GSK-3β Axis Modulation. *Saudi J. Biol. Sci.* **2022**, *29*, 103308. [CrossRef]
10. Guo, C.; Zheng, L.; Chen, S.; Liang, X.; Song, X.; Wang, Y.; Hua, B.; Qiu, L. Thymol Ameliorates Ethanol-Induced Hepatotoxicity via Regulating Metabolism and Autophagy. *Chem. Biol. Interact.* **2023**, *370*, 110308. [CrossRef]
11. Mahran, Y.F.; Al-Kharashi, L.A.; Atawia, R.T.; Alanazi, R.T.; Dhahi, A.M.B.; Alsubaie, R.; Badr, A.M. Radioprotective Effects of Carvacrol and/or Thymol against Gamma Irradiation-Induced Acute Nephropathy: In Silico and In Vivo Evidence of the Involvement of Insulin-like Growth Factor-1 (IGF-1) and Calcitonin Gene-Related Peptide. *Biomedicines* **2023**, *11*, 2521. [CrossRef]
12. Güvenç, M.; Cellat, M.; Gökçek, İ.; Yavaş, İ.; Özsoy, Ş.Y. Effects of Thymol and Carvacrol on Sperm Quality and Oxidant/Antioxidant Balance in Rats. *Arch. Physiol. Biochem.* **2019**, *125*, 396–403. [CrossRef]
13. Botelho, M.A.; Barros, G.; Queiroz, D.B.; Carvalho, C.F.; Gouvea, J.; Patrus, L.; Bannet, M.; Patrus, D.; Rego, A.; Silva, I.; et al. Nanotechnology in Phytotherapy: Antiinflammatory Effect of a Nanostructured Thymol Gel from Lippia Sidoides in Acute Periodontitis in Rats. *Phytother. Res.* **2016**, *30*, 152–159. [CrossRef] [PubMed]
14. Chamanara, M.; Abdollahi, A.; Rezayat, S.M.; Ghazi-Khansari, M.; Dehpour, A.; Nassireslami, E.; Rashidian, A. Thymol Reduces Acetic Acid-Induced Inflammatory Response through Inhibition of NF-kB Signaling Pathway in Rat Colon Tissue. *Inflammopharmacology* **2019**, *27*, 1275–1283. [CrossRef]
15. Al-Khrashi, L.A.; Badr, A.M.; Al-Amin, M.A.; Mahran, Y.F. Thymol Ameliorates 5-Fluorouracil-Induced Intestinal Mucositis: Evidence of down-Regulatory Effect on TGF-β/MAPK Pathways through NF-κB. *J. Biochem. Mol. Toxicol.* **2022**, *36*, e22932. [CrossRef] [PubMed]
16. Badr, A.M.; Alkharashi, L.A.; Sherif, I.O.; Alanteet, A.A.; Alotaibi, H.N.; Mahran, Y.F. IL-17/Notch1/STAT3 Pathway Contributes to 5-Fluorouracil-Induced Intestinal Mucositis in Rats: Amelioration by Thymol Treatment. *Pharmaceuticals* **2022**, *15*, 1412. [CrossRef]
17. Ibrahim, D.; Abdelfattah-Hassan, A.; Badawi, M.; Ismail, T.A.; Bendary, M.M.; Abdelaziz, A.M.; Mosbah, R.A.; Mohamed, D.I.; Arisha, A.H.; El-Hamid, M.I.A. Thymol Nanoemulsion Promoted Broiler Chicken's Growth, Gastrointestinal Barrier and Bacterial Community and Conferred Protection against Salmonella Typhimurium. *Sci. Rep.* **2021**, *11*, 7742. [CrossRef] [PubMed]
18. Ye, X.; Ling, T.; Xue, Y.; Xu, C.; Zhou, W.; Hu, L.; Chen, J.; Shi, Z. Thymol Mitigates Cadmium Stress by Regulating Glutathione Levels and Reactive Oxygen Species Homeostasis in Tobacco Seedlings. *Molecules* **2016**, *21*, 1339. [CrossRef]
19. Omonijo, F.A.; Liu, S.; Hui, Q.; Zhang, H.; Lahaye, L.; Bodin, J.-C.; Gong, J.; Nyachoti, M.; Yang, C. Thymol Improves Barrier Function and Attenuates Inflammatory Responses in Porcine Intestinal Epithelial Cells during Lipopolysaccharide (LPS)-Induced Inflammation. *J. Agric. Food Chem.* **2019**, *67*, 615–624. [CrossRef]
20. Dou, X.; Yan, D.; Liu, S.; Gao, L.; Shan, A. Thymol Alleviates LPS-Induced Liver Inflammation and Apoptosis by Inhibiting NLRP3 Inflammasome Activation and the AMPK-mTOR-Autophagy Pathway. *Nutrients* **2022**, *14*, 2809. [CrossRef]
21. Jafari, A.; Rasmi, Y.; Hajaghazadeh, M.; Karimipour, M. Hepatoprotective Effect of Thymol against Subchronic Toxicity of Titanium Dioxide Nanoparticles: Biochemical and Histological Evidences. *Environ. Toxicol. Pharmacol.* **2018**, *58*, 29–36. [CrossRef]
22. Rayasam, G.V.; Tulasi, V.K.; Sodhi, R.; Davis, J.A.; Ray, A. Glycogen Synthase Kinase 3: More than a Namesake. *Br. J. Pharmacol.* **2009**, *156*, 885–898. [CrossRef] [PubMed]
23. Jacobs, K.M.; Bhave, S.R.; Ferraro, D.J.; Jaboin, J.J.; Hallahan, D.E.; Thotala, D. GSK-3β: A Bifunctional Role in Cell Death Pathways. *Int. J. Cell Biol.* **2012**, *2012*, 930710. [CrossRef]
24. Abu-Elfotuh, K.; Abdel-Sattar, S.A.; Abbas, A.N.; Mahran, Y.F.; Alshanwani, A.R.; Hamdan, A.M.E.; Atwa, A.M.; Reda, E.; Ahmed, Y.M.; Zaghlool, S.S.; et al. The Protective Effect of Thymoquinone or/and Thymol against Monosodium Glutamate-Induced Attention-Deficit/Hyperactivity Disorder (ADHD)-like Behavior in Rats: Modulation of Nrf2/HO-1, TLR4/NF-κB/NLRP3/Caspase-1 and Wnt/β-Catenin Signaling Pathways in Rat Model. *Biomed. Pharmacother.* **2022**, *155*, 113799. [CrossRef]
25. Wang, Q.; Qi, G.; Zhou, H.; Cheng, F.; Yang, X.; Liu, X.; Wang, R. Protective Effect of Thymol on Glycerol-Induced Acute Kidney Injury. *Ren. Fail.* **2023**, *45*, 2227728. [CrossRef]
26. Yao, L.; Swartz, P.; Hamilton, P.T.; Clark, A.C. Remodeling Hydrogen Bond Interactions Results in Relaxed Specificity of Caspase-3. *Biosci. Rep.* **2021**, *41*, BSR20203495. [CrossRef]
27. Martinez, A.; Castro, A.; Dorronsoro, I.; Alonso, M. Glycogen Synthase Kinase 3 (GSK-3) Inhibitors as New Promising Drugs for Diabetes, Neurodegeneration, Cancer, and Inflammation. *Med. Res. Rev.* **2002**, *22*, 373–384. [CrossRef] [PubMed]
28. Mohammad, M.K.; Al-Masri, I.M.; Taha, M.O.; Al-Ghussein, M.A.S.; Alkhatib, H.S.; Najjar, S.; Bustanji, Y. Olanzapine Inhibits Glycogen Synthase Kinase-3β: An Investigation by Docking Simulation and Experimental Validation. *Eur. J. Pharmacol.* **2008**, *584*, 185–191. [CrossRef]
29. Taha, M.O.; Bustanji, Y.; Al-Ghussein, M.A.S.; Mohammad, M.; Zalloum, H.; Al-Masri, I.M.; Atallah, N. Pharmacophore Modeling, Quantitative Structure–Activity Relationship Analysis, and in Silico Screening Reveal Potent Glycogen Synthase Kinase-3β Inhibitory Activities for Cimetidine, Hydroxychloroquine, and Gemifloxacin. *J. Med. Chem.* **2008**, *51*, 2062–2077. [CrossRef] [PubMed]
30. Alonso, M.; Martinez, A. GSK-3 Inhibitors: Discoveries and Developments. *Curr. Med. Chem.* **2004**, *11*, 755–763. [CrossRef]

31. Borek: Antioxidants and Radiation Therapy—Google Scholar. Available online: https://scholar.google.com/scholar_lookup?title=Antioxidants%20and%20radiation%20therapy&publication_year=2004&author=C.%20Borek (accessed on 6 December 2023).
32. Minami, M.; Matsumoto, S.; Horiuchi, H. Cardiovascular Side-Effects of Modern Cancer Therapy. *Circ. J.* **2010**, *74*, 1779–1786. [CrossRef] [PubMed]
33. Abou-Zeid, N.R.A. Ameliorative Effect of Vitamin C against 5-Fuorouracil-Induced Hepatotoxicity in Mice: A Light and Electron Microscope Study. *J. Basic Appl. Zool.* **2014**, *67*, 109–118. [CrossRef]
34. Yaegashi, A.; Yoshida, K.; Suzuki, N.; Shimada, I.; Tani, Y.; Saijo, Y.; Toyama, A. A Case of Severe Hepatotoxicity Induced by Cisplatin and 5-Fluorouracil. *Int. Cancer Conf. J.* **2019**, *9*, 24–27. [CrossRef] [PubMed]
35. Ali, N. Protective Effect of Captopril against 5-Fluorouracil-Induced Hepato and Nephrotoxicity in Male Albino Rats. *J. Am. Sci.* **2012**, *8*, 680–685.
36. Zeng, D.; Wang, Y.; Chen, Y.; Li, D.; Li, G.; Xiao, H.; Hou, J.; Wang, Z.; Hu, L.; Wang, L.; et al. Angelica Polysaccharide Antagonizes 5-FU-Induced Oxidative Stress Injury to Reduce Apoptosis in the Liver Through Nrf2 Pathway. *Front. Oncol.* **2021**, *11*, 720620. [CrossRef] [PubMed]
37. Liu, Y.; Wen, P.-H.; Zhang, X.-X.; Dai, Y.; He, Q. Breviscapine Ameliorates CCl4-induced Liver Injury in Mice through Inhibiting Inflammatory Apoptotic Response and ROS Generation. *Int. J. Mol. Med.* **2018**, *42*, 755–768. [CrossRef]
38. Choudhury, S.; Ghosh, S.; Mukherjee, S.; Gupta, P.; Bhattacharya, S.; Adhikary, A.; Chattopadhyay, S. Pomegranate Protects against Arsenic-Induced P53-Dependent ROS-Mediated Inflammation and Apoptosis in Liver Cells. *J. Nutr. Biochem.* **2016**, *38*, 25–40. [CrossRef]
39. Mohammadi, A.; Mahjoub, S.; Ghafarzadegan, K.; Nouri, H.R. Immunomodulatory Effects of Thymol through Modulation of Redox Status and Trace Element Content in Experimental Model of Asthma. *Biomed. Pharmacother.* **2018**, *105*, 856–861. [CrossRef]
40. Zhao, J.-A.; Peng, L.; Geng, C.-Z.; Liu, Y.-P.; Wang, X.; Yang, H.-C.; Wang, S.-J. Preventive Effect of Hydrazinocurcumin on Carcinogenesis of Diethylnitrosamine-Induced Hepatocarcinoma in Male SD Rats. *Asian Pac. J. Cancer Prev.* **2014**, *15*, 2115–2121. [CrossRef]
41. Stockham, S.L.; Scott, M.A. *Fundamentals of Veterinary Clinical Pathology*; John Wiley & Sons: Hoboken, NJ, USA, 2013; ISBN 978-1-118-68607-2.
42. Sugarbaker, P.H.; Gianola, F.J.; Speyer, J.C.; Wesley, R.; Barofsky, I.; Meyers, C.E. Prospective, Randomized Trial of Intravenous versus Intraperitoneal 5-Fluorouracil in Patients with Advanced Primary Colon or Rectal Cancer. *Surgery* **1985**, *98*, 414–422.
43. Ray, S.; Roy, K.; Sengupta, C. In Vitro Evaluation of Protective Effects of Ascorbic Acid and Water Extract of Spirulina Plantesis (Blue Green Algae) on 5-Fluorouracil-Induced Lipid Peroxidation. *Acta Pol. Pharm.* **2007**, *64*, 335–344. [PubMed]
44. Rashid, S.; Ali, N.; Nafees, S.; Hasan, S.K.; Sultana, S. Mitigation of 5-Fluorouracil Induced Renal Toxicity by Chrysin via Targeting Oxidative Stress and Apoptosis in Wistar Rats. *Food Chem. Toxicol.* **2014**, *66*, 185–193. [CrossRef]
45. Llana-Ruiz-Cabello, M.; Gutiérrez-Praena, D.; Puerto, M.; Pichardo, S.; Jos, Á.; Cameán, A.M. In Vitro Pro-Oxidant/Antioxidant Role of Carvacrol, Thymol and Their Mixture in the Intestinal Caco-2 Cell Line. *Toxicol. In Vitro* **2015**, *29*, 647–656. [CrossRef]
46. Elgaml, S.A.; Hashish, E. Clinicopathological Studies of *Thymus vulgaris* Extract against Cadmium Induced Hepatotoxicity in Albino Rats. *Glob. J. Pharmacol.* **2014**, *8*, 501–509.
47. Chun, K.-S.; Joo, S.H. Modulation of Reactive Oxygen Species to Overcome 5-Fluorouracil Resistance. *Biomol. Ther.* **2022**, *30*, 479–489. [CrossRef] [PubMed]
48. Richter, C.; Gogvadze, V.; Laffranchi, R.; Schlapbach, R.; Schweizer, M.; Suter, M.; Walter, P.; Yaffee, M. Oxidants in Mitochondria: From Physiology to Diseases. *Biochim. Biophys. Acta BBA Mol. Basis Dis.* **1995**, *1271*, 67–74. [CrossRef] [PubMed]
49. Alfaradhi, M.Z.; Fernandez-Twinn, D.S.; Martin-Gronert, M.S.; Musial, B.; Fowden, A.; Ozanne, S.E. Oxidative Stress and Altered Lipid Homeostasis in the Programming of Offspring Fatty Liver by Maternal Obesity. *Am. J. Physiol. Regul. Integr. Comp. Physiol.* **2014**, *307*, R26–R34. [CrossRef] [PubMed]
50. Barzilai, A.; Yamamoto, K.-I. DNA Damage Responses to Oxidative Stress. *DNA Repair* **2004**, *3*, 1109–1115. [CrossRef] [PubMed]
51. El-Sayyad, H.I.; Ismail, M.F.; Shalaby, F.M.; Abou-El-Magd, R.F.; Gaur, R.L.; Fernando, A.; Raj, M.H.G.; Ouhtit, A. Histopathological Effects of Cisplatin, Doxorubicin and 5-Flurouracil (5-FU) on the Liver of Male Albino Rats. *Int. J. Biol. Sci.* **2009**, *5*, 466–473. [CrossRef]
52. Rodriguez, I.; Matsuura, K.; Khatib, K.; Reed, J.C.; Nagata, S.; Vassalli, P. A Bcl-2 Transgene Expressed in Hepatocytes Protects Mice from Fulminant Liver Destruction but Not from Rapid Death Induced by Anti-Fas Antibody Injection. *J. Exp. Med.* **1996**, *183*, 1031–1036. [CrossRef] [PubMed]
53. Nagoor Meeran, M.F.; Jagadeesh, G.S.; Selvaraj, P. Thymol Attenuates Altered Lipid Metabolism in β-Adrenergic Agonist Induced Myocardial Infarcted Rats by Inhibiting Tachycardia, Altered Electrocardiogram, Apoptosis and Cardiac Hypertrophy. *J. Funct. Foods* **2015**, *14*, 51–62. [CrossRef]
54. Bai, P.; Nagy, L.; Fodor, T.; Liaudet, L.; Pacher, P. Poly(ADP-Ribose) Polymerases as Modulators of Mitochondrial Activity. *Trends Endocrinol. Metab.* **2015**, *26*, 75–83. [CrossRef] [PubMed]
55. Kraus, W.L.; Hottiger, M.O. PARP-1 and Gene Regulation: Progress and Puzzles. *Mol. Asp. Med.* **2013**, *34*, 1109–1123. [CrossRef] [PubMed]
56. Mukhopadhyay, P.; Horváth, B.; Rajesh, M.; Varga, Z.V.; Gariani, K.; Ryu, D.; Cao, Z.; Holovac, E.; Park, O.; Zhou, Z.; et al. PARP Inhibition Protects against Alcoholic and Non-Alcoholic Steatohepatitis. *J. Hepatol.* **2017**, *66*, 589–600. [CrossRef]

57. Gobeil, S.; Boucher, C.C.; Nadeau, D.; Poirier, G.G. Characterization of the Necrotic Cleavage of Poly(ADP-Ribose) Polymerase (PARP-1): Implication of Lysosomal Proteases. *Cell Death Differ.* **2001**, *8*, 588–594. [CrossRef] [PubMed]
58. Curtin, N.J.; Szabo, C. Therapeutic Applications of PARP Inhibitors: Anticancer Therapy and Beyond. *Mol. Asp. Med.* **2013**, *34*, 1217–1256. [CrossRef]
59. Erzurumlu, Y.; Dogan, H.; Çatakli, D. Thymol Reduces the Lipopolysaccharide-Induced Acute Kidney Inflammation by Modulating Lysosomal Stress. *J. Res. Pharm.* **2023**, *27*, 375–385. [CrossRef]
60. Sampey, B.P.; Stewart, B.J.; Petersen, D.R. Ethanol-Induced Modulation of Hepatocellular Extracellular Signal-Regulated Kinase-1/2 Activity via 4-Hydroxynonenal. *J. Biol. Chem.* **2007**, *282*, 1925–1937. [CrossRef]
61. Agoglia, A.E.; Sharko, A.C.; Psilos, K.E.; Holstein, S.E.; Reid, G.T.; Hodge, C.W. Alcohol Alters the Activation of ERK1/2, a Functional Regulator of Binge Alcohol Drinking in Adult C57BL/6J Mice. *Alcohol. Clin. Exp. Res.* **2015**, *39*, 463–475. [CrossRef]
62. Xia, Z.; Dickens, M.; Raingeaud, J.; Davis, R.J.; Greenberg, M.E. Opposing Effects of ERK and JNK-P38 MAP Kinases on Apoptosis. *Science* **1995**, *270*, 1326–1331. [CrossRef]
63. Kummer, J.L.; Rao, P.K.; Heidenreich, K.A. Apoptosis Induced by Withdrawal of Trophic Factors Is Mediated by P38 Mitogen-Activated Protein Kinase. *J. Biol. Chem.* **1997**, *272*, 20490–20494. [CrossRef] [PubMed]
64. Marsh, H.N.; Scholz, W.K.; Lamballe, F.; Klein, R.; Nanduri, V.; Barbacid, M.; Palfrey, H.C. Signal Transduction Events Mediated by the BDNF Receptor Gp 145trkB in Primary Hippocampal Pyramidal Cell Culture. *J. Neurosci.* **1993**, *13*, 4281–4292. [CrossRef] [PubMed]
65. Mattson, M.P.; Scheff, S.W. Endogenous Neuroprotection Factors and Traumatic Brain Injury: Mechanisms of Action and Implications for Therapy. *J. Neurotrauma* **1994**, *11*, 3–33. [CrossRef] [PubMed]
66. Wang, Z.; Yao, T.; Song, Z. Involvement and Mechanism of DGAT2 Upregulation in the Pathogenesis of Alcoholic Fatty Liver Disease. *J. Lipid Res.* **2010**, *51*, 3158–3165. [CrossRef]
67. He, Y.; Zhou, A.; Jiang, W. Toll-like Receptor 4-Mediated Signaling Participates in Apoptosis of Hippocampal Neurons. *Neural Regen. Res.* **2013**, *8*, 2744–2753. [CrossRef]
68. Yang, W.; Liu, Y.; Xu, Q.-Q.; Xian, Y.-F.; Lin, Z.-X. Sulforaphene Ameliorates Neuroinflammation and Hyperphosphorylated Tau Protein via Regulating the PI3K/Akt/GSK-3β Pathway in Experimental Models of Alzheimer's Disease. *Oxid. Med. Cell. Longev.* **2020**, *2020*, 4754195. [CrossRef]
69. Ivánovics, G.; Horváth, S. Raphanin, an Antibacterial Principle of the Radish (*Raphanus sativus*). *Nature* **1947**, *160*, 297–298. [CrossRef]
70. Li, C.S.; Van Nguyen, T.; Chai, O.H.; Park, B.H.; Lee, J.-S.; Kim, S.M. 3,3′-Diindolylmethane Augments 5-Fluorouracil-InducedGrowth Suppression in Gastric Cancer Cells through Suppression of the Akt/GSK-3β and WNT/Beta-Catenin. *J. Oncol.* **2023**, *2023*, 8268955. [CrossRef]
71. Fresno Vara, J.A.; Casado, E.; de Castro, J.; Cejas, P.; Belda-Iniesta, C.; González-Barón, M. PI3K/Akt Signalling Pathway and Cancer. *Cancer Treat. Rev.* **2004**, *30*, 193–204. [CrossRef]
72. Han, Z.; Hong, L.; Han, Y.; Wu, K.; Han, S.; Shen, H.; Li, C.; Yao, L.; Qiao, T.; Fan, D. Phospho Akt Mediates Multidrug Resistance of Gastric Cancer Cells through Regulation of P-Gp, Bcl-2 and Bax. *J. Exp. Clin. Cancer Res.* **2007**, *26*, 261–268.
73. Sun, Y.; Jiang, Y.; Huang, J.; Chen, H.; Liao, Y.; Yang, Z. CISD2 Enhances the Chemosensitivity of Gastric Cancer through the Enhancement of 5-FU-Induced Apoptosis and the Inhibition of Autophagy by AKT/mTOR Pathway. *Cancer Med.* **2017**, *6*, 2331–2346. [CrossRef]
74. Jope, R.S.; Johnson, G.V.W. The Glamour and Gloom of Glycogen Synthase Kinase-3. *Trends Biochem. Sci.* **2004**, *29*, 95–102. [CrossRef]
75. Eldar-Finkelman, H. Glycogen Synthase Kinase 3: An Emerging Therapeutic Target. *Trends Mol. Med.* **2002**, *8*, 126–132. [CrossRef] [PubMed]
76. Shinohara, M.; Ybanez, M.D.; Win, S.; Than, T.A.; Jain, S.; Gaarde, W.A.; Han, D.; Kaplowitz, N. Silencing Glycogen Synthase Kinase-3β Inhibits Acetaminophen Hepatotoxicity and Attenuates JNK Activation and Loss of Glutamate Cysteine Ligase and Myeloid Cell Leukemia Sequence 1. *J. Biol. Chem.* **2010**, *285*, 8244–8255. [CrossRef]
77. Abalo, R.; Uranga, J.A.; Pérez-García, I.; de Andrés, R.; Girón, R.; Vera, G.; López-Pérez, A.E.; Martín-Fontelles, M.I. May Cannabinoids Prevent the Development of Chemotherapy-Induced Diarrhea and Intestinal Mucositis? Experimental Study in the Rat. *Neurogastroenterol. Motil.* **2017**, *29*, e12952. [CrossRef]
78. Javed, H.; Azimullah, S.; Meeran, M.F.N.; Ansari, S.A.; Ojha, S. Neuroprotective Effects of Thymol, a Dietary Monoterpene Against Dopaminergic Neurodegeneration in Rotenone-Induced Rat Model of Parkinson's Disease. *Int. J. Mol. Sci.* **2019**, *20*, 1538. [CrossRef] [PubMed]
79. Badr, A.M.; Bassiouni, Y.A.; Alqarni, I. Implication of Sphingosine-1-P/Sphingosine Kinase Pathway in Non-Alcoholic Fatty Liver Disease. *Adv. Res. Gastroenterol. Hepatol.* **2019**, *13*, 555855. [CrossRef]
80. Bancroft, J.; Stevens, M.A.; Bancroft, J.D. *Theory and Practice of Histological Techniques*; Elsevier: Amsterdam, The Netherlands, 1996.
81. Ellman, G.L.; Lysko, H. Disulfide and Sulfhydryl Compounds in TCA Extracts of Human Blood and Plasma. *J. Lab. Clin. Med.* **1967**, *70*, 518–527.
82. Ohkawa, H.; Ohishi, N.; Yagi, K. Assay for Lipid Peroxides in Animal Tissues by Thiobarbituric Acid Reaction. *Anal. Biochem.* **1979**, *95*, 351–358. [CrossRef] [PubMed]

83. Nishikimi, M.; Rao, N.A.; Yagi, K. The Occurrence of Superoxide Anion in the Reaction of Reduced Phenazine Methosulfate and Molecular Oxygen. *Biochem. Biophys. Res. Commun.* **1972**, *46*, 849–854. [CrossRef]
84. Badr, A.M.; Al-Kharashi, L.A.; Attia, H.; Alshehri, S.; Alajami, H.N.; Ali, R.A.; Mahran, Y.F. TLR4/Inflammasomes Cross-Talk and Pyroptosis Contribute to N-Acetyl Cysteine and Chlorogenic Acid Protection against Cisplatin-Induced Nephrotoxicity. *Pharmaceuticals* **2023**, *16*, 337. [CrossRef] [PubMed]

pharmaceuticals

MDPI

Article

Evaluation of Crocetin as a Protective Agent in High Altitude Hypoxia-Induced Organ Damage

Jun Yang [1,2,†], Kai Luo [1,2,†], Ziliang Guo [3,†], Renjie Wang [1,2], Qingyuan Qian [2,3], Shuhe Ma [1,2], Maoxing Li [1,2,3,4,*] and Yue Gao [2,4,*]

[1] College of Pharmacy, Gansu University of Chinese Medicine, Lanzhou 730000, China; yangjunzy@163.com (J.Y.); 18294623280@163.com (K.L.); wangrenjiegy@163.com (R.W.); mclsxka@163.com (S.M.)

[2] Department of Pharmaceutical Sciences, Beijing Institute of Radiation Medicine, Beijing 100850, China; q15888906749@163.com

[3] College of Pharmacy, Lanzhou University, Lanzhou 730000, China; guozl20@lzu.edu.cn

[4] National Key Laboratory of Kidney Diseases, Beijing 100850, China

[*] Correspondence: limaox2020@aliyun.com (M.L.); gaoyue@bmi.ac.cn (Y.G.); Tel.: +86-010-6693-1225 (M.L. & Y.G.)

[†] These authors contributed equally to this work.

Abstract: Crocetin is an aglycone of crocin naturally occurring in saffron and has been proved to have antioxidant, anti-inflammatory, and antibacterial activities. In this experiment, the protective effect of crocetin on vital organs in high-altitude hypoxia rats was studied. Crocetin was prepared from gardenia by the alkaline hydrolysis method, and its reducing ability and free radical scavenging ability were tested. The in vitro anti-hypoxia vitality was studied on PC_{12} cells. The anti-hypoxic survival time of mice was determined in several models. The acute hypoxic injury rat model was established by simulating the hypoxic environment of 8000 m-high altitude for 24 h, and the anti-hypoxia effect of crocetin was evaluated by intraperitoneal injection with the doses of 10, 20, and 40 mg/kg. The water contents of the brain and lung were determined, and the pathological sections in the brain, lung, heart, liver, and kidney were observed by HE staining. The levels of oxidative stress (SOD, CAT, H_2O_2, GSH, GSH-Px, MDA) and inflammatory factors (IL-1β, IL-6, TNF-α, VEGF) in rat brain, lung, heart, liver, and kidney tissues were detected by ELISA. The results indicated that crocetin exhibited strong reducing ability and free radical scavenging ability and could improve the activity of PC_{12} cells under hypoxia. After intraperitoneal injection with crocetin, the survival time of mice was prolonged, and the pathological damage, oxidative stress, and inflammation in rats' tissue were ameliorated. The protective activity of crocetin on vital organs in high-altitude hypoxia rats may be related to reducing oxidative stress and inhibiting inflammatory response.

Keywords: crocetin; anti-hypoxia; antioxidant; anti-inflammatory

1. Introduction

High-altitude regions attract millions of people each year for recreational reasons, such as sightseeing, trekking, climbing, and skiing, or even to escape heat waves. In 2014 alone, >15 million tourists travelled to Lhasa, Tibet, which is at 3658 m above sea level. In addition, many thousands of workers, soldiers, and pilgrims are temporarily exposed to high altitudes, and >80 million people live permanently in places above 2500 m [1]. The air pressure decreases exponentially with the increase of altitude. The exposure to the plateau environment will lead to hypoxia in tissues, organs, and bodies, which will lead to energy metabolism disorders, mitochondrial damage, cell apoptosis, oxidative stress, and inflammation outbreak. The main physiological responses of the body's acute hypoxia exposure include hyperventilation [2] triggered by the hypoxic ventilatory response, which causes sympathetic activation with an increase in heart rate and cardiac output [3], pulmonary vasoconstriction, and elevated pulmonary artery pressure [4]. Overloaded and long-term physiological responses may contribute to the occurrence of high-altitude diseases, including acute mountain sickness (AMS), high-altitude hypertension (HAH), high-altitude heart disease (HAHD), high-altitude cerebral edema (HACE), and high-altitude pulmonary edema (HAPE) [5].

Plenty of studies have proved that acute or chronic high-altitude hypoxia may induce the decrease of the activity of antioxidant capacity biomarkers, such as superoxide dismutase (SOD), catalase (CAT), glutathione peroxidase/reductase (GSH-Px), peroxiredoxin/thioredoxin (PRX/Trx), and metalloproteases (MMPs), and then lead to the increase of oxidative stress biomarkers, such as malondialdehyde (MDA) and reactive oxygen species (ROS) [6–9]. Oxidative stress and inflammation are mutual influences. Hypoxia causes oxidative stress, which in turn leads to the production of many inflammatory cytokines such as cytokine interleukin-6 (IL-6), cytokine interleukin-1β (IL-1β), tumor necrosis factor-α (TNF-α), vascular endothelial cell growth factor (VEGF), hypoxia inducible factor-1 α (HIF-1α), etc. [10,11]. It should be emphasized that systemic oxidative stress and inflammatory outbreaks caused by high-altitude hypoxia are important factors leading to damage of important tissues and organs, which manifests as various diseases related to high-altitude exposure.

Saffron (*Crocus sativus* L.) is a valuable traditional medicine of Persia and China, which has been used for thousands of years. Crocin and its aglycone crocetin are characteristic pigment components in saffron, which have been proved with cardioprotective, hepatoprotective, neuroprotective, antinociceptive, antidepressant, antiviral, anticancer, atherosclerotic, antidiabetic, and memory enhancing properties [12].

Miraculously, the fruit of traditional Chinese medicine *Gardenia jasminoides* J. Ellis also contains a large amount of crocin [12]. In the past decade, our group established enrichment and purification technology for the first time to obtain gardenia yellow pigment with high content of crocin. In vitro and in vivo experiments proved this gardenia yellow pigment had strong radical scavenging ability, antioxidant activity, and anti-hypoxia and anti-fatigue effects with mechanisms to reduce the accumulation of bad metabolites, increase energy reserves, improve free radical scavenging capacity, increase related metabolic enzyme activities, inhibit the infiltration of inflammatory cells, and reduce apoptosis under simulated high-altitude hypoxic environments [13]. Preliminary studies of our group have found that after 400 mg/kg administration of crocin-I to normoxic and hypoxic rats, not only crocin-I, but also crocetin can be detected with considerable content in the liver, lung, spleen, testis, kidney, heart, and brain tissue. Crocin-I may be absorbed and hydrolyzed by intestinal flora and liver into crocetin [14].

Based on our group's study of crocin-I's metabolism in rats under normoxic and hypoxic conditions, we propose that crocetin may be the ultimate anti-hypoxia material basis of crocin-I, gardenia yellow pigment, and saffron. This paper investigates the anti-hypoxia effects of crocetin through various in vivo and in vitro experiments and examines its protective effects on vital organs in rats subjected to simulated high-altitude hypoxia, thereby providing a theoretical foundation for the use of crocetin in combating high-altitude hypoxia.

2. Results

2.1. Reducing Ability and Radical Scavenging Ability

As shown in Figure 1A, the inhibitory effect of crocetin on $\bullet O_2^-$ increased, and the effect of the system was much higher than that of ascorbic acid. Before 180 μg/mL, the luminescence inhibitory effect of crocetin on the system was much greater than the ascorbic acid.

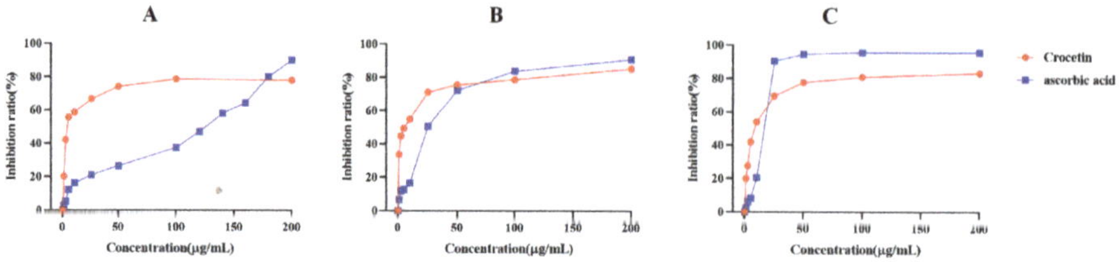

Figure 1. Reducing ability and radical scavenging ability of crocetin. (**A**) Inhibition of $\bullet O_2^-$, (**B**) inhibition of H_2O_2, (**C**) inhibition of $\bullet OH^-$.

As shown in Figure 1B, the inhibition rate of crocetin increased rapidly with increasing concentration. In the range of 1.00 to 50.00 μg/mL, the inhibition rate of crocetin on H_2O_2 was greater than ascorbic acid, and the inhibition rate of ascorbic acid over 50.00 μg/mL was greater than that of crocetin after 50.00 μg/mL.

The experiments found that the IC_{50} of crocetin on $\bullet O_2^-$, H_2O_2, and $\bullet OH^-$ were 6.39, 4.67, and 8.63 μg/mL, respectively (Table 1). The results showed that crocetin had strong antioxidant activities, and compared with the control group ascorbic acid, there was a very significant difference ($p < 0.001$).

Table 1. Half concentration of crocetin for each radical group IC50 ($n = 3$).

Group	IC_{50} (μg/mL)		
	$\bullet O_2^-$	H_2O_2	$\bullet OH^-$
ascorbic acid	89.29 ± 1.26	23.71 ± 0.10	14.82 ± 0.05
Crocetin	6.39 ± 0.15 *	4.67 ± 0.12 *	8.63 ± 0.05

Note: Compared with the ascorbate control group, * $p < 0.001$.

2.2. *Effect of Crocetin on PC_{12} Cell Viability*

As shown in Figure 2, compared with the normoxic control group, the viability of PC_{12} cells decreased significantly in the hypoxia model group ($p < 0.01$). After administration with crocetin, both the CRT-M group and the CRT-H group could significantly increase PC_{12} cell viability ($p < 0.01$). The results showed that crocetin could improve the viability of PC_{12} cells under hypoxia.

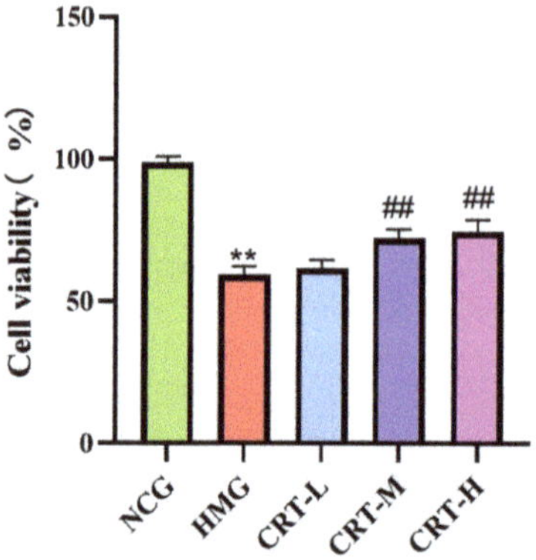

Figure 2. Effect of crocetin on hypoxic injury activity of PC_{12} cell. Data are expressed as mean ± SD (n = 3/group). Note: Compared to the NC, ** $p < 0.01$; compared with HM, ## $p < 0.01$. NCG: normoxic control group; HMG: hypoxia model group; CRT-L: crocetin low-dose group (25 μmol/L); CRT-M: crocetin medium-dose group (50 μmol/L); CRT-H: crocetin high-dose group (100 μmol/L).

2.3. *Effect of Crocetin on Hypoxic Mice*

As shown in Figure 3A, the result of normobaric hypoxia test indicate that low, medium, and high CRT doses can effectively prolong the survival time of mice in a dose-dependent manner; prolonged rates were 5.56%, 13.57% ($p < 0.05$), and 22.90% ($p < 0.01$), respectively.

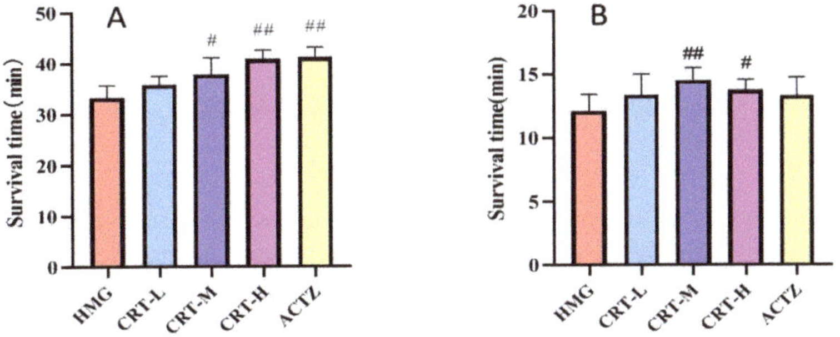

Figure 3. Effect on the survival time of hypoxia mice by intraperitoneal injection crocetin. Data are expressed as mean ± SD (n = 10/group). Note: compared with HM, # $p < 0.05$, ## $p < 0.01$. HMG: hypoxia model group; CRT-L: crocetin low-dose group; CRT-M: crocetin medium-dose group; CRT-H: crocetin high-dose group; ACTZ: positive control group. (**A**) The close normobaric hypoxia experiment. (**B**) The sodium nitrite hypoxia experiment.

The results of the sodium nitrite hypoxia experiment are shown in Figure 3B. Compared with the HM group, the prolongation rates of CRT-L, CRT-M, and CRT-H groups are 10.30%, 19.88% ($p < 0.01$), and 13.52%, respectively. The prolongation rate of the ACTZ group is 9.58%. Among them, the CRT-M group and CRT-H group ($p < 0.05$) can significantly prolong the time to live of hypoxic mice, indicating that crocetin can significantly improve the hypoxia tolerance of mice and has certain anti-hypoxia activity.

2.4. *Protective Effect of Crocetin on High Altitude Hypoxia Rats*

2.4.1. Observation on Survival State of Hypoxia Rats

During the whole process of hypoxia injury, the respiration amplitude of rats decreased, and the respiration frequency increased significantly. Rats in the HMG manifested significant changes, including less food and water intake, hair disorder, slow movement, and the death of two rats.

Except for one rat that died in the CRT-L group, the rats in other crocetin administration groups and ACTZ had relatively less food and water intake, better activity state, slightly disordered hair, and rapid breathing. The rats in the NCG had normal feeding, water intake, and other activities.

2.4.2. Effect of Crocetin on Brain and Lung Water Content in Hypoxic Rats

The results of crocetin anti-hypoxia activity are shown in Figure 4; compared with NCG, the brain water content of rats with HMG increased by 3.32%, and the lung water content increased by 5.23%, but the difference was not significant ($p > 0.05$). Compared with HMG, the brain and lung water contents in crocetin treatment groups and the acetazolamide group had a certain downward trend; the brain water content decreased by 1.32%, 2.74%, 2.78%, and 3.13% in the CRT-L, CRT-M, CRT-H, and ACTZ groups, respectively. The lung water content decreased by 2.26%, 2.32%, 3.22%, and 3.85% in the CRT-L, CRT-M, CRT-H, and ACTZ group groups, respectively, but there was no significant difference between the above groups ($p > 0.05$).

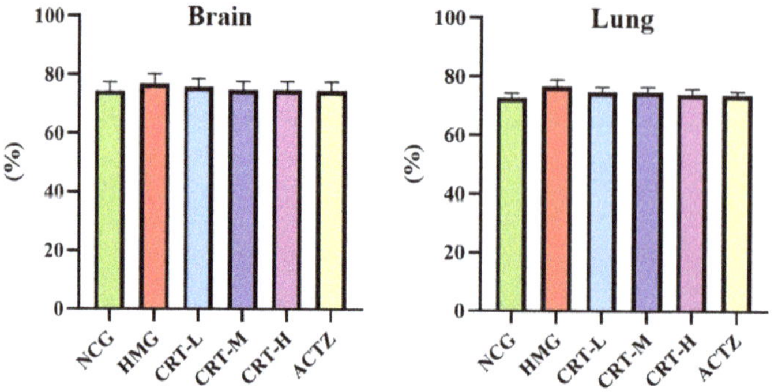

Figure 4. The effect of crocetin on brain and lung water content in high-altitude hypoxia rats. Data are expressed as mean ± SD (n = 10/group). Note: NCG: normal oxygen control group; HMG: hypoxia model group; CRT-L: crocetin low-dose group; CRT-M: crocetin medium-dose group; CRT-H: crocetin high-dose group; ACTZ: positive control group.

2.4.3. Effect of Crocetin on Pathological Structure of Tissues in Hypoxic Rats

The histopathological effects of crocetin on simulated high-altitude hypoxia rats are shown in Figure 5, compared with NCG, the arrangement of hippocampus cells was disordered, the number of hippocampus cells decreased, the gap of nuclear-cytoplasmic increased, and the nucleus showed pyknosis into an irregular shape in HMG. After CRT and ACTZ drug intervention, the pathological structure of brain tissue was improved to a certain extent; the cell structure tended to be normal, the number of neurons increased, and the nuclear staining decreased.

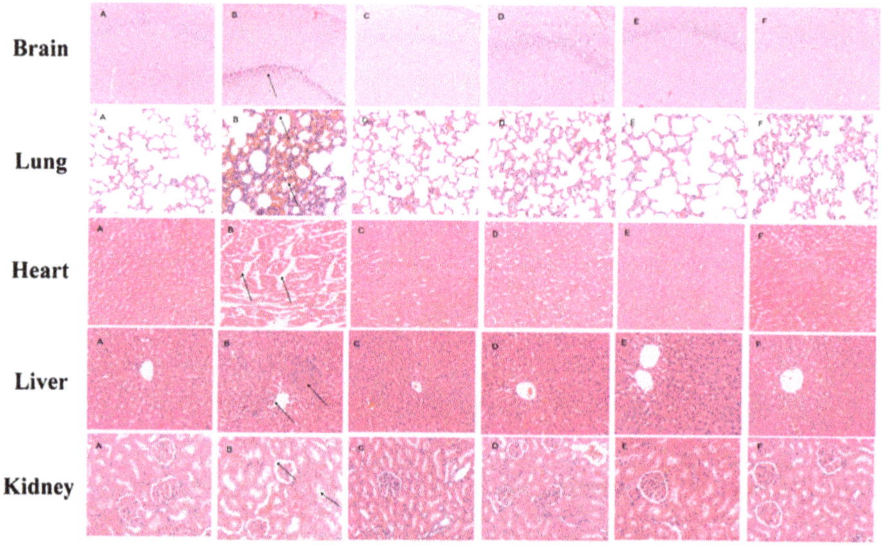

Figure 5. Histopathological changes of vital organs in high-altitude hypoxia rats (×400). (**A**) Normoxic control group (NCG), (**B**) hypoxia model group (HMG), (**C**) crocetin low-dose group (CRT-L, 10 mg/kg), (**D**) crocetin medium-dose group (CRT-M, 20 mg/kg), (**E**) crocetin high-dose group (CRT-H, 40 mg/kg), (**F**) acetazolamide group (ACTZ, 70 mg/kg).

The structure of lung tissue was regular, the alveolar cavity was clear, and there was no obvious edema, inflammation, or other pathological damage in NCG. Compared with NCG, the lung tissue of HMG rats was significantly damaged, the structural integrity was destroyed, the alveolar wall was obviously thickened, and the pulmonary interstitium was seriously congested. Correspondingly, the pathological structure of lung tissue was improved, the alveolar wall was slightly thickened, the alveolar cavity was dilated and tended to be normal, and the inflammatory reaction was reduced in the drug intervention group.

The myocardial cells of NCG group rats have clear boundaries, visible myofibrils and striations, and clear nuclei. Compared with NCG, the heart tissue of HMG rats was accompanied by a small amount of inflammatory cell infiltration. Correspondingly, the pathological structure of the heart tissue in the drug intervention group was alleviated, and myocardial cells tended to be normal without significant inflammatory cell infiltration.

The hepatocytes of NCG were arranged in a radial and compact manner with the central vein as the center, the morphology and structure of cells were clear and complete without pathological damage. The hepatocytes of HMG were swollen and loosely arranged, the structure of hepatic lobules was abnormal, central veins were disordered, inflammatory cells infiltrated in the portal area, and fibrous tissue proliferated. After drug intervention, the pathological structure of rat liver tissue was improved. The hepatocytes were arranged in an orderly fashion and tended to be normal, accompanied by mild granular degeneration.

The kidney tissue cells in NCG were clear, the structure was neat, and the shape of glomerulus was regular. Meanwhile, there was obvious glomerular basement membrane hyperplasia and interstitial swelling in HMG. Compared with HMG, the structure of the administration group was orderly arranged, the cell swelling was reduced, and the proliferation of the glomerular basement membrane was alleviated.

2.4.4. Inhibition of Crocetin on Tissues Peroxidation Damage in Hypoxic Rats

Effect of Crocetin on Oxidative Stress Markers in Brain Tissue of Hypoxic Rats

As shown in Figure 6, compared with NCG, the content of MDA and H_2O_2 in the brains of HMG rats was significantly increased, reaching 41.10% and 40.45% ($p < 0.01$), respectively. The content of GSH ($p < 0.01$) and the activity of GSH-Px ($p < 0.01$), SOD ($p < 0.01$), CAT ($p < 0.05$) in the brain of HMG rats was significantly decreased by 24.27%, 13.42%, 20.55%, and 27.61%, respectively.

After giving crocetin intervention, compared with HMG, the content of MDA in CRT-M, CRT-H, and ACTZ groups decreased by 13.10%, 18.82%, and 21.42%, respectively. There were significant differences ($p < 0.05$). The content of H_2O_2 in CRT-M, CRT-H, and ACTZ groups decreased by 14.56%, 19.69%, 18.40%, respectively. There were significant differences ($p < 0.05$). The content of GSH in CRT-M, CRT-H, and ACTZ groups increased by 16.02%, 28.83%, and 15.43%, respectively. There were significant differences ($p < 0.05$ or $p < 0.01$). The activity of GSH-Px in CRT-H and ACTZ groups increased by 14.63% and 14.01%, respectively. There were significant differences ($p < 0.05$). The activity of SOD in CRT-L, CRT-M, CRT-H, and ACTZ groups increased by 1.09%, 7.58%, 14.49%, and 17.47%, respectively. However, there was no significant difference ($p > 0.05$). The activity of CAT in CRT-M, CRT-H, and ACTZ groups increased by 39.19%, 46.47%, and 44.62%, respectively. There were significant differences ($p < 0.05$ or $p < 0.01$).

Effect of Crocetin on Oxidative Stress Markers in Lung Tissue of Hypoxic Rats

As shown in Figure 7, compared with NCG, the content of MDA and H_2O_2 in the lungs of HMG rats was significantly increased, reaching 40.73% and 49.39% ($p < 0.01$), respectively. The content of GSH ($p < 0.05$) and the activity of GSH-Px ($p < 0.01$), SOD ($p < 0.01$), and CAT ($p > 0.05$) in the brain of HMG rats was significantly decreased by 28.64%, 20.82%, 39.65%, and 7.53%, respectively.

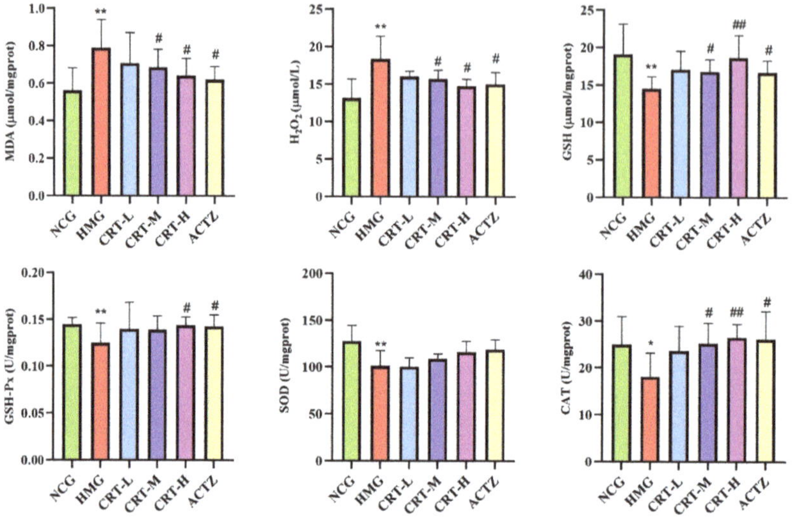

Figure 6. Crocetin regulated the oxidative stress index in hypoxic-injured brain tissue. Data are expressed as mean ± SD (n = 8/group). Note: * $p < 0.05$ NCG vs. HMG; ** $p < 0.01$ NCG vs. HMG; ## $p < 0.01$, # $p < 0.05$, HMG vs. medication groups. NCG: normal oxygen control group; HMG: hypoxia model group; CRT-L: crocetin low-dose group; CRT-M: crocetin medium-dose group; CRT-H: crocetin high-dose group; ACTZ: positive control group.

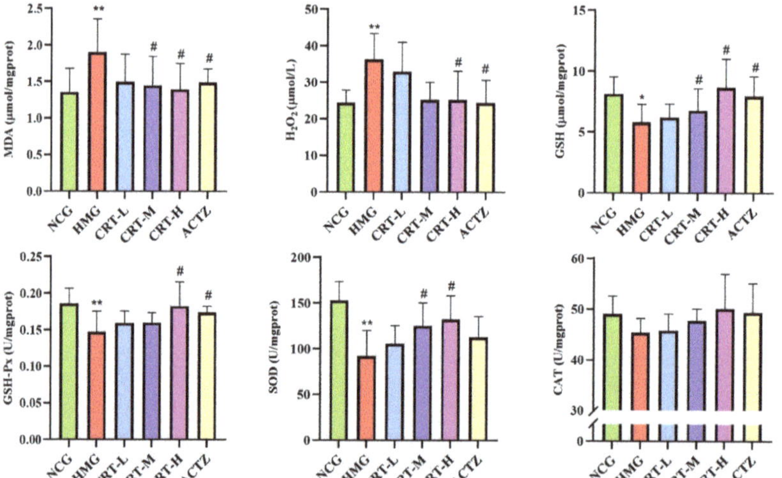

Figure 7. Crocetin regulated the oxidative stress index in hypoxic-injured lung tissue. Data are expressed as mean ± SD (n = 8/group). Note: * $p < 0.05$ NCG vs. HMG; ** $p < 0.01$ NCG vs. HMG; # $p < 0.05$, HMG vs. medication groups. NCG: normal oxygen control group; HMG: hypoxia model group; CRT-L: crocetin low-dose group; CRT-M: crocetin medium-dose group; CRT-H: crocetin high-dose group; ACTZ: positive control group.

After giving crocetin intervention, compared with HMG, the content of MDA in CRT-M, CRT-H, and ACTZ groups decreased by 24.16%, 26.79%, and 21.96%, respectively. There were significant differences ($p < 0.05$). The content of H_2O_2 in CRT-H and ACTZ groups decreased by 30.71% and 32.82%, respectively. There were significant differences ($p < 0.05$). The content of GSH in CRT-M, CRT-H, and ACTZ groups increased by 16.69%, 49.33%, and 37.39%, respectively. There were significant differences ($p < 0.05$). The activity of GSH-Px in CRT-H and ACTZ groups increased by 24.00% and 16.98%, respectively, and there were significant differences ($p < 0.05$).The activity of SOD in CRT-M and CRT-H groups increased by 35.69% and 43.54%, respectively. There were significant differences ($p < 0.05$). The activity of CAT in rat lung tissue increased; however, none of them were significant ($p > 0.05$).

Effect of Crocetin on Oxidative Stress Markers in Heart Tissue of Hypoxic Rats

As shown in Figure 8, compared with NCG, the content of MDA and H_2O_2 in the hearts of HMG rats was significantly increased, reaching 35.63% and 14.35% ($p < 0.01$ or $p < 0.05$), respectively. The content of GSH ($p < 0.01$) and the activity of GSH-Px ($p < 0.01$), SOD ($p < 0.05$), and CAT ($p < 0.05$) in the brain of HMG rats was significantly decreased by 39.21%, 15.74%, 18.26%, and 22.91%, respectively.

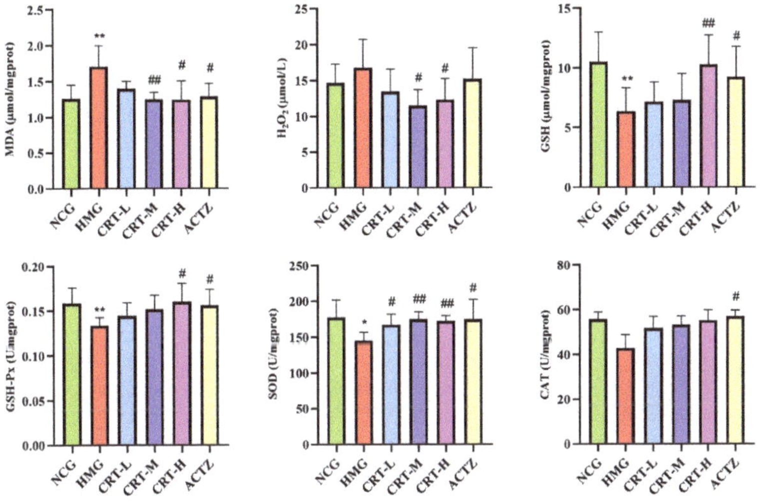

Figure 8. Crocetin regulated the oxidative stress index in hypoxic-injured heart tissue. Data are expressed as mean ± SD ($n = 8$/group). Note: * $p < 0.05$ NCG vs. HMG; ** $p < 0.01$ NCG vs. HMG; ## $p < 0.01$, # $p < 0.05$, HMG vs. medication groups. NCG: normal oxygen control group; HMG: hypoxia model group; CRT-L: crocetin low-dose group; CRT-M: crocetin medium-dose group; CRT-H: crocetin high-dose group; ACTZ: positive control group.

After giving crocetin intervention, compared with HMG, the content of MDA in CRT-M, CRT-H, and ACTZ groups decreased by 26.86%, 27.13%, and 24.75%, respectively. There were significant differences ($p < 0.05$ or $p < 0.01$). The content of H_2O_2 in CRT-M and CRT-H groups decreased by 31.57% and 26.68%, respectively. There were significant differences ($p < 0.05$). The content of GSH in CRT-H and ACTZ groups increased by 60.68% and 44.62%, respectively. There were significant differences ($p < 0.05$ or $p < 0.01$). The activity of GSH-Px in CRT-H and ACTZ groups increased by 19.58% and 16.60%, respectively. There were significant differences ($p < 0.05$). The activity of SOD in CRT-L, CRT-M, CRT-H, and ACTZ groups increased by 15.43%, 20.85%, 18.86%, and 20.78, respectively. There were significant differences ($p < 0.05$ or $p < 0.01$). The activity of CAT in ACTZ groups increased by 32.75%, respectively. There were significant differences ($p < 0.05$).

Effect of Crocetin on Oxidative Stress Markers in Liver Tissue of Hypoxic Rats

As shown in Figure 9, compared with NCG, the content of MDA and H_2O_2 in the livers of HMG rats was significantly increased, reaching 150.52% and 33.29% ($p < 0.01$ or $p < 0.05$), respectively. The content of GSH and the activity of GSH-Px, SOD, and CAT in the brains of HMG rats was significantly decreased by 28.01%, 16.78%, 22.74%, and 17.61% ($p < 0.05$), respectively.

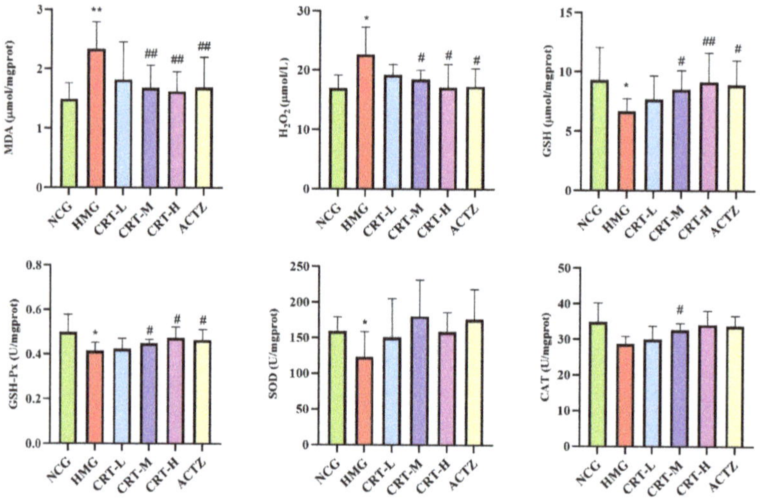

Figure 9. Crocetin regulated the oxidative stress index in hypoxic-injured liver tissue. Data are expressed as mean ± SD ($n = 8$/group). Note: * $p < 0.05$ NCG vs. HMG; ** $p < 0.01$ NCG vs. HMG; ## $p < 0.01$, # $p < 0.05$, HMG vs. medication groups. NCG: normal oxygen control group; HMG: hypoxia model group; CRT-L: crocetin low-dose group; CRT-M: crocetin medium-dose group; CRT-H: crocetin high-dose group; ACTZ: positive control group.

After giving crocetin intervention, compared with HMG, the content of MDA in CRT-M, CRT-H, and ACTZ groups decreased by 37.75%, 50.46%, and 48.92%, respectively. There were significant differences ($p < 0.01$). The content of H_2O_2 in CRT-M, CRT-H, and ACTZ groups decreased by 18.61%, 24.33%, and 23.44%, respectively. There were significant differences ($p < 0.05$). The content of GSH in CRT-M, CRT-H, and ACTZ groups increased by 27.10%, 36.69%, and 33.32%, respectively. There were significant differences ($p < 0.05$). The activity of GSH-Px in CRT-M, CRT-H, and ACTZ groups increased by 8.03%, 14.08%, and 11.88%, respectively. There were significant differences ($p < 0.05$). The activity of SOD in CRT-L, CRT-M, CRT-H, and ACTZ groups increased by 22.28%, 46.48%, 28.63%, and 43.21%, respectively. However, there was no significant difference ($p > 0.05$). The activity of CAT in CRT-M groups increased by 13.66% ($p < 0.05$).

Effect of Crocetin on Oxidative Stress Markers in Kidney Tissue of Hypoxic Rats

As shown in Figure 10, compared with NCG, the content of MDA and H_2O_2 in the kidneys of HMG rats was significantly increased, reaching 56.64% and 49.38% ($p < 0.01$), respectively. The content of GSH ($p < 0.01$) and the activity of GSH-Px ($p < 0.01$), SOD ($p < 0.05$), and CAT ($p > 0.05$) in the brains of HMG rats was significantly decreased by 30.96%, 16.02%, 9.17%, and 13.58% ($p < 0.05$), respectively.

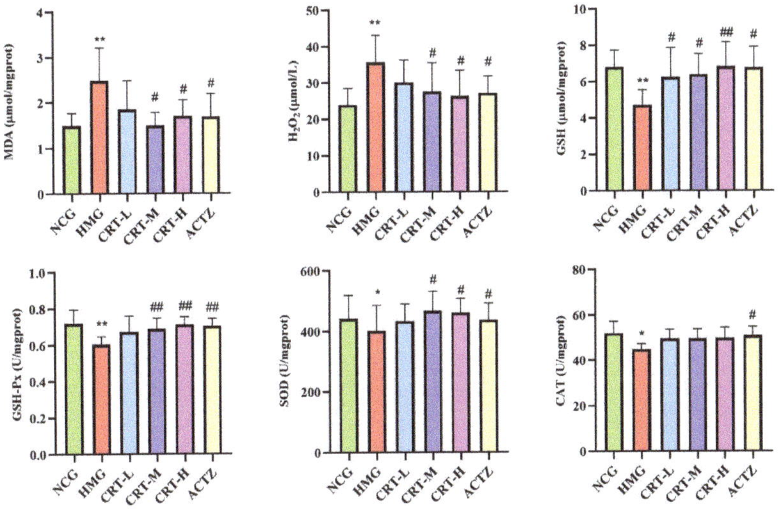

Figure 10. Crocetin regulated the oxidative stress index in hypoxic-injured kidney tissue. Data are expressed as mean ± SD (n = 8/group). Note: * $p < 0.05$ NCG vs. HMG; ** $p < 0.01$ NCG vs. HMG; ## $p < 0.01$, # $p < 0.05$, HMG vs. medication groups. NCG: Normal oxygen control group; HMG: hypoxia model group; CRT-L: crocetin low-dose group; CRT-M: crocetin medium-dose group; CRT-H: crocetin high-dose group; ACTZ: positive control group.

After giving crocetin intervention, compared with HMG, the content of MDA in CRT-M, CRT-H, and ACTZ groups decreased by 28.01%, 30.41%, and 27.51%, respectively. There were significant differences ($p < 0.01$). The content of H_2O_2 in CRT-M, CRT-H, and ACTZ groups decreased by 23.23%, 26.87%, and 24.37%, respectively. There were significant differences ($p < 0.05$). The content of GSH in CRT-M, CRT-H, and ACTZ groups increased by 35.97%, 45.01%, and 44.16%, respectively. There were significant differences ($p < 0.05$ or $p < 0.01$). The activity of GSH-Px in CRT-M, CRT-H, and ACTZ groups increased by 13.79%, 17.86%, and 16.46%, respectively. There were significant differences ($p < 0.01$). The activity of SOD in CRT-L, CRT-M, CRT-M, CRT-H, and ACTZ groups increased by 8.15%, 16.32%, 14.89%, and 8.95, respectively. However, there was no significant difference ($p > 0.05$). The activity of CAT in CRT-M groups increased by 10.52% ($p < 0.05$).

2.4.5. Anti-Inflammatory Effect of Crocetin on Tissue of Hypoxic Rats

Effect of Crocetin on Inflammatory Factors in Brain Tissue of Hypoxic Rats

As shown in Figure 11, compared with NCG, the content of IL-1β ($p < 0.01$), IL-6 ($p < 0.05$), TNF-α ($p < 0.05$), and VEGF ($p < 0.01$) in the brains of HMG rats was significantly increased by 56.96%%, 37.44%, 38.64%, and 46.12%, respectively.

After drug intervention, compared with HMG, the content of IL-1β in CRT-M, CRT-H, and ACTZ groups decreased by 30.27%, 32.22%, and 29.67%, respectively. There were significant differences ($p < 0.05$ or $p < 0.01$). The content of IL-6 in CRT-M, CRT-H, and ACTZ groups decreased by 25.27%, 27.44%, and 31.17%, respectively. There were significant differences ($p < 0.05$). The content of TNF-α in CRT-H and ACTZ groups decreased by 23.23% and 27.69%, respectively. There were significant differences ($p < 0.05$). The content of VEGF in CRT-L, CRT-H, and ACTZ groups decreased by 24.01%, 27.19%, and 23.28%, respectively. There were significant differences ($p < 0.05$).

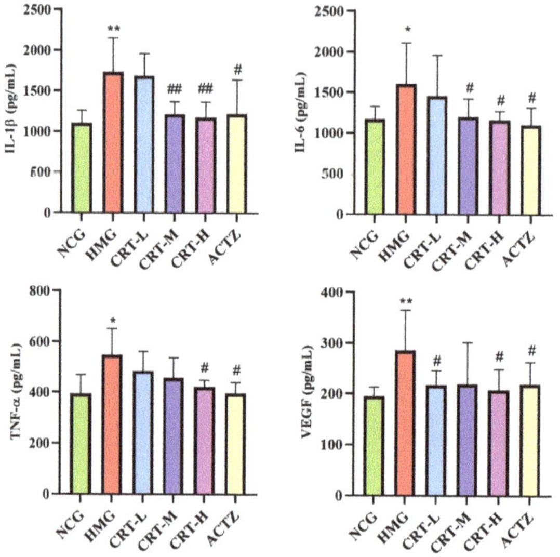

Figure 11. Crocetin reduces inflammatory factor in acute hypoxic injury in rats' brain tissues. Data are expressed as mean ± SD (n = 8/group) Note: ** $p < 0.01$, * $p < 0.05$, NCG vs. HMG; ## $p < 0.01$, # $p < 0.05$, HMG vs. medication groups; NCG: normal oxygen control group; HMG: hypoxia model group; CRT-L: crocetin low-dose group; CRT-M: crocetin medium-dose group; CRT-H: crocetin high-dose group; ACTZ: positive control group.

Effect of Crocetin on Inflammatory Factors in Lung Tissue of Hypoxic Rats

As shown in Figure 12, compared with NCG, the content of IL-1β ($p < 0.01$), IL-6 ($p < 0.01$), TNF-α ($p < 0.01$), and VEGF ($p < 0.05$) in the lung of HMG rats was significantly increased by 56.96%, 79.98%, 51.71%, and 38.84%, respectively.

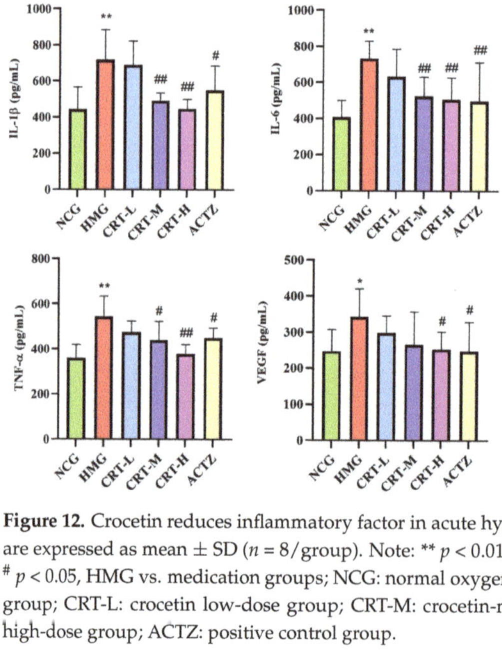

Figure 12. Crocetin reduces inflammatory factor in acute hypoxic injury in rats' lung tissues. Data are expressed as mean ± SD (n = 8/group). Note: ** $p < 0.01$, * $p < 0.05$, NCG vs. HMG; ## $p < 0.01$, # $p < 0.05$, HMG vs. medication groups; NCG: normal oxygen control group; HMG: hypoxia model group; CRT-L: crocetin low-dose group; CRT-M: crocetin-medium dose group; CRT-H: crocetin high-dose group; ACTZ: positive control group.

After drug intervention, compared with HMG, the content of IL-1β in CRT-M, CRT-H, and ACTZ groups decreased by 30.27%, 32.22%, and 29.67%, respectively. There were significant differences ($p < 0.05$ or $p < 0.01$). The content of IL-6 in CRT-M, CRT-H, and ACTZ groups decreased by 28.57%, 31.15%, and 32.02%, respectively. There were significant differences ($p < 0.01$). The content of TNF-α in CRT-M, CRT-H, and ACTZ groups decreased by 19.13%, 30.65%, and 17.42%, respectively. There were significant differences ($p < 0.05$ or $p < 0.01$). The content of VEGF in CRT-H and ACTZ groups decreased by 26.40% and 27.69%, respectively. There were significant differences ($p < 0.05$).

Effect of Crocetin on Inflammatory Factors in Heart Tissue of Hypoxic Rats

As shown in Figure 13, Compared with NCG, the content of IL-1β ($p < 0.01$), IL-6 ($p < 0.01$), TNF-α ($p < 0.01$), and VEGF ($p < 0.01$) in the hearts of HMG rats was significantly increased by 27.46%, 45.83%, 15.93%, and 6.19%, respectively.

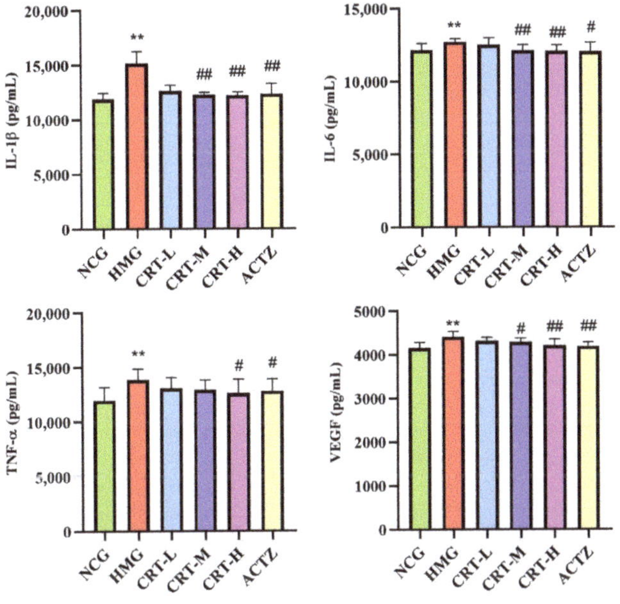

Figure 13. Crocetin reduces inflammatory factor in acute hypoxic injury in rats' heart tissues. Data are expressed as mean ± SD (n = 8/group) Note: ** $p < 0.01$, NCG vs. HMG; ## $p < 0.01$, # $p < 0.05$, HMG vs. medication groups; NCG: normal oxygen control group; HMG: hypoxia model group; CRT-L: crocetin low-dose group; CRT-M: crocetin medium-dose group; CRT-H: crocetin high-dose group; ACTZ: positive control group.

After drug intervention, compared with HMG, the content of IL-1β in CRT-M, CRT-H, and ACTZ groups decreased by 19.21%, 19.58%, and 18.59%, respectively. There were significant differences ($p < 0.01$). The content of IL-6 in CRT-M, CRT-H, and ACTZ groups decreased by 4.68%, 5.04%, and 5.30%, respectively. There were significant differences ($p < 0.05$ or $p < 0.01$). The content of TNF-α in CRT-H and ACTZ groups decreased by 9.16% and 7.79%, respectively. There were significant differences ($p < 0.05$). The content of VEGF in CRT-M, CRT-H, and ACTZ groups decreased by 2.75%, 4.66%, and 5.04%, respectively. There were significant differences ($p < 0.05$ or $p < 0.01$).

Effect of Crocetin on Inflammatory Factors in Liver Tissue of Hypoxic Rats

As shown in Figure 14, compared with NCG, the content of IL-1β ($p < 0.01$), IL-6 ($p < 0.01$), TNF-α ($p < 0.01$), and VEGF ($p < 0.05$) in the liver of HMG rats was significantly increased by 37.85%, 11.19%, 35.72%, and 10.43%.

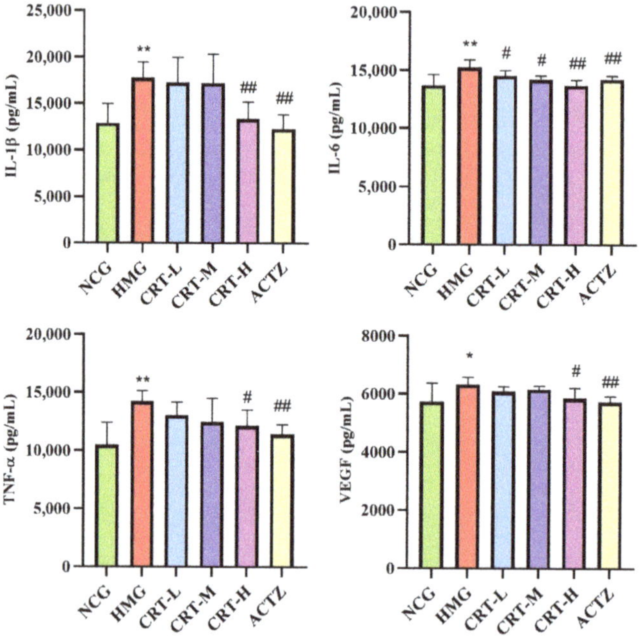

Figure 14. Crocetin reduces inflammatory factor in acute hypoxic injury in rats' liver tissues. Data are expressed as mean ± SD ($n = 8$/group). Note: ** $p < 0.01$, * $p < 0.05$, NCG vs. HMG; ## $p < 0.01$, # $p < 0.05$, HMG vs. medication groups; NCG: normal oxygen control group; HMG: hypoxia model group; CRT-L: crocetin low-dose group; CRT-M: crocetin medium-dose group; CRT-H: crocetin high-dose group; ACTZ: positive control group.

After drug intervention, compared with HMG, the content of IL-1β in CRT-H and ACTZ groups decreased by 24.79% and 30.79%, respectively, and there were significant differences ($p < 0.01$). The content of IL-6 in CRT-L, CRT-M, CRT-H, and ACTZ groups decreased by4.45, 6.73%, 9.97%, and 6.52%, respectively ($p < 0.05$). The content of TNF-α in CRT-H and ACTZ groups decreased by 14.70% and 19.67%, respectively. There were significant differences ($p < 0.05$ or $p < 0.01$). The content of VEGF in CRT-H and ACTZ groups decreased by 7.51% and 9.28%, respectively. There were significant differences ($p < 0.05$).

Effect of Crocetin on Inflammatory Factors in Kidney Tissue of Hypoxic Rats

As shown in Figure 15, compared with NCG, the content of IL-1β ($p < 0.01$), IL-6 ($p < 0.01$), TNF-α ($p < 0.01$), and VEGF ($p < 0.05$) in the kidney of HMG rats was significantly increased by 66.17%, 9.10%, 35.95%, and 12.83%.

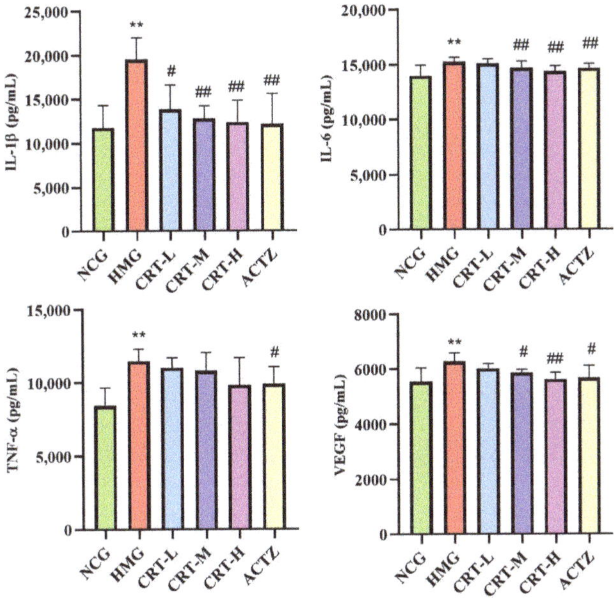

Figure 15. Crocetin reduces inflammatory factor in acute hypoxic injury in rats' kidney tissues. Data are expressed as mean ± SD (n = 8/group). Note: ** $p < 0.01$, NCG vs. HMG; ## $p < 0.01$, # $p < 0.05$, HMG vs. medication groups; NCG: normal oxygen control group; HMG: hypoxia model group; CRT-L: crocetin low-dose group; CRT-M: crocetin medium-dose group; CRT-H: crocetin high-dose group; ACTZ: positive control group.

After drug intervention, compared with HMG, the content of IL-1β in CRT-H, and ACTZ groups decreased by 36.85% and 37.95%, respectively. There were significant differences ($p < 0.01$). The content of IL-6 in CRT-H and ACTZ groups decreased by 6.03% and 3.97%, respectively. There were significant differences ($p < 0.05$). The content of TNF-α in ACTZ groups decreased by 13.68%, ($p < 0.05$). The content of VEGF in CRT-M, CRT-H, and ACTZ groups decreased by 6.57%, 10.33%, and 9.54%, respectively. There were significant differences ($p < 0.05$ or $p < 0.01$).

3. Discussion

Crocetin is the main active ingredient of *Crocus sativus* L. and mainly exists in the stigma of its plants. Crocetin is a polyunsaturated conjugated enoic acid structure with seven conjugated double bonds, which can form glycosidic bonds with gentian disaccharides or glucose to generate different crocin. Its solubility is poor in water and most organic solvents (except pyridine and dimethyl sulfoxide) [15]. According to reports, the fruit of gardenia also contains crocetin [16]. In this study, we prepared crocetin from the fruit of *Gardenia jasminoides* Ellis (content and yield were tested as 96.18% and 1.36%, respectively). In the reducing ability and free radical scavenging ability test, crocetin was found with strong scavenging ability for $\bullet O_2^-$, H_2O_2, and $\bullet OH^-$, and strong antioxidant activity. In vitro anti-hypoxia tests with PC_{12} cell, normobaric hypoxia, and sodium nitrite hypoxia tests with mice proved crocetin had a strong anti-hypoxia effect.

In this experiment, the acute hypoxic injury rat model was established by simulating the plateau environment at an altitude of 8000 m. The water content of the brain and lung, the pathological changes, and the levels of oxidative stress indexes and inflammatory factors in the brain, lung, heart, liver, and kidney were tested to prove the protective effect of crocetin on high-altitude hypoxia rats. The results showed that the oxidative stress indicators and inflammatory factors in important tissues and organs of the HM group rats were significantly increased, indicating that high-altitude hypoxia can lead to systemic oxidative stress and inflammation outbreaks and cause pathological damage to the brain, lungs, liver, and kidney tissues. Due to the different tolerances of different tissues to high altitude hypoxia, the degree of pathological damage in each tissue also varies. Among them, brain and lung damage is more obvious, while heart tissue is less obvious. The intervention of crocetin could ameliorate the pathological damage in brain, lung, liver, and kidney, reduce the water content of the brain and lung, reduce the content of MDA, and H_2O_2, increase the content of GSH, increase the activity of GSH-Px, and reduce IL-6, IL-1β, TNF-α, and VEGF levels in acute hypoxic injury rats. It was suggested that crocetin could relieve oxidative stress and inflammatory response to alleviate hypoxic impairment on vital organs in high-altitude hypoxia rats (Figure 16).

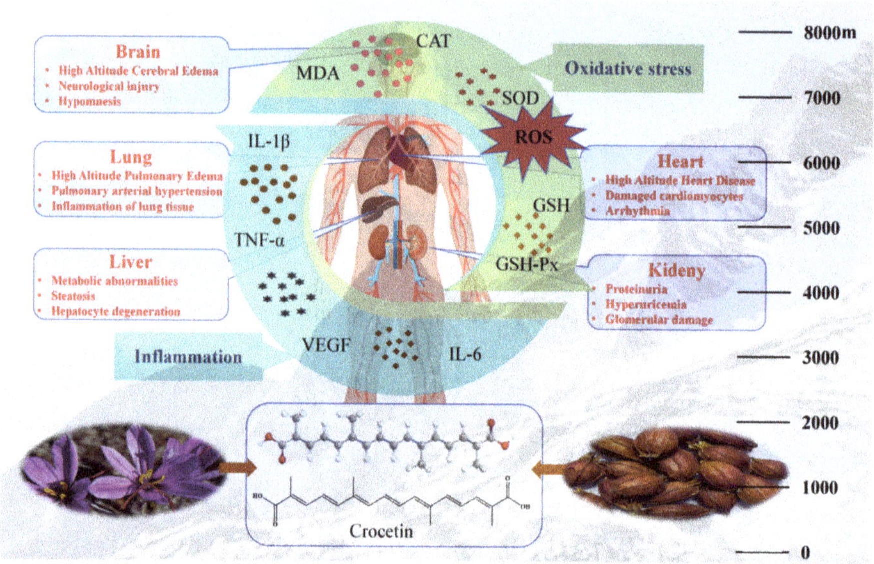

Figure 16. The damage of high-altitude hypoxia to vital organs and the protective effect of crocetin on various tissues. High altitude hypoxia can lead to oxidative stress and inflammation outbreaks, which in turn cause damage to the brain, lungs, heart, liver, and kidney organs, manifested as corresponding high-altitude hypoxic diseases in various tissues. Crocetin exists in the stigma of saffron and the fruit of traditional Chinese medicine *Gardenia jasminoides* and has a good inhibitory effect on oxidative stress and inflammation of various organs and tissues caused by high-altitude hypoxia.

In the past decade, crocetin has been reported with potential antioxidant and anti-inflammatory activity [17,18]. Peng et al. found that crocetin pretreatment can effectively protect the uterus from I/R injury and inhibit oxidative stress. The mechanism may be related to the activation of Nrf2/HO-1 signaling pathway [19]. The effects of crocetin on oxidative stress include reducing MDA and NO levels, increasing GSH content, and increasing the activity of antioxidant enzymes (SOD, CAT, GPx).

More and more studies have proved that oxidative stress and inflammation played essential roles in diseases that are caused by high-altitude hypoxia [12,20,21]. ROS refers to the general term for peroxides that are related to oxygen metabolism in living organisms, including oxygen-containing free radicals and those that are prone to forming free radicals, including peroxides (H_2O_2), superoxides (O_2^-), hydroxyl radicals (OH^-), etc. Oxidative phosphorylation is optimal at physiological oxygen concentrations, and any change in the direction of oxygen availability may lead to an increase in ROS production [3].

Upon reaching high altitude, the hypoxic environment causes an imbalance between oxidation and antioxidation, leading to an overproduction of free radicals and intensifying oxidative stress. As our experimental results reveal, following hypoxia, the levels of antioxidants like SOD, CAT, GSH, and GSH-Px in rats' tissues decreased, whereas the levels of oxidative stress markers MDA and H_2O_2 increased. The current study is in agreement with the research of Xiong Y, et al. [22], who observed that hypoxia causes an increase in serum and liver pro-inflammatory cytokine release, liver ROS production, and MDA content in rats, as well as a decrease in liver SOD, CAT, and GSH-Px activity. The copious free radicals from oxidative stress attack biomolecules such as cell membranes, proteins, and nucleic acids, causing oxidative damage and triggering cell apoptosis and inflammatory responses, which ultimately worsen tissue damage and the incidence of high-altitude illnesses.

Furthermore, hypoxia can also lead to the outbreak of inflammation, and it has been reported that the contents of inflammatory factors TNF-α, IL-6, and IL-1β in the brain tissue of hypoxia rats were significantly increased [23]. A similar study showed that the levels of proinflammatory factors iNOS, IL-6, and IL-1β increased for 30 consecutive days in Wistar rats at an altitude of 3658 m [24].

Abnormal expression of inflammatory factors (TNF-α, IL-1, IL-6) and chemokines (IL-8, CXC-4), induction of cyclooxygenase-2 (COX-2) and inducible nitric oxide synthase (iNOS), and changes in microRNA expression play a key role in oxidative stress-induced inflammation [25]. VEGF is a vascular endothelial growth factor that can promote vascular permeability, vascular endothelial cell migration, proliferation, and angiogenesis. Studies have shown that the VEGF promoter contains HRE, which can bind to the transcription factor-HIF-1α, and hypoxia exposure can promote cell VEGF expression [26,27]. Our experimental results showed that after hypoxia, the levels of TNF-α, IL-1 β, IL-6, and VEGF in various tissues of rats significantly increased, indicating that there were inflammatory reactions in all tissues of rats after hypoxia.

Crocetin, a carotenoid, possesses potent antioxidant properties, confirmed by our free radical scavenging experiments. Following intraperitoneal injections in simulated high-altitude hypoxia rats, crocetin notably reduced oxidative stress and inflammatory factors in the brain, lungs, heart, liver, and kidney tissues, showcasing its effective antioxidant and anti-inflammatory properties. It presents as a promising potential treatment for high-altitude hypoxia. Despite crocetin's excellent anti-hypoxia activity, its specific polyunsaturated conjugated enoic acid structure contributes to its instability, insolubility, and low bioavailability, thereby limiting its application potential. The solubility and oral bioavailability issues have also influenced the administration method of crocetin. In this study, we used intraperitoneal injections. Future research could focus on enhancing the dosage form, such as integrating crocetin with nano-delivery systems, to enhance its solubility, stability, and bioavailability, thus better leveraging its anti-hypoxia properties. Modifying the dosage form can also alter the administration method of crocetin, rendering it safer and more convenient for the prevention and treatment of high-altitude hypoxia injuries.

4. Materials and Methods

4.1. Materials and Reagents

The fruit of *Gardenia jasminoides* Ellis was purchased from the medicinal materials market of An-Guo and was authenticated by professor Jinhui Wang of the Department of Pharmacy, Affiliated Hospital of Gansu University of Chinese Medicine, Lanzhou, China.

Polyamide (30 mesh) was purchased from Huangyan Resin Chemical Co., Ltd. (Taizhou, China). All other chemicals were of analytical grade or purchased from Rionlon Bohua (Tianjin, China) Pharmaceutical & Chemical Co., Ltd. The superoxide dismutase (SOD, No:A001-1-2), glutathione peroxidase (GSH-Px, No:A005-1-2), hydrogen peroxide (H_2O_2, No:E004-1-1), and catalase (CAT, No:A007-1-1) kits were purchased from Biyuntian Biotechnology Co., Ltd. (Shanghai, China).

The malondialdehyde (MDA, No:A003-1-1) and glutathione (GSH, No:A006-1-1) kits were purchased from Jiancheng Bioengineering Research Institute (Nanjing, China). IL-1β (No:SEKR-0002), IL-6 (No:SEKR-0005), VEGF (No:SEKR-0032), and TNF-α (No:SEKR-0009) ELISA kits for rats were purchased from Xinbosheng Biotechnology Co., Ltd. (Shenzheng, China). The TaKaRa MiniBEST Universal RNA Extraction Kit, PrimeScript™ RT Master Mix, TB Green™ Premix EX Taq™ II, and primers were bought from TaKaRa Biotechnology (Dalian, China).

4.2. Equipment

DYC-9070 simulated plateau hypobaric and hypoxic animal experimental cabin (Fenglei Aviation Ordnance Co., Ltd., Anshun, China); 3K15 High-Speed Refrigerated Centrifuge (Sigma, Livonia, MI, USA); SpectraMax® i3 Automatic Fluorescence Microplate Reader (Molecular Devices, San Jose, CA, USA); BP210S Electronic Balance (Sartorius, Göttingen, Germany); DK-8A Electric Constant Temperature Bath (Jinghong Experimental Equipment Co., Ltd., Shanghai, China); E200 Optical Microscope (Nikon, Tokyo, Japan); Electric Homogenizer (Polytron@PT 1200E, Kinematica AG, Malters, Switzerland); Freeze dryer (Telster LyoQuest-55 plus type in Spain).

4.3. Prepared Crocetin from the Fruit of Gardenia Jasminoides Ellis and Its Content Determination

An amount of 500 g of powder of the fruit of *Gardenia jasminoides* Ellis was extracted at 100 °C with 5000 mL water three times. The aqueous extract was cooled, filtered, and flowed through polyamide chromatographic column (500 g, Φ 8 cm × 35 cm), which had been depurated with 95% alcohol and distilled water. The polyamide column was eluted with distilled water until the Molish reaction of elution was negative. Next, 1000 mL of 90% alcohol was used to elute the polyamide column, and the gardenia yellow pigment was obtained after the alcohol elution was vacuum-dried at 60 °C. An amount of 3 mol/L NaOH solution was added into the gardenia yellow pigment with a material-to-liquid ratio of 1:6. This reacted at a constant temperature of 55 °C for 60 min, then was cooled to room temperature and filtered with suction. The filter cake was washed with purified water 2~3 times and then dissolved in an appropriate amount of purified water, then filtered with the microporous membrane; 20% hydrochloric acid was add to the filtrate to adjust the pH to 2–3, and this was filtered to obtain crocetin.

The chromatographic conditions were determined: the chromatographic column was a Waters Symmetry C18 liquid chromatographic column (4.6 mm × 150 mm, 5 μm); the gradient elution was performed with acetonitrile (A)–0.6% formic acid aqueous solution (B) as the mobile phase, and the elution procedure was as follows: 0~12 min, 10%→70% A; 12~16 min, 70%→85% A; 16~25 min, 85% A; 25–26 min, 85%→100% A; 26–29 min, 100% A; 29–32 min, 100%→10% A; 32–35 min, 10% A. The flow rate was 1.0 mL/min; the detection wavelength was 423 nm; the column temperature was 37.0 °C; the injection volume was 20 μL; and the analysis time was 35 min.

According to the high-performance liquid chromatography (Figures 17 and 18), it can be seen that the prepared crocetin sample and crocetin standard have the same retention time under the same chromatographic conditions. And the manual integration result shows that the relative peak area of the sample is 96.18%, indicating that the purity of the sample is greater than 95%.

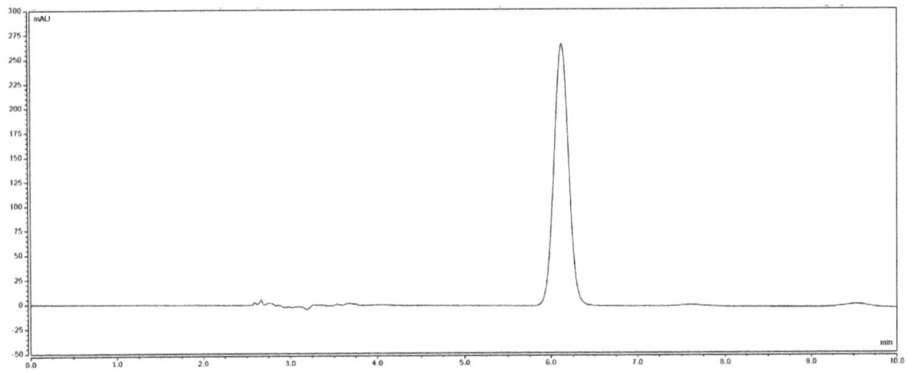

Figure 17. High-performance liquid chromatogram of the crocetin standard.

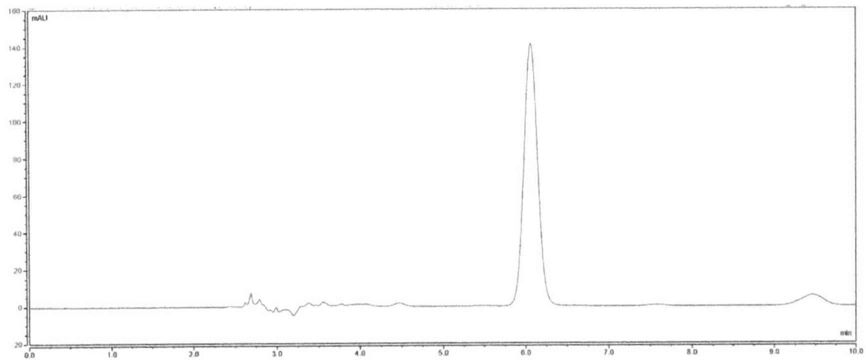

Figure 18. High-performance liquid chromatogram of the crocetin samples.

4.4. Reducing Ability and Radical Scavenging Ability Test

An amount of 10.00 mg crocetin was dissolved with 0.5 mL DMSO and diluted with distilled water in a 50 mL volumetric flask to obtain 200.00 μg/mL crocetin solution. This solution was further diluted with distilled water to 1.00, 2.50, 5.00, 10.00, 25.00, 50.00, 100.00, and 200.00 μg/mL series solution, respectively. The series solution of ascorbic acid was prepared with the same method.

The in vitro reducing ability of crocetin was determined by the Prussian blue reaction. The luminol dimethyl sulfoxide sodium hydroxide luminescence system was used to determine the superoxide anion scavenging capacity of crocetin, the luminol H_2O_2 chemiluminescence system was used to determine the H_2O_2 scavenging capacity of crocetin, and the luminol $FeSO_4$-H_2O_2 chemiluminescence system was used to determine the OH^- scavenging capacity of crocetin. The inhibition rate and half-inhibitory concentration (IC_{50}) were calculated to evaluate the reducing ability and scavenging ability of $\bullet O_2^-$, H_2O_2, and $\bullet OH^-$.

4.5. In Vitro Anti-Hypoxia Test with PC_{12} Cell

The PC_{12} cell experiment was divided into a normal control group (NC), a hypobaric hypoxia group (HH), and a low dose of crocetin group (CRT-L, 25 μMol/L), medium dose of crocetin group (CRT-M, 50 μMol/L), and high dose of crocetin group (CRT-H, 100 μMol/L). Among them, crocetin was soluted with DMSO and added in medium for crocetin groups. The NC group was cultured in a normoxia constant temperature incubator for 36 h. The other groups were cultured in a hypoxic constant temperature incubator (1%

O_2, 5% CO_2, and 37°C) for 36 h. Then, the culture medium was discarded, and 100 μL 100% CCK-8 medium was added and cultured for another 2 h. The absorbance at 450 nm was measured using an enzyme-linked immunosorbent assay (ELISA) to calculate cell viability.

4.6. Animals

SPF male BALB/C mice (aged 4–5 weeks with an average body weight of 20 ± 2 g) and Wistar rats (aged 6–8 weeks with an average body weight of 200 ± 20 g) were purchased from the Beijing Vital River Laboratory Animal Technology Co., Ltd. (Beijing, China, License No. SCXK (Jing) 2021-0011). The animals were fed in the rearing room with a temperature of 20–25 °C and a relative humidity of 40–70%. Alternating light and darkness every 12 h in the rearing room, the rats freely fed and drank water. The adaptation period was 1 week before the start of the investigation.

The experimental protocol used in this study was approved by the 940th Hospital of Joint Logistic Support Force of Chinese People's Liberation Army, with approval number: 2022KYLL031.

4.7. Normobaric Hypoxia and Sodium Nitrite Hypoxia Tests

A total of 50 BALB/c mice were randomly divided into the control group (sterile water, 10 mL/Kg), positive control group (acetazolamide, 100 mg/kg/d), crocetin low-dose group (15 mg/kg/d), crocetin medium-dose group (30 mg/kg/d), and crocetin high-dose group (60 mg/kg/d). The drugs were given twice, at 12 h and 30 min before normobaric hypoxia. All mice were placed in a 200 mL jar with 5 g of soda lime (absorption of carbon dioxide and water). The bottles were covered tightly with Vaseline, and time was counted immediately. The mice were observed, and the time when the mice died due to lack of oxygen was recorded.

The animals were divided into groups and administered as described in the normobaric hypoxia test. One hour after the last administration, 300 mg/kg sodium nitrite solution was injected into the abdominal cavity. The mice were observed, and the time when the mice died due to lack of oxygen was recorded.

4.8. Establishment of High Altitude Hypoxia Rat Model and Administration

The 72 experimental rats were randomly divided into the normoxic control group (NCG, 0.5% CMC-Na, 10 mL/kg), hypoxia model group (HMG, 0.5% CMC-Na, 10 mL/kg), crocetin-low dose group (CRT-L,10 mg/kg), crocetin-medium dose group (CRT-M, 20 mg/kg), crocetin-high dose group (CRT-H, 40 mg/kg), and acetazolamide group (ACTZ, 70 mg/kg). Under the condition of an SPF environment, the rats began the experiment after 3 days of adaptive feeding.

The DYC-9070 simulated altitude hypoxia animal experimental cabin used in the experiment consists of three parts: control system, experimental cabin, and simulation cabin. The experimental cabin was the one where the rats were dissected after the hypoxia model was established, and the simulated altitude is 4000 m; the simulation cabin is a place where experimental animals were exposed to hypoxia and could simulate altitudes above 8000 m; the control system controlled them. There were independent valves between the experimental cabin and the simulation cabin, as well as between the experimental cabin and the external environment, that is, internal valves and external valves.

The specific administration methods of the six groups of rats were as follows: the rats in the normoxic control group (NCG) and the hypoxia model group (HMG) were intraperitoneally injected with 0.5% CMC-Na, and the other four groups were intraperitoneally injected with the corresponding doses, respectively, 30 min before hypoxia, 12 h after hypoxia, and 24 h after hypoxia. A total of three times were administered, and the hypoxia exposure time was 24 h. During this period, the rats were fed and drank freely. Within 24 h of hypoxia, the on-duty personnel were arranged to observe the food intake and active state of the rats by monitoring.

The normoxia control group (NCG) was raised in the experimental animal department during the experiment, and the other five groups of rats were placed in a simulated cabin at an altitude of 8000 m after the first administration. After 12 h of hypoxia in the experimental rats, the experimenters entered the experimental cabin. The extravehicular experimenters used the control system to rise at a constant speed of 4 m/s to the altitude of 4000 m in the experimental cabin, and at the same time, they dropped at a constant speed of 20 m/s to the altitude of 4000 m in the simulation cabin. After the two cabins became stable, the experimenters could open the inner valve and enter the simulation cabin for the second intraperitoneal injection. After 24 h of hypoxia in the experimental rats, the experimenters entered the cabin for the third administration. After 30 min of administration, the rats were decapitated and killed to take tissues. At the same time, the extravehicular experimenters handled NCG rats in the same way (Figure 19).

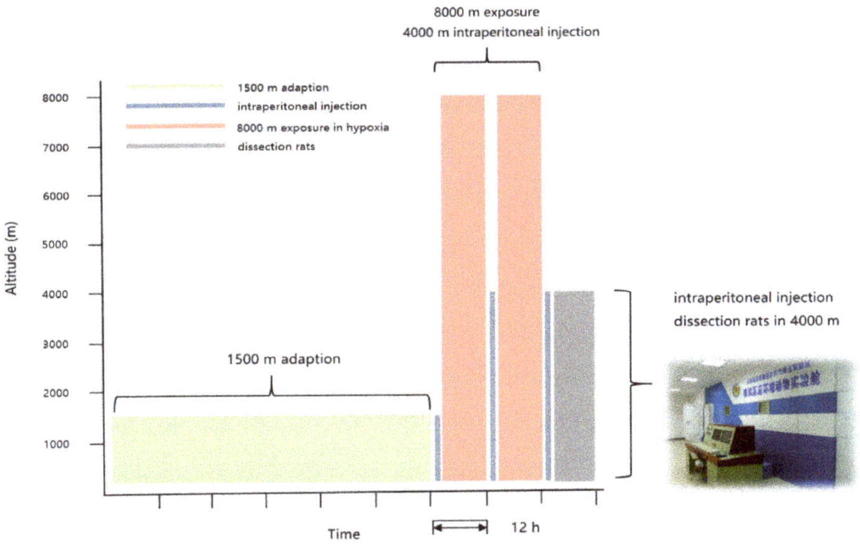

Figure 19. Establishment of high-altitude hypoxia rat model and administration.

4.9. Determination of Brain and Lung Water Content

The 1/2 tissue of the upper part of the left brain and the upper lobe of the left lung were placed on the weighing paper to weigh the wet weight. After weighing, they were placed in a constant temperature blast oven at 60 °C for more than 72 h until the difference between the two weighing dry weights did not exceed 0.002 g. The water content of rat brain and lung tissue was calculated according to Formula (1):

$$\text{Water content } (\%) = \frac{\text{wet weight} - \text{dry weight}}{\text{wet weight}} \times 100\% \tag{1}$$

4.10. HE Staining

After the high-altitude hypoxia model was established, rats were decapitated, and the right half brain was fixed in 4% paraformaldehyde solution, embedded, and sectioned for HE staining. The histopathologic changes were observed under the microscope (×400).

4.11. Biochemical Analysis and Enzyme-Linked Immunosorbent Assay (ELISA)

An amount of 180–220 mg tissue was weighed to make 10% homogenate with cold 1×PBS. The supernatant was taken after centrifugation (10,000 r/min, 10 min, 4 °C).

Followed the kit instructions, MDA, H_2O_2, GSH, GSH-Px, SOD, CAT, IL-1β, IL-6, TNF-α, and VEGF were determined.

4.12. Statistical Analysis

Statistical analysis was performed using SPSS 26.0 software. The data were expressed as the mean ± standard deviation (SD) ($\overline{x} \pm$ SD), and one-way analysis of variance (ANOVA) was used for further pairwise comparison using the LSD-*t* test. $p < 0.05$ was considered a significant difference.

5. Conclusions

In summary, the current findings demonstrate that crocetin exhibits good anti-hypoxia effects in both in vitro and in vivo models. In this regard, crocetin has strong free radical scavenging ability and can enhance the vitality of PC_{12} cells under hypoxic conditions and prolong the survival time of mice with different hypoxia models. More importantly, crocetin restored the oxidative and antioxidant balance in important organs of simulated high-altitude hypoxia rats, reducing oxidative stress and inflammatory reactions, thereby protecting the important organs of simulated high-altitude hypoxia rats from damage caused by hypoxia. Therefore, we recommend using crocetin as a protective agent to combat tissue damage caused by high-altitude hypoxia. The prevention and treatment of high-altitude diseases are based on our understanding of the physiological and pathological changes in people and bodies in high-altitude areas. Further research on the pathophysiological mechanisms of high-altitude diseases can improve our understanding of their precise therapeutic effects. However, crocetin has not yet been applied clinically to treat altitude illnesses due to its unique structure. Therefore, while studying the anti-hypoxic effects of crocetin, attention should also be paid to the drug's administration method, dosage form, and safety. It is of great significance for it to enter clinical research as soon as possible.

Author Contributions: Data curation, Z.G., R.W. and Q.Q.; Investigation, S.M.; Writing—original draft, J.Y., Z.G. and K.L.; Writing—review and editing, J.Y., M.L. and Y.G.; Supervision, M.L. and Y.G.; Project Administration, M.L.; Funding Acquisition, Y.G. All authors have read and agreed to the published version of the manuscript.

Funding: Traditional Chinese Medicine Innovation Team and Talent Support Program Project from National Administration of Traditional Chinese Medicine (ZYYCXTDD-202207).

Institutional Review Board Statement: The experimental protocol used in this study was approved by the 940th Hospital of Joint Logistic Support Force of Chinese People's Liberation Army, with approval number: 2022KYLL031 (30 March 2022).

Informed Consent Statement: Not applicable.

Data Availability Statement: The data used to support the findings of this study are available from the corresponding author upon request.

Conflicts of Interest: The authors declare that they do not have any conflicts of interest related to the contents of this article.

References

1. Hannes Gatterer, F.C.V.; Ulrich, S.; Bhandari, S.S.; Keyes, L.E.; Burtscher, M. Altitude illnesses. *Nat. Rev. Dis. Primers* **2024**, *10*, 44. [CrossRef]
2. Weil, J.V.; Byrne-Quinn, E.; Sodal, I.E.; Friesen, W.O.; Underhill, B.; Filley, G.F.; Grover, R.F. Hypoxic ventilatory drive in normal man. *J. Clin. Investig.* **1970**, *49*, 1061–1072. [CrossRef]
3. Burtscher, M.; Faulhaber, M.; Flatz, M.; Likar, R.; Nachbauer, W. Effects of short-term acclimatization to altitude (3200 m) on aerobic and anaerobic exercise performance. *Int. J. Sports Med.* **2006**, *27*, 629–635. [CrossRef]
4. Bärtsch, P.; Maggiorini, M.; Ritter, M.; Noti, C.; Vock, P.; Oelz, O. Prevention of high-altitude pulmonary edema by nifedipine. *N. Engl. J. Med.* **1991**, *325*, 1284–1289. [CrossRef]
5. Luks, A.M.; Hackett, P.H. Medical Conditions and High-Altitude Travel. *N. Engl. J. Med.* **2022**, *386*, 364–373. [CrossRef]
6. Askew, E.W. Work at high altitude and oxidative stress: Antioxidant nutrients. *Toxicology* **2002**, *180*, 107–119. [CrossRef]

7. Jefferson, J.A.; Simoni, J.; Escudero, E.; Hurtado, M.E.; Swenson, E.R.; Wesson, D.E.; Schreiner, G.F.; Schoene, R.B.; Johnson, R.J.; Hurtado, A. Increased oxidative stress following acute and chronic high altitude exposure. *High. Alt. Med. Biol.* **2004**, *5*, 61–69. [CrossRef]
8. Pena, E.; El Alam, S.; Siques, P.; Brito, J. Oxidative Stress and Diseases Associated with High-Altitude Exposure. *Antioxidants* **2022**, *11*, 267. [CrossRef]
9. Sarada, S.; Himadri, P.; Mishra, C.; Geetali, P.; Ram, M.S.; Ilavazhagan, G. Role of oxidative stress and NFkB in hypoxia-induced pulmonary edema. *Exp. Biol. Med.* **2008**, *233*, 1088–1098. [CrossRef]
10. Burtscher, J.; Mallet, R.T.; Pialoux, V.; Millet, G.P.; Burtscher, M. Adaptive Responses to Hypoxia and/or Hyperoxia in Humans. *Antioxid. Redox Signal.* **2022**, *37*, 887–912. [CrossRef]
11. Burtscher, M.; Hefti, U.; Hefti, J.P. High-altitude illnesses: Old stories and new insights into the pathophysiology, treatment and prevention. *Sports Med. Health Sci.* **2021**, *3*, 59–69. [CrossRef] [PubMed]
12. Chen, L.; Li, M.; Yang, Z.; Tao, W.; Wang, P.; Tian, X.; Li, X.; Wang, W. *Gardenia jasminoides* Ellis: Ethnopharmacology, phytochemistry, and pharmacological and industrial applications of an important traditional Chinese medicine. *J. Ethnopharmacol.* **2020**, *257*, 112829. [CrossRef] [PubMed]
13. Li, M.; Tian, X.; Li, X.; Mao, T.; Liu, T. Anti-fatigue activity of gardenia yellow pigment and Cistanche phenylethanol glycosides mixture in hypoxia. *Food Biosci.* **2021**, *40*, 100902. [CrossRef]
14. Wang, P.; Li, M.; Guo, Z.; Wang, W.; Li, X.; Yan, N.; Liu, T. Comparison of the pharmacokinetics of Crocin-I in normoxic and hypoxic rats. *Toxicol. Appl. Pharmacol.* **2022**, *447*, 116088. [CrossRef] [PubMed]
15. Yang, Z. Preparation and Plasma Kinetics Study of Cis/Trans Crocetin. Master's Thesis, Gansu University of Traditional Chinese Medicine, Lanzhou, China, 2022. Available online: https://link.cnki.net/doi/10.27408/d.cnki.gxmzc.2022.000294 (accessed on 1 June 2022).
16. Zhang, L.; Ai, Y.; Chen, Y.; Li, C.; Li, P.; Chen, J.; Jiang, L.; Pan, Y.; Sun, A.; Yang, Y.; et al. Elucidation of Geniposide and Crocin Accumulation and Their Biosysnthsis-Related Key Enzymes during *Gardenia jasminoides* Fruit Growth. *Plants* **2023**, *12*, 2209. [CrossRef] [PubMed]
17. Dong, N.; Dong, Z.; Chen, Y.; Gu, X. Crocetin Alleviates Inflammation in MPTP-Induced Parkinson's Disease Models through Improving Mitochondrial Functions. *Park. Dis.* **2020**, *2020*, 9864370. [CrossRef] [PubMed]
18. Xu, Z.; Lin, S.; Tong, Z.; Chen, S.; Cao, Y.; Li, Q.; Jiang, Y.; Cai, W.; Tong, Y.; Zahra, B.S.; et al. Crocetin ameliorates non-alcoholic fatty liver disease by modulating mitochondrial dysfunction in L02 cells and zebrafish model. *J. Ethnopharmacol.* **2022**, *285*, 114873. [CrossRef] [PubMed]
19. Peng, S.; Wu, Y.; Wang, Y. Crocetin Suppresses Uterine Ischemia/Reperfusion-induced Inflammation and Apoptosis through the Nrf-2/HO-1 Pathway. *Curr. Mol. Med.* **2023**, *23*, 527–535. [CrossRef]
20. Fagenholz, P.J.; Gutman, J.A.; Murray, A.F.; Harris, N.S. Treatment of high altitude pulmonary edema at 4240 m in Nepal. *High Alt. Med. Biol.* **2007**, *8*, 139–146. [CrossRef]
21. Nieto Estrada, V.H.; Molano Franco, D.; Medina, R.D.; Gonzalez Garay, A.G.; Martí-Carvajal, A.J.; Arevalo-Rodriguez, I. Interventions for preventing high altitude illness: Part 1. Commonly-used classes of drugs. *Cochrane Database Syst. Rev.* **2017**, *6*, Cd009761. [CrossRef]
22. Xiong, Y.; Wang, Y.; Xiong, Y.; Teng, L. Protective effect of Salidroside on hypoxia-related liver oxidative stress and inflammation via Nrf2 and JAK2/STAT3 signaling pathways. *Food Sci. Nutr.* **2021**, *9*, 5060–5069. [CrossRef] [PubMed]
23. Wu, C.; Li, X.; Yan, Y.; Wang, D.; Wang, M.; Hou, Z. Effects of plaster acupuncture pretreatment on the expression of NF-κB and related inflammatory factors in the lung tissue of rats with acute low-pressure hypoxic pulmonary edema. *China J. Tradit. Chin. Med. Pharm.* **2022**, *37*, 5904–5907.
24. Gong, G.; Pu, Z.; Reng, Z.; Sun, J.; Xie, H.; Ba, L.; Shi, Y. Protective effects of salidroside on the injured heart of rats migratedfrom plain to high altitude. *Immunol. J.* **2021**, *37*, 939–946. [CrossRef]
25. Wang, J.; Reng, X.; Li, X.; Ma, J.; Chen, L.; Li, M.; Qiu, J. Protective Effect of *Hypericum perforatum* L. Extract on Rats with High-altitude Pulmonary Edema. *Med. Pharm. J. Chin. People's Lib. Army* **2022**, *34*, 1–6.
26. Breen, E.; Tang, K.; Olfert, M.; Knapp, A.; Wagner, P. Skeletal muscle capillarity during hypoxia: VEGF and its activation. *High. Alt. Med. Biol.* **2008**, *9*, 158–166. [CrossRef]
27. Melincovici, C.S.; Boşca, A.B.; Şuşman, S.; Mărginean, M.; Mihu, C.; Istrate, M.; Moldovan, I.M.; Roman, A.L.; Mihu, C.M. Vascular endothelial growth factor (VEGF)—Key factor in normal and pathological angiogenesis. *Rom. J. Morphol. Embryol.* **2018**, *59*, 455–467.

pharmaceuticals

Article

Garcinia brasiliensis Leaves Extracts Inhibit the Development of Ascitic and Solid Ehrlich Tumors

Lucas Sylvestre Silva [1], Eduardo Cavallini [1], Rafael André da Silva [2], Monielle Sant'Ana [1], Ariane Harumi Yoshikawa [3], Thiago Salomão [3], Bianca Huang [3], Paula Craice [3], Luiz Philipe de Souza Ferreira [1], Heitor Pedro Della Matta [3], Cristiane Damas Gil [1,2], Maria de Lourdes Gomes Pereira [4] and Ana Paula Girol [1,2,3,*]

[1] Post Graduate Program in Structural and Functional Biology, Paulista School of Medicine (UNIFESP-EPM), Federal University of São Paulo, São Paulo 04023-062, SP, Brazil; lucas.sylvestre@icloud.com (L.S.S.); educavallini01@gmail.com (E.C.); monibiologia@yahoo.com.br (M.S.); luiz.philipe@unifesp.br (L.P.d.S.F.); cristiane.gil@unifesp.br (C.D.G.)

[2] Department of Biology, Institute of Biosciences, Humanities and Exact Sciences (Ibilce), São Paulo State University (UNESP), São José do Rio Preto 15054-000, SP, Brazil; rafael.andre@unesp.br

[3] Experimental and Clinical Research Center (CEPEC), Padre Albino University Center (UNIFIPA), Catanduva 15809-144, SP, Brazil; ariane.yoshikawa@unifipa.com.br (A.H.Y.); thi_salomao@hotmail.com (T.S.); biancafameca@gmail.com (B.H.); paulacraice@outlook.com (P.C.); heitorpedm@gmail.com (H.P.D.M.)

[4] CICECO-Aveiro Institute of Materials, Department of Medical Sciences, University of Aveiro, 3810-193 Aveiro, Portugal; mlourdespereira@ua.pt

* Correspondence: anapaula.girol@unifipa.com.br; Tel.: +55-(17)-3311-3340

Abstract: Background: *Garcinia brasiliensis* is traditionally known for its medicinal properties. Objectives: Here, we investigated the effects of crude extract (CE) and ethyl acetate fraction (EAF) obtained from *G. brasiliensis* leaves on the ascitic (EA) and solid (ES) forms of Ehrlich tumors. **Methods**: Induced and uninduced BALB/c mice were treated intramuscularly, for 7 or 14 days, with saline solution or CE and EAF, both at a 10% concentration, based on in vitro cytotoxicity assessment. Biochemical analyses were also performed to evaluate in vivo cytotoxicity. In relation to tumor-induced animals, morphological changes, plasma enzymes, inflammatory mediators and the induction of apoptosis were analyzed, in addition to histopathological studies, to evaluate the inhibition of tumor growth. **Results**: Alanine aminotransferase (ALT), aspartate aminotransferase (AST) and gamma glutamyl transferase (GGT) were regulated by CE and EAF administration. Furthermore, both treatments were effective in inhibiting tumor growth in EA and ES by modulating the levels of interleukin (IL)-6 and tumor necrosis factor (TNF)-α, decreasing mast cells numbers and inducing apoptosis. **Conclusions**: This research indicates that both CE and EAF from *G. brasiliensis* leaves have potential antitumor effects with low cytotoxicity.

Keywords: *Garcinia brasiliensis*; antitumor; Ehrlich tumor; antioxidant

1. Introduction

Cancer is a malignant disease characterized by the rapid and uncontrolled formation/division of abnormal cells that can form tumor nodules or proliferate elsewhere in the body [1]. The disease, which is considered one of the most devastating human pathologies, presents a versatile range of striking clinical features leading to millions of deaths each year with major negative implications for social, economic and health levels [2].

One of the biggest challenges in developing new drugs for cancer is the inhibition or activation of the target without interfering with normal cellular functions. Therefore, it is necessary to characterize the actions of the new therapeutic proposals and establish safe and effective dosages. Preclinical studies are indispensable, and an interesting model is the Ehrlich tumor, which originates from female mouse breast adenocarcinoma. Ehrlich tumors resemble human tumors that are more sensitive to chemotherapy, as they are undifferentiated and fast growing [3].

The experimental model of cancer using Ehrlich tumor cells is widely used to understand tumorigenic, immunological and physiological processes, and also to evaluate new diagnostic methods and therapeutic actions of drugs, since the model is similar to pathological and behavioral processes related to tumors in humans [4].

Ehrlich tumors can develop into two forms, depending on where the tumor cells are inoculated. The ascitic form develops after peritoneal inoculation where ascites is formed as a consequence of tumor-induced inflammation due to increased peritoneal vascular permeability [5]. In the solid form, in which inoculation occurs subcutaneously, the tumors are circumscribed by a defined capsule and are composed of connective tissue infiltrated by lymphocytes, polymorphonuclear and neoplastic cells. They have significant heterogeneity in cell composition and many necrotic zones, predominantly in the central areas. Projections of connective tissue from the capsule to the tumor mass are common findings [5].

Several treatments are proposed for cancer, such as chemotherapy, radiation therapy and surgery. Chemotherapy is considered an effective method for treatment; however, its success is limited due to its hepatotoxic, nephrotoxic, cardiotoxic, myelosuppressive, immunosuppressive and other cytotoxic effects [6]. Despite the advances in medical research related to cancer treatment, the development of tumor resistance against the available therapies, as well as the various side effects of chemotherapy drugs, encourages research for newer, safer and more effective drugs.

In Brazil, therapies based on medicinal plants are regulated by the National Policy on Medicinal Plants and Herbal Medicines and by the National Policy on Integrative and Complementary Practices of the Brazilian Unified Health System [7]. In view of this, there is scientific interest in investigating the effectiveness of medicinal herbs and developing herbal medicines or isolating bioactive compounds for different clinical conditions, including cancer.

In this study, we highlight a native Brazilian plant with great medicinal potential, *Garcinia brasiliensis* (Family Clusiaceae), popularly known as "Bacupari". This arboreal and fruitful plant, with sweet, astringent and refreshing fruits, is widely distributed throughout Brazil, and is used in popular and traditional medicine to treat inflammations, infections and allergies [8–10].

The fruit, as well as other organs of *G. brasiliensis*, has already been the subject of studies in the last two decades, used in crude extracts, fractions, oil and/or isolated components [11]. These studies showed that G. *brasiliensis* contains important phytochemical components such as phenols and flavonoids with anti-inflammatory, anti-allergic, antioxidant, antimicrobial, antitumorigenic and photoprotective properties. The protective effects of *G. brasiliensis* were investigated in Chagas disease, schistosomiasis, leishmaniasis, wound closure, pain and inflammation modulation in obese rats [8,12–18].

However, its effect as an antineoplastic and pro-apoptotic potential is still little explored. The effects of the bioactive compound 7-epiclusianone isolated from *G. brasiliensis* were investigated in vitro in lung cancer cells and glioblastoma, and it was demonstrated that the compound is able to stop the cell cycle of cancer cells [19,20].

Therefore, we conducted a study on the herbal properties and cytotoxicity of extract solutions from *G. brasiliensis* leaves. We evaluated the effects of their administration on ascitic and solid Ehrlich tumors to determine whether treatment with the crude extract and ethyl acetate fraction of *G. brasiliensis* alters crucial biological processes in tumorigenesis, such as apoptosis, inflammation and cytotoxicity.

2. Results

2.1. Assessment of Total Phenolic and Flavonoid Content and Free Radical Scavenging Capacity of G. brasiliensis Leaf Extract

Phytochemical analyses were carried out in order to quantify the total content of flavonoids and phenolic compounds in the crude extract (CE) at a 10% concentration and also in the ethyl acetate fraction (EAF) at a 10% concentration.

The total flavonoid content was 94.9 μg/mL in CE and 61.21 μg/mL in EAF (Figure 1A). In turn, the polyphenol content was 10.85 μg/mL for EC and 8.42 μg/mL for EAF (Figure 1B).

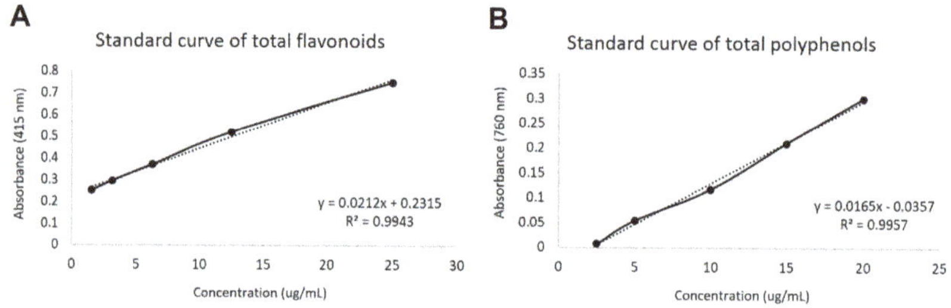

Figure 1. Standard curves for phytochemical analyses. (**A**) Standard curve for total flavonoid content, constructed using quercetin as standard, from a serial dilution of 25 μg/mL to 1.56 μg/mL (R^2 = 0.9943). (**B**) Standard curve for total polyphenol content, constructed using gallic acid as standard, from different concentrations (2; 1.5; 1.0; 0.5; and 0.25 μg/mL—R^2 = 0.9957). Solid lines represent measurements and the dashed lines represent the linear trend line.

In addition, through the 2,2-diphenyl-1-picryl-hydrazyl (DPPH) assay, CE at a 10% concentration and EAF at a 10% concentration showed high scavenging capacities, respectively, 83.52% ± 5.62% and 87.43% ± 0.75%, with no significant differences between them (Figure 2A,B).

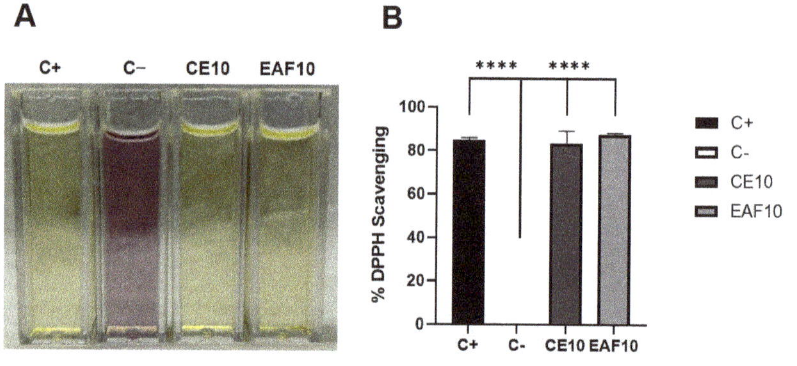

Figure 2. Scavenging capacity against DPPH. (**A**) DPPH assay visual result. C+: positive control (standard antioxidant, butylhydroxytoluene-BHT); C−: negative control; CE10: crude extract at a 10% concentration; and EAF10: ethyl acetate fraction at a 10% concentration. (**B**) Comparisons of total antioxidant activity among controls and CE at a 10% concentration and EAF at a 10% concentration. Statistical analysis was conducted using one-way ANOVA, followed by Tukey's multiple comparison test. Significance levels are indicated as **** $p < 0.0001$.

2.2. Cytotoxicity Profile of G. brasiliensis CE and EAF

Before proceeding with the model of ascitic and solid Ehrlich tumors, it was important to determine the cytotoxicity profile of the crude extract (CE) and ethyl acetate fraction (EAF) obtained from *G. brasiliensis* leaves.

The hemolysis assay indicated that CE and EAF have low cytotoxicity at 5% and 10% concentration ($p < 0.0001$) (Figure 3A–F). The half-maximum inhibitory concentrations (IC_{50}) for CE and EAF were calculated, resulting in 28.32% and 33.19%, respectively.

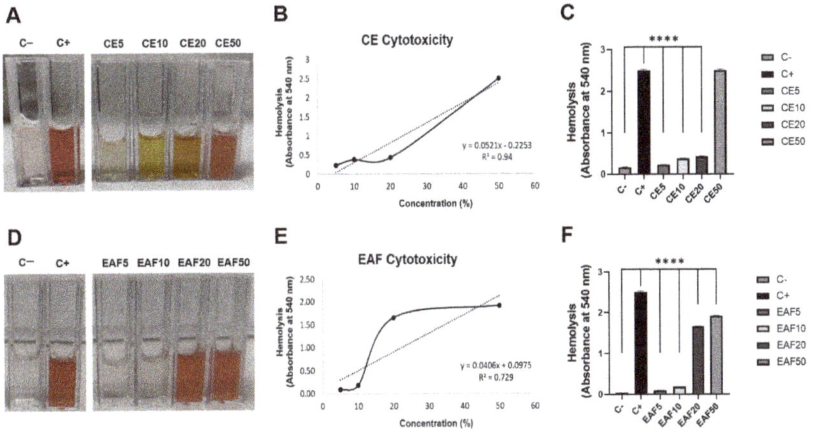

Figure 3. In vitro cytotoxicity test by hemolysis. (**A**) Visual result of the hemolysis test for the CE. Negative control (C−), positive control (C+), CE samples at 5% concentration (CE5), 10% concentration (CE10), 20% concentration (CE20) and 50% concentration (CE50). (**B**) Graphic of cytotoxicity in red blood cells from the CE samples. Solid line represents measurements and the dashed line represents the linear trend line. (**C**) Comparisons of cytotoxicity among controls and samples of CE. (**D**) Visual result of the hemolysis test for the EAF. Negative control (C−), positive control (C+), CE samples at 5% concentration (CE5), 10% concentration (CE10), 20% concentration (CE20) and 50% concentration (CE50). (**E**) Graphic of cytotoxicity in red blood cells from the EAF samples. Solid line represents measurements and the dashed line represents the linear trend line (**F**) Comparisons of cytotoxicity among controls and samples of EAF. Statistical analysis was conducted using one-way ANOVA, followed by Tukey's multiple comparison test. Significance levels are indicated as **** $p < 0.0001$.

In this way, a concentration of 10% for CE and EAF was selected for the treatment protocols.

2.3. Biochemical Profile of Non-Induced and Ehrlich Tumor-Induced Animals

To evaluate the occurrence of metabolic changes caused by the administration of the extract, biochemical analyses were performed in non-induced and induced animals to ascitic and solid Ehrlich tumors. In these analyses, the treatments comprised CE at a 10% concentration and EAF at a 10% concentration and lasted 7 days for the ascitic tumor and 14 days for the solid tumor.

In this way, the plasma levels of alanine aminotransferase (ALT), aspartate aminotransferase (AST), gamma glutamyl transferase (Gamma GT), creatinine, urea, albumin, alkaline phosphatase, uric acid and blood glucose were measured.

In non-induced animals but treated with CE or EAF for 7 days (CE7 and EAF7) there were no significant changes in the levels of the evaluated markers compared to group C. (Figure 4A–I). In contrast, non-induced animals and animals treated with CE for 14 days (CE14 group) showed elevated levels of ALT ($p < 0.05$) compared to those in group C (Figure 5A). However, treatment with EAF did not change the levels of markers evaluated in relation to group C (Figure 5A–I).

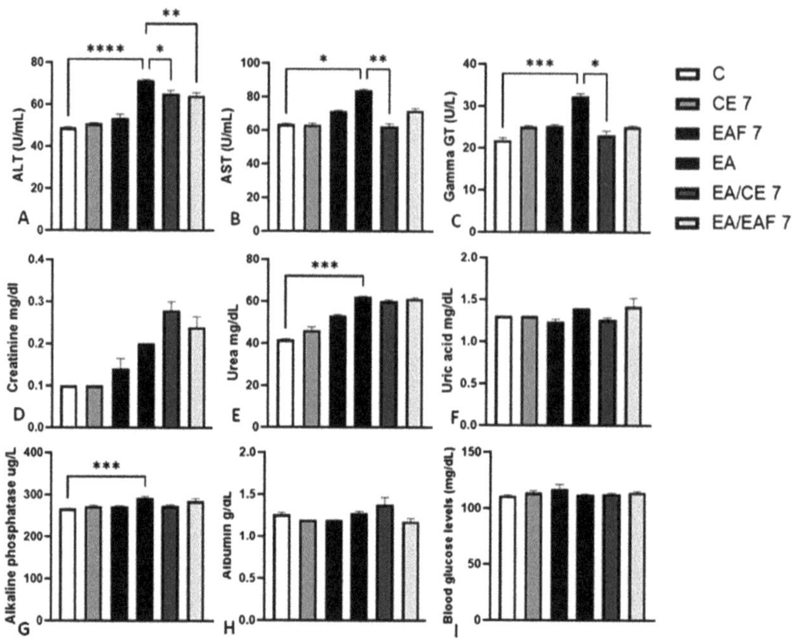

Figure 4. Blood biochemical analyses of ascitic Ehrlich tumor-induced animals and non-induced animals treated with CE at 10% concentration and EAF at 10% concentration for 7 days. The dosages of (**A**) ALT, (**B**) AST, (**C**) Gamma GT, (**D**) creatinine, (**E**) urea, (**F**) albumin, (**G**) alkaline phosphatase, (**H**) uric acid and (**I**) blood glucose levels were measured in blood plasma. Results presented as mean ± S.E.M ($n = 8$/group). Statistical analysis was conducted using one-way ANOVA, followed by Tukey's multiple comparison test. Significance levels are indicated as * $p < 0.05$; ** $p < 0.01$; *** $p < 0.001$; and **** $p < 0.0001$.

With regard to animals induced with ascitic Ehrlich tumors without treatment (EA group), the analyses indicated a significant increase in plasma levels of ALT ($p < 0.0001$), AST ($p < 0.05$), Gamma GT ($p < 0.001$), urea ($p < 0.001$) and alkaline phosphatase ($p < 0.001$) compared to non-induced animals (group C) (Figure 4A–C,E,G). Creatinine, uric acid, albumin and glucose dosages did not show significant changes between groups EA and C (Figure 4D,F,H,I).

Animals induced with solid Ehrlich tumors (ES group) that were not treated showed a significant increase in the plasma levels of ALT ($p < 0.0001$), when compared with animals in the control group (C) (Figure 5A), while the levels of other markers did not show significant differences between groups (Figure 5B–I).

When observing the effects of the treatments, the group induced with ascitic Ehrlich tumors and treated with CE for 7 days (EA/CE7 group) showed a reduction in ALT ($p < 0.05$), AST ($p < 0.01$) and Gamma GT ($p < 0.05$), compared to the EA group, while the other markers did not show significant changes between these groups (Figure 4A,C). On the other hand, the group induced and treated with EAF (EA/EAF7) showed a reduction only in ALT levels ($p < 0.01$), compared to the EA group (Figure 4A).

Regarding the treatment of animals induced with solid Ehrlich tumors, the group treated with CE (ES/CE14) showed a reduction in AST ($p < 0.05$) and Gamma GT ($p < 0.01$) levels, compared to the ES group (Figure 5B,C). Urea levels had a significant increase in the ES/CE14 group compared to the CE14 group (Figure 5E). On the other hand, the group induced and treated with EAF (ES/EAF14) showed a reduction in Gamma GT levels ($p < 0.01$), compared to the ES group (Figure 5C).

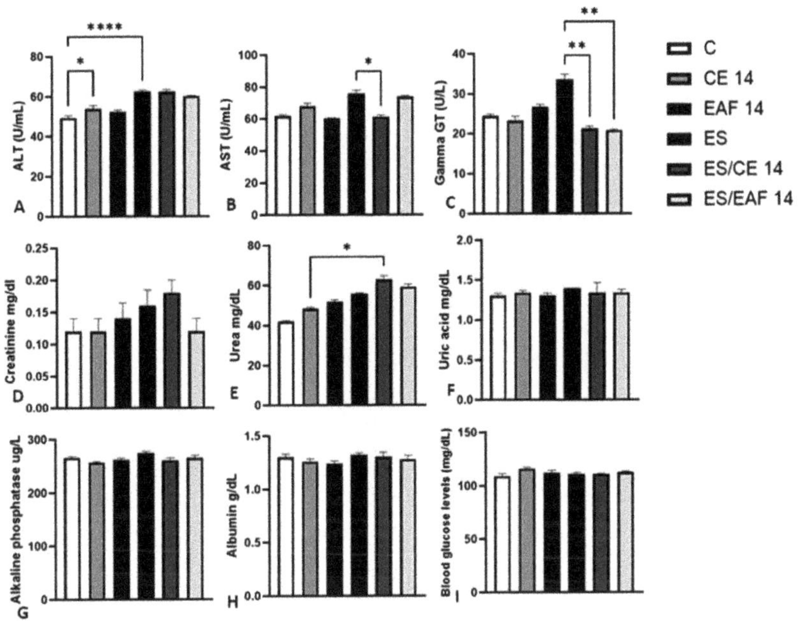

Figure 5. Blood biochemical analyses of solid Ehrlich tumor-induced animals and non-induced animals treated with CE and EAF for 14 days. The dosages of (**A**) ALT, (**B**) AST, (**C**) Gamma GT, (**D**) creatinine, (**E**) urea, (**F**) albumin, (**G**) alkaline phosphatase, (**H**) uric acid and (**I**) blood glucose levels were measured in blood plasma. Results presented as mean ± S.E.M ($n = 8$/group. Statistical analysis was conducted using one-way ANOVA, followed by Tukey's multiple comparison test. Significance levels are indicated as * $p < 0.05$; ** $p < 0.01$; and **** $p < 0.0001$.

Finally, no differences were observed in any of the evaluated markers between the EA/CE7 and EA/EAF7 groups (Figure 4A–I) and the ES/CE14 and ES/EAF14 groups (Figure 5A–I).

2.4. Inhibition of the Development of Ascitic Ehrlich Tumors in Treated Animals

The animals were weighed at the beginning and at the end of the experiments to obtain their relative weights, with no significant differences between the groups (Figure 6E). However, when the tumor inhibition rate due to weight variation was calculated, the results were 45% in CE-treated animals (EA/CE group) and 59.09% in EAF-treated animals (EA/EAF group), considering moderate and high inhibition rates, respectively.

After 7 consecutive days of treatment with CE and EAF, a reduction in abdominal circumference was observed in the EA/CE ($p < 0.05$) and EA/EAF ($p < 0.05$) groups compared to the EA group (Figure 6D). The rate of tumor growth reduction in relation to abdominal circumference was 66.66% in the CE group and 67.69% in the EAF, both considered high.

Regarding the ascitic fluid, the animals in the EA/EAF group also showed a reduction in total fluid (Figure 6F) ($p < 0.05$) and ascitic cells after centrifugation (%) (Figure 6G) ($p < 0.05$) when compared to the animals in the EA group.

After counting the number of cells in the ascitic fluid, both treatments with CE (EA/CE group) and EAF (EA/EAF group) significantly decreased the number of cells ($p < 0.0001$) compared to animals of the EA group (Figure 6H).

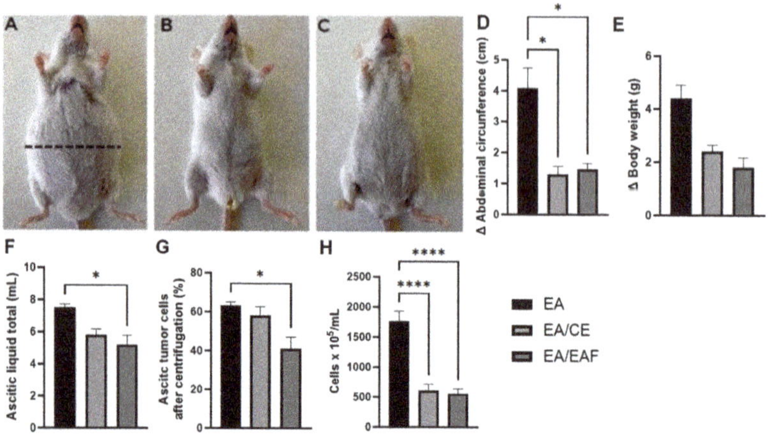

Figure 6. Analysis of the development of ascitic Ehrlich tumors and effects of treatments. Animals induced with ascitic Ehrlich tumors: (**A**) untreated. Dashed line represents the abdominal circumference measurement, (**B**) treated with CE for 7 days and (**C**) treated with EAF for 7 days. (**D**) Abdominal circumference (cm), (**E**) body weight (g), (**F**) ascitic liquid total (mL), (**G**) ascitic tumor cells after centrifugation (%) and (**H**) cell count $\times 10^5$/mL. Results presented as mean ± S.E.M. (n = 8/group). Statistical analysis was conducted using one-way ANOVA, followed by Tukey's multiple comparison test. Significance levels are indicated as * $p < 0.05$; and **** $p < 0.0001$.

2.5. Inhibition of Solid Ehrlich Tumor Development Mediated by CE and EAF Administration

The animals with solid Ehrlich tumors were treated for 14 consecutive days. The macroscopic analysis evidenced the reduction in the development of the tumor treated with CE and EAF in comparison to ES animals (Figure 7A–F).

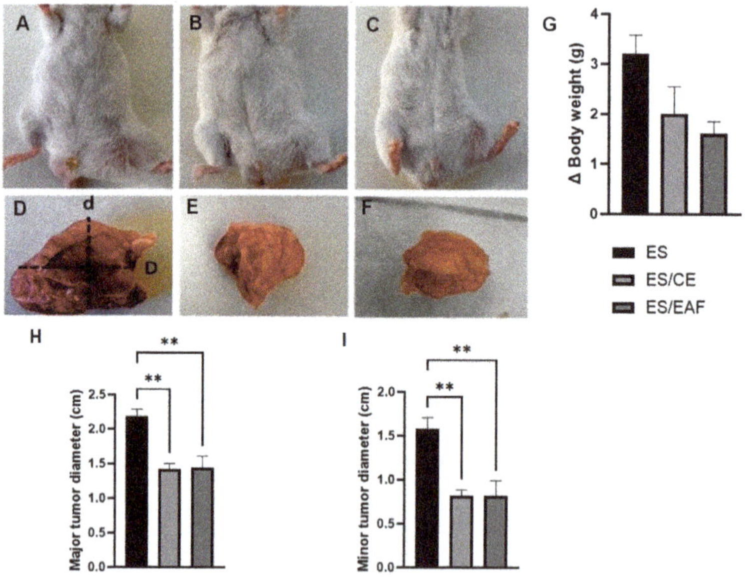

Figure 7. Analysis of solid Ehrlich tumor development and effects of treatments. Macroscopic analysis showing the tumors in the animals' bodies (**A–C**) and after excision (**D–F**), with the measured axes (major D and minor d), (**G**) Δ body weight, (**H**) major tumor diameter and (**I**) minor tumor diameter

of untreated solid Ehrlich tumor-induced mice (ES) indicated in induced mice treated with crude extract (ES/CE) and induced mice treated with ethyl acetate fraction (ES/EAF). Results are presented as means ± S.E.M. (n = 8/group). Statistical analysis was conducted using one-way ANOVA, followed by Tukey's multiple comparison test. Significance levels are indicated as ** $p < 0.01$.

The analysis of weight variation did not show a significant decrease when comparing the treated groups and the untreated animals (Figure 7G). However, in the animals induced and treated with CE, the rate of inhibition of tumor growth was 50%, while those treated with EAF had the tumor reduced by 35.7%, with percentages of inhibition being considered high and moderate, respectively.

Both treatments with CE at 10% concentration and EAF at 10% concentration reduced the major (Figure 7H) ($p < 0.01$) and minor (Figure 7I) ($p < 0.01$) tumor diameters in relation to the ES group. Likewise, the analysis of tumor showed significant differences with reduction ($p < 0.05$) in the groups treated with CE (0.7448 ± 0.04857 mm^3) and EAF (0.7700 ± 0.1879 mm^3) compared to the treated animals (2.684 ± 0.6847 mm^3).

2.6. Histopathology Studies of Solid Ehrlich Tumors

Histopathological analysis revealed the characteristics of poorly differentiated invasive carcinoma with rapidly progressing tumor masses, frequent mitotic figures and anaplastic cells evidenced by nuclear pleomorphism, with variations in shape, size and chromatin, as well as changes in the nucleus/cytoplasm ratio, prominence and quantity of nucleoli (Figure 8C).

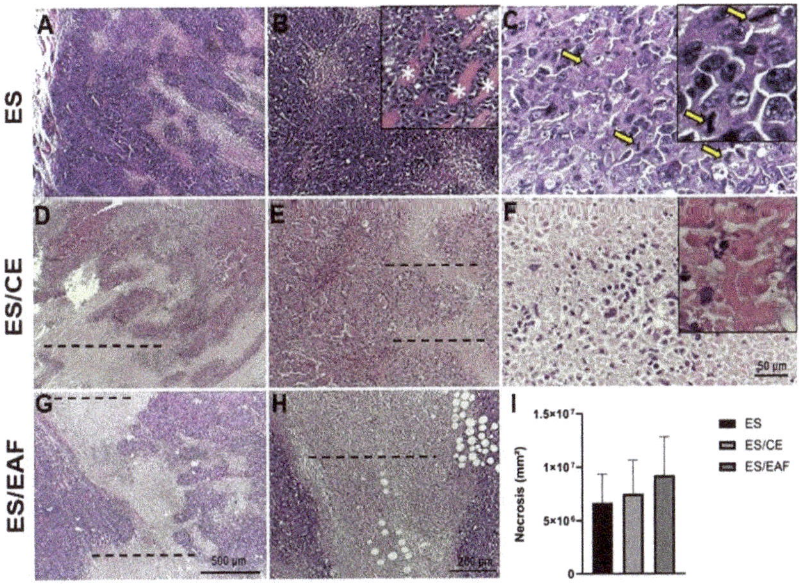

Figure 8. Histopathological analysis of solid Ehrlich tumors. Tumor masses of untreated animals (**A–C**), treated with CE (**D–F**) and treated with EAF (**G–I**). Dashed lines indicate regions of necrosis. Yellow arrows show mitosis figures. White asterisks indicate skeletal striated muscle. The detailed magnifications show mitosis figures (**C**) and necrosis regions (**F**). Bars of 500 µm (**A**,**D**,**G**), 200 µm (**B**,**E**,**H**) and 50 µm (**C**,**F**). Staining, Hematoxylin–Eosin. Statistical analysis was conducted using one-way ANOVA, followed by Tukey's multiple comparison test.

The invasion of the underlying skeletal muscle, leukocyte infiltration, cells in apoptosis with pycnotic nuclei and appearance of fat cells, as well as regions of necrosis presenting cells with karyolitic nuclei and acidophilus cytoplasm, were also observed (Figure 8A–C).

In the groups treated with CE (ES/CE group) and EAF (ES/EAF group), which demonstrated a macroscopic reduction in tumor masses, it was possible to observe an increase in the area of necrosis when compared to the untreated group (ES); however, the results were not statistically significant (Figure 8D–I).

2.7. *Quantification of Mast Cells and Evaluation of Mast Cell Protease-6 (Mcpt6) Expression in Solid Ehrlich Tumors*

To investigate the presence and interaction of mast cells in the development of the solid form of Ehrlich tumors, these cells were identified by histological staining with toluidine blue and quantified. Also, Mcpt6 expression was evaluated in the tumor macerate using Western blotting.

Several mast cells were observed in the tumor tissues of untreated animals. In treated groups, few cells could be identified (Figure 9A–C). Animals induced with solid tumor and treated with CE and EAF (ES/CE and ES/EAF groups) showed a reduction ($p < 0.05$) of mast cells in tumor tissue, compared to animals induced but without treatment (ES group) (Figure 9D). Similarly, decreased Mcpt6 expression ($p < 0.001$) was observed in animals induced with solid tumor and treated with CE and EAF (ES/CE and ES/EAF groups) (Figure 9E,F).

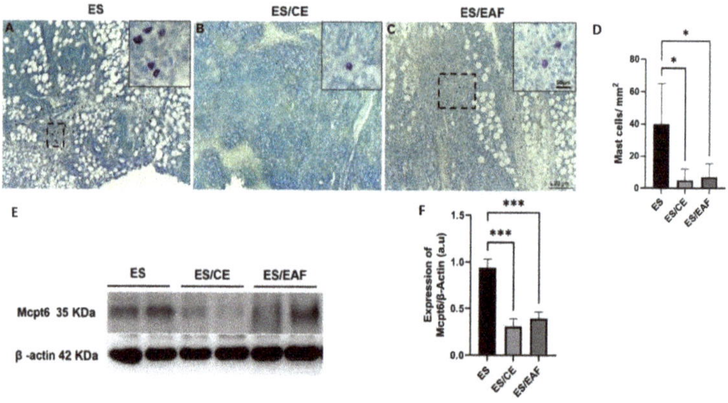

Figure 9. Analysis of mast cells and Mcpt6 levels in animals induced with solid Ehrlich tumor. (**A**) Various mast cells were present in animals induced with tumors without treatment. But fewer mast cells were present in animals induced with tumors and treated (**B**) with CE or (**C**) EAF. The insets represent enlargements of the dashed areas. Bars of 50 μm. Staining, Toluidine blue. (**D**) Statistical analysis was conducted using one-way ANOVA, followed by Tukey's multiple comparison test. Significance levels are indicated as * $p < 0.05$. (**E**) Western blotting for Mcpt6 expression in animals treated with CE and EAF. (**F**) Statistical analysis was conducted using one-way ANOVA, followed by Tukey's multiple comparison test. Significance levels are indicated as * $p < 0.05$ and *** $p < 0.001$.

2.8. *Evaluation of Bax Expression in Ascitic and Solid Ehrlich Tumors Through Western Blotting*

Higher levels of Bax were observed in animals induced with ascitic Ehrlich tumors and treated with CE at a 10% concentration (EA/CE group, $p < 0.01$) and EAF at a 10% concentration (EA/EAF group, $p < 0.05$) for 7 days, compared to untreated animals in the EA group (Figure 10A,C).

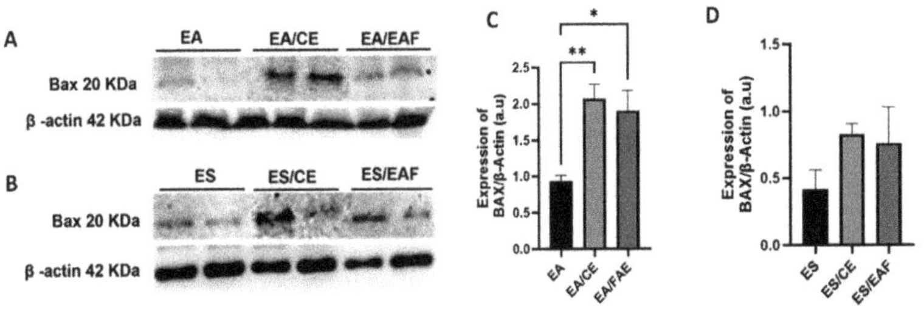

Figure 10. Analysis of Bax levels. Animals induced with ascitic Ehrlich tumors and treated with CE 10% concentration and EAF 10% concentration for 7 days (**A**,**C**). Animals induced with solid Ehrlich tumors and treated with CE 10% concentration and EAF 10% concentration for 14 days (**B**,**D**). Statistical analysis was conducted using one-way ANOVA, followed by Tukey's multiple comparison test. Significance levels are indicated as * $p < 0.05$. and ** $p < 0.01$.

Animals induced with solid Ehrlich tumors, both the 14-day CE and 14-day EAF treatment groups, also showed an increase in Bax levels—without statistical significance, however (Figure 10B,D).

2.9. Measurement of Cytokine Levels IL-6, TNF-α and IFN-γ in Ascitic and Solid Ehrlich Tumors

To evaluate the influence of CE and EAF treatments on the expression of pro-inflammatory cytokines, the levels of IL-6, IFN-γ and TNF-α were measured in the ascitic fluid and tumor tissue of animals induced with ascitic and solid Ehrlich tumors.

In the EA/CE group, treated for 7 days, the levels of IFN-γ (Figure 11B) and TNF-α (Figure 11C) did not change significantly, while the levels of IL-6 (Figure 11A) were significantly increased ($p < 0.05$) after treatment, in comparison with the levels of such cytokines in the EA group. On the other hand, the EA/EAF group, treated for 7 days, did not present significant alterations in cytokine levels when compared with the EA group (Figure 11A–C). There was no statistically significant difference in the expression of the cytokines studied between the EA/CE and EA/EAF groups.

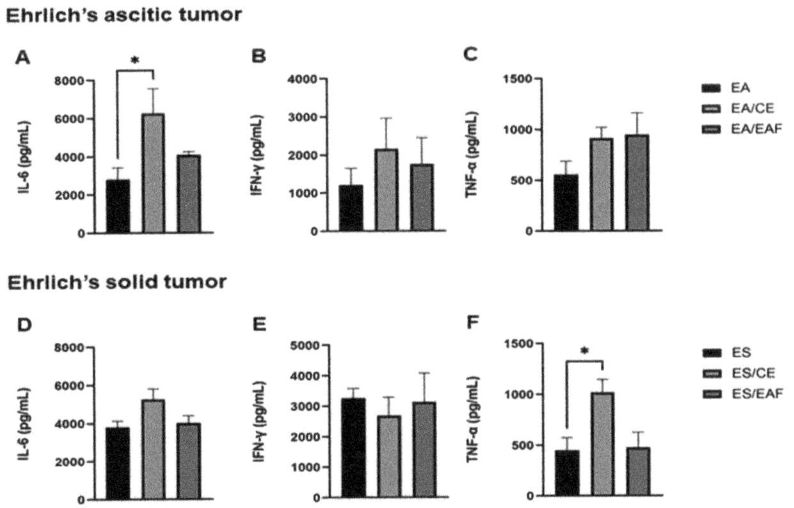

Figure 11. Measurement of IL-6, IFN-γ and TNF-α cytokine levels in ascitic (**A**–**C**) and solid (**D**–**F**) Ehrlich tumors. Statistical analysis was conducted using one-way ANOVA, followed by Tukey's multiple comparison test. Significance levels are indicated as * $p < 0.05$.

In the ES/CE group, treated for 14 days, the levels of IL-6 (Figure 11D) and IFN-γ (Figure 11E) did not show significant changes, while the levels of TNF-α (Figure 11F) were significantly increased ($p < 0.05$) in relation to the levels of such cytokines in the ES group. On the other hand, the ES/EAF group, treated for 14 days, did not present significant differences in cytokine levels when compared with the ES group (Figure 11D–F). Finally, there were no statistically significant differences in the expressions of the cytokines between the ES/CE and ES/EAF groups.

3. Discussion

Considering the impact of cancer on global health, as well as the importance of medicinal plants in the search for new therapies, in this investigation, we studied the effects of the administration of crude extract (CE) and ethyl acetate fraction (EAF) of *G. brasiliensis* leaves in the ascitic and solid forms of Ehrlich's tumor. Figure 12 summarizes all the results found in this investigation.

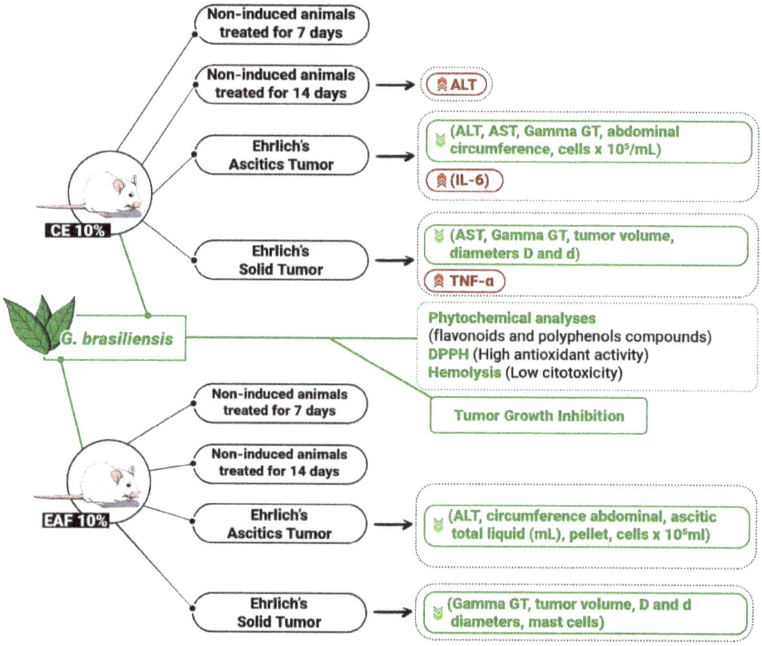

Figure 12. Representative scheme of the results obtained by the administration of CE at 10% concentration and EAF 10% concentration in mice non-induced and induced with ascitic and solid Ehrlich tumors. Both extractive solutions showed potential for tumor growth inhibition. Upward-facing red arrows indicate increased levels. Downward-facing green arrows indicate reduced levels.

Initially, the total content of flavonoids and polyphenols was measured, and we observed that CE and EAF at a 10% concentration exhibited high concentrations of total flavonoids and polyphenols. Furthermore, we observed that CE and EAF, both at a 10% concentration, exhibited high degrees of free radical-scavenging activity. In previous investigations, the same DPPH assay was used to assess the antioxidant potential of extracts from several plants of industrial interest [21,22]. Although it has some limitations regarding the specific conditions of the reaction, this assay can be standardized and used on a large scale, with high reproducibility between different laboratories [22,23].

We also evaluated CE and EAF through cytotoxicity analysis. The in vitro hemolysis test demonstrated that CE and EAF at a concentration of 10% had low cytotoxicity. In a previous investigation, the absence of toxicity at a concentration of 10% was also demonstrated by both hemolysis and the chorioallantoic membrane assay [18], reinforcing its safety. Therefore, a concentration of 10% for CE and EAF was selected for subsequent experiments.

Natural antioxidant components present in functional foods can protect the human body against free radical damage, which may be the reason behind several chronic diseases, including cancer [24]. The biological properties of these natural antioxidants are mostly due to their high levels of various phenolic compounds, such as flavonoids and phenolic acids [25,26].

Plants of the *Garcinia* genus are sources of important bioactive compounds, related to diverse therapeutic properties. As reviewed by Espirito Santo et al. (2020), the species *G. brasiliensis* has a high content of compounds from the classes of sesquiterpenes, biflavonoids, benzophenones, organic acids, flavonoids and xanthones, which can be obtained from leaves, fruits, fruit peels, pulp and seeds. Such compounds are especially related to anti-inflammatory, antioxidant, antiparasitic and antitumor properties [8].

The processing of plant material can be carried out using different methodologies, each with the potential to extract specific compounds. Using the high-performance liquid chromatography diode-array detection (HPLC-DAD) methodology to compare four extraction methods of bioactive compounds from the epicarp of *G. brasiliensis* fruits, it was observed that the highest levels of 7-epiclusianone and gutiferone-A were identified from the N-hexane fraction, obtained by the maceration extraction method, while higher levels of fukugetin and noratiriol were found in the ethyl acetate fraction, obtained by the extraction method with Soxhlet equipment [27].

The phenolic composition of the ethyl acetate fraction of the methanolic extract of *G. brasiliensis* leaves has also been previously studied, indicating the presence of twelve flavonoids, with emphasis on morelloflavone-7″-O-glucoside (fukugeside) and GB-2AA glucoside, which were associated with high antioxidant, antimicrobial and anti-inflammatory activity [28]. Additionally, antioxidant activity has also been characterized in the immature pulp and epicarp of *G. brasiliensis* [13,29].

In a previous investigation, our group demonstrated through phytochemical and chromatographic analyses that the CE and EAF of *G. brasiliensis* present products of plant metabolism of pharmacological interest such as polyphenols and flavonoids, comprising catechin, quercetin and garcinol as well as high antioxidant capacity [18]. Another research group demonstrated that the leaf extract of *G. brasiliensis* has a higher content of phenolic compounds and flavonoids compared to the bark and seed of *G. brasiliensis* extracts [11].

After phytochemical analyses and the selection of the CE and EAF concentration, in vivo tests were carried out. First, enzymes related to hepatic metabolism and glycemia were measured in non-induced and tumor-induced animals. Our results indicate that animals induced with ascitic Ehrlich tumors have increased plasma levels of ALT, AST, Gamma GT, alkaline phosphatase and urea. However, treatment with CE from *G. brasiliensis* promoted a reduction in ALT, AST and Gamma GT levels in these animals, indicating that the treatment can modulate the activity of important enzymes of hepatic metabolism against the development of Ehrlich's ascitic tumor. Furthermore, treatment with EAF also promoted the reduction in ALT levels in induced animals. However, no statistically significant difference was observed in ALT levels between animals induced and treated with CE or EAF, indicating that both treatments modulate the activity of this enzyme similarly.

With regard to solid Ehrlich tumors, it was observed that the induced animals had higher levels of ALT. CE treatment promoted a reduction in AST and Gamma GT levels, but not in ALT. Furthermore, EAF treatment also reduced Gamma GT levels. Similarly to the treatment of animals with ascitic tumors, we did not observe a significant difference in the levels of the studied markers between groups of animals induced with solid tumors and treated with CE or EAF.

During the development of Ehrlich tumors, the occurrence of a metabolic imbalance is common, increasing the levels of AST, ALT, urea and creatinine [30]. One of the frequently used therapies in the treatment of tumors is radiation therapy. In the solid Ehrlich model, exposure to ionizing radiation led to increased ALT and AST levels; however, it promoted pyroptotic cell death at lower and higher doses and ferroptosis at higher doses with marked tumor reduction, which may support its use as an anti-cancer strategy [31].

Among the enzymes, ALT is more precise for liver disease than AST, as AST may also be related to muscle injuries [32], which may explain the observed effect of the treatment on the levels of such enzymes. Due to its anatomical location, the liver can be more easily affected in the development of ascitic Ehrlich tumors, which can lead to increased ALT levels. On the other hand, in the development of the solid form, the invasion of muscle tissue by the tumor occurs, which can lead to increased AST levels. Our results indicate that the proposed treatments, especially using CE, reduced ALT levels in animals induced with Ehrlich's ascitic tumor, as well as decreased AST levels in animals induced with solid Ehrlich tumor.

The search for natural compounds that could be efficient for neoplasms face the challenge of proposing a safe treatment with less toxicity. Although some natural compounds, such as *Capsicum annuum*, show antitumor action, they can lead to metabolic imbalance, increasing AST and ALT [33]. Similarly to our findings, other researchers have verified the reduction in liver enzyme levels in the Ehrlich model after treatment with natural products such as scorpion venom [34], *Annona squamosa* extract-loaded niosome [35] and royal jelly [36].

In addition to the modulation of AST and ALT levels, we also observed that animals induced with ascitic and solid Ehrlich tumors and treated with CE showed a reduction in Gamma GT levels, as well as animals induced with solid tumors and treated with EAF, in comparison with animals induced without treatment. As reviewed by Hanigan (1998), Gamma GT levels can be increased in different types of developing tumors [37]. In a study with ascitic Ehrlich tumor models, hepatic levels of Gamma GT were reduced after treatment with alpha-lipoic acid [38]. Similarly, our results indicate that the considered treatments modulate Gamma GT levels.

After verifying the biochemical markers, we evaluated the effects of CE and EAF administration in controlling tumor growth. Our analyses indicated that treatment with CE and EAF were effective in inhibiting tumor growth in the ascitic and solid forms of Ehrlich tumors. In the ascitic model, there was a reduction in abdominal circumference and ascitic fluid volume as well as in the ascitic tumor cells numbers.

In Ehrlich tumors, the production of ascitic fluid is associated with proliferation and migration of inflammatory cells [39]. In this context, quercetin, a flavonoid with antioxidant and anti-inflammatory properties, has stood out due to its ability to inhibit the recruitment of neutrophils associated with the inflammatory process [39]. In agreement with our findings, Islam et al. (2020) also observed the inhibition of ascitic Ehrlich tumor growth, evidenced by reduced number and viability of tumor cells after treatment with leaf and bark extracts of *Morus latifolia* [40].

In the solid Ehrlich tumor model, we observed a reduction in tumor volume and major and minor tumor diameters, with a significant rate of tumor growth inhibition in the animals treated with CE and EAF. In a randomized double-blind clinical trial [41], researchers revealed that oral administration of royal jelly considerably reduced tumor size. In another study conducted by Zhang et al. (2017), results showed that royal jelly also decreased tumor weight in mice with breast tumor [42]. In addition, the use of chalcones, a bioactive compound belonging to the flavonoid family, in the treatment of Ehrlich tumors was able to reduce tumor volume [43]. Another study using mice with Ehrlich tumors, demonstrated that flavonoids, especially quercetin present in royal jelly, showed their anticancer effects through the induction of apoptosis, the reduction in animal weight and tumor volume and the inhibition of elevated serum markers such as AST and ALT [36]. In a previous study by our group, quercetin was observed in the CE and EAF extracts of leaves of *G. brasiliensis* [18].

Following our studies with solid Ehrlich tumors, we undertook the histological analyses of tumor masses, which showed anaplastic cells with invasion in skeletal muscle and necrosis regions. Although not statistically significant, the presence of large areas of necrotic tissue was observed after treatments. In addition, the increased levels of Bax in treated animals also reinforce the pro-apoptotic effect of the proposed treatments on tumor cells. The reduction in tumor masses with increased necrotic regions and apoptosis was observed in other investigations using the solid Ehrlich tumor model and treatments with extracts and bioactive compounds of medicinal plants [33,43,44]. Moreover, the modulation of apoptosis was indicated by the up-regulation of the proapoptotic genes p53, Bax [43,44] and caspase 3 as well as down-regulation of the antiapoptotic gene Bcl2 [44].

To explore the effects of treatments with CE and EAF of *G. brasiliensis* on the tumor microenvironment, the levels of pro-inflammatory cytokines IL-6, IFN-γ and TNF-α in ascitic fluid and tumor macerate were evaluated. As reviewed by Feitosa et al. (2021), the inflammatory response and the consequent expression profile of pro-inflammatory and anti-inflammatory cytokines may be variable between the two forms of Ehrlich tumors, according to the number of inoculated cells, anatomical location and other biological processes associates [5].

Our results indicated that treatment of ascitic Ehrlich tumors with CE led to increased IL-6 levels in the ascitic fluid of induced animals. Similarly, Da Cunha Leal et al. (2019) observed that the administration of high doses of gabapentin for 7 days in animals induced with ascitic Ehrlich tumors resulted in increased levels of IL-6 in the ascitic fluid compared to that in animals without treatment [45]. Another study demonstrated that natural phenolic compounds derived from bee honey, such as gallic acid and caffeic acid, induced an increase in IL-6 and IFN-γ levels in the ascitic fluid of induced animals, which contributed to the reduction in volume of the tumor and the number of viable tumor cells [46]. In line with these findings, it has already been shown that IL-6 plays an important role in the course of ascitic Ehrlich tumor.

IL-6 knockout animals induced with the disease showed greater weight gain and did not develop cachexia, compared to wild animals, indicating that cachexia induced by IL-6 secretion may be a mechanism of adaptation to cancer, leading to the increased life expectancy of animals [47]. However, some studies indicate that IL-6 levels tend to be increased after 14 days of induction of ascitic Ehrlich tumors and be reduced in the same period after treatment with *Bothrops jararaca* venom [48] and indomethacin [49]. Gentile et al. (2015) propose that IL-6 can be produced by tumor cells themselves or by cells involved in the late immune response, which justifies the increase in its secretion on day 14 after induction [49]. In the present study, we only evaluated the response to the treatment of ascitic Ehrlich tumors for 7 days; thus, the effect of prolonged treatment with CE and EAF of *G. brasiliensis* on the microenvironment of ascitic Ehlich tumor should still be investigated.

Regarding solid Ehrlich tumors, it was observed that treatment with CE induced a significant increase in TNF-α levels in the tumor. Regarding TNF-α levels, a study demonstrated that the treatment of solid Ehrlich tumors with ethanolic extract of *Salvia lachnostachys* Benth leaves also induced increased levels of this cytokine in tumor tissue, which contributed to the induction of inflammation in the tumor tissue, with consequent increase in necrosis and reduction in tumor volume and weight [50]. In contrast, using the methanolic extract of *Arthrocnemum machrostachyum* for the treatment of solid Ehrlich tumors, Sharawi (2020) observed that TNF-α levels were reduced after treatment, suggesting that such a reduction is important to prevent tumor cell survival [44]. In a review conducted by Cruceriu et al. (2020), the role of TNF-α in breast cancer was emphasized, since this cytokine can act by stimulating or inhibiting tumor progression, depending on the cellular context in which it is involved [51].

To investigate the participation of mast cells in the development of solid Ehrlich tumor, we evaluated the levels of Mcpt6; in addition, histological studies were performed with toluidine blue. In animals treated with CE and EAF, as seen through histological analysis, a reduction in the number of mast cells was observed, compared to animals that were not sujected to treatment. In addition, our results indicate that both treatments were able to reduce the levels of Mcpt6 in the tumor.

In the tumor context, mast cells can modulate several events in the tumor microenvironment, such as cell proliferation and survival, angiogenesis, invasiveness and metastasis. The increase in mast cell density may be associated with both the inhibition and stimulation of tumor progression, which demonstrates its dual role [52]. As reviewed by Ribatti et al. (2021) and Majorini et al. (2022), mast cells play an ambiguous role, depending on the type of tumor and stage of development, and is still little studied in breast tumors, with no consensus regarding their activity in these types of tumors [53,54]. Thus, mast cells have already been associated with favorable or unfavorable prognoses, in different contexts of tumor development [53,54].

Considering advances in research related to the application of natural products in diseases, including cancer, Gou et al. (2021) conducted a review regarding the relationship between mast cells, macrophages and breast cancer, proposing an investigation of the activity of natural products in inhibiting such cell types, and their relationship with breast tumor development [55]. Several studies have demonstrated the in vitro inhibition of mast cells (HMC-1 and LAD2) by various natural products. However, the authors point out that there is a lack of in vivo studies in this field [55].

Likewise, only one study indirectly investigated the participation of mast cells in solid Ehrlich tumors, through the analysis of histamine levels in the tumor microenvironment after treatment with cimetidine and/or vitamin C [56]. The researchers noted that the combined treatment of cimetidine and vitamin C, in particular, was responsible for the reduction in histamine in the tumor microenvironment, and they proposed that such a treatment, by reducing histamine levels, may reduce the activity of the PI3K/AKT/mTOR signaling pathway, which is related to the survival of breast tumor cells, with the consequent inhibition of tumor progression [56]. Similarly, our results indicate that the modulation of mast cell activity, evidenced by the reduction in these cells in the tumor tissue, is important to inhibit the growth of solid Ehrlich tumors. However, further studies are needed to better understand the role of mast cells in this type of tumor.

In summary, in this investigation, the inflammatory processes induced by the treatment, represented by the increase in IL-6 in the ascitic fluid and of TNF-α in the tumor tissue, in addition to the induction of apoptosis, represented by the increase in Bax levels, act as tumor cell inhibition mechanisms, preventing tumor progression. The inhibition of tumor growth was indicated by the reduction in abdominal circumference, total ascitic fluid volume, in addition to the number of tumor cells in animals induced with the ascitic form, as well as a reduction in volume and larger and smaller diameters of the tumor in animals induced with solid Ehrlich tumors.

Furthermore, the histopathological analysis demonstrated extensive necrosis regions in the tumor tissue of the treated animals, corroborating the proposal that the induction of inflammation, in this model, may contribute to the inhibition of tumor progression. However, we also observed a reduction in Mcpt6 levels in the microenvironment of solid Ehrlich tumors, indicating a reduction in mast cell activity in the tumors. Thus, apparently, the observed inhibitory effect from inflammation may be associated with the increased activity of other cell types that make up the immune system, which may be the target of future investigations.

4. Materials and Methods

4.1. Standardization of the Herbal Extract and Obtaining Fractions

The research is registered in the National Genetic Heritage and Associated Traditional Knowledge Management System (SisGen), Brazil, Registration AD8BA6B.

The leaves of *G. brasiliensis* were collected for exsiccates and deposited in the herbarium Irina Delanova Gemtchujnicov (BOTU nº 33511). After cleaning and drying the material, the extracts were obtained by percolation with 20 g of crushed leaves in 100 mL of 70% alcohol for 24 h [18]. The alcohol was rotaevaporated at 45 °C at reduced pressure, avoiding loss of material properties and obtaining the crude extract (CE). The extract was then diluted to a concentration of 10% (10 μg/mL) and stored in an amber vial. The solvent, ethyl acetate, was mixed with the CE at a 1:1 ratio for 24 h to obtain the organic fraction. The solvent was eliminated by evaporation and the organic portion of the fraction was re-eluted in filtered water, obtaining the ethyl acetate fraction (EAF) at a 10% concentration (7.5 μg/mL).

4.2. In Vitro Cytotoxicity Analysis (Hemolysis Assay)

The cytotoxicities of CE and EAF were evaluated in this investigation by the study of hemolysis. Glycosylated solution (5%) of human blood (4%) was mixed with CE and EAF at concentrations of 5%, 10%, 20% and 50%. For the positive control, 1 mL of the red blood cell suspension and 1 mL of 10% triton were added, and, for the negative control, 1 mL of the red blood cell suspension and 1 mL of glycosylated solution were added. Samples and controls were taken to the water bath at 37 °C for 15 min with subsequent centrifugation at 1500 rpm for 5 min. Finally, the samples were read in the spectrophotometer (Kasuaki IL-592-LC, Wuxi, Jiangsu, China) at 540 nm after zeroing the equipment with glycosylated solution [18]. Determinations were performed in triplicate. The IC_{50} of EC and EAF was calculated using the average of the measurements for each sample.

4.3. Free Radical Scavenging Capacity

DPPH was used to determine the free radical scavenging capacity of the extracts [11,18,21–23]. For this analysis, CE and EAF were used, both at a 10% concentration. After adding DPPH solution at 2.4 mg/100 mL, the samples were kept protected from light for 30 min for later reading in a spectrophotometer (Kasuaki IL-592-LC) at 520 nm. As a positive control, the standard antioxidant BHT was used. In the negative control, BHT, CE and EAF were omitted. Determinations were performed in triplicate. The percentage of DPPH radical elimination was estimated, according to the expression below.

$$\text{DPPH Scavenging (\%)} = \frac{\text{negative control absorbance} - \text{sample absorbance}}{\text{negative control absorbance}} \times 100$$

4.4. Analysis of Total Flavonoid and Total Polyphenol Content

To determine the total flavonoid content in CE at 10% concentration and EAF at 10% concentration, quercetin (Q4951—Sigma Aldrich, Cotia, São Paulo, Brazil) was used to generate the standard curve (serial dilution from 25 µg/mL to 1.56 µg/mL). A mixture of 1 mL of different concentrations of the curve or 1 mL of the samples added to 1 mL of 2% aluminum chloride ($AlCl_3$) alcoholic solution was read at 415 nm in the spectrophotometer (Kasuaki IL-592-LC) [12,57].

The total polyphenol content in CE at 10% concentration and EAF at 10% concentration, was evaluated with Folin–Ciocalteu reagent [12,57], using galic acid (1274—Dinâmica, Indaiatuba, São Paulo, Brazil) for the construction of the standard curve (20; 15; 10; 5; 2.5 µg/mL). Sodium carbonate ($NaCO_3$) (1.5 mL) and Folin–Ciocalteu reagent (0.5 mL) were added to the samples, and the absorbance was read at 760 nm using the spectrophotometer (Kasuaki IL-592-LC).

4.5. Ehrlich Tumors and Treatments

Male Balb/c mice aged six to eight weeks (weight between 20 and 30 g) were obtained from the Didatic and Experimental Research Unit of the Padre Albino University Center (UNIFIPA). The animals were kept in cages in an environment with controlled temperature (24° to 25 °C) with water and food ad libitum. The experimental procedures were carried out in accordance with the rules of the Ethics Committees for the Use of Animals (CEUA-UNIFESP, certificate of approval nº 7189031221, and CEUA-UNIFIPA, certificate of approval nº 15/21) and under veterinary supervision.

The animals were divided into 12 groups (n = 8/group) as follows: control animals treated with saline solution 0,9% for 7 (C 7) and 14 (C 14) days; non-induced animals treated with CE at 10% concentration and EAF at 10% concentration for 7 days (CE 7, EAF 7) and 14 days (CE 14, EAF 14); animals induced with ascitic Ehrlich tumors treated with saline solution 0.9% for 7 days (EA); animals with solid Ehrlich tumors treated with saline solution 0.9% for 14 days (ES); animals induced with ascitic Ehrlich tumors treated with CE at a 10% concentration (EA/CE) and EAF at a 10% concentration (EA/EAF) for 7 days; and animals induced with solid Ehrlich tumors treated with CE at a 10% concentration (ES/CE) and EAF at a 10% concentration (ES/EAF) for 14 days (Figure 13).

For the induction of the tumor in its ascitic form, the animals were inoculated intraperitoneally with ascitic fluid from previously induced animals. The injection was applied into the left lower quadrant and the cells amount inoculated was 0.5 mL (2×10^6 cell/mL) [58]. For the solid form of the Ehrlich tumor, the inoculation of neoplastic cells was subcutaneous above the thigh in the same amount of 0.5 mL (2×10^6 cell/mL) [59].

The induced animals were treated intramuscularly with 0.5 mL of CE or EAF 10% concentration, selected according to a previous study by our research group [18] and corroborated in this investigation by hemolysis assay. The treatments were started on the same day as the induction of the tumors and were continued through daily applications into the thigh region until the seventh day for the ascitic tumors [60,61] and fourteenth day for the solid tumors [62].

The animals were euthanized by an overdose of anesthetic one day after the end of the treatment protocols. Figure 14 summarizes the analyses used in this investigation.

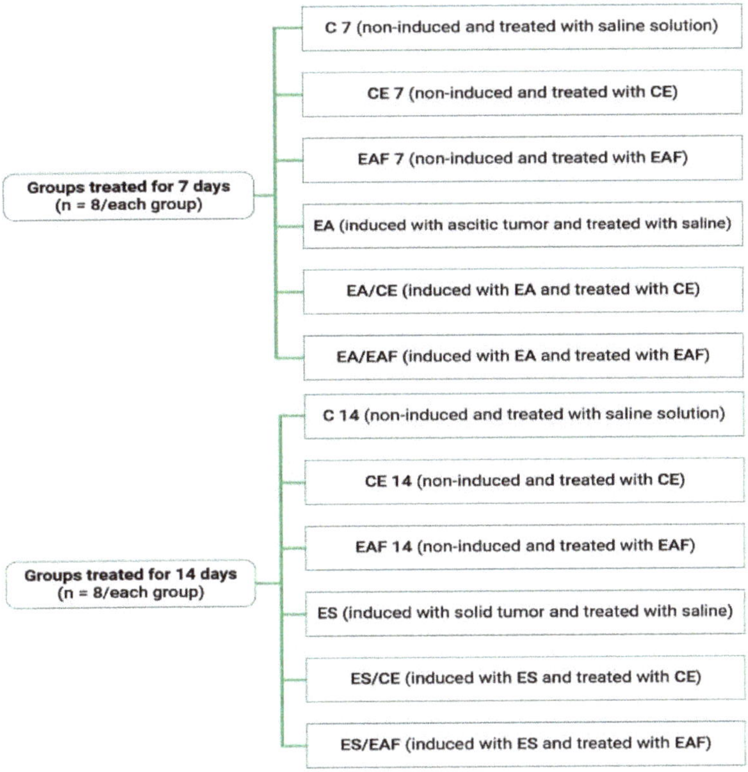

Figure 13. Groups of animals that were non-induced and induced with Ehrlich ascitic and solid tumors and were treated for 7 days and 14 days.

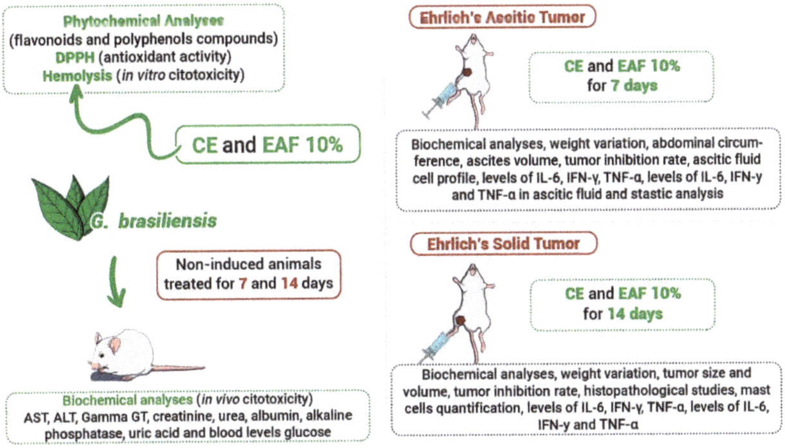

Figure 14. Schematic summary of the assessments used in this investigation.

4.6. In Vivo Cytotoxicity Analysis (Biochemical Analysis of Blood)

To evaluate the in vivo cytotoxicity of CE and EAF treatments in non-induced and tumor-induced animals, the levels of alanine aminotransferase (ALT), aspartate aminotransferase (AST), gamma glutamyl transferase (Gamma GT), creatinine, urea, albumin, alkaline phosphatase, uric acid and blood glucose were measured. After euthanasia, blood was collected by cardiac puncture in heparinized syringes. After that, it was centrifuged at 7000 rpm for 15 min and the blood plasma was separated into aliquots for the analyses with commercial kits (Ortho Clinical Diagnostics, Vitros Chemistry System, San Diego, CA, USA), according to the manufacturer's instructions.

4.7. Evaluation of Tumor Growth by Body Weight Variation in Ascitic and Solid Tumor

The variation in body weight was given by the difference between the final measurement (after the last day of treatment) and the initial measurement (before the start of treatment). The results are expressed in grams [62]. The percentage of inhibition of tumor growth is determined by the formula below:

$$\%\text{ Tumor Growth Inhibition} = \frac{\Delta\text{BW tumor group} - \Delta\text{BW treated group}}{\Delta\text{BW tumor group}} \times 100$$

where ΔBW is the variation in body weight.

4.8. Evaluation of Tumor Growth by Abdominal Circumference Variation in Ascitic Tumor

The variation in the abdominal circumference measurement was calculated by the difference between the final measurement and the initial measurement, and the results were expressed in centimeters [62]. The percentage of inhibition of tumor growth is calculated according to the formula below:

$$\%\text{ Tumor Growth Inhibition} = \frac{\Delta\text{CA tumor group} - \Delta\text{CA treated group}}{\Delta\text{CA tumor group}} \times 100$$

where ΔCA is the variation in abdominal circumference

For both growth evaluation techniques, the antitumor activity was classified according to the percentage of tumor growth inhibition as follows: absent = percentage of tumor inhibition is equal to 0; mild = percentage of tumor inhibition is $\leq$30%; moderate = percentage of tumor inhibition is $\geq$30–50%; high = percentage of tumor inhibition is >50% [62].

4.9. Evaluation of Tumor Growth by Ascites Volume

After euthanasia, ascitic fluid was aspirated from the peritoneal cavity of mice with ascitic tumors using a 5 mL syringe, and the volume was measured using a graduated centrifuge tube in mL [62].

4.10. Evaluation of Tumor Volume in Solid Tumors

The animals were weighed daily, and the size of the tumor measured with a caliper was determined by the following formula:

Tumor volume: $0.5 \times D \times d^2$ mm^3. Here, D is the major diameter of the tumor and d the minor measured thickness [63,64].

4.11. Fixation, Processing and Inclusion for Light Microscopy and Histopathological Analyses

After the excision of the tumor mass, the fragments were fixed in 4% formaldehyde for 24 h and dehydrated in increasing series of ethanol, then diaphanized with xylol and included in paraffin (Lupetec, São Carlos, São Paulo, Brazil). The 3 µm sections were obtained by microtome (MRP2016SA, Lupetec, São Carlos, São Paulo, Brazil) and stained with Hematoxylin–Eosin for histopathological analyses.

The areas of necrosis were measured in different fields in the 10× objective (Leica microscope, DM500, Wetzlar, Germany), using the Leica Image Analysis software (LAS V4.0). Values are presented as mean ± SEM of the mm^2 area obtained in the different experimental groups.

For the microscopic analysis of mast cells, 3 μm sections were stained with Toluidine blue. Mast cells were identified due to their metachromatic cytoplasmic granules. The quantification of mast cells was performed in different images per slide obtained by 10× objective and the values are expressed as number of cells per mm^2.

4.12. Levels of the Cytokines IL-6, INF-γ and TNF-α by Magpix Assay

Inflammatory mediators (IL-6, INF-γ, TNF-α) were assessed using the MILLIPLEX MAP MCYTOMAG 70K kit and the LUMINEX xMAP MAGPIX instrument (Luminex, Austin, TX, USA) for the quantitative multiplex detection of multiple analytes, with speed and specificity, by means of magnetic beads. Tissue samples underwent processing, with tumor fragments macerated in liquid nitrogen for ES analysis. The ascitic fluid was centrifuged for EA analysis. Additionally, samples were treated with protease inhibitors and phosphatases. Components, including magnetic beads, controls, buffer, serum and standards, were prepared following kit instructions.

In a 96-well magnetic plate, 25 μL of standards, controls and samples were added, along with assay buffer, standards medium and magnetic beads coated with antibodies. The plate was sealed and incubated for 2 h at room temperature with agitation. Subsequent steps involved washing, incubation with detection antibodies, the addition of phycoerythrin conjugated to streptavidin and additional washing before incubation with fluid. Plate readings were performed using the LUMINEX xMAP MAGPIX, and analyte concentrations were determined using the MAGPIX xPONENT software (V4.2 NCM, Luminex, Austin, Texas, USA).

4.13. Western Blotting

Proteins from both EA tumor cells and ES tumor tissue were extracted using RIPA buffer (Thermo Fisher Scientific #89900, Waltham, MA, USA), supplemented with protease inhibitor (Roche #CO-RO, Basileia, Suíça) and phosphatase inhibitor (Roche #PHOSS-RO) to prevent protein degradation. The protein concentration of each sample was determined using the Qubit system (#Q33211 Quanti-iT Protein Assay Kit, Thermo Fisher Scientific). Samples containing 30 μg of total protein were separated using SDS-PAGE on a 12% gel and subsequently transferred to a nitrocellulose membrane. To prevent nonspecific binding, the membranes were blocked using a 5% solution of bovine serum albumin (BSA, Sigma-Aldrich) for a duration of 2 h. Following blocking, the membranes were incubated overnight at 4 °C with primary antibodies: goat anti-Mcpt6 Clone 286820 (R&DSystem #MAB3736, Mineápolis, MN, USA, 1:1000), rabbit anti-Bax (Abclonal #A0207, Woburn, MA, USA 1:500), and mouse anti-β-actin, clone AC-74 (Sigma-Aldrich #A2228, 1:2000). The β-actin marker was used to normalize the experiment. After incubation with primary antibodies, the membranes were washed thrice with T-TBS for 10 min each time. Subsequently, they were incubated at room temperature for 2 h with horseradish peroxidase-conjugated secondary antibodies: goat, mouse or rabbit IgG (1:3000), used for chemiluminescence detection (SuperSignal West Pico Chemiluminescent Substrate, Thermo Fisher Scientific #34578). The chemiluminescent signal was captured using UVITEC equipment (UVITEC, Cambridge, UK). For quantification, the density of the bands was analyzed utilizing ImageJ 1.53k (NIH). The ratio of the protein of interest to the housekeeping protein B-actin was calculated in order to determine relative expression levels.

4.14. Statistical Analysis

The results obtained were previously submitted to descriptive analysis and determination of normality. Data are presented as means ± SEM for normally distributed data and medians for non-normally distributed data. To assess normality, the Shapiro–Wilk test was performed. As the groups showed normal distribution, an ANOVA with Tukey's post-test for multiple comparisons was employed. Data analysis was conducted using GraphPad Prism 9.0.0, utilizing either the mean or median as appropriate. Statistical significance was considered to be $p < 0.05$. Figure 14 summarizes the analyses used in this investigation.

5. Conclusions

Our results indicate that treatments with CE and EAF, both at a 10% concentration, were able to regulate the metabolic imbalance caused by the tumor and inhibit the growth of ascitic and solid Ehrlich tumors by inducing apoptosis and modulating mast cells and the cytokines IL-6 and TNF-α. These findings will encourage the development of new studies to deepen the understanding of the antitumor effects of *G. brasiliensis* extracts.

Author Contributions: Conceptualization, L.S.S. and A.P.G.; methodology, validation, formal analyses, investigation, L.S.S., E.C., R.A.d.S., M.S., A.H.Y., T.S., B.H., P.C., L.P.d.S.F., H.P.D.M., C.D.G. and A.P.G.; writing—original draft preparation L.S.S., E.C., R.A.d.S., M.S., A.H.Y., L.P.d.S.F., C.D.G. and A.P.G.; writing—review and editing, L.S.S., M.d.L.G.P. and A.P.G.; resources, funding acquisition, A.P.G. All authors have read and agreed to the published version of the manuscript.

Funding: This research was funded by the Padre Albino University Center (UNIFIPA), grant numbers PESQMED2022996 and PESQPIN20221010 (A.P.G.); and Project CICECO-Aveiro Institute of Materials, UIDB/50011/2020, UIDP/50011/2020, and LA/P/0006/2020, financed by national funds through the FCT/MEC (PIDDAC).

Institutional Review Board Statement: The local Institutional Review Board approved the study protocol and was performed in accord with the Ethics Committees for the Use of Animals (CEUA-UNIFESP, certificate of approval nº 7189031221, and CEUA-UNIFIPA, certificate of approval nº 15/21).

Informed Consent Statement: Not applicable.

Data Availability Statement: The data used and analyzed in this study are available from the corresponding authors upon reasonable requests. The data are not publicly available due to institutional policy.

Acknowledgments: The authors thank the Multiuser Laboratory of the Faculty of Medicine of São José do Rio Preto (FAMERP)/SP for permission and support in the use of the Equipment LUMINEX xMAP MAGPIX; Vítor Afonso Favaretto for his assistance in histopathological analyses Andressa Fernanda Araújo Ferreira for her assistance in the handling of the animals.

Conflicts of Interest: The authors declare no conflicts of interest.

References

1. Meera, R.; Chidambaranathan, N. Anticancer Activity of Ethanolic Extract of *Crataeva magna* Lour (DC) against Ehrlich Ascitic Carcinoma Cell Lines in Mice. *J. Pharm. Sci. Res.* **2017**, *9*, 1869–1873.
2. Hassapour, S.H.; Dehghani, M. Review of cancer from perspective of molecular. *J. Cancer Res. Pract.* **2017**, *4*, 27–129.
3. Ozaslan, M.; Karagoz, I.D.; Kilic, I.H.; Guldur, M.E. Ehrlich ascites carcinoma. *Afr. J. Biotechnol.* **2011**, *10*, 2375–2378.
4. Doroshow, J.H. Mechanisms of Anthracycline-Enhanced Reactive Oxygen Metabolism in Tumor Cells. *Oxidative Med. Cell. Longev.* **2019**, *2019*, 9474823. [CrossRef] [PubMed]
5. Feitosa, I.B.; Mori, B.; Teles, C.B.G.; da Costa, A.G. What are the immune responses during the growth of Ehrlich's tumor in ascitic and solid form? *Life Sci.* **2021**, *264*, 118578. [CrossRef] [PubMed]
6. Nurgali, K.; Jagoe, R.T.; Abalo, R. Editorial: Adverse effects of cancer chemotherapy: Anything new to improve tolerance and reduce sequelae? *Front. Pharmacol.* **2018**, *9*, 245. [CrossRef] [PubMed]
7. Boccolini, P.d.M.M.; Boccolini, C.S. Prevalence of complementary and alternative medicine (CAM) use in Brazil. *BMC Complement. Med. Ther.* **2020**, *20*, 51.
8. Santo, B.L.S.d.E.; Santana, L.F.; Junior, W.H.K.; de Araújo, F.d.O.; Bogo, D.; Freitas, K.d.C.; Guimarães, R.d.C.A.; Hiane, P.A.; Pott, A.; Filiú, W.F.d.O.; et al. Medicinal Potential of Garcinia Species and Their Compounds. *Molecules* **2020**, *25*, 4513. [CrossRef]
9. Hemshekhar, M.; Sunitha, K.; Santhosh, M.S.; Devajara, S.; Kemparaju, K.; Vishwanath, B.S.; Niranjana, S.R.; Girish, K.S. An overview on genus garcinia: Phytochemical and therapeutical aspects. *Phytochem. Rev.* **2011**, *10*, 325–351. [CrossRef]

10. Kumar, S.; Sharma, S.; Chattopadhyay, S.K. The potential health benefit of polyisoprenylated benzophenones from Garcinia and related genera: Ethnobotanical and therapeutic importance. *Fitoterapia* **2013**, *89*, 86–125. [CrossRef]
11. Naves, V.M.L.; dos Santos, M.H.; Ribeiro, I.S.; da Silva, C.A.; Silva, N.C.; da Silva, G.A.; Dias, A.L.T.; Ionta, M.; Dias, D.F. Antimicrobial and antioxidant activity of *Garcinia brasiliensis* extracts. *S. Afr. J. Bot.* **2019**, *124*, 244–250. [CrossRef]
12. Figueiredo, S.A.; Vilela, F.M.P.; da Silva, C.A.; Cunha, T.M.; dos Santos, M.H.; Fonseca, M.J.V. In vitro and in vivo photoprotective/photochemopreventive potential of *Garcinia brasiliensis* epicarp extract. *J. Photochem. Photobiol. B Biol.* **2014**, *131*, 65–73. [CrossRef]
13. Gontijo, V.S.; de Souza, T.C.; Rosa, I.A.; Soares, M.G.; da Silva, M.A.; Vilegas, W.; Júnior, C.V.; dos Santos, M.H. Isolation and evaluation of the antioxidant activity of phenolic constituents of the *Garcinia brasiliensis* epicarp. *Food Chem.* **2012**, *132*, 1230–1235. [CrossRef]
14. Moreira, M.E.d.C.; Araújo, F.d.O.; de Sousa, A.R.; Toledo, R.C.L.; Benjamin, L.d.A.; Veloso, M.P.; Reis, K.d.S.; dos Santos, M.H.; Martino, H.S.D. Bacupari peel extracts (*Garcinia brasiliensis*) reduces the biometry, lipogenesis and hepatic steatosis in obese rats. *Food Res. Int.* **2018**, *114*, 169–177. [CrossRef] [PubMed]
15. Naldoni, F.J.; Claudino, A.L.R.; Cruz, J.W., Jr.; Chavasco, J.K.; Faria e Silva, P.M.; Veloso, M.P.; dos Santos, M.H. Antimicrobial activity of benzophenones and extracts from the fruits of *Garcinia bras. J. Med. Food* **2009**, *12*, 403–407. [CrossRef] [PubMed]
16. Pereira, I.O.; Assis, D.M.; Juliano, M.A.; Cunha, R.L.O.R.; Barbieri, C.L.; do Sacramento, L.V.S.; Marques, M.J.; dos Santos, M.H. Natural products from *Garcinia brasiliensis* as Leishmania protease inhibitors. *J. Med. Food* **2011**, *14*, 557–562. [CrossRef]
17. Santa-Cecília, F.V.; Vilela, F.C.; da Rocha, C.Q.; Dias, D.F.; Cavalcante, G.P.; Freitas, L.A.S.; dos Santos, M.H.; Giusti-Paiva, A. Anti-inflammatory and antinociceptive effects of *Garcinia brasiliensis*. *J. Ethnopharmacol.* **2011**, *133*, 467–473. [CrossRef] [PubMed]
18. Souza, H.R.; Zucoloto, A.R.; Francisco, I.T.P.; Rays, H.P.; Tinti, N.P.; Matta, N.J.D.; Guandalini, R.B.; Yoshikawa, A.H.; da Silva, J.M.; Possebon, L.; et al. Evaluation of the healing properties of *Garcinia brasiliensis* extracts in a cutaneous wound model. *J. Ethnopharmacol.* **2022**, *295*, 115334. [CrossRef]
19. Ionta, M.; Ferreira-Silva, G.A.; Niero, E.L.; Costa, E.D.M.; Martens, A.A.; Rosa, W.; Soares, M.G.; Machado-Santelli, G.M.; Lago, J.H.G.; dos Santos, M.H. 7-Epiclusianone, a benzophenone extracted from *Garcinia brasiliensis* (Clusiaceae), induces cell cycle arrest in G1/S transition in A549 cells. *Molecules* **2015**, *20*, 12804–12816. [CrossRef] [PubMed]
20. Sales, L.; Pezuk, J.A.; Borges, K.S.; Brassesco, M.S.; Scrideli, C.A.; Tone, L.G.; dos Santos, M.H.; Ionta, M.; de Oliveira, J.C. Anticancer activity of 7-epiclusianone, a benzophenone from *Garcinia brasiliensis*, in glioblastoma. *BMC Complement. Altern. Med.* **2015**, *15*, 393. [CrossRef]
21. Dudonné, S.; Vitrac, X.; Coutière, P.; Woillez, M.; Mérillon, J.M. Comparative study of antioxidant properties and total phenolic content of 30 plant extracts of industrial interest using DPPH, ABTS, FRAP, SOD, and ORAC assays. *J. Agric. Food Chem.* **2009**, *57*, 1768–1774. [CrossRef] [PubMed]
22. Yamauchi, M.; Kitamura, Y.; Nagano, H.; Kawatsu, J.; Gotoh, H. DPPH Measurements and Structure-Activity Relationship Studies on the Antioxidant Capacity of Phenols. *Antioxidants* **2024**, *13*, 309. [CrossRef]
23. Rumpf, J.; Burger, R.; Schulze, M. Statistical evaluation of DPPH, ABTS, FRAP, and Folin-Ciocalteu assays to assess the antioxidant capacity of lignins. *Int. J. Biol. Macromol.* **2023**, *233*, 123470. [CrossRef]
24. Chikara, S.; Nagaprashantha, L.D.; Singhal, J.; Horne, D.; Awasthi, S.; Singhal, S.S. Oxidative stress and dietary phytochemicals: Role in cancer chemoprevention and treatment. *Cancer Lett.* **2018**, *413*, 122–134. [CrossRef] [PubMed]
25. Dias, M.C.; Pinto, D.C.G.A.; Silva, A.M. Plant flavonoids: Chemical characteristics and biological activity. *Molecules* **2021**, *26*, 5377. [CrossRef]
26. Shen, N.; Wang, T.; Gan, Q.; Liu, S.; Wang, L.; Jin, B. Plant flavonoids: Classification, distribution, biosynthesis, and antioxidant activity. *Food Chem.* **2022**, *383*, 132531. [CrossRef] [PubMed]
27. da Silva, C.A.; Rosa, I.A.; de Souza, T.C.; dos Santos, M.H. Evaluating four modes of extraction to analyze bioactive compounds in *Garcinia brasiliensis* (bacupari) by high-performance liquid chromatography diode-array detection (HPLC-DAD). *Nat. Prod. Res.* **2020**, *35*, 4073–4077. [CrossRef] [PubMed]
28. Zan, R.A.; Fernandes, A.; Jedoz, S.; Oludemi, T.; Calhelha, R.C.; Pires, T.C.S.P.; Alves, M.J.; Martins, R.C.C.; Barros, L.; Ferreira, I.C.F.R. Bioactive properties and phytochemical assessment of Bacupari-anão (*Garcinia brasiliensis* Mart.) leaves native to Rondônia, Brazil. *Food Funct.* **2018**, *9*, 5621–5628. [CrossRef]
29. de Melo, A.M.; Costa, B.P.; Ikeda, M.; Ribani, R.H. Identification of bioactive compounds, morphology, and nutritional composition of bacupari (*Garcinia brasiliensis* (Mart)) pulp powder in two stages of maturation—A short communication. *Food Chem.* **2022**, *391*, 133279. [CrossRef] [PubMed]
30. Medhat, D.; Hussein, J.; El-Naggar, M.E.; Attia, M.F.; Anwar, M.; Latif, Y.A.; Booles, H.F.; Morsy, S.; Farrag, A.R.; Khalil, W.K.B.; et al. Effect of Au-dextran NPs as anti-tumor agent against EAC and solid tumor in mice by biochemical evaluations and histopathological investigations. *Biomed. Pharmacother.* **2017**, *91*, 1006–1016. [CrossRef]

31. El-Benhawy, S.A.; Fahmy, E.I.; Mahdy, S.M.; Khedr, G.H.; Sarhan, A.S.; Nafady, M.H.; Selim, Y.A.Y.; Salem, T.M.; Abu-Samra, N.; El-Khadry, H.A. Assessment of thyroid gland hormones and ultrasonographic abnormalities in medical staff occupationally exposed to ionizing radiation. *BMC Endocr. Disord.* **2022**, *22*, 287. [CrossRef] [PubMed]
32. Sookoian, S.; Pirola, C.J. Systematic review with meta-analysis: Risk factors for non-alcoholic fatty liver disease suggest a shared altered metabolic and cardiovascular profile between lean and obese patients. *Aliment. Pharmacol. Ther.* **2017**, *46*, 85–95. [CrossRef] [PubMed]
33. Adami, E.R.; Corso, C.R.; Turin-Oliveira, N.M.; Galindo, C.M.; Milani, L.; Stipp, M.C.; do Nascimento, G.E.; Chequin, A.; da Silva, L.M.; de Andrade, S.F.; et al. Antineoplastic effect of pectic polysaccharides from green sweet pepper (*Capsicum annuum*) on mammary tumor cells in vivo and in vitro. *Carbohydr. Polym.* **2018**, *201*, 280–292. [CrossRef] [PubMed]
34. Salem, M.L.; Shoukry, N.M.; Teleb, W.K.; Abdel-Daim, M.M.; Abdel-Rahman, M.A. In vitro and in vivo antitumor effects of the Egyptian scorpion *Androctonus amoreuxi* venom in an Ehrlich ascites tumor model. *Springerplus* **2016**, *10*, 570. [CrossRef] [PubMed]
35. Abd-Elghany, A.A.; Mohamad, E.A.; El-Sakhawy, M.A.; Mansouri, S.; Ismail, S.H.; Elneklawi, M.S. Enhancement of mechanical properties of chitosan film by doping with sage extract-loaded niosomes. *Mater. Res. Express* **2022**, *9*, 035006. [CrossRef]
36. Albalawi, A.E.; Althobaiti, N.A.; Alrdahe, S.S.; Alhasani, R.H.; Alaryani, F.S.; BinMowyna, M.N. Antitumor Activity of Royal Jelly and Its Cellular Mechanisms against Ehrlich Solid Tumor in Mice. *BioMed Res. Int.* **2022**, *11*, 7233997. [CrossRef]
37. Hanigan, M.H. Gamma-Glutamyl transpeptidase, a glutathionase: Its expression and function in carcinogenesis. *Chem. -Biol. Interact.* **1998**, *111–112*, 333–342. [CrossRef]
38. Al Abdan, M. Alfa-lipoic acid controls tumor growth and modulates hepatic redox state in Ehrlich-ascites-carcinoma-bearing mice. *Sci. World J.* **2012**, *2012*, 509838. [CrossRef]
39. Calixto-Campos, C.; Corrêa, M.P.; Carvalho, T.T.; Zarpelon, A.C.; Hohmann, M.S.N.; Rossaneis, A.C.; Coelho-Silva, L.; Pavanelli, W.R.; Pinge-Filho, P.; Crespigio, J.; et al. Quercetin Reduces Ehrlich Tumor-Induced Cancer Pain in Mice. *Anal. Cell. Pathol.* **2015**, *2015*, 285708. [CrossRef] [PubMed]
40. Islam, M.S.; Jahangir, C.A.; Rahi, M.S.; Hasan, M.M.; Sajib, S.A.; Hoque, K.M.F.; Reza, M.A. In-vivo antiproliferative activity of *Morus latifolia* leaf and bark extracts against Ehrlich's ascites carcinoma. *Toxicol. Res.* **2020**, *36*, 79–88. [CrossRef] [PubMed]
41. Miyata, Y.; Araki, K.; Ohba, K.; Mastuo, T.; Nakamura, Y.; Yuno, T.; Mukai, Y.; Otsubo, A.; Mitsunari, K.; Mochizuki, Y.; et al. Oral intake of royal jelly improves anti-cancer effects and suppresses adverse events of molecular targeted therapy by regulating tnf-α and tgf-β in renal cell carcinoma: A preliminary study based on a randomized double-blind clinical trial. *Mol. Clin. Oncol.* **2020**, *13*, 1–8. [CrossRef] [PubMed]
42. Zhang, S.; Shao, Q.; Geng, H.; Su, S. The effect of royal jelly on the growth of breast cancer in mice. *Oncol. Lett.* **2017**, *14*, 7615–7621. [CrossRef] [PubMed]
43. Walyeldeen, A.A.; El-Shorbagy, H.M.; Hassaneen, H.M.; Abdelhamid, I.A.; Sabet, S.; Ibrahim, S.A. [1,2,4] Triazolo [3,4-a]isoquinoline chalcone derivative exhibits anticancer activity via induction of oxidative stress, DNA damage, and apoptosis in Ehrlich solid carcinoma-bearing mice. *Naunyn-Schmiedeberg's Arch. Pharmacol.* **2022**, *395*, 1225–1238. [CrossRef]
44. Sharawi, Z.W. Therapeutic effect of arthrocnemum machrostachyum methanolic extract on ehrlich solid tumor in mice. *BMC Complement. Med. Ther.* **2020**, *20*, 153. [CrossRef]
45. Leal, P.d.C.; Moura, E.C.R.; Cosseti, R.J.D.; do Nascimento, J.R.; Serra, I.C.P.B.; Ribeiro, B.d.P.; Vale, A.A.M.; dos Santos, A.P.S.d.A.; do Nascimento, F.R.F.; Sakata, R.K. High dose gabapentin does not alter tumor growth in mice but reduces arginase activity and increases superoxide dismutase, IL-6 and MCP-1 levels in Ehrlich ascites. *BMC Res. Notes* **2019**, *12*, 59.
46. Orsolic, N.; Kunstíc, M.; Kukolj, M.; Odeh, D.; Ancíc, D. Natural phenolic acid, product of the honey bee, for the control of oxidative stress, peritoneal angiogenesis, and tumor growth in mice. *Molecules* **2011**, *25*, 5583. [CrossRef]
47. Molotkov, A.; Satoh, M.; Tohyama, C. Tumor growth and food intake in interleukin-6 gene knock-out mice. *Cancer Lett.* **1998**, *132*, 187–192. [CrossRef]
48. da Silva, R.J.; da Silva, M.G.; Vilela, L.C.; Fecchio, D. Cytokine profile of Ehrlich ascites tumor treated with Bothrops jararaca venom. *Res. Commun.* **2002**, *11*, 197–201. [CrossRef] [PubMed]
49. Gentile, L.B.; Queiroz-Hazarbassanov, N.; Massoco, C.d.O.; Fecchio, D. Modulation of cytokines production by indomethacin acute dose during the evolution of ehrlich ascites tumor in mice. *Mediat. Inflamm.* **2015**, *2015*, 924028. [CrossRef]
50. Corso, C.R.; Stipp, M.C.; Adami, E.R.; da Silva, L.M.; Mariott, M.; de Andrade, S.F.; Ramos, E.A.d.S.; Klassen, G.; Beltrame, O.C.; Queiroz-Telles, J.E.; et al. *Salvia lachnostachys* Benth has antitumor and chemopreventive effects against solid *Ehrlich carcinoma*. *Mol. Biol. Rep.* **2019**, *46*, 4827–4841. [CrossRef] [PubMed]
51. Cruceriu, D.; Baldasici, O.; Balacescu, O.; Berindan-Neagoe, I. The dual role of tumor necrosis factor-alpha (TNF-α) in breast cancer: Molecular insights and therapeutic approaches. *Cell. Oncol.* **2020**, *43*, 1–18. [CrossRef] [PubMed]
52. Aponte-López, A.; Muñoz-Cruz, S. Mast Cells in the Tumor Microenvironment. *Adv. Exp. Med. Biol.* **2020**, *1273*, 159–173. [PubMed]

53. Ribatti, D.; Annese, T.; Tamma, R. Controversial role of mast cells in breast cancer tumor progression and angiogenesis. *Clin. Breast Cancer* **2021**, *21*, 486–491. [CrossRef]
54. Majorini, M.T.; Colombo, M.P.; Lecis, D. Few, but Efficient: The Role of Mast Cells in Breast Cancer and Other Solid Tumors. *Cancer Res.* **2022**, *82*, 1439–1447. [CrossRef] [PubMed]
55. Gou, L.; Yue, G.G.-L.; Puno, P.T.; Lau, C.B.S. A review on the relationship of mast cells and macrophages in breast cancer—Can herbs or natural products facilitate their anti-tumor effects? *Pharmacol. Res.* **2021**, *164*, 105321. [CrossRef]
56. Ibrahim, S.S.A.; El-Aal, S.A.A.; Reda, A.M.; El-Alchy, S.; Shahine, Y. Anti-neoplastic action of Cimetidine/Vitamin C on histamine and the PI3K/AKT/mTOR pathway in Ehrlich breast cancer. *Sci. Rep.* **2022**, *12*, 11514. [CrossRef]
57. Arwa, P.S.; Zeraik, M.L.; Ximenes, V.F.; da Fonseca, L.M.; Bolzani, V.d.S.; Silva, D.H.S. Redox-active biflavonoids from Garcinia brasiliensis as inhibitors of neutrophil oxidative burst and human erythrocyte membrane damage. *J. Ethnopharmacol.* **2015**, *174*, 415–418.
58. Barua, A.; Choudhury, P.; Maity, J.K.; Mandal, S.B.; Mandal, S.; Saha, P. Chemotherapeutic potential of novel non-toxic nucleoside analogues on EAC ascitic tumour cells. *Free Radic. Res.* **2019**, *53*, 57–67. [CrossRef] [PubMed]
59. Morgan, H.J.N.; Delgado, A.Q.; Saldanha, L.L.; Camaforte, N.A.d.P.; Dokkedal, A.L.; Bosqueiro, J.R. *Vochysia tucanorum* Mart. butanol fraction presents antitumoral activity in vivo and prevents the installation of cachexia in solid Ehrlich tumor model. *BMC Complement. Med. Ther.* **2012**, *21*, 20. [CrossRef]
60. Yilmaz, S.; Ülger, H.; Ertekin, T.; Yay, A.H.; Nisari, M.; Alpa, S.; Acer, N. Investigating the anti-tumoral effect of curcumin on the mice in which Ehrlich ascites and solid tumor is created. *Iran. J. Basic Med. Sci.* **2019**, *22*, 418–425. [PubMed]
61. Bari, M.W.; Islam, A.; Islam, M.M.; Sultana, M.J.; Afroz, R.; Khan, M.M.R.; Parul, S.S.; Swaraz, A.M.; Hossain, M.I.; Islam, M.A. Determination of in vitro antioxidant activity and in vivo antineoplastic effects against Ehrlich ascites carcinoma of methanolic extract of *Sphagneticola calendulacea* (L.). *Pruski. Heliyon* **2021**, *7*, e07228. [CrossRef]
62. Saleh, N.; Allam, T.; Korany, R.M.S.; Abdelfattah, A.M.; Omran, A.M.; Eldaim, M.A.A.; Hassan, A.M.; El-Borai, N.B. Protective and Therapeutic Efficacy of Hesperidin versus Cisplatin against Ehrlich Ascites Carcinoma-Induced Renal Damage in Mice. *Pharmaceuticals* **2022**, *15*, 294. [CrossRef] [PubMed]
63. Jaganathan, S.K.; Mondhe, D.; Wani, Z.A.; Pal, H.C.; Mandal, M. Effect of honey and eugenol on Ehrlich ascites and solid carcinoma. *J. Biomed. Biotechnol.* **2010**, *2010*, 989163. [CrossRef]
64. Frajacomo, F.T.T.; Padilha, C.d.S.; Marinello, P.C.; Guarnier, F.A.; Cecchini, R.; Duarte, J.A.R.; Deminice, R. Solid Ehrlich carcinoma reproduces functional and biological characteristics of cancer cachexia. *Life Sci.* **2016**, *162*, 47–53. [CrossRef]

pharmaceuticals

MDPI

Review

The Dynamic Role of Curcumin in Mitigating Human Illnesses: Recent Advances in Therapeutic Applications

Md Shamshir Alam [1,*], Md Jamir Anwar [2,*], Manish Kumar Maity [3], Faizul Azam [4], Mariusz Jaremko [5] and Abdul-Hamid Emwas [6]

1 Department of Pharmacy Practice, College of Pharmacy, National University of Science and Technology, P.O. Box 620, Bosher, Muscat 130, Oman
2 Department of Pharmacology and Toxicology, College of Pharmacy, Qassim University, Buraydah 51452, Saudi Arabia
3 Department of Pharmacy Practice, MM College of Pharmacy, Maharishi Markandeshwar (Deemed to be University), Mullana, Ambala 133207, Haryana, India
4 Department of Medicinal Chemistry and Pharmacognosy, College of Pharmacy, Qassim University, Buraydah 51452, Saudi Arabia
5 Smart-Health Initiative (SHI) and Red Sea Research Center (RSRC), Division of Biological and Environmental Sciences and Engineering (BESE), King Abdullah University of Science and Technology (KAUST), Thuwal 23955, Saudi Arabia
6 Core Labs, King Abdullah University of Science and Technology (KAUST), Thuwal 23955, Saudi Arabia
* Correspondence: shamshir_pharma@yahoo.com (M.S.A.); m.anwar@qu.edu.sa (M.J.A.)

Abstract: Herbal medicine, particularly in developing regions, remains highly popular due to its cost-effectiveness, accessibility, and minimal risk of adverse effects. *Curcuma longa* L., commonly known as turmeric, exemplifies such herbal remedies with its extensive history of culinary and medicinal applications across Asia for thousands of years. Traditionally utilized as a dye, flavoring, and in cultural rituals, turmeric has also been employed to treat a spectrum of medical conditions, including inflammatory, bacterial, and fungal infections, jaundice, tumors, and ulcers. Building on this longstanding use, contemporary biochemical and clinical research has identified curcumin—the primary active compound in turmeric—as possessing significant therapeutic potential. This review hypothesizes that curcumin's antioxidant properties are pivotal in preventing and treating chronic inflammatory diseases, which are often precursors to more severe conditions, such as cancer, and neurological disorders, like Parkinson's and Alzheimer's disease. Additionally, while curcumin demonstrates a favorable safety profile, its anticoagulant effects warrant cautious application. This article synthesizes recent studies to elucidate the molecular mechanisms underlying curcumin's actions and evaluates its therapeutic efficacy in various human illnesses, including cancer, inflammatory bowel disease, osteoarthritis, atherosclerosis, peptic ulcers, COVID-19, psoriasis, vitiligo, and depression. By integrating diverse research findings, this review aims to provide a comprehensive perspective on curcumin's role in modern medicine and its potential as a multifaceted therapeutic agent.

Keywords: curcumin; turmeric; anti-inflammatory; anticancer; antibacterial; antifungal; antioxidant

1. Introduction

The utilization of plants as medicinal remedies has been a cornerstone of human health across diverse societies and civilizations throughout history [1,2]. *Curcuma longa* (*C. longa*), commonly known as turmeric, belongs to the *Zingiberaceae* family and is widely recognized for its diverse applications worldwide. Native to tropical South Asia, turmeric has been traditionally used as a dye, a cleansing agent (e.g., before marriage), a food additive (spice), and a medicine [3].

The structure of curcumin, supported by its synthesis, was published as early as 1910 by Miłobędzka and coworkers [4]. Later, Lampe [5] introduced another synthetic method in 1918. This multi-step process began with ethyl acetoacetate and carbomethoxyferuloyl as the primary reagents. Later, Pabon [6] developed a more efficient and straightforward synthesis with improved yields (Scheme 1). His method involved reacting acetyl acetone with boron trioxide (B_2O_3), substituted aromatic aldehydes, primary amine, and alkyl borate. With minor modifications, Pabon's synthetic approach has been widely adopted by researchers worldwide, forming the basis for most curcumin syntheses [7–10].

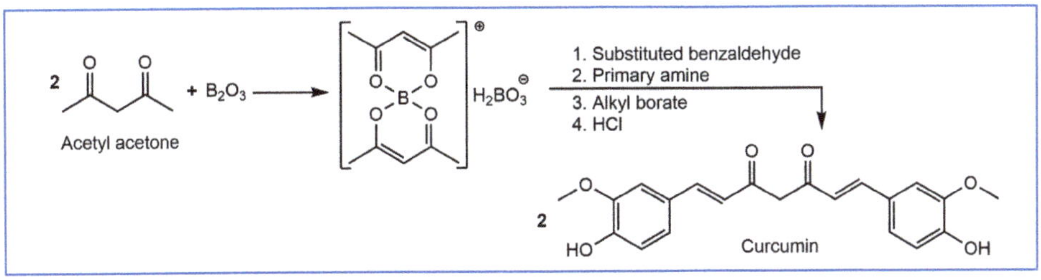

Scheme 1. Chemical synthesis of curcumin reported by Pabon [6].

Modern studies have confirmed that turmeric is very rich in antioxidants, which is in line with its historically known anti-inflammatory properties. Curcumin, the primary active compound in turmeric, along with other curcuminoids, such as dihydrocurcumin, tetrahydrocurcumin, bis-demethoxycurcumin, and demethoxycurcumin (Figure 1), has attracted considerable attention for its therapeutic potential [11–14]. These compounds have been extensively studied for their efficacy in preventing and treating a wide array of illnesses, including inflammatory diseases, cancer, diabetes, bacterial and fungal infections, ulcers, and liver and circulatory disorders, and as an anticoagulant agent (Figure 2) [11–14]. In addition, curcumin has been tested in clinical studies both alone and in conjunction with several other medications, including sulfasalazine, quercetin, piperine, lactoferrin, docetaxel, prednisone, gemcitabine, and pantoprazole [15].

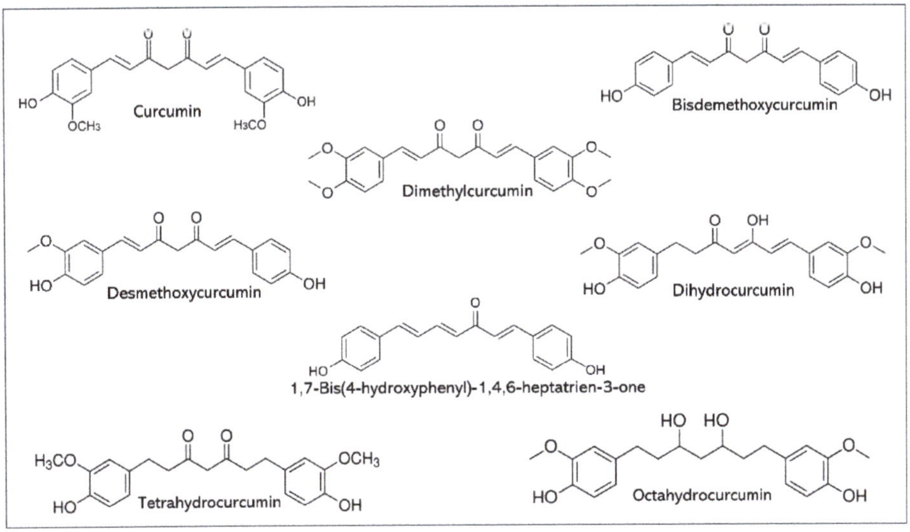

Figure 1. Chemical structure of curcuminoids isolated from turmeric.

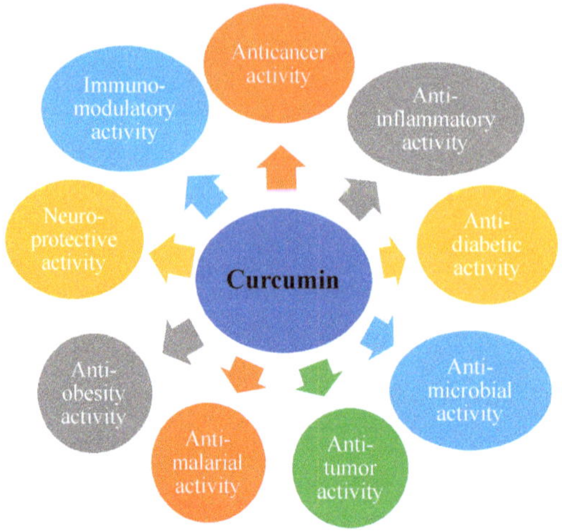

Figure 2. Summary overview of the pharmacological activities of curcumin.

Despite the promising therapeutic benefits demonstrated in both preclinical and clinical studies, the exact molecular mechanisms through which curcumin exerts its effects remain only partially understood. Curcumin's ability to modulate multiple cellular signaling pathways suggests a multifaceted mechanism of action, which may contribute to its effectiveness as both an adjuvant and alternative therapy [14,16]. For instance, clinical trials have shown that curcumin can decrease inflammatory markers and enhance antioxidant capacities in healthy individuals [17], improve circulation [18], chelate metals [19,20], and support neurogenesis [21], among other benefits.

This review hypothesizes that the diverse pharmacological characteristics of curcumin, especially its antioxidant and anti-inflammatory properties, are critical in influencing the fundamental disease mechanisms involved in a variety of human illnesses. By targeting multiple cellular pathways, curcumin has the potential to improve therapeutic outcomes when used alone or in combination with other therapies.

To explore this hypothesis, the following sections will provide an in-depth analysis of recent studies on curcumin, focusing on its molecular mechanisms of action and therapeutic applications in various human diseases, including cancer, inflammatory bowel disease, osteoarthritis, atherosclerosis, peptic ulcers, COVID-19, psoriasis, vitiligo, and depression. Additionally, the review will examine synergistic responses and the implications of curcumin in diverse pathogenesis by modulating a variety of biomolecules and mediators.

2. Preclinical and Clinical Evidence for Therapeutic Applications of Curcumin

2.1. Cancer

Curcumin demonstrates significant anticancer properties by modulating key molecular signaling pathways, leading to apoptosis and inhibiting tumor growth and metastasis [22]. It effectively suppresses NF-κB by inhibiting IkBs, thereby reducing the expression of pro-inflammatory genes, like TNF-α (Figure 3) [23,24]. Additionally, curcumin downregulates AP-1, which is associated with anti-apoptotic proteins, promoting cancer cell death [25]. By targeting the IL-6/STAT3 pathway, curcumin disrupts oncogenic signaling, further inhibiting tumorigenesis [26,27]. These mechanisms underscore curcumin's dual role as an anti-inflammatory and pro-apoptotic agent, enhancing its potential as both a standalone and adjunctive therapy across various cancer types, including pancreatic, prostate, breast, oral, lung, colorectal cancers, and multiple myeloma [28–30].

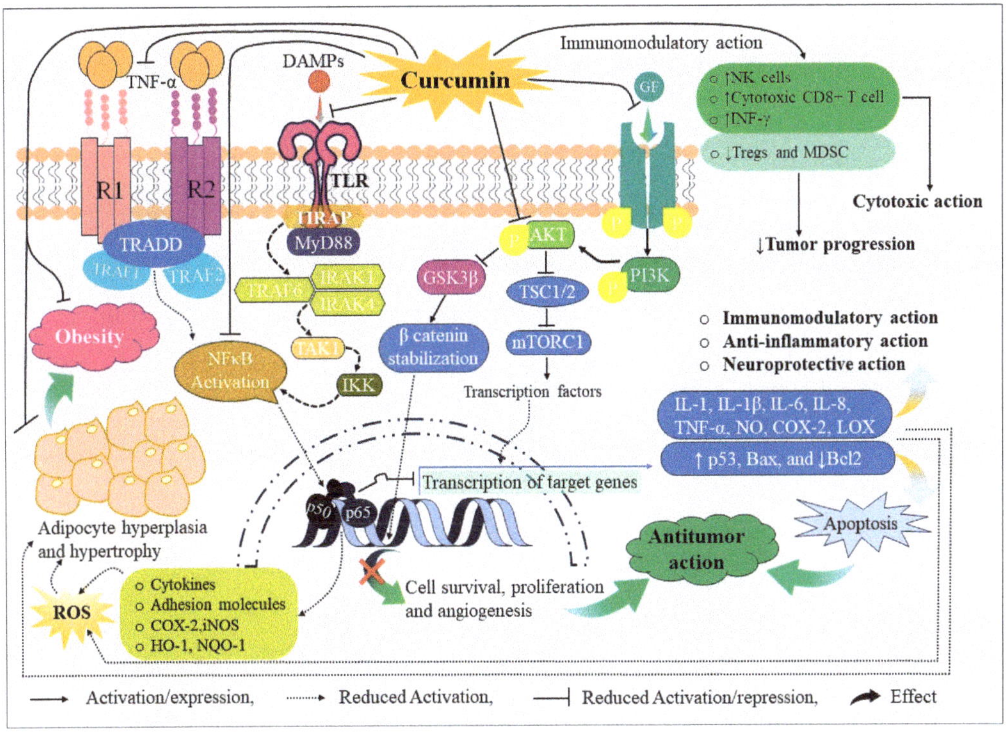

Figure 3. Multifaceted mechanism of action of curcumin in human illnesses. **Abbreviations:** AKT: protein kinase B; COX-2: cyclooxygenase-2; GF: growth factors; GSK 3β: glycogen synthase kinase-3 beta; HO-1: heme oxygenase-1; NQO-1: NAD(P)H quinone oxidoreductase 1; IL-1: interleukin-1 family, INF-γ: interferon gamma; iNOS: inducible nitric oxide synthase; LOX: lipoxygenases; MDSC: myeloid-derived suppressor cells; mTORC1: mammalian target of rapamycin complex 1; NFκB: nuclear factor kappa B; NK cells: natural killer cells; PI3K: phosphoinositide 3-kinase; TRADD: TNFR1-associated death domain protein; TRAF1/2: TNF receptor-associated factor 1 and 2; Tregs: regulatory T cells; TSC1/2: tuberous sclerosis proteins 1 and 2; DAMPs: damage-associated molecular patterns; TLR: Toll-like receptors; IRAK1/4: interleukin-1 receptor-associated kinase 1/4 protein; TRAF6: tumor necrosis factor receptor-associated factor 6; TAK1: transforming growth factor-β (TGF-β)-activated kinase 1; IKK: inhibitor of nuclear factor-κB.

In colorectal cancer, curcumin addresses the complex etiology involving genetic, environmental, and inflammatory factors [31,32]. Clinical trials have shown that standardized curcuma extracts achieve pharmacologically active levels in colorectal tissues, reducing polyp size and number in familial adenomatous polyposis patients and preventing precancerous lesions in smokers without significant toxicity [15,33–35]. For instance, a dose-escalation study administering up to 3.6 g/day of curcumin demonstrated effective tissue concentrations and safety, while combinations with quercetin further enhanced therapeutic outcomes [19,33,35]. These findings highlight curcumin's efficacy and safety, emphasizing the need for larger, randomized clinical trials to optimize its bioavailability and fully validate its therapeutic benefits in colorectal cancer treatment.

2.2. Inflammatory Bowel Disease

Curcumin demonstrates substantial anti-inflammatory effects by interacting with toll-like receptors and regulating mediators, such as MAPK and NF-κB, making it a promising therapeutic agent for inflammatory bowel disease (IBD) [36,37]. Clinical trials have shown that curcumin effectively induces and maintains remission in IBD patients. For example, studies report significant reductions in the inflammatory markers ESR and CRP in patients with ulcerative proctitis and Crohn's disease following curcumin administration [38]. Additionally, maintenance therapy combining curcumin with sulfasalazine or mesalamine results in lower recurrence rates compared to a placebo [39], and case reports indicate that curcumin alongside prednisone can achieve clinical and endoscopic remission [40]. Another clinical trial demonstrated that curcumin supplementation at 1500 mg per day for eight weeks significantly improves clinical conditions and reduces inflammatory markers in individuals with mild-to-moderate ulcerative colitis [41]. Dose-dependent studies reveal that curcumin lowers levels of MAPK, NF-κB, and MMP3 while increasing IL-10 and reducing IL-1beta [42], and in vivo research supports its role in inhibiting the NLRP3 inflammasome [43]. However, curcumin's inhibition of hepcidin may exacerbate anemia in IBD patients, necessitating careful monitoring [44,45]. These findings underscore curcumin's potential as a complementary therapy for IBD, warranting further large-scale randomized trials to confirm its efficacy and safety.

2.3. Osteoarthritis

Osteoarthritis (OA) is a chronic inflammatory condition marked by joint degradation and cartilage damage, driven by dysregulated pro-inflammatory markers and cytokines, such as IL-1 and TNF-alpha. Curcumin emerges as a promising candidate due to its ability to modulate key inflammatory and catabolic pathways involved in OA pathogenesis. Preclinical studies demonstrate that curcumin reduces the expression of pro-inflammatory cytokines and matrix metalloproteinases, thereby protecting cartilage integrity and inhibiting disease progression [46–50]. Formulations, such as Advanced Ultrasol Curcumin and curcumin-loaded nanoparticles, have improved its bioavailability and therapeutic efficacy in animal models [51]. In addition, nanoparticles loaded with curcumin alleviated type II collagen loss, resulting in the reversal of elevated malondialdehyde levels in monosodium iodoacetate-induced knee OA in rodents [52]. Clinically, proprietary formulations, like Meriva™, have shown significant improvements in pain, joint function, and inflammatory markers in OA patients, while reducing the need for NSAIDs and minimizing adverse effects [53–56]. These outcomes suggest that curcumin not only addresses symptomatic relief but may also influence the underlying disease mechanisms. Integrating curcumin into OA management could offer a multifaceted approach by targeting inflammation, protecting cartilage, and enhancing patient quality of life [57]. Further large-scale randomized trials are warranted to fully establish its efficacy, optimize dosing regimens, and confirm its role as a viable adjunct therapy in osteoarthritis treatment protocols.

2.4. Atherosclerosis

Atherosclerosis is a chronic inflammatory condition of the vascular tissues and a major risk factor for cardiovascular diseases, primarily driven by oxidative stress that damages the vascular endothelium, triggering disease development [58]. Curcumin has emerged as a promising therapeutic agent due to its potent anti-inflammatory and antioxidant properties, which influence inflammatory cells and enzymes involved in atherosclerosis [59,60]. By scavenging reactive oxygen species (ROS) and enhancing the activity of endogenous antioxidant enzymes, such as glutathione peroxidase and superoxide dismutase, curcumin mitigates oxidative stress and protects vascular integrity [61–65]. Furthermore, curcumin modulates the TLR4/MAPK/NF-κB pathway, reducing the activity of pro-inflammatory M1 macrophages and lowering overall inflammation, thereby inhibiting the progression of atherosclerosis [66–69]. Clinical studies reinforce curcumin's cardiovascular benefits. Randomized controlled trials have shown that curcumin supplementation improves lipid profiles by increasing high-density lipoprotein cholesterol (HDL-C) and decreasing plasma triglycerides (TGs) [70]. Additionally, curcumin (Theracurmin®) significantly decreased LDL-C levels in patients with chronic obstructive pulmonary disease (COPD), highlighting its role in reducing atherosclerotic risk factors [71]. However, some meta analyses report no significant changes in total cholesterol or low-density lipoprotein cholesterol (LDL-C), indicating the need for more comprehensive research [72]. These findings underscore curcumin's potential as a multifaceted adjunct therapy for atherosclerosis by targeting oxidative stress, inflammation, and lipid metabolism. Nonetheless, further large-scale randomized trials are essential to validate its efficacy and optimize dosing strategies for cardiovascular disease management.

2.5. Peptic Ulcer

Peptic ulcer disease arises from the disruption of the gastrointestinal (GI) tract protective barrier, primarily due to increased gastric acid secretion or decreased duodenal bicarbonate production. This disruption leads to mucosal injury and inflammation. Curcumin offers a promising therapeutic approach by reinforcing the mucosal barrier through its anti-apoptotic and antioxidant properties. Inhibition of caspase-3 by curcumin reduces gastric acid secretion and mitigates oxidative stress, thereby protecting the gastric mucosa [73]. Curcumin also exhibits antisecretory activity against nonsteroidal anti-inflammatory drugs (NSAIDs), enhancing gastroprotective effects [74]. Studies demonstrate that curcumin and bisdemethoxycurcumin decrease inducible nitric oxide synthase (iNOS) expression without affecting tumor necrosis factor-alpha (TNF-α), thereby reducing inflammation and acid secretion [75]. In rodent models, curcumin administration increases gastric juice pH, reduces neutrophil activity, and lowers oxidative stress markers, showcasing anti-ulcer efficacy [76]. Several formulations, such as chitosan–curcumin mixtures and omeprazole–curcumin-loaded hydrogel beads, further improve curcumin's therapeutic outcomes by enhancing its antioxidant and anti-inflammatory activities [77–79]. Additionally, curcumin has demonstrated anti-Helicobacter pylori effects in mouse models, evidenced by significant reductions in serum IL-4, IFN-γ, somatostatin, gastrin, lipid peroxide, myeloperoxidase, and bacterial counts, alongside increased anti-H. pylori antibodies [80]. Clinically, turmeric supplementation has shown significant ulcer remission and symptom improvement, although antacids remain more effective in some cases [81,82]. The potential of curcumin as a complementary therapy for peptic ulcer disease is emphasized by these findings, which demonstrate that it can protect and repair the gastric mucosa through multifaceted mechanisms. However, larger randomized trials are necessary to fully validate its efficacy and optimize dosing regimens for clinical application.

2.6. COVID-19

COVID-19 is characterized by a hyperinflammatory state marked by elevated levels of colony-stimulating factors (G-CSF and GM-CSF), inflammatory markers (IL-1β, IL-6, IL-8, and TNF-α), and activated cytokine-tracing agents [83]. Central to its pathogenesis is the activation of the NOD-like receptor pyrin domain-containing 3 (NLRP3) inflammasome, which contributes to the catastrophic cytokine storm leading to acute respiratory distress syndrome (ARDS) and increased mortality, especially in patients with comorbidities, like diabetes and obesity [84–87]. Curcumin presents a multifaceted therapeutic potential by modulating these inflammatory pathways. It inhibits the NLRP3 inflammasome, thereby reducing the excessive inflammatory response [88]. Additionally, curcumin regulates Treg and Th17 cell populations, lowering inflammatory markers and mitigating immune dysregulation in COVID-19 patients [89].

Preclinical studies demonstrate curcumin's ability to inhibit SARS-CoV-2 entry into cells, impede viral replication, and reduce inflammatory mediator production, which collectively diminish disease severity [90]. Clinical trials further support these findings, showing that curcumin supplementation improves oxygen levels, reduces hospital stays, and accelerates recovery in COVID-19 patients [91,92]. Moreover, combination therapies involving curcumin and other agents, such as piperine, have been shown to enhance clinical outcomes and reduce mortality rates [92]. Recent research also highlights specific curcuminoids, like Me08 and Me23, for their antiviral and anti-inflammatory effects, suggesting their potential in targeting both the virus and the host's inflammatory response [93].

These integrated actions of curcumin underscore its potential as an effective adjuvant therapy for COVID-19, addressing both viral replication and the detrimental hyperinflammatory response. However, further large-scale randomized clinical trials are essential to validate curcumin's efficacy, optimize dosing regimens, and fully integrate it into COVID-19 treatment protocols.

2.7. Psoriasis

Psoriasis is a chronic inflammatory skin condition characterized by scaly, red, and thick plaques that can affect any part of the body. Current treatments, such as UVB therapy and systemic medications, like methotrexate and cyclosporine, are often time-consuming and may pose risks to vital organs. Curcumin, renowned for its anti-inflammatory, antioxidant, and antimicrobial properties, emerges as an ideal herbal compound for managing psoriasis [94]. Curcumin exerts its therapeutic effects by modulating key inflammatory pathways, including the inhibition of NF-κB and the reduction of pro-inflammatory cytokines, like TNF-alpha, IL-17, and IL-22, thereby alleviating the inflammatory environment associated with psoriasis [95–98]. Additionally, curcumin inhibits the Kv1.3 potassium channel, which is crucial for T cell activation and proliferation, further mitigating psoriatic inflammation [99–101]. Moreover, the Lineweaver–Burk plot analysis demonstrated that curcumin is a non-competitive inhibitor of PhK with an inhibition constant (Ki) of 0.075 mM [102]. Advanced formulations, such as curcumin-loaded nanoparticles and SmartPearls, enhance skin penetration and therapeutic efficacy, resulting in improved anti-keratinization and a reduction in inflammatory markers [103–106]. Clinical studies demonstrate that curcumin supplementation significantly reduces psoriasis severity scores and inflammatory markers, though some trials indicate the necessity for larger, placebo-controlled studies to confirm these benefits [107,108]. These findings highlight curcumin's potential as a multifaceted adjunct therapy for psoriasis, targeting both symptom relief and underlying inflammatory processes, warranting further comprehensive clinical research.

2.8. Vitiligo

Vitiligo is a chronic inflammatory skin condition characterized by the loss of melanocytes, resulting in white patches on the skin. Oxidative stress plays a significant role in melanocyte destruction, contributing to the disease's etiology [109,110]. Curcumin, with its potent antioxidant and anti-inflammatory properties, emerges as a promising therapeutic agent for vitiligo. By reducing oxidative stress and modulating inflammatory pathways, curcumin helps protect melanocytes and promote skin repigmentation [111,112].

Preclinical research highlights curcumin's ability to decrease advanced glycation end-products and activate the NRF2 antioxidant pathway, enhancing cellular protection against oxidative damage [111,112]. These findings underscore curcumin's potential as a complementary therapy for vitiligo, addressing both oxidative stress and inflammation to restore skin pigmentation. Further large-scale randomized trials are essential to validate curcumin's efficacy and optimize treatment protocols for vitiligo patients.

Clinical studies support curcumin's efficacy in managing vitiligo. In a trial with ten patients, the combination of tetrahydrocurcuminoid cream and narrowband UVB (NB-UVB) therapy resulted in significant repigmentation compared to baseline, with enhanced outcomes observed in the combination group [109]. Additionally, turmeric cream applied twice daily for four months significantly reduced lesion size and improved vitiligo scores compared to placebo controls [113]. A case study further illustrated spontaneous repigmentation following the consumption of a curcumin-based herbal remedy [114].

2.9. Depression

Depression is increasingly recognized as being closely linked to inflammation, where dysregulated innate and adaptive immune responses contribute to its onset [115,116]. Curcumin, renowned for its anti-inflammatory and antioxidant properties, presents a promising therapeutic option for alleviating depressive symptoms. By inhibiting the NLRP3 inflammasome, curcumin reduces the expression of pro-inflammatory cytokines, thereby mitigating the inflammatory processes associated with depression [117]. Preclinical studies demonstrate that curcumin administration reverses depressive-like behaviors in stressed rodents by restoring neurotransmitter levels, including serotonin, norepinephrine, and dopamine, and modulating the serotonergic system through 5-HT receptors [118–122]. Additionally, curcumin enhances the brain-derived neurotrophic factor (BDNF) pathway, promoting neuronal survival and synaptic plasticity, which are critical for mood regulation [123,124].

Enhanced formulations, such as curcumin-coated nanoparticles, have further improved its bioavailability and therapeutic efficacy, resulting in significant behavioral and biochemical improvements in animal models of depression [125–127]. Clinical trials support these findings, with curcumin supplementation showing reductions in inflammatory markers and improvements in depressive symptoms [128–130]. However, some studies highlight the need for larger, randomized controlled trials to confirm curcumin's antidepressant efficacy and optimize dosing strategies [129,130]. These integrated actions of curcumin underscore its potential as a multifaceted adjunct therapy for depression, targeting both inflammatory pathways and neurochemical imbalances to enhance mental health outcomes.

2.10. Diabetes Mellitus

Diabetes mellitus, particularly type 2 diabetes (T2DM), is a chronic metabolic disorder characterized by impaired glucose metabolism, insulin resistance, and associated complications, such as neuropathy, cardiovascular, and renal damage. Curcumin, with its multifaceted bioactive properties, has been extensively investigated for its potential to manage diabetes and its complications through mechanisms including improved lipid metabolism, reduced inflammation, antioxidant effects, and prevention of cell death [131–133].

Curcumin administration has demonstrated significant benefits in clinical trials. In a randomized, double-blind, placebo-controlled study, nano-curcumin (80 mg/day) for three months in T2DM patients resulted in notable reductions in glycosylated hemoglobin (HbA1c), fasting blood glucose (FBG), triglycerides (TG), and body mass index (BMI), along with improvements in low-density lipoprotein cholesterol (LDL-C) levels [134]. Additionally, curcumin administration at 300 mg/kg for three months in diabetic obese patients significantly reduced fasting blood sugar, insulin resistance, HbA1c, serum triglycerides, and free fatty acids (FFAs), while increasing lipoprotein lipase activity, highlighting its efficacy in lipid metabolism modulation [135]. Proprietary formulations, like Theracurmin®, have shown efficacy in reducing α1-antitrypsin-LDL levels and increasing adiponectin in non-insulin-dependent diabetic patients [136]. Additionally, combining curcumin with piperine significantly improved glycemic control and hepatic parameters, although effects on high-sensitivity C-reactive protein (hs-CRP) were inconclusive due to study limitations [137].

Curcumin also plays a role in mitigating diabetic complications. Topical application of curcumin ointments significantly reduced the size of diabetic foot ulcers, enhancing wound healing through sustained local concentrations and anti-inflammatory effects [138,139]. These findings underscore curcumin's potential as a comprehensive adjunct therapy for managing diabetes and its complications, although further large-scale, long-term randomized trials are necessary to fully establish its efficacy and optimize dosing strategies.

2.11. Malaria

Malaria, caused by *Plasmodium* species, remains a significant global health challenge, particularly due to the emergence of drug-resistant strains. Curcumin, a polyphenolic compound from turmeric, has shown promising antimalarial potential through multiple mechanisms. Preclinical studies indicate that curcumin inhibits the histone acetyl transferase (HAT) enzyme and generates reactive oxygen species (ROS) within the malaria parasite, leading to cellular damage and reduced parasitemia [140,141]. Notably, curcumin effectively targets chloroquine-resistant *Plasmodium falciparum* with an IC_{50} of approximately 5 μM and significantly decreases parasitic loads and increases survival rates in *Plasmodium berghei*-infected mice [142]. Additionally, curcumin enhances the efficacy of traditional antimalarial drugs, like α,β-arteether, resulting in 100% survival and protection against recrudescence when combined [142,143].

Mechanistically, curcumin mitigates cerebral malaria by inhibiting pro-inflammatory cytokines, such as TNF-α, IL-1β, IL-6, and IFN-γ, thereby preventing blood–brain barrier disruption and neuronal injury [144,145]. Several curcumin formulations, including PLGA nanoparticles [146], nano-emulsions [147], hydrogel nanoparticles [148], solid–lipid dispersions [149], chitosan nanoparticles [150], polymeric capsules [151], and lipoidal drug delivery systems [152], have demonstrated improved bioavailability and greater efficacy in reducing inflammatory markers, preventing infected red blood cell sequestration in the brain, and exhibiting antimalarial activity in experimental animals. Furthermore, combinations of curcumin with bioavailability enhancers, like piperine, have shown enhanced antimalarial effects by increasing ROS production, which is cytotoxic to *Plasmodium* parasites [153].

Despite the promising preclinical outcomes, clinical studies are limited. Future research should focus on comprehensive clinical trials to validate curcumin's antimalarial efficacy, optimize dosing regimens, and explore its potential to counteract drug resistance, thereby contributing to sustained malaria control and eradication efforts.

2.12. Antimicrobial Properties

Curcumin, the primary curcuminoid in turmeric, has long been recognized for its antimicrobial properties, complementing its well-documented anti-inflammatory and antioxidant effects [154,155]. Curcumin combats bacterial infections through multiple mechanisms, including the inhibition of FtsZ, a crucial enzyme for bacterial cell division, and the disruption of bacterial cell membranes due to its amphipathic nature [156,157]. These actions render curcumin effective against both Gram-positive and Gram-negative bacteria, such as *Escherichia coli* and *Staphylococcus aureus* [156,157]. Additionally, curcumin impedes biofilm formation in pathogens, like *Pseudomonas aeruginosa*, enhancing the efficacy of conventional antibiotics and offering a promising strategy against antibiotic-resistant strains [158,159].

Beyond antibacterial effects, curcumin exhibits antiviral activity, demonstrated by its ability to interfere with viral entry and replication processes in *Herpes Simplex Virus type 1* (HSV-1), thereby reducing viral load and infection severity [160]. Curcumin also shows potential against *Helicobacter pylori*, effectively lowering bacterial counts and mitigating infection-related inflammation in preclinical models [161].

However, the clinical application of curcumin is limited by its poor bioavailability, rapid metabolism, and systemic elimination. Advances in nanotechnology have led to the development of nanocurcumin formulations, which significantly enhance curcumin's stability, absorption, and therapeutic efficacy [162]. These innovative delivery systems not only improve antimicrobial activity but also enable synergistic interactions with existing antimicrobial agents, reducing the required dosages and minimizing side effects [163,164].

Despite the promising preclinical outcomes, comprehensive clinical studies are necessary to fully establish curcumin's efficacy and safety as an antimicrobial agent. Future research should focus on optimizing curcumin formulations and exploring its potential as an adjunct therapy to overcome the growing challenge of antimicrobial resistance.

2.13. Neuroprotective Properties

Neurodegenerative disorders (NDs), such as Alzheimer's disease (AD) and Parkinson's disease (PD), are characterized by the progressive loss of neurons and impaired neural function, significantly impacting the aging population [165]. Current pharmacological treatments for NDs are limited by their inability to halt disease progression and their adverse side effects, prompting the exploration of alternative therapeutic strategies. Curcumin, a bioactive compound from turmeric, has emerged as a promising neuroprotective agent due to its multifaceted mechanisms of action.

Curcumin mitigates neuronal degeneration by suppressing oxidative stress, inflammation, cell death, and mitochondrial dysfunction [165]. It activates the NRF2 pathway by dissociating from Keap1, leading to the increased expression of antioxidant enzymes, such as heme oxygenase-1 (HO1) and NAD(P)H–quinone oxidoreductase 1 (NQO1), while inhibiting pro-inflammatory cytokines, like TNF-alpha, IL-6, and IL-1beta [166]. This dual action enhances neuronal survival and plasticity, critical for combating neurodegeneration.

In animal models, curcumin has demonstrated significant neuroprotective effects. For instance, chronic administration of curcumin in stressed rats reduced IL-1beta expression and neuronal death in the ventromedial prefrontal cortex, correlating with decreased depressive behavior [167]. Additionally, curcumin enhanced neurotransmitter levels and modulated the serotonergic system, contributing to its antidepressant effects [168]. Nanotechnology-based formulations, such as curcumin-coated nanoparticles, have further improved its bioavailability and efficacy, leading to enhanced behavioral and biochemical outcomes in rodent models of neurodegeneration [169–171].

In PD models induced by 6-hydroxydopamine, curcumin protected dopaminergic neurons, improved memory function, and increased dopamine and acetylcholine levels in the substantia nigra, while reducing oxidative stress and upregulating neurotrophic factors, like BDNF and TrkB [172–174]. Similarly, in AD models, curcumin reduced beta-amyloid plaque formation, oxidative stress, and neuronal damage, demonstrating its potential to slow disease progression [175–178]. Furthermore, the transcriptional modification of dysfunctional microglial miR-155 reduced retinal inflammation and related vasculopathy by decreasing the generation of Clec7a/Galectin-3+ microglia, which led to neurodegenerative outcomes [179]. Interestingly, curcumin at a lower dose stimulated microglial migration to and phagocytosis of amyloid plaques, decreased miR-155-mediated neurodegenerative phenotype, and reduced amyloid stress in mouse brains [180]. Clinical studies in humans have shown that bioavailable curcumin formulations, such as Theracurmin® and CurQfen®, improve cognitive function and reduce biomarkers of neuronal degeneration, although some studies report inconclusive results, highlighting the need for larger trials [181–183].

Overall, curcumin's ability to enhance antioxidant defenses, suppress inflammatory pathways, and promote neuronal health underscores its potential as a neuroprotective agent. Continued research, particularly large-scale clinical trials, is essential to fully establish curcumin's efficacy and optimize its therapeutic applications in neurodegenerative diseases.

3. Curcumin's Bioavailability: Challenges and Innovative Formulations

Despite the numerous advantageous effects of curcumin, its oral bioavailability continues to be a significant constraint in curcumin therapy, necessitating further research to resolve this problem. Curcumin has been demonstrated to have an exceptionally poor bioavailability, as evidenced by numerous studies that have demonstrated either undetectable or extremely low concentrations in plasma and other tissues [184]. The primary factors contributing to low bioavailability are insufficient absorption, swift first-pass metabolism, limited tissue penetration, chemical instability, and rapid elimination [185].

To overcome these obstacles, various strategies have been employed to enhance curcumin's bioavailability. These includes the formulations of curcumin as nanoparticles, lipid formulations, drug complexation, and the use of structural analogs, such as turmeric oil [186,187]. Combining curcumin with 20 mg of piperine significantly boosts its bioavailability, increasing absorption by 2000%, resulting in a raised plasma concentration within 1 h of co-administration in both rats and humans without producing adverse effects [188]. The stability of curcumin complexes with metals was improved, which contributed to the enhancement of biological activities, including antioxidant, anti-inflammatory, antimicrobial, antineoplastic, neuroprotective, and anti-ulcer activity, in comparison to unformulated curcumin [189].

Nanotechnology-based formulations have shown promise in increasing the bioavailability and therapeutic efficacy of curcumin. For example, N-carboxymethyl chitosan-coated solid lipid nanoparticles of curcumin exhibited a 6.3-fold increase in oral bioavailability and a 9.5-fold increase in lymphatic absorption when contrasted with curcumin solution [190]. These findings suggest that NCC-SLN could serve as an effective oral delivery system for curcumin, improving both absorption and distribution. Currently, a variety of formulations, including BioCurc, Cavacurcmin, CurcuWIN, Hydrocurc, Meriva, Nanocurcumin, Novasol, Theracurmin, and Turmipure Gold, are available in the global market with the potential to enhance bioavailability and solubility. Emulsifiers, such as polyethoxylated hydrogenated castor oil, carbohydrate complexes, lipoidal/phospholipid complexes, and polysorbates, are commonly used in these preparations to further improve bioavailability and solubility [191]. In addition, poloxamers offer an intriguing approach to enhance the steric stability and assimilation of conventional liposomes. Curcumin's bioavailability was elevated to 43.3% in the pluronic-modified liposomal formulation, as compared to 26.9% with the standard liposomal formulation [192]. These formulations have been shown to significantly enhance the bioavailability of curcumin, making it more effective for therapeutic use in various chronic diseases.

4. Safety Profile of Curcumin

According to the results of safety investigations, curcumin is generally considered safe for human consumption. It has also been revealed by several studies that curcuminoids, including curcumin, and the extracts of Curcuma longa do not elevate the incidence of adverse events [193,194]. Curcumin is safe for human consumption, even at comparatively high doses, as support from studies conducted in humans indicate that healthy volunteers can tolerate doses of up to 8 g/d and even 12 g/d. Furthermore, a meta-analysis of 6 human studies including 172 participants found that curcuminoids substantially reduced circulating C-reactive protein levels when compared to placebo, with no adverse effects [195]. Studies on its potential toxicity indicated that it is generally safe, even at larger quantities (up to 12 g in human) [196,197]. According to toxicological studies, curcumin does not cause any discernible mutagenic, teratogenic, or subchronic toxicity damage [193,198]. Furthermore, research conducted by a study group stated that the administration of 8 g per day of curcumin plus gemcitabine to pancreatic cancer patients was found to be well-tolerated and safe [20,21]. However, curcumin and its derivative, bisdemethoxycurcumin, have been reported to prolong the aPTT and PT, and inhibited the activity of thrombin and factor Xa [199]. Therefore, curcumin should be used cautiously in patients with bleeding disorders and in pregnant and nursing women. Curcumin's advantageous effects are evident; however, it is crucial to evaluate its antiplatelet properties, as it has the potential to enhance the efficacy of other antiplatelet medications, including ginkgo biloba, garlic, and other anticoagulants [200], which could result in a significant risk of hemorrhagic complications. Notably, the inappropriate bioavailability of the administered formulation could also be considered, as the various formulations achieved varying plasma concentrations, which may also affect these interactions. Despite its anti-inflammatory properties, it has been recognized as an allergen causing contact dermatitis in some individuals [201]. Consequently, it is imperative that patients and dermatologists remain vigilant regarding potential allergic reactions.

5. Probable Mechanisms of Action of Curcumin

Curcumin's efficacy in preventing the development of disease is shown, e.g., by its ability to efficiently counteract the effects of reactive oxygen species (ROS) and nitrogen species [202]. Curcumin inhibits lipid peroxidation and peroxide-induced DNA damage via the inhibition of oxidative stress by reducing the production of ROS, including the generation of highly reactive free radicals, such as hydroxyl groups, univalent anion oxygen, and singlet oxygen, etc. [203]. Nevertheless, the inflammatory response can be induced by oxidative stress, which in turn generates a greater proportion of free radicals that can further exacerbate oxidative stress. Cardiovascular ailments, diabetes, and arthritic conditions are among the conditions that can result from this cycle, as chronic inflammation can be induced by oxidative stress [204]. Curcumin modulates many signaling molecules to exert powerful anti-inflammatory and anti-carcinogenic effects [205]. Numerous crucial elements in cellular signal transduction pathways connected to proliferation, differentiation, and malignant transformations have been demonstrated to be inhibited by curcumin (Table 1) [206].

Furthermore, a multitude of studies have reported the implications of increased prostaglandin biosynthesis following upregulated cyclooxygenase-2 (COX-2) expression, which leads to activation of c-Jun/AP-1 and protein kinases in inflammatory conditions [207]. However, reports suggest that curcumin's anti-inflammatory properties contribute to its inhibitory effect on enzymes, like 5-lipooxygenase and COX-2 [208]. In addition, curcumin has been reported to suppress lipopolysaccharide-induced increased expression of inflammatory genes, such as COX-2 and iNOS, in RAW 264.7 macrophages cells [209]. Furthermore, curcumin alleviated the carrageenan-induced increase in inflammatory cytokines, such as IFN-γ, IL-1β, IL-6, IL-13, and IL-17, through suppressing the NF-κB/COX-2 pathway and inhibiting iNOS expression [210].

Table 1. Summary of the mechanisms/actions of curcumin and the main findings from the studies.

S. No.	Pathway/Methods	Study Type	Main Findings	References
1.	DPPH scavenging method	In vitro	Curcumin and nanosuspension exhibited more potency in scavenging of superoxide free radicals followed by demethoxycurcumin and bisdemethoxycurcumin.	[211–213]
2.	Radiation-induced lipid peroxidation DFT studies	In vitro, in vivo, and in silico	Curcumin inhibited lipid peroxidation by 82% and dimethoxy curcumin by 24%. In curcumin, the hydrogen of -OH is more labile for separation than the hydrogen of -CH(2).	[214]
3.	ABTS and DMPD radical scavenging assay	In vitro	Curcumin exhibited free radical scavenging activity against DPPH, ABTS, DMPD, superoxide anion free radical, and H_2O_2, as well as for ferrous (Fe^{2+}) ion chelation and ferric ion (Fe^{3+}) reduction.	[62]
4.	Styrene oxidation assay	In vitro	Curcumin produced phenolic chain-breaking antioxidant activity.	[203]
5.	Phosphomolybdenum peroxidation and linoleic acid peroxidation assay	In vitro	Curcumin exhibited maximum antioxidant activity followed by demethoxycurcumin and then bisdemethoxycurcumin.	[215]
6.	Keap1/Nrf2/ARE signaling pathway	In vitro	Curcumin demonstrated resistance to oxidizing agents by activating the Nrf2-Keap1 pathway and boosting the activity of antioxidant enzymes.	[216]
		In vivo	Curcumin demonstrated Nrf2 activation by inhibiting the upregulation of Keap1 induced by inflammatory signals, thereby contributing to its antioxidant benefits and alleviating insulin resistance in high-fat-diet obese mice.	[217]
7.	PI3K/Akt-1/mTOR signaling pathway	In vitro	Curcumin stimulates autophagy by inhibiting the PI3K/AKT/mTOR signaling pathway, which is achieved by at least partially inhibiting the phosphorylation of both Akt and mTOR.	[218,219]
8.	Modulation of inflammatory cytokines	In vivo	A curcuminoid preparation (180 mg/day) produces a significant reduction in TNFα, IL-6, substance P, hs-CRP, CGRP, and TGF-β as compared to a placebo control.	[220,221]
		In vivo	In patients with metabolic syndrome, the administration of curcumin (1 g/day) once daily results in a substantial decrease in serum levels of inflammatory cytokines.	[222]
		In vitro	Curcumin inhibited the release of inflammatory cytokines, including IL-8, monocyte inflammatory protein-1 (MIP-1α), monocyte chemotactic protein-1 (MCP-1), interleukin-1β (IL-1β), and tumor necrosis factor-α (TNF-α), from lipopolysaccharide-induced monocytes and macrophages extracted from the peripheral blood and alveoli of humans, respectively.	[223]
		In vitro	Curcumin reduces LPS-induced NO and pro-inflammatory cytokine production in microglial cells.	[224]
		In vitro	Curcumin suppresses PHA-induced T-cell growth, production of IL-2, NO generation, and LPS-induced NF-κB, while increasing NK cell cytotoxicity.	[225]

Table 1. *Cont.*

S. No.	Pathway/Methods	Study Type	Main Findings	References
9.	Modulation of growth factors	In vitro	Curcumin suppressed the EGF/EGFR signaling pathway, which in turn prevented hyperglycemia-driven EGF-induced pancreatic cancer from migrating and invading by downregulating the ERK and Akt signaling molecules.	[226]
		In vitro	Curcumin suppresses angiogenesis by inhibiting FGF-induced neovascularization in cultured corneal cells.	[227]
		In vivo and in vitro	Both in vitro and in vivo models exhibited the angiogenesis-inhibiting effects of curcumin through its inhibitory action on VEGF and VEGFR2.	[228,229]
10.	Modulation of growth factor receptors	In vitro	Curcumin induces autophagy in both AR-positive and AR-negative prostate cancer cells by reducing the activity and expression of the androgen receptor (AR) and related cofactors AP-1, NF-κB, and CBP.	[230,231]
		In vitro	The Her2-Akt signaling pathway is suppressed by curcumin (18 μmol/L), resulting in the inhibition of cell proliferation in the human breast cancer cell line. Furthermore, the low-dose (1.5 μmol/L) combination of curcumin and lapatinib resulted in a more potentiated inhibitory effect on the Her2-Akt signaling pathway and the inhibition of cancer cell growth.	[232]
		In vitro	Curcumin inhibits EGFR by repressing the expression of genes and proteins in the EGFR-PI3K-AKT pathway, thereby overcoming Lenvatinib's resistance in hepatocellular carcinoma cells.	[233]
		In vivo and in vitro	Curcumin enhanced the degradation of EGFR protein, thereby suppressing its activation. This, in turn, resulted in the reversal of gefitinib in non-small cell lung cancer in both in vitro and in vivo conditions.	[234]
11.	Modulation of enzymes	In vitro and in vivo	Curcumin treatment produces inhibition of NO production, reduced expression of iNOS and COX-2 by inhibiting ERK 1/2, and p38 activation in RAW 264.7 macrophages. Additionally, curcumin produces reversal of CPA-induced changes in body weight, immunoglobulins, and NK cell activity in mice.	[235]
		In vitro and in vivo	Addition of curcumin (5–10 microM) to epidermal microsomes produces inhibition of arachidonic acid metabolism into PGE2, PGF2α, and PGD2. Topically applied curcumin results in inhibition of the activity of LOX and COX in epidermal inflammation.	[236]
		In vivo	Curcumin is less ulcerogenic than phenylbutazone and exerts anti-inflammatory activity that is comparable to that of phenylbutazone. It also impeded the increased levels of SGOT and SGPT that were induced by inflammation.	[237]
		In vitro	Curcumin inhibits the AMPK-MAPK (mitogen-activated protein kinase) and PKC pathways by reversing PMA-induced PKC activation and suppressing chronic AMPK activation, resulting in decreased synthesis of EMMPRIN, MMP-9, and MMP-13.	[238]

Table 1. *Cont.*

S. No.	Pathway/Methods	Study Type	Main Findings	References
12.	Modulation of adhesion molecules	In vitro	Curcumin demonstrated anti-inflammatory activity by suppressing monocytic THP-1 adhesiveness by inhibiting the TNF-α induced ICAM-1 expression in the human keratinocyte cell line.	[239]
		In vivo	Curcumin inhibited the formation of glial scars by preventing the production of MIP1α, IL-2, and CCL5 and by reducing NF-κB activation.	[240]
		In vitro	Curcumin modulates the PI3K/Akt/MAPK/NF-B pathway to suppress the expression of VCAM-1 induced by tumour necrosis factor-α (TNFα)/lipopolysaccharide (LPS) in human intestinal microvascular endothelial cell culture.	[241]
13.	Modulation of apoptosis-related proteins	In vitro	Increased apoptosis and growth inhibition were observed in HT-29 cells that were treated with curcumin. This was accompanied by corresponding changes in apoptosis-related proteins, including a decrease in the expression of Bcl-2, Bcl-xL, and survivin, as well as an increase in Bax and Bad.	[242]
14.	Modulation of cell cycle proteins	In vitro	The expression levels of PCNA, cyclin D1, and Bcl-xL were reduced by curcumin, which prevented human keratinocyte cell differentiation by arresting them in the G1/S phase.	[243]
		In vitro	Curcumin nanoparticles triggers cellular arrest at the G1/S and G2/M phases, as well as cell death by inhibiting several cell cycle proteins, including cyclin E in MDA-MB-231 cells.	[244]
15.	Modulation of transcription factors and their signaling pathways	In vivo	Curcumin demonstrated an antidepressant effect by inhibiting the activation of NF-κB and reducing the expression of pro-inflammatory cytokines.	[119]
		In vitro	Curcumin suppresses inflammation induced by LPS by controlling microglia polarization (M1/M2), balancing TREM2/TLR4, and inhibiting NF-κB activity.	[37]
		In vitro	Curcumin lowers cellular viability in human and rat glioma cell lines, which is associated with the suppression of the AP-1 and NFkappaB signaling pathways by preventing JNK and Akt activation	[245]
16.	Ca2+/CaN/NFAT/IL-2 signaling pathway	In vitro	Curcumin reduced inflammation by inhibiting T cell-mediated Ca2+ mobilization and NFAT-regulated IL-2 and NF-κB production in freshly separated T cells and the Jurkat T leukemia cell line.	[246]
17.	CD95/CD95L apoptotic signaling pathway	In vitro	Curcumin induces apoptosis in colorectal cancer cells via altering the Fas-regulated extrinsic pathway, activating caspase 8 and TRAIL binding to death receptors (DR), and upregulating DR5 proteins.	[247]
18.	c-Jun N-terminal kinases 1/2 (JNK1/2) pathways	In vitro	Curcumin inhibits MEKK1-induced JNK activation via interfering with upstream signaling molecules, resulting in the inhibition of AP-1 and NF-kappaB signaling and significant anti-inflammatory and anticancer effects.	[248]
19.	FABP5/ PPARβ/δ pathway	In vitro	Curcumin suppresses the expression of FABP5 and PPARβ/δ, thereby overcoming the resistance to retinoic acid in MDA-MB-231 and MD-MB-468 cell lines (triple-negative breast cancer).	[249]

Table 1. *Cont.*

S. No.	Pathway/Methods	Study Type	Main Findings	References
20.	Modulation of PPARγ/NF-κB signaling pathway	In vitro and in vivo	Curcumin prevents cigarette smoke extract (CSE)-induced inflammation both in vivo and in vitro, possibly by upregulating PPARγ and inhibiting NF-κB activation.	[250]
		In vitro and in vivo	In in vitro and in vivo models, curcumin suppresses PPAR activation, inhibits NF-κB p65 translocation, and improves the increased expression of MCP-1 and MUC5AC induced by OVA and IL-4.	[251]

Abbreviations: ABTS, 2,2′-azino-bis(3-ethylbenzothiazoline-6-sulfonic acid); Akt-1, alpha serine/threonine-protein kinase-1; AMPK, 5′ AMP-activated protein kinase; AP-1, activator protein 1; AR, androgen receptor; ARE, antioxidant response element; Bcl-2, B-cell lymphoma-2; CaN, calcineurin; CBP, CREB binding protein; CCL5, chemokine (C-C motif) ligand 5; CGRP, calcitonin gene-related peptide; COX-2, cyclooxy-genase-2; CPA, cyclophosphamide; DFT, discrete Fourier transform; DMPD, N,N-Dimethyl-p-phenylene diamine; DPPH, 2,2-Diphenyl-1-picrylhydrazyl; EGF/EGFR, epidermal growth factor (EGF) receptor (EGFR); EMMPRIN, extracellular matrix metalloproteinase inducer; ERK1/2, extracellular signal-regulated protein kinases 1 and 2; FABP5, fatty acid binding protein 5; FGF, fibroblast growth factor; Her2, human epidermal growth factor receptor 2; hs-CRP, high-sensitivity C-reactive protein; ICAM-1, intercellular adhesion molecule 1; IL-1/6/8, interleukin-1/6/8; iNOS, inducible nitric oxide synthase; Keap1, Kelch-like ECH-associated protein 1; LOX, lysyl oxidase; LPS, lipopolysaccharide; MAPK, mitogen-activated protein kinases; MCP-1, monocyte chemoattractant protein 1; MIP-1α, macrophage inflammatory protein-1 alpha; MMP-9/13, matrix metalloproteinase-9/13; mTOR, mammalian target of rapamycin; NFAT, nuclear factor of activated T-cells; NF-kB, nuclear factor kappa-light-chain-enhancer of activated B cells; NO, nitric oxide; Nrf2, nuclear factor-erythroid 2-related factor 2; PCNA, proliferating cell nuclear antigen; PHA, phytohaemagglutinin; PI3K, phosphatidylinositide 3-kinases; PKC, protein kinase C; PMA, phorbol 12-myristate 13-acetate; PPARβ/δ, peroxisome-proliferator-activated receptor β/δ; PPARγ, peroxisome-proliferator-activated receptor γ; SGOT, serum glutamic oxaloacetic transaminase; SGPT, serum glutamate pyruvate transaminase; TGF-β, transforming growth factor beta; THP-1, human leukemia monocytic cell line; TLR4, Toll-like receptor 4; TNFα, tumor necrosis factor alpha; TRAIL, tumor necrosis factor (TNF)-related apoptosis-inducing ligand; TREM2, triggering receptor expressed on myeloid cells 2; VEGF, vascular endothelial growth factor; VEGFR2, vascular endothelial growth factor receptor-2.

Figure 3, illustrates the action mechanisms of curcumin in diverse pathologic conditions. Nuclear factor-kappa B (NF-kB) is a transcription factor that regulates the expression of numerous genes, including pro-inflammatory genes. It is a critical mediator between inflammation and the development of a variety of human diseases. Its activity is strictly regulated by a variety of mechanisms (Figure 3) and it functions in the regulation, activation, and maintenance of innate white blood cells, such as T- and B lymphocytes [86]. Tumor necrosis factor alpha (TNF-α) is a pleiotropic cytokine that is a significant regulator of inflammatory processes [252]. It is implicated in the pathogenesis of a wide range of pathologic conditions, including neurologic [253], autoimmune [254], and endocrine disorders [255], as well as obesity [256]. As shown in Figure 3, curcumin inhibits the expression of inflammatory genes by direct inhibitory action on NF-κB [257] and also by inhibiting the TNFα signal transduction pathway [258]. In addition, curcumin inhibits TLR4 homodimerization required for activation of the MyD88 adaptor protein. This suppresses downstream signaling molecules, like IRAK1 and IRAK4 kinases, preventing TAK1-mediated activation of the IKK complex and activation of NF-κB [259]. The inhibition of NF-κB pathways exerts modulatory action on cellular oxidative stress by regulating the production of cytokines, adhesion molecules, COX-2, iNOS [260], HO-1, and NQO-1 [261], which is crucial for the adipocyte hyperplasia and hypertrophy leading to obesity. NAD(P)H–quinone oxidoreductase 1 (NQO1) is a key enzyme in the antioxidative system, catalyzing the reduction of two electrons, which takes place in different endogenous and exogenous quinones where flavin adenine nucleotides (FAD) acts as a cofactor. The promoter domain of the NQO1 gene encodes antioxidant response element (ARE) sequences, which have been shown to be regulated by nuclear factor (erythroid-derived 2)-like 2 (NRF2) [262]. Curcumin may activate the NRF2 pathway, which may reduce the expression of cytokines that promote inflammation, such as MCP-1, TNF-a, IL-6, and IL-1β, and induce antioxidant enzymes [263,264]. Furthermore, curcumin exerts direct inhibitory action on adipocyte hyperplasia and hypertrophy [265]. The vast majority of tumor therapies rely on the direct destruction of cancer cells or promoting the action of antitumor immune cells, such as natural killer (NK) cells and cytotoxic CD8+ T lymphocytes (CTLs) [266]. Interestingly, curcumin exerts direct antitumor and cytotoxic action by elevating NK cells [267], cytotoxic CD8+ T cells [268], and INFγ [269], and by reducing the activity of Tregs and MDSC in tumor cells [270]. Also, curcumin suppresses tumor progression by reducing Tregs and MDSC [271]. It directly suppresses the phosphorylation of AKT, leading to a reduction in cellular survival, differentiation, and angiogenesis through the inhibition of GSK3β-mediated stabilization of β-catenin. Further inhibition of AKT activation leads to the inhibition of transcription factors for inflammatory genes through TSC1/2 and mTORC1 inhibition, thus contributing to the immunomodulatory, anti-inflammatory, and neuroprotective actions of curcumin [272].

Furthermore, curcumin has been shown to inhibit the adherence of *Streptococcus* mutants to human dental surfaces and the extracellular matrix protein [273]. Curcumin suppresses the expression of *Pseudomonas aeruginosa* (PAO1) virulence factors, including biofilm formation, pyocyanin biosynthesis, elastase/protease activity, and acyl homoserine lactone (HSL) production [274]. The antimicrobial action of curcumin is multifactorial, including the disruption of cell membrane function, the inhibition of bacterial cell division by binding to FtsZ, the induction of bacterial apoptosis, and the induction of phototoxicity due to a photosensitizer under blue-light irradiation [275]. As shown in Figure 4, curcumin reduces the bacterial virulence due to the instability of the biofilm structure, increased susceptibility to antibiotics, and the host immune system through the inhibition of a biofilm promotor gene [276]. In addition, it also prevents bacterial growth by disrupting the membrane structures and inhibits DNA gyrase, which in turn leads to bacterial lysis. Curcumin's several antibacterial modes of action have made it a promising candidate for overcoming bacterial resistance and serving as an effective addition to antimicrobial therapy. However, the issues of its instability and low oral bioavailability from conventional dosage forms must be overcome in order to achieve the appropriate outcomes for therapeutic purposes.

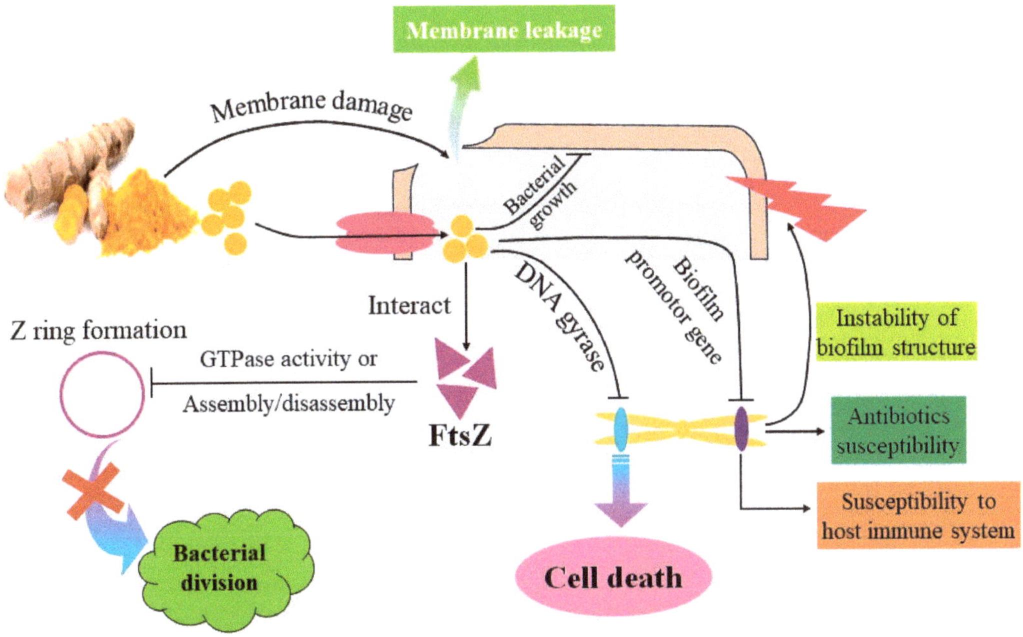

Figure 4. Schematic summary of mechanism of antimicrobial activity of curcumin.

6. Future Perspectives

While curcumin has demonstrated extensive therapeutic potential across various chronic diseases, several critical areas require further investigation to fully harness its benefits. Enhancing bioavailability remains a paramount challenge; innovative delivery systems, such as nanotechnology-based formulations, liposomal encapsulations, and curcumin–piperine combinations, show promise in overcoming curcumin's poor absorption and rapid metabolism. Future studies should focus on optimizing these formulations to maximize bio-efficacy and ensure consistent therapeutic outcomes.

Large-scale clinical trials are essential to validate the promising preclinical findings and establish standardized dosing regimens. Most existing clinical studies on curcumin are limited by small sample sizes and short durations. Comprehensive, multi-center trials are necessary to assess curcumin's long-term safety, efficacy, and role as an adjunct therapy in managing diseases, like cancer, diabetes, neurodegenerative disorders, and inflammatory conditions.

Combination therapies represent a promising avenue, where curcumin is used alongside conventional medications to enhance efficacy and reduce side effects. Investigating synergistic effects with existing drugs could lead to more effective treatment protocols, particularly in combating antibiotic resistance and enhancing antimalarial strategies.

Standardization and quality control of curcumin supplements are important to ensure consistency and reliability in clinical outcomes. Establishing standardized extraction methods and formulation protocols will enhance the reproducibility of research findings and facilitate regulatory approval.

Taken together, bridging the existing knowledge gaps through targeted research initiatives, innovative formulation strategies, and rigorous clinical evaluations will significantly advance curcumin's role in modern medicine. These efforts will not only validate curcumin's therapeutic efficacy but also pave the way for its integration into mainstream treatment protocols for a wide array of chronic diseases.

7. Conclusions

The health-promoting effects of curcumin are well recognized and have been in practice in traditional medicine since ancient times. Curcumin is used in traditional system-based medicinal products for diseases management because it is non-toxic and has only slight side effects. Numerous in vitro and in vivo laboratory based studies, as well as human clinical trials, have demonstrated the effectiveness of turmeric and its constituents as a favorable modulator of biological processes. Curcumin has shown a diverse range of effects in inflammatory disorders, perhaps by influencing multiple genes, signaling molecules, and enzymes. However, additional research is necessary to enlighten ourselves with the knowledge of curcumin's wide-ranging benefits, efficiency, plausible uses, and working mechanisms, especially in terms of its usage in the prevention and treatment of human illnesses. The combination of curcumin with other potential therapeutic reagents should further be explored and tested in controlled clinical studies.

Funding: This research received no external funding.

Conflicts of Interest: The authors declare no conflicts of interest.

References

1. El-Saadony, M.T.; Yang, T.; Korma, S.A.; Sitohy, M.; Abd El-Mageed, T.A.; Selim, S.; Al Jaouni, S.K.; Salem, H.M.; Mahmmod, Y.; Soliman, S.M.; et al. Impacts of Turmeric and Its Principal Bioactive Curcumin on Human Health: Pharmaceutical, Medicinal, and Food Applications: A Comprehensive Review. *Front. Nutr.* **2022**, *9*, 1040259. [CrossRef] [PubMed]
2. Hewlings, S.J.; Kalman, D.S. Curcumin: A Review of Its Effects on Human Health. *Foods* **2017**, *6*, 92. [CrossRef] [PubMed]
3. Fuloria, S.; Mehta, J.; Chandel, A.; Sekar, M.; Rani, N.N.I.M.; Begum, M.Y.; Subramaniyan, V.; Chidambaram, K.; Thangavelu, L.; Nordin, R. A Comprehensive Review on the Therapeutic Potential of Curcuma Longa Linn. in Relation to Its Major Active Constituent Curcumin. *Front. Pharmacol.* **2022**, *13*, 820806. [CrossRef] [PubMed]
4. Miłobędzka, J.; Kostanecki, S.V.; Lampe, V. Zur Kenntnis Des Curcumins. *Berichte Dtsch. Chem. Ges.* **1910**, *43*, 2163–2170. [CrossRef]
5. Lampe, V.; Milobedzka, J. Studien Über Curcumin. *Berichte Dtsch. Chem. Ges.* **1913**, *46*, 2235–2240. [CrossRef]
6. Pabon, H.J.J. A Synthesis of Curcumin and Related Compounds. *Recl. Trav. Chim. des Pays-Bas* **1964**, *83*, 379–386. [CrossRef]
7. Grynkiewicz, G.; Ślifirski, P. Curcumin and Curcuminoids in Quest for Medicinal Status. *Acta Biochim. Pol.* **2012**, *59*, 201–212. [CrossRef]
8. Esatbeyoglu, T.; Huebbe, P.; Ernst, I.M.A.; Chin, D.; Wagner, A.E.; Rimbach, G. Curcumin—From Molecule to Biological Function. *Angew. Chem. Int. Ed.* **2012**, *51*, 5308–5332. [CrossRef]
9. Venkateswarlu, S.; Ramachandra, M.S.; Subbaraju, G.V. Synthesis and Biological Evaluation of Polyhydroxycurcuminoids. *Bioorg. Med. Chem.* **2005**, *13*, 6374–6380. [CrossRef]
10. Priyadarsini, K.I. The Chemistry of Curcumin: From Extraction to Therapeutic Agent. *Molecules* **2014**, *19*, 20091–20112. [CrossRef]
11. Chattopadhyay, I.; Biswas, K.; Bandyopadhyay, U.; Banerjee, R.K. Turmeric and Curcumin: Biological Actions and Medicinal Applications. *Curr. Sci.* **2004**, *87*, 44–53.
12. Anand, P.; Thomas, S.G.; Kunnumakkara, A.B.; Sundaram, C.; Harikumar, K.B.; Sung, B.; Tharakan, S.T.; Misra, K.; Priyadarsini, I.K.; Rajasekharan, K.N. Biological Activities of Curcumin and Its Analogues (Congeners) Made by Man and Mother Nature. *Biochem. Pharmacol.* **2008**, *76*, 1590–1611. [CrossRef] [PubMed]
13. Aggarwal, B.B.; Harikumar, K.B. Potential Therapeutic Effects of Curcumin, the Anti-Inflammatory Agent, against Neurodegenerative, Cardiovascular, Pulmonary, Metabolic, Autoimmune and Neoplastic Diseases. *Int. J. Biochem. Cell Biol.* **2009**, *41*, 40–59. [CrossRef] [PubMed]
14. Witkin, J.M.; Li, X. Curcumin, an Active Constiuent of the Ancient Medicinal Herb Curcuma Longa L.: Some Uses and the Establishment and Biological Basis of Medical Efficacy. *CNS Neurol. Disord. Drug Targets* **2013**, *12*, 487–497. [CrossRef]
15. Sharma, R.A.; McLelland, H.R.; Hill, K.A.; Ireson, C.R.; Euden, S.A.; Manson, M.M.; Pirmohamed, M.; Marnett, L.J.; Gescher, A.J.; Steward, W.P. Pharmacodynamic and Pharmacokinetic Study of Oral Curcuma Extract in Patients with Colorectal Cancer. *Clin. Cancer Res.* **2001**, *7*, 1894–1900.
16. Aggarwal, B.B.; Sung, B. Pharmacological Basis for the Role of Curcumin in Chronic Diseases: An Age-Old Spice with Modern Targets. *Trends Pharmacol. Sci.* **2009**, *30*, 85–94. [CrossRef]
17. DiSilvestro, R.A.; Joseph, E.; Zhao, S.; Bomser, J. Diverse Effects of a Low Dose Supplement of Lipidated Curcumin in Healthy Middle Aged People. *Nutr. J.* **2012**, *11*, 79. [CrossRef]
18. Ide, H.; Tokiwa, S.; Sakamaki, K.; Nishio, K.; Isotani, S.; Muto, S.; Hama, T.; Masuda, H.; Horie, S. Combined Inhibitory Effects of Soy Isoflavones and Curcumin on the Production of Prostate-specific Antigen. *Prostate* **2010**, *70*, 1127–1133. [CrossRef]

19. Sharma, R.A.; Euden, S.A.; Platton, S.L.; Cooke, D.N.; Shafayat, A.; Hewitt, H.R.; Marczylo, T.H.; Morgan, B.; Hemingway, D.; Plummer, S.M. Phase I Clinical Trial of Oral Curcumin: Biomarkers of Systemic Activity and Compliance. *Clin. Cancer Res.* **2004**, *10*, 6847–6854. [CrossRef]
20. Dhillon, N.; Aggarwal, B.B.; Newman, R.A.; Wolff, R.A.; Kunnumakkara, A.B.; Abbruzzese, J.L.; Ng, C.S.; Badmaev, V.; Kurzrock, R. Phase II Trial of Curcumin in Patients with Advanced Pancreatic Cancer. *Clin. Cancer Res.* **2008**, *14*, 4491–4499. [CrossRef]
21. Kanai, M.; Yoshimura, K.; Asada, M.; Imaizumi, A.; Suzuki, C.; Matsumoto, S.; Nishimura, T.; Mori, Y.; Masui, T.; Kawaguchi, Y. A Phase I/II Study of Gemcitabine-Based Chemotherapy plus Curcumin for Patients with Gemcitabine-Resistant Pancreatic Cancer. *Cancer Chemother. Pharmacol.* **2011**, *68*, 157–164. [CrossRef] [PubMed]
22. Islam, M.R.; Rauf, A.; Akash, S.; Trisha, S.I.; Nasim, A.H.; Akter, M.; Dhar, P.S.; Ogaly, H.A.; Hemeg, H.A.; Wilairatana, P. Targeted Therapies of Curcumin Focus on Its Therapeutic Benefits in Cancers and Human Health: Molecular Signaling Pathway-Based Approaches and Future Perspectives. *Biomed. Pharmacother.* **2024**, *170*, 116034. [CrossRef] [PubMed]
23. He, Z.-Y.; Shi, C.-B.; Wen, H.; Li, F.-L.; Wang, B.-L.; Wang, J. Upregulation of P53 Expression in Patients with Colorectal Cancer by Administration of Curcumin. *Cancer Invest.* **2011**, *29*, 208–213. [CrossRef] [PubMed]
24. Shanmugam, M.K.; Rane, G.; Kanchi, M.M.; Arfuso, F.; Chinnathambi, A.; Zayed, M.E.; Alharbi, S.A.; Tan, B.K.H.; Kumar, A.P.; Sethi, G. The Multifaceted Role of Curcumin in Cancer Prevention and Treatment. *Molecules* **2015**, *20*, 2728–2769. [CrossRef]
25. Sivani, B.M.; Azzeh, M.; Patnaik, R.; Pantea Stoian, A.; Rizzo, M.; Banerjee, Y. Reconnoitering the Therapeutic Role of Curcumin in Disease Prevention and Treatment: Lessons Learnt and Future Directions. *Metabolites* **2022**, *12*, 639. [CrossRef]
26. Moon, D.-O. Curcumin in Cancer and Inflammation: An In-Depth Exploration of Molecular Interactions, Therapeutic Potentials, and the Role in Disease Management. *Int. J. Mol. Sci.* **2024**, *25*, 2911. [CrossRef]
27. Fetoni, A.R.; Paciello, F.; Mezzogori, D.; Rolesi, R.; Eramo, S.L.M.; Paludetti, G.; Troiani, D. Molecular Targets for Anticancer Redox Chemotherapy and Cisplatin-Induced Ototoxicity: The Role of Curcumin on PSTAT3 and Nrf-2 Signalling. *Br. J. Cancer* **2015**, *113*, 1434–1444. [CrossRef]
28. Zoi, V.; Galani, V.; Lianos, G.D.; Voulgaris, S.; Kyritsis, A.P.; Alexiou, G.A. The Role of Curcumin in Cancer Treatment. *Biomedicines* **2021**, *9*, 1086. [CrossRef]
29. Mansouri, K.; Rasoulpoor, S.; Daneshkhah, A.; Abolfathi, S.; Salari, N.; Mohammadi, M.; Rasoulpoor, S.; Shabani, S. Clinical Effects of Curcumin in Enhancing Cancer Therapy: A Systematic Review. *BMC Cancer* **2020**, *20*, 791. [CrossRef]
30. Aggarwal, B.B.; Kumar, A.; Bharti, A.C. Anticancer Potential of Curcumin: Preclinical and Clinical Studies. *Anticancer Res.* **2003**, *23*, 363–398.
31. Screening, P.D.Q.; Board, P.E. Colorectal Cancer Screening (PDQ®). In *PDQ Cancer Information Summaries [Internet]*; National Cancer Institute (US): Bethesda, MD, USA, 2023.
32. Sharma, N.; Alam, M.S.; Sharma, A.; Garg, S.; Maity, M.K. Colorectal Cancer in Young Adults: Epidemiology, Risk Factors, Development, Symptoms, Traditional Herbal Therapy And Prevention. *J. Pharm. Negat. Results* **2022**, *14*, 1370–1382.
33. Garcea, G.; Berry, D.P.; Jones, D.J.L.; Singh, R.; Dennison, A.R.; Farmer, P.B.; Sharma, R.A.; Steward, W.P.; Gescher, A.J. Consumption of the Putative Chemopreventive Agent Curcumin by Cancer Patients: Assessment of Curcumin Levels in the Colorectum and Their Pharmacodynamic Consequences. *Cancer Epidemiol. Biomark. Prev.* **2005**, *14*, 120–125. [CrossRef]
34. Carroll, R.E.; Benya, R.V.; Turgeon, D.K.; Vareed, S.; Neuman, M.; Rodriguez, L.; Kakarala, M.; Carpenter, P.M.; McLaren, C.; Meyskens, F.L., Jr. Phase IIa Clinical Trial of Curcumin for the Prevention of Colorectal Neoplasia. *Cancer Prev. Res.* **2011**, *4*, 354–364. [CrossRef] [PubMed]
35. Cruz–Correa, M.; Shoskes, D.A.; Sanchez, P.; Zhao, R.; Hylind, L.M.; Wexner, S.D.; Giardiello, F.M. Combination Treatment with Curcumin and Quercetin of Adenomas in Familial Adenomatous Polyposis. *Clin. Gastroenterol. Hepatol.* **2006**, *4*, 1035–1038. [CrossRef]
36. Gao, Y.; Zhuang, Z.; Lu, Y.; Tao, T.; Zhou, Y.; Liu, G.; Wang, H.; Zhang, D.; Wu, L.; Dai, H. Curcumin Mitigates Neuro-Inflammation by Modulating Microglia Polarization through Inhibiting TLR4 Axis Signaling Pathway Following Experimental Subarachnoid Hemorrhage. *Front. Neurosci.* **2019**, *13*, 496029. [CrossRef]
37. Zhang, J.; Zheng, Y.; Luo, Y.; Du, Y.; Zhang, X.; Fu, J. Curcumin Inhibits LPS-Induced Neuroinflammation by Promoting Microglial M2 Polarization via TREM2/TLR4/NF-KB Pathways in BV2 Cells. *Mol. Immunol.* **2019**, *116*, 29–37. [CrossRef]
38. Holt, P.R.; Katz, S.; Kirshoff, R. Curcumin Therapy in Inflammatory Bowel Disease: A Pilot Study. *Dig. Dis. Sci.* **2005**, *50*, 2191–2193. [CrossRef]
39. Hanai, H.; Iida, T.; Takeuchi, K.; Watanabe, F.; Maruyama, Y.; Andoh, A.; Tsujikawa, T.; Fujiyama, Y.; Mitsuyama, K.; Sata, M. Curcumin Maintenance Therapy for Ulcerative Colitis: Randomized, Multicenter, Double-Blind, Placebo-Controlled Trial. *Clin. Gastroenterol. Hepatol.* **2006**, *4*, 1502–1506. [CrossRef]
40. Lahiff, C.; Moss, A.C. Curcumin for Clinical and Endoscopic Remission in Ulcerative Colitis. *Inflamm. Bowel Dis.* **2011**, *17*, E66. [CrossRef]
41. Sadeghi, N.; Mansoori, A.; Shayesteh, A.; Hashemi, S.J. The Effect of Curcumin Supplementation on Clinical Outcomes and Inflammatory Markers in Patients with Ulcerative Colitis. *Phyther. Res.* **2020**, *34*, 1123–1133. [CrossRef]
42. Epstein, J.; Docena, G.; MacDonald, T.T.; Sanderson, I.R. Curcumin Suppresses P38 Mitogen-Activated Protein Kinase Activation, Reduces IL-1β and Matrix Metalloproteinase-3 and Enhances IL-10 in the Mucosa of Children and Adults with Inflammatory Bowel Disease. *Br. J. Nutr.* **2010**, *103*, 824–832. [CrossRef] [PubMed]

43. Karthikeyan, A.; Young, K.N.; Moniruzzaman, M.; Beyene, A.M.; Do, K.; Kalaiselvi, S.; Min, T. Curcumin and Its Modified Formulations on Inflammatory Bowel Disease (IBD): The Story so Far and Future Outlook. *Pharmaceutics* **2021**, *13*, 484. [CrossRef] [PubMed]
44. Kaitha, S.; Bashir, M.; Ali, T. Iron Deficiency Anemia in Inflammatory Bowel Disease. *World J. Gastrointest. Pathophysiol.* **2015**, *6*, 62–72. [CrossRef] [PubMed]
45. Jiao, Y.; Wilkinson, J., IV; Di, X.; Wang, W.; Hatcher, H.; Kock, N.D.; D'Agostino, R., Jr.; Knovich, M.A.; Torti, F.M.; Torti, S.V. Curcumin, a Cancer Chemopreventive and Chemotherapeutic Agent, Is a Biologically Active Iron Chelator. *Blood J. Am. Soc. Hematol.* **2009**, *113*, 462–469. [CrossRef] [PubMed]
46. Nicoliche, T.; Maldonado, D.C.; Faber, J.; da Silva, M.C.P. Evaluation of the Articular Cartilage in the Knees of Rats with Induced Arthritis Treated with Curcumin. *PLoS ONE* **2020**, *15*, e0230228. [CrossRef]
47. Yan, D.; He, B.; Guo, J.; Li, S.; Wang, J. Involvement of TLR4 in the Protective Effect of Intra-Articular Administration of Curcumin on Rat Experimental Osteoarthritis. *Acta Cirúrgica Bras.* **2019**, *34*, e201900604. [CrossRef]
48. Sun, Y.; Liu, W.; Zhang, H.; Li, H.; Liu, J.; Zhang, F.; Jiang, T.; Jiang, S. Curcumin Prevents Osteoarthritis by Inhibiting the Activation of Inflammasome NLRP3. *J. Interf. Cytokine Res.* **2017**, *37*, 449–455. [CrossRef]
49. Guo, C.; Fu, R.; Wang, S.; Huang, Y.; Li, X.; Zhou, M.; Zhao, J.; Yang, N. NLRP3 Inflammasome Activation Contributes to the Pathogenesis of Rheumatoid Arthritis. *Clin. Exp. Immunol.* **2018**, *194*, 231–243. [CrossRef]
50. Martinon, F.; Pétrilli, V.; Mayor, A.; Tardivel, A.; Tschopp, J. Gout-Associated Uric Acid Crystals Activate the NALP3 Inflammasome. *Nature* **2006**, *440*, 237–241. [CrossRef]
51. Sahin, K.; Orhan, C.; Er, B.; Durmus, A.S.; Ozercan, I.H.; Sahin, N.; Padigaru, M.; Morde, A.; Rai, D. Protective Effect of a Novel Highly Bioavailable Formulation of Curcumin in Experimentally Induced Osteoarthritis Rat Model. *Curr. Dev. Nutr.* **2020**, *4*, 1765. [CrossRef]
52. Hamdalla, H.M.; Ahmed, R.R.; Galaly, S.R.; Naguib, I.A.; Alghamdi, B.S.; Ahmed, O.M.; Farghali, A.; Abdul-Hamid, M. Ameliorative Effect of Curcumin Nanoparticles against Monosodium Iodoacetate-Induced Knee Osteoarthritis in Rats. *Mediat. Inflamm.* **2022**, *2022*, 8353472. [CrossRef] [PubMed]
53. Paultre, K.; Cade, W.; Hernandez, D.; Reynolds, J.; Greif, D.; Best, T.M. Therapeutic Effects of Turmeric or Curcumin Extract on Pain and Function for Individuals with Knee Osteoarthritis: A Systematic Review. *BMJ Open Sport Exerc. Med.* **2021**, *7*, e000935. [CrossRef] [PubMed]
54. Chandran, B.; Goel, A. A Randomized, Pilot Study to Assess the Efficacy and Safety of Curcumin in Patients with Active Rheumatoid Arthritis. *Phyther. Res.* **2012**, *26*, 1719–1725. [CrossRef]
55. Belcaro, G.; Cesarone, M.R.; Dugall, M.; Pellegrini, L.; Ledda, A.; Grossi, M.G.; Togni, S.; Appendino, G. Efficacy and Safety of Meriva®, a Curcumin-Phosphatidylcholine Complex, during Extended Administration in Osteoarthritis Patients. *Altern. Med. Rev.* **2010**, *15*, 337–344.
56. Belcaro, G.; Cesarone, M.R.; Dugall, M.; Pellegrini, L.; Ledda, A.; Grossi, M.G.; Togni, S.; Appendino, G. Product-Evaluation Registry of Meriva®, a Curcumin-Phosphatidylcholine Complex, for the Complementary Management of Osteoarthritis. *Panminerva Med.* **2010**, *52*, 55–62.
57. Saber, M.M.; Mahmoud, M.M.; Amin, H.M.; Essam, R.M. Therapeutic Effects of Combining Curcumin and Swimming in Osteoarthritis Using a Rat Model. *Biomed. Pharmacother.* **2023**, *166*, 115309. [CrossRef]
58. Singh, L.; Sharma, S.; Xu, S.; Tewari, D.; Fang, J. Curcumin as a Natural Remedy for Atherosclerosis: A Pharmacological Review. *Molecules* **2021**, *26*, 4036. [CrossRef]
59. Chen, Y.; Chai, Y.; Xie, K.; Yu, F.; Wang, C.; Lin, S.; Yang, Y.; Xu, F. Curcumin Promotes the Expression of IL-35 by Regulating Regulatory T Cell Differentiation and Restrains Uncontrolled Inflammation and Lung Injury in Mice. *Inflammation* **2020**, *43*, 1913–1924. [CrossRef]
60. Cox, F.F.; Misiou, A.; Vierkant, A.; Ale-Agha, N.; Grandoch, M.; Haendeler, J.; Altschmied, J. Protective Effects of Curcumin in Cardiovascular Diseases—Impact on Oxidative Stress and Mitochondria. *Cells* **2022**, *11*, 342. [CrossRef]
61. Sun, Y.; Hu, X.; Hu, G.; Xu, C.; Jiang, H. Curcumin Attenuates Hydrogen Peroxide-Induced Premature Senescence via the Activation of SIRT1 in Human Umbilical Vein Endothelial Cells. *Biol. Pharm. Bull.* **2015**, *38*, 1134–1141. [CrossRef]
62. Ak, T.; Gülçin, I. Antioxidant and Radical Scavenging Properties of Curcumin. *Chem. Biol. Interact.* **2008**, *174*, 27–37. [CrossRef] [PubMed]
63. Jovanovic, S.V.; Steenken, S.; Boone, C.W.; Simic, M.G. H-Atom Transfer Is a Preferred Antioxidant Mechanism of Curcumin. *J. Am. Chem. Soc.* **1999**, *121*, 9677–9681. [CrossRef]
64. Menon, V.P.; Sudheer, A.R. Antioxidant and Anti-Inflammatory Properties of Curcumin. *Adv. Exp. Med. Biol.* **2007**, *595*, 105–125. [PubMed]
65. Faten, R.A.; Ibrahim, A.E.; Khaled, A.E. Protective and Modulatory Effects of Curcumin and L-Carnitine against Methotrexate-Induced Oxidative Stress in Albino Rats. *Res. J. Pharm. Biol. Chem. Sci.* **2013**, *4*, 744–754.
66. Gao, S.; Zhang, W.; Zhao, Q.; Zhou, J.; Wu, Y.; Liu, Y.; Yuan, Z.; Wang, L. Curcumin Ameliorates Atherosclerosis in Apolipoprotein E Deficient Asthmatic Mice by Regulating the Balance of Th2/Treg Cells. *Phytomedicine* **2019**, *52*, 129–135. [CrossRef]
67. Momtazi-Borojeni, A.A.; Abdollahi, E.; Nikfar, B.; Chaichian, S.; Ekhlasi-Hundrieser, M. Curcumin as a Potential Modulator of M1 and M2 Macrophages: New Insights in Atherosclerosis Therapy. *Heart Fail. Rev.* **2019**, *24*, 399–409. [CrossRef]

68. Zhang, S.; Zou, J.; Li, P.; Zheng, X.; Feng, D. Curcumin Protects against Atherosclerosis in Apolipoprotein E-Knockout Mice by Inhibiting Toll-like Receptor 4 Expression. *J. Agric. Food Chem.* **2018**, *66*, 449–456. [CrossRef]
69. Han, Y.; Sun, H.-J.; Tong, Y.; Chen, Y.-Z.; Ye, C.; Qiu, Y.; Zhang, F.; Chen, A.-D.; Qi, X.-H.; Chen, Q. Curcumin Attenuates Migration of Vascular Smooth Muscle Cells via Inhibiting NFκB-Mediated NLRP3 Expression in Spontaneously Hypertensive Rats. *J. Nutr. Biochem.* **2019**, *72*, 108212. [CrossRef]
70. Simental-Mendía, L.E.; Pirro, M.; Gotto, A.M., Jr.; Banach, M.; Atkin, S.L.; Majeed, M.; Sahebkar, A. Lipid-Modifying Activity of Curcuminoids: A Systematic Review and Meta-Analysis of Randomized Controlled Trials. *Crit. Rev. Food Sci. Nutr.* **2019**, *59*, 1178–1187. [CrossRef]
71. Funamoto, M.; Sunagawa, Y.; Katanasaka, Y.; Miyazaki, Y.; Imaizumi, A.; Kakeya, H.; Yamakage, H.; Satoh-Asahara, N.; Komiyama, M.; Wada, H.; et al. Highly Absorptive Curcumin Reduces Serum Atherosclerotic Low-Density Lipoprotein Levels in Patients with Mild COPD. *Int. J. Chron. Obstruct. Pulmon. Dis.* **2016**, *11*, 2029–2034. [CrossRef]
72. Sahebkar, A. A Systematic Review and Meta-Analysis of Randomized Controlled Trials Investigating the Effects of Curcumin on Blood Lipid Levels. *Clin. Nutr.* **2014**, *33*, 406–414. [CrossRef] [PubMed]
73. Czekaj, R.; Majka, J.; Magierowska, K.; Sliwowski, Z.; Magierowski, M.; Pajdo, R.; Ptak-Belowska, A.; Surmiak, M.; Kwiecien, S.; Brzozowski, T. Mechanisms of Curcumin-Induced Gastroprotection against Ethanol-Induced Gastric Mucosal Lesions. *J. Gastroenterol.* **2018**, *53*, 618–630. [CrossRef] [PubMed]
74. Mei, X.; Xu, D.; Xu, S.; Zheng, Y.; Xu, S. Novel Role of Zn (II)–Curcumin in Enhancing Cell Proliferation and Adjusting Proinflammatory Cytokine-Mediated Oxidative Damage of Ethanol-Induced Acute Gastric Ulcers. *Chem. Biol. Interact.* **2012**, *197*, 31–39. [CrossRef] [PubMed]
75. Mahattanadul, S.; Nakamura, T.; Panichayupakaranant, P.; Phdoongsombut, N.; Tungsinmunkong, K.; Bouking, P. Comparative Antiulcer Effect of Bisdemethoxycurcumin and Curcumin in a Gastric Ulcer Model System. *Phytomedicine* **2009**, *16*, 342–351. [CrossRef]
76. Tuorkey, M.; Karolin, K. Anti-Ulcer Activity of Curcumin on Experimental Gastric Ulcer in Rats and Its Effect on Oxidative Stress/Antioxidant, IL-6 and Enzyme Activities. *Biomed. Environ. Sci.* **2009**, *22*, 488–495. [CrossRef]
77. Mahattanadul, S.; Mustafa, M.W.; Kuadkaew, S.; Pattharachayakul, S.; Ungphaiboon, S.; Sawanyawisuth, K. Oral Ulcer Healing and Anti-Candida Efficacy of an Alcohol-Free Chitosan-Curcumin Mouthwash. *Eur. Rev. Med. Pharmacol. Sci.* **2018**, *22*, 7020–7023.
78. Kuadkaew, S.; Ungphaiboon, S.; Phdoongsombut, N.; Kaewsuwan, S.; Mahattanadul, S. Efficacy of a Chitosan-Curcumin Mixture in Treating Indomethacininduced Acute Gastric Ulcer in Rats. *Curr. Pharm. Biotechnol.* **2021**, *22*, 1919–1931. [CrossRef]
79. Heikal, E.J.; Kaoud, R.M.; Gad, S.; Mokhtar, H.I.; Aldahish, A.A.; Alzlaiq, W.A.; Zaitone, S.A.; Moustafa, Y.M.; Hammady, T.M. Design and Optimization of Omeprazole-Curcumin-Loaded Hydrogel Beads Coated with Chitosan for Treating Peptic Ulcers. *Pharmaceuticals* **2023**, *16*, 795. [CrossRef]
80. Vetvicka, V.; Vetvickova, J.; Fernandez-Botran, R. Effects of Curcumin on Helicobacter Pylori Infection. *Ann. Transl. Med.* **2016**, *4*, 479. [CrossRef]
81. Kositchaiwat, C.; Kositchaiwat, S.; Havanondha, J. Curcuma Longa Linn. in the Treatment of Gastric Ulcer Comparison to Liquid Antacid: A Controlled Clinical Trial. *J. Med. Assoc. Thail.* **1993**, *76*, 601–605.
82. Prucksunand, C.; Indrasukhsri, B.; Leethochawalit, M.; Hungspreugs, K. Phase II Clinical Trial on Effect of the Long Turmeric (*Curcuma Longa* Linn.) on Healing of Peptic Ulcer. *Southeast Asian J. Trop. Med. Public Health* **2001**, *32*, 208–215. [PubMed]
83. Huang, C.; Wang, Y.; Li, X.; Ren, L.; Zhao, J.; Hu, Y.; Zhang, L.; Fan, G.; Xu, J.; Gu, X. Clinical Features of Patients Infected with 2019 Novel Coronavirus in Wuhan, China. *Lancet* **2020**, *395*, 497–506. [CrossRef] [PubMed]
84. Jiang, H.; He, H.; Chen, Y.; Huang, W.; Cheng, J.; Ye, J.; Wang, A.; Tao, J.; Wang, C.; Liu, Q. Identification of a Selective and Direct NLRP3 Inhibitor to Treat Inflammatory Disorders. *J. Exp. Med.* **2017**, *214*, 3219. [CrossRef] [PubMed]
85. Sahoo, M.; Ceballos-Olvera, I.; del Barrio, L.; Re, F. Role of the Inflammasome, IL-1beta, and IL-18 in Bacterial Infections. *Sci. World J.* **2011**, *11*, 2037–2050. [CrossRef]
86. Liu, T.; Zhang, L.; Joo, D.; Sun, S.-C. NF-KB Signaling in Inflammation. *Signal Transduct. Target. Ther.* **2017**, *2*, 17023. [CrossRef]
87. Marín-Palma, D.; Tabares-Guevara, J.H.; Zapata-Cardona, M.I.; Flórez-Álvarez, L.; Yepes, L.M.; Rugeles, M.T.; Zapata-Builes, W.; Hernandez, J.C.; Taborda, N.A. Curcumin Inhibits in Vitro SARS-CoV-2 Infection in Vero E6 Cells through Multiple Antiviral Mechanisms. *Molecules* **2021**, *26*, 6900. [CrossRef]
88. Rattis, B.A.C.; Ramos, S.G.; Celes, M. Curcumin as a Potential Treatment for COVID-19. *Front. Pharmacol.* **2021**, *12*, 675287. [CrossRef]
89. Tahmasebi, S.; Saeed, B.Q.; Temirgalieva, E.; Yumashev, A.V.; El-Esawi, M.A.; Navashenaq, J.G.; Valizadeh, H.; Sadeghi, A.; Aslani, S.; Yousefi, M. Nanocurcumin Improves Treg Cell Responses in Patients with Mild and Severe SARS-CoV2. *Life Sci.* **2021**, *276*, 119437. [CrossRef]
90. Golpour-Hamedani, S.; Pourmasoumi, M.; Askari, G.; Bagherniya, M.; Majeed, M.; Guest, P.C.; Sahebkar, A. Antiviral Mechanisms of Curcumin and Its Derivatives in Prevention and Treatment of COVID-19: A Review. *Adv. Exp. Med. Biol.* **2023**, *1412*, 397–411. [CrossRef]
91. Saber-Moghaddam, N.; Salari, S.; Hejazi, S.; Amini, M.; Taherzadeh, Z.; Eslami, S.; Rezayat, S.M.; Jaafari, M.R.; Elyasi, S. Oral Nano-curcumin Formulation Efficacy in Management of Mild to Moderate Hospitalized Coronavirus Disease-19 Patients: An Open Label Nonrandomized Clinical Trial. *Phyther. Res.* **2021**, *35*, 2616–2623. [CrossRef]

92. Kahkhaie, K.R.; Mirhosseini, A.; Aliabadi, A.; Mohammadi, A.; Mousavi, M.J.; Haftcheshmeh, S.M.; Sathyapalan, T.; Sahebkar, A. Curcumin: A Modulator of Inflammatory Signaling Pathways in the Immune System. *Inflammopharmacology* **2019**, *27*, 885–900. [CrossRef] [PubMed]
93. Nicoliche, T.; Bartolomeo, C.S.; Lemes, R.M.R.; Pereira, G.C.; Nunes, T.A.; Oliveira, R.B.; Nicastro, A.L.M.; Soares, É.N.; da Cunha Lima, B.F.; Rodrigues, B.M. Antiviral, Anti-Inflammatory and Antioxidant Effects of Curcumin and Curcuminoids in SH-SY5Y Cells Infected by SARS-CoV-2. *Sci. Rep.* **2024**, *14*, 10696. [CrossRef] [PubMed]
94. Kasprzak-Drozd, K.; Niziński, P.; Hawrył, A.; Gancarz, M.; Hawrył, D.; Oliwa, W.; Pałka, M.; Markowska, J.; Oniszczuk, A. Potential of Curcumin in the Management of Skin Diseases. *Int. J. Mol. Sci.* **2024**, *25*, 3617. [CrossRef] [PubMed]
95. Bahraini, P.; Rajabi, M.; Mansouri, P.; Sarafian, G.; Chalangari, R.; Azizian, Z. Turmeric Tonic as a Treatment in Scalp Psoriasis: A Randomized Placebo-Control Clinical Trial. *J. Cosmet. Dermatol.* **2018**, *17*, 461–466. [CrossRef]
96. Zhang, S.; Wang, J.; Liu, L.; Sun, X.; Zhou, Y.; Chen, S.; Lu, Y.; Cai, X.; Hu, M.; Yan, G.; et al. Efficacy and Safety of Curcumin in Psoriasis: Preclinical and Clinical Evidence and Possible Mechanisms. *Front. Pharmacol.* **2022**, *13*, 903160. [CrossRef]
97. Jain, A.; Doppalapudi, S.; Domb, A.J.; Khan, W. Tacrolimus and Curcumin Co-Loaded Liposphere Gel: Synergistic Combination towards Management of Psoriasis. *J. Control. Release* **2016**, *243*, 132–145. [CrossRef]
98. Mao, K.-L.; Fan, Z.-L.; Yuan, J.-D.; Chen, P.-P.; Yang, J.-J.; Xu, J.; ZhuGe, D.-L.; Jin, B.-H.; Zhu, Q.-Y.; Shen, B.-X.; et al. Skin-Penetrating Polymeric Nanoparticles Incorporated in Silk Fibroin Hydrogel for Topical Delivery of Curcumin to Improve Its Therapeutic Effect on Psoriasis Mouse Model. *Colloids Surf. B Biointerfaces* **2017**, *160*, 704–714. [CrossRef]
99. Kim, H.; Choi, M.R.; Jeon, S.H.; Jang, Y.; Yang, Y.D. Pathophysiological Roles of Ion Channels in Epidermal Cells, Immune Cells, and Sensory Neurons in Psoriasis. *Int. J. Mol. Sci.* **2024**, *25*, 2756. [CrossRef]
100. Tabeshpour, J.; Banaeeyeh, S.; Eisvand, F.; Sathyapalan, T.; Hashemzaei, M.; Sahebkar, A. Effects of Curcumin on Ion Channels and Pumps: A Review. *IUBMB Life* **2019**, *71*, 812–820. [CrossRef]
101. Kang, D.; Li, B.; Luo, L.; Jiang, W.; Lu, Q.; Rong, M.; Lai, R. Curcumin Shows Excellent Therapeutic Effect on Psoriasis in Mouse Model. *Biochimie* **2016**, *123*, 73–80. [CrossRef]
102. Reddy, S.; Aggarwal, B.B. Curcumin Is a Non-Competitive and Selective Inhibitor of Phosphorylase Kinase. *FEBS Lett.* **1994**, *341*, 19–22. [CrossRef] [PubMed]
103. Li, L.; Liu, C.; Fu, J.; Wang, Y.; Yang, D.; Peng, B.; Liu, X.; Han, X.; Meng, Y.; Feng, F.; et al. CD44 Targeted Indirubin Nanocrystal-Loaded Hyaluronic Acid Hydrogel for the Treatment of Psoriasis. *Int. J. Biol. Macromol.* **2023**, *243*, 125239. [CrossRef] [PubMed]
104. Zhang, Y.; Xia, Q.; Li, Y.; He, Z.; Li, Z.; Guo, T.; Wu, Z.; Feng, N. CD44 Assists the Topical Anti-Psoriatic Efficacy of Curcumin-Loaded Hyaluronan-Modified Ethosomes: A New Strategy for Clustering Drug in Inflammatory Skin. *Theranostics* **2019**, *9*, 48–64. [CrossRef] [PubMed]
105. Sun, L.; Liu, Z.; Wang, L.; Cun, D.; Tong, H.H.Y.; Yan, R.; Chen, X.; Wang, R.; Zheng, Y. Enhanced Topical Penetration, System Exposure and Anti-Psoriasis Activity of Two Particle-Sized, Curcumin-Loaded PLGA Nanoparticles in Hydrogel. *J. Control. Release Off. J. Control. Release Soc.* **2017**, *254*, 44–54. [CrossRef]
106. Jin, N.; Lin, J.; Yang, C.; Wu, C.; He, J.; Chen, Z.; Yang, Q.; Chen, J.; Zheng, G.; Lv, L.; et al. Enhanced Penetration and Anti-Psoriatic Efficacy of Curcumin by Improved SmartPearls Technology with the Addition of Glycyrrhizic Acid. *Int. J. Pharm.* **2020**, *578*, 119101. [CrossRef]
107. Heng, M.C.Y.; Song, M.K.; Harker, J.; Heng, M.K. Drug-induced Suppression of Phosphorylase Kinase Activity Correlates with Resolution of Psoriasis as Assessed by Clinical, Histological and Immunohistochemical Parameters. *Br. J. Dermatol.* **2000**, *143*, 937–949. [CrossRef]
108. Kurd, S.K.; Smith, N.; VanVoorhees, A.; Troxel, A.B.; Badmaev, V.; Seykora, J.T.; Gelfand, J.M. Oral Curcumin in the Treatment of Moderate to Severe Psoriasis Vulgaris: A Prospective Clinical Trial. *J. Am. Acad. Dermatol.* **2008**, *58*, 625–631. [CrossRef]
109. Asawanonda, P.; Klahan, S.-O. Tetrahydrocurcuminoid Cream plus Targeted Narrowband UVB Phototherapy for Vitiligo: A Preliminary Randomized Controlled Study. *Photomed. Laser Surg.* **2010**, *28*, 679–684. [CrossRef]
110. Vaccaro, M.; Bagnato, G.; Cristani, M.; Borgia, F.; Spatari, G.; Tigano, V.; Saja, A.; Guarneri, F.; Cannavò, S.P.; Gangemi, S. Oxidation Products Are Increased in Patients Affected by Non-Segmental Generalized Vitiligo. *Arch. Dermatol. Res.* **2017**, *309*, 485–490. [CrossRef]
111. Sun, Y.P.; Gu, J.F.; Tan, X.B.; Wang, C.F.; Jia, X.B.; Feng, L.; Liu, J.P. Curcumin Inhibits Advanced Glycation End Product-Induced Oxidative Stress and Inflammatory Responses in Endothelial Cell Damage via Trapping Methylglyoxal. *Mol. Med. Rep.* **2016**, *13*, 1475–1486. [CrossRef]
112. Ashrafizadeh, M.; Ahmadi, Z.; Mohammadinejad, R.; Farkhondeh, T.; Samarghandian, S. Curcumin Activates the Nrf2 Pathway and Induces Cellular Protection against Oxidative Injury. *Curr. Mol. Med.* **2020**, *20*, 116–133. [PubMed]
113. Jalalmanesh, S.; Mansouri, P.; Rajabi, M.; Monji, F. Therapeutic Effects of Turmeric Topical Cream in Vitiligo: A Randomized, Double-Blind, Placebo-Controlled Pilot Study. *J. Cosmet. Dermatol.* **2022**, *21*, 4454–4461. [CrossRef] [PubMed]
114. Alshaikh, A.A.; Bharti, R.K. Spontaneous Reversal of Vitiligo, a Rare Phenomenon Reported in a Case in Saudi Arabia with an Insight into Metabolic Biochemical Derangements. *Medicina* **2023**, *59*, 427. [CrossRef] [PubMed]
115. Miller, A.H.; Raison, C.L. The Role of Inflammation in Depression: From Evolutionary Imperative to Modern Treatment Target. *Nat. Rev. Immunol.* **2016**, *16*, 22–34. [CrossRef] [PubMed]

116. Beurel, E.; Toups, M.; Nemeroff, C.B. The Bidirectional Relationship of Depression and Inflammation: Double Trouble. *Neuron* **2020**, *107*, 234–256. [CrossRef]
117. Rahimifard, M.; Maqbool, F.; Moeini-Nodeh, S.; Niaz, K.; Abdollahi, M.; Braidy, N.; Nabavi, S.M.; Nabavi, S.F. Targeting the TLR4 Signaling Pathway by Polyphenols: A Novel Therapeutic Strategy for Neuroinflammation. *Ageing Res. Rev.* **2017**, *36*, 11–19. [CrossRef]
118. Fan, C.; Song, Q.; Wang, P.; Li, Y.; Yang, M.; Liu, B.; Yu, S.Y. Curcumin Protects against Chronic Stress-Induced Dysregulation of Neuroplasticity and Depression-like Behaviors via Suppressing IL-1β Pathway in Rats. *Neuroscience* **2018**, *392*, 92–106. [CrossRef]
119. Zhang, W.; Guo, Y.; Han, W.; Yang, M.; Wen, L.; Wang, K.; Jiang, P. Curcumin Relieves Depressive-like Behaviors via Inhibition of the NLRP3 Inflammasome and Kynurenine Pathway in Rats Suffering from Chronic Unpredictable Mild Stress. *Int. Immunopharmacol.* **2019**, *67*, 138–144. [CrossRef]
120. Fattore, L.; Amchova, P.; Fadda, P.; Ruda-Kucerova, J. Olfactory Bulbectomy Model of Depression Lowers Responding for Food in Male and Female Rats: The Modulating Role of Caloric Restriction and Response Requirement. *Biomedicines* **2023**, *11*, 2481. [CrossRef]
121. Xu, Y.; Ku, B.-S.; Yao, H.-Y.; Lin, Y.-H.; Ma, X.; Zhang, Y.-H.; Li, X.-J. Antidepressant Effects of Curcumin in the Forced Swim Test and Olfactory Bulbectomy Models of Depression in Rats. *Pharmacol. Biochem. Behav.* **2005**, *82*, 200–206. [CrossRef]
122. Wang, R.; Xu, Y.; Wu, H.-L.; Li, Y.-B.; Li, Y.-H.; Guo, J.-B.; Li, X.-J. The Antidepressant Effects of Curcumin in the Forced Swimming Test Involve 5-HT1 and 5-HT2 Receptors. *Eur. J. Pharmacol.* **2008**, *578*, 43–50. [CrossRef] [PubMed]
123. Yang, T.; Nie, Z.; Shu, H.; Kuang, Y.; Chen, X.; Cheng, J.; Yu, S.; Liu, H. The Role of BDNF on Neural Plasticity in Depression. *Front. Cell. Neurosci.* **2020**, *14*, 82. [CrossRef] [PubMed]
124. Hurley, L.L.; Akinfiresoye, L.; Nwulia, E.; Kamiya, A.; Kulkarni, A.A.; Tizabi, Y. Antidepressant-like Effects of Curcumin in WKY Rat Model of Depression Is Associated with an Increase in Hippocampal BDNF. *Behav. Brain Res.* **2013**, *239*, 27–30. [CrossRef] [PubMed]
125. Bhutani, M.K.; Bishnoi, M.; Kulkarni, S.K. Anti-Depressant like Effect of Curcumin and Its Combination with Piperine in Unpredictable Chronic Stress-Induced Behavioral, Biochemical and Neurochemical Changes. *Pharmacol. Biochem. Behav.* **2009**, *92*, 39–43. [CrossRef]
126. Khadrawy, Y.A.; Hosny, E.N.; Magdy, M.; Mohammed, H.S. Antidepressant Effects of Curcumin-Coated Iron Oxide Nanoparticles in a Rat Model of Depression. *Eur. J. Pharmacol.* **2021**, *908*, 174384. [CrossRef]
127. Fahmy, H.M.; Aboalasaad, F.A.; Mohamed, A.S.; Elhusseiny, F.A.; Khadrawy, Y.A.; Elmekawy, A. Evaluation of the Therapeutic Effect of Curcumin-Conjugated Zinc Oxide Nanoparticles on Reserpine-Induced Depression in Wistar Rats. *Biol. Trace Elem. Res.* **2024**, *202*, 2630–2644. [CrossRef]
128. Chen, J.; Wei, Y.; Li, N.; Pi, C.; Zhao, W.; Zhong, Y.; Li, W.; Shen, H.; Yang, Y.; Zheng, W. Preliminary Investigation Into the Antidepressant Effects of a Novel Curcumin Analogue (CACN136) In Vitro and In Vivo. *Mol. Neurobiol.* **2024**, 1–24. [CrossRef]
129. Ng, Q.X.; Koh, S.S.H.; Chan, H.W.; Ho, C.Y.X. Clinical Use of Curcumin in Depression: A Meta-Analysis. *J. Am. Med. Dir. Assoc.* **2017**, *18*, 503–508. [CrossRef]
130. Kanchanatawan, B.; Tangwongchai, S.; Sughondhabhirom, A.; Suppapitiporn, S.; Hemrunrojn, S.; Carvalho, A.F.; Maes, M. Add-on Treatment with Curcumin Has Antidepressive Effects in Thai Patients with Major Depression: Results of a Randomized Double-Blind Placebo-Controlled Study. *Neurotox. Res.* **2018**, *33*, 621–633. [CrossRef]
131. Abu-Taweel, G.M.; Attia, M.F.; Hussein, J.; Mekawi, E.M.; Galal, H.M.; Ahmed, E.I.; Allam, A.A.; El-Naggar, M.E. Curcumin Nanoparticles Have Potential Antioxidant Effect and Restore Tetrahydrobiopterin Levels in Experimental Diabetes. *Biomed. Pharmacother.* **2020**, *131*, 110688. [CrossRef]
132. Noorafshan, A.; Ashkani-Esfahani, S. A Review of Therapeutic Effects of Curcumin. *Curr. Pharm. Des.* **2013**, *19*, 2032–2046. [PubMed]
133. Yallapu, M.M.; Nagesh, P.K.B.; Jaggi, M.; Chauhan, S.C. Therapeutic Applications of Curcumin Nanoformulations. *AAPS J.* **2015**, *17*, 1341–1356. [CrossRef] [PubMed]
134. Rahimi, H.R.; Mohammadpour, A.H.; Dastani, M.; Jaafari, M.R.; Abnous, K.; Mobarhan, M.G.; Oskuee, R.K. The Effect of Nano-Curcumin on HbA1c, Fasting Blood Glucose, and Lipid Profile in Diabetic Subjects: A Randomized Clinical Trial. *Avicenna J. Phytomedicine* **2016**, *6*, 567.
135. Na, L.; Li, Y.; Pan, H.; Zhou, X.; Sun, D.; Meng, M.; Li, X.; Sun, C. Curcuminoids Exert Glucose-lowering Effect in Type 2 Diabetes by Decreasing Serum Free Fatty Acids: A Double-blind, Placebo-controlled Trial. *Mol. Nutr. Food Res.* **2013**, *57*, 1569–1577. [CrossRef]
136. Funamoto, M.; Shimizu, K.; Sunagawa, Y.; Katanasaka, Y.; Miyazaki, Y.; Kakeya, H.; Yamakage, H.; Satoh-Asahara, N.; Wada, H.; Hasegawa, K.; et al. Effects of Highly Absorbable Curcumin in Patients with Impaired Glucose Tolerance and Non-Insulin-Dependent Diabetes Mellitus. *J. Diabetes Res.* **2019**, *2019*, 8208237. [CrossRef]
137. Panahi, Y.; Khalili, N.; Sahebi, E.; Namazi, S.; Simental-Mendía, L.E.; Majeed, M.; Sahebkar, A. Effects of Curcuminoids plus Piperine on Glycemic, Hepatic and Inflammatory Biomarkers in Patients with Type 2 Diabetes Mellitus: A Randomized Double-Blind Placebo-Controlled Trial. *Drug Res.* **2018**, *68*, 403–409. [CrossRef]
138. Agharazi, M.; Gazerani, S.; Huntington, M.K. Topical Turmeric Ointment in the Treatment of Diabetic Foot Ulcers: A Randomized, Placebo-Controlled Study. *Int. J. Low. Extrem. Wounds* **2022**, 15347346221143222. [CrossRef]

139. Mokhtari, M.; Razzaghi, R.; Momen-Heravi, M. The Effects of Curcumin Intake on Wound Healing and Metabolic Status in Patients with Diabetic Foot Ulcer: A Randomized, Double-blind, Placebo-controlled Trial. *Phyther. Res.* **2021**, *35*, 2099–2107. [CrossRef]
140. Cui, L.; Miao, J.; Cui, L. Cytotoxic Effect of Curcumin on Malaria Parasite Plasmodium Falciparum: Inhibition of Histone Acetylation and Generation of Reactive Oxygen Species. *Antimicrob. Agents Chemother.* **2007**, *51*, 488–494. [CrossRef]
141. Reddy, R.C.; Vatsala, P.G.; Keshamouni, V.G.; Padmanaban, G.; Rangarajan, P.N. Curcumin for Malaria Therapy. *Biochem. Biophys. Res. Commun.* **2005**, *326*, 472–474. [CrossRef]
142. Nandakumar, D.N.; Nagaraj, V.A.; Vathsala, P.G.; Rangarajan, P.; Padmanaban, G. Curcumin-Artemisinin Combination Therapy for Malaria. *Antimicrob. Agents Chemother.* **2006**, *50*, 1859–1860. [CrossRef] [PubMed]
143. Tjahjani, S.; Tjokropranoto, R. Interaction of Alphamangostin and Curcumin with Dihydroartemisinin as Antimalaria in Vitro. In Proceedings of the IOP Conference Series: Earth and Environmental Science; IOP Publishing: Bristol, UK, 2018; Volume 125, p. 12017.
144. Akide Ndunge, O.B.; Kilian, N.; Salman, M.M. Cerebral Malaria and Neuronal Implications of Plasmodium Falciparum Infection: From Mechanisms to Advanced Models. *Adv. Sci.* **2022**, *9*, e2202944. [CrossRef] [PubMed]
145. Aggarwal, B.B.; Gupta, S.C.; Sung, B. Curcumin: An Orally Bioavailable Blocker of TNF and Other pro-Inflammatory Biomarkers. *Br. J. Pharmacol.* **2013**, *169*, 1672–1692. [CrossRef] [PubMed]
146. Dende, C.; Meena, J.; Nagarajan, P.; Nagaraj, V.A.; Panda, A.K.; Padmanaban, G. Nanocurcumin Is Superior to Native Curcumin in Preventing Degenerative Changes in Experimental Cerebral Malaria. *Sci. Rep.* **2017**, *7*, 10062. [CrossRef]
147. Ghosh, A.; Banerjee, T.; Bhandary, S.; Surolia, A. Formulation of Nanotized Curcumin and Demonstration of Its Antimalarial Efficacy. *Int. J. Nanomed.* **2014**, *9*, 5373–5387. [CrossRef]
148. Dandekar, P.P.; Jain, R.; Patil, S.; Dhumal, R.; Tiwari, D.; Sharma, S.; Vanage, G.; Patravale, V. Curcumin-Loaded Hydrogel Nanoparticles: Application in Anti-Malarial Therapy and Toxicological Evaluation. *J. Pharm. Sci.* **2010**, *99*, 4992–5010. [CrossRef]
149. Rashidzadeh, H.; Salimi, M.; Sadighian, S.; Rostamizadeh, K.; Ramazani, A. In Vivo Antiplasmodial Activity of Curcumin-Loaded Nanostructured Lipid Carriers. *Curr. Drug Deliv.* **2019**, *16*, 923–930. [CrossRef]
150. Akhtar, F.; Rizvi, M.M.A.; Kar, S.K. Oral Delivery of Curcumin Bound to Chitosan Nanoparticles Cured Plasmodium Yoelii Infected Mice. *Biotechnol. Adv.* **2012**, *30*, 310–320. [CrossRef]
151. Dos Santos, R.B.; Nakama, K.A.; Pacheco, C.O.; de Gomes, M.G.; de Souza, J.F.; de Souza Pinto, A.C.; de Oliveira, F.A.; da Fonseca, A.L.; Varotti, F.; Fajardo, A.R. Curcumin-Loaded Nanocapsules: Influence of Surface Characteristics on Technological Parameters and Potential Antimalarial Activity. *Mater. Sci. Eng. C* **2021**, *118*, 111356. [CrossRef]
152. Memvanga, P.B.; Coco, R.; Préat, V. An Oral Malaria Therapy: Curcumin-Loaded Lipid-Based Drug Delivery Systems Combined with β-Arteether. *J. Control. Release* **2013**, *172*, 904–913. [CrossRef]
153. Khairani, S.; Fauziah, N.; Wiraswati, H.L.; Panigoro, R.; Setyowati, E.Y.; Berbudi, A. The Potential Use of a Curcumin-Piperine Combination as an Antimalarial Agent: A Systematic Review. *J. Trop. Med.* **2021**, *2021*, 9135617. [CrossRef] [PubMed]
154. Schraufstätter, E.; Bernt, H. Antibacterial Action of Curcumin and Related Compounds. *Nature* **1949**, *164*, 456–457. [CrossRef] [PubMed]
155. Mitra, A.K. Chemistry and Biomedical Applications of Cumin and Turmeric: A Review, Challenge and Perspective. *Chem. Afr.* **2022**, *5*, 1191–1213. [CrossRef]
156. Rai, D.; Singh, J.K.; Roy, N.; Panda, D. Curcumin Inhibits FtsZ Assembly: An Attractive Mechanism for Its Antibacterial Activity. *Biochem. J.* **2008**, *410*, 147–155. [CrossRef]
157. Tyagi, P.; Singh, M.; Kumari, H.; Kumari, A.; Mukhopadhyay, K. Bactericidal Activity of Curcumin I Is Associated with Damaging of Bacterial Membrane. *PLoS ONE* **2015**, *10*, e0121313. [CrossRef]
158. Sharifian, P.; Yaslianifard, S.; Fallah, P.; Aynesazi, S.; Bakhtiyari, M.; Mohammadzadeh, M. Investigating the Effect of Nano-Curcumin on the Expression of Biofilm Regulatory Genes of Pseudomonas Aeruginosa. *Infect. Drug Resist.* **2020**, *13*, 2477–2484. [CrossRef]
159. Teow, S.-Y.; Liew, K.; Ali, S.A.; Khoo, A.S.-B.; Peh, S.-C. Antibacterial Action of Curcumin against Staphylococcus Aureus: A Brief Review. *J. Trop. Med.* **2016**, *2016*, 2853045. [CrossRef]
160. Zandi, K.; Ramedani, E.; Mohammadi, K.; Tajbakhsh, S.; Deilami, I.; Rastian, Z.; Fouladvand, M.; Yousefi, F.; Farshadpour, F. Evaluation of Antiviral Activities of Curcumin Derivatives against HSV-1 in Vero Cell Line. *Nat. Prod. Commun.* **2010**, *5*, 1934578X1000501220. [CrossRef]
161. De, R.; Kundu, P.; Swarnakar, S.; Ramamurthy, T.; Chowdhury, A.; Nair, G.B.; Mukhopadhyay, A.K. Antimicrobial Activity of Curcumin against Helicobacter Pylori Isolates from India and during Infections in Mice. *Antimicrob. Agents Chemother.* **2009**, *53*, 1592–1597. [CrossRef]
162. Hettiarachchi, S.S.; Perera, Y.; Dunuweera, S.P.; Dunuweera, A.N.; Rajapakse, S.; Rajapakse, R.M.G. Comparison of Antibacterial Activity of Nanocurcumin with Bulk Curcumin. *ACS Omega* **2022**, *7*, 46494–46500. [CrossRef]
163. Mun, S.-H.; Joung, D.-K.; Kim, Y.-S.; Kang, O.-H.; Kim, S.-B.; Seo, Y.-S.; Kim, Y.-C.; Lee, D.-S.; Shin, D.-W.; Kweon, K.-T. Synergistic Antibacterial Effect of Curcumin against Methicillin-Resistant Staphylococcus Aureus. *Phytomedicine* **2013**, *20*, 714–718. [CrossRef] [PubMed]
164. Teow, S.-Y.; Ali, S.A. Synergistic Antibacterial Activity of Curcumin with Antibiotics against Staphylococcus Aureus. *Pak. J. Pharm. Sci.* **2015**, *28*, 2109–2111. [PubMed]

165. Olufunmilayo, E.O.; Gerke-Duncan, M.B.; Holsinger, R.M.D. Oxidative Stress and Antioxidants in Neurodegenerative Disorders. *Antioxidants* **2023**, *12*, 517. [CrossRef] [PubMed]
166. Wang, S.; Wu, P.; Fan, Z.; He, X.; Liu, J.; Li, M.; Chen, F. Dandelion Polysaccharide Treatment Protects against Dextran Sodium Sulfate-induced Colitis by Suppressing NF-κB/NLRP3 Inflammasome-mediated Inflammation and Activating Nrf2 in Mouse Colon. *Food Sci. Nutr.* **2023**, *11*, 7271–7282. [CrossRef]
167. Fan, C.; Song, Q.; Wang, P.; Li, Y.; Yang, M.; Yu, S.Y. Neuroprotective Effects of Curcumin on IL-1β-Induced Neuronal Apoptosis and Depression-like Behaviors Caused by Chronic Stress in Rats. *Front. Cell. Neurosci.* **2019**, *12*, 516. [CrossRef]
168. Wu, J.; Li, Q.; Wang, X.; Yu, S.; Li, L.; Wu, X.; Chen, Y.; Zhao, J.; Zhao, Y. Neuroprotection by Curcumin in Ischemic Brain Injury Involves the Akt/Nrf2 Pathway. *PLoS ONE* **2013**, *8*, e59843. [CrossRef]
169. Qi, X.-J.; Liu, X.-Y.; Tang, L.-M.-Y.; Li, P.-F.; Qiu, F.; Yang, A.-H. Anti-Depressant Effect of Curcumin-Loaded Guanidine-Chitosan Thermo-Sensitive Hydrogel by Nasal Delivery. *Pharm. Dev. Technol.* **2020**, *25*, 316–325. [CrossRef]
170. Zbarsky, V.; Datla, K.P.; Parkar, S.; Rai, D.K.; Aruoma, O.I.; Dexter, D.T. Neuroprotective Properties of the Natural Phenolic Antioxidants Curcumin and Naringenin but Not Quercetin and Fisetin in a 6-OHDA Model of Parkinson's Disease. *Free Radic. Res.* **2005**, *39*, 1119–1125. [CrossRef]
171. Agrawal, S.S.; Gullaiya, S.; Dubey, V.; Singh, V.; Kumar, A.; Nagar, A.; Tiwari, P. Neurodegenerative Shielding by Curcumin and Its Derivatives on Brain Lesions Induced by 6-OHDA Model of Parkinson's Disease in Albino Wistar Rats. *Cardiovasc. Psychiatry Neurol.* **2012**, *2012*, 942981. [CrossRef]
172. Song, S.; Nie, Q.; Li, Z.; Du, G. Curcumin Improves Neurofunctions of 6-OHDA-Induced Parkinsonian Rats. *Pathol. Res. Pract.* **2016**, *212*, 247–251. [CrossRef]
173. Yang, J.; Song, S.; Li, J.; Liang, T. Neuroprotective Effect of Curcumin on Hippocampal Injury in 6-OHDA-Induced Parkinson's Disease Rat. *Pathol. Res. Pract.* **2014**, *210*, 357–362. [CrossRef] [PubMed]
174. Liu, X.; Zhang, H.; Li, C.; Chen, Z.; Gao, Q.; Han, M.; Zhao, F.; Chen, D.; Chen, Q.; Hu, M.; et al. The Dosage of Curcumin to Alleviate Movement Symptoms in a 6-Hydroxydopamine-Induced Parkinson's Disease Rat Model. *Heliyon* **2023**, *9*, e16921. [CrossRef] [PubMed]
175. Armstrong, R.A. Risk Factors for Alzheimer's Disease. *Folia Neuropathol.* **2019**, *57*, 87–105. [CrossRef] [PubMed]
176. Cummings, J.; Osse, A.M.L.; Cammann, D.; Powell, J.; Chen, J. Anti-Amyloid Monoclonal Antibodies for the Treatment of Alzheimer's Disease. *BioDrugs* **2024**, *38*, 5–22. [CrossRef]
177. Yang, F.; Lim, G.P.; Begum, A.N.; Ubeda, O.J.; Simmons, M.R.; Ambegaokar, S.S.; Chen, P.P.; Kayed, R.; Glabe, C.G.; Frautschy, S.A.; et al. Curcumin Inhibits Formation of Amyloid Beta Oligomers and Fibrils, Binds Plaques, and Reduces Amyloid in Vivo. *J. Biol. Chem.* **2005**, *280*, 5892–5901. [CrossRef]
178. Ye, J.; Zhang, Y. Curcumin Protects against Intracellular Amyloid Toxicity in Rat Primary Neurons. *Int. J. Clin. Exp. Med.* **2012**, *5*, 44–49.
179. Shi, H.; Yin, Z.; Koronyo, Y.; Fuchs, D.-T.; Sheyn, J.; Davis, M.R.; Wilson, J.W.; Margeta, M.A.; Pitts, K.M.; Herron, S.; et al. Regulating Microglial MiR-155 Transcriptional Phenotype Alleviates Alzheimer's-Induced Retinal Vasculopathy by Limiting Clec7a/Galectin-3(+) Neurodegenerative Microglia. *Acta Neuropathol. Commun.* **2022**, *10*, 136. [CrossRef]
180. Teter, B.; Morihara, T.; Lim, G.P.; Chu, T.; Jones, M.R.; Zuo, X.; Paul, R.M.; Frautschy, S.A.; Cole, G.M. Curcumin Restores Innate Immune Alzheimer's Disease Risk Gene Expression to Ameliorate Alzheimer Pathogenesis. *Neurobiol. Dis.* **2019**, *127*, 432–448. [CrossRef]
181. Small, G.W.; Siddarth, P.; Li, Z.; Miller, K.J.; Ercoli, L.; Emerson, N.D.; Martinez, J.; Wong, K.-P.; Liu, J.; Merrill, D.A. Memory and Brain Amyloid and Tau Effects of a Bioavailable Form of Curcumin in Non-Demented Adults: A Double-Blind, Placebo-Controlled 18-Month Trial. *Am. J. Geriatr. Psychiatry* **2018**, *26*, 266–277. [CrossRef]
182. Das, S.S.; Gopal, P.M.; Thomas, J.V.; Mohan, M.C.; Thomas, S.C.; Maliakel, B.P.; Krishnakumar, I.M.; Pulikkaparambil Sasidharan, B.C. Influence of CurQfen®-Curcumin on Cognitive Impairment: A Randomized, Double-Blinded, Placebo-Controlled, 3-Arm, 3-Sequence Comparative Study. *Front. Dement.* **2023**, *2*, 1222708. [CrossRef]
183. Rainey-Smith, S.R.; Brown, B.M.; Sohrabi, H.R.; Shah, T.; Goozee, K.G.; Gupta, V.B.; Martins, R.N. Curcumin and Cognition: A Randomised, Placebo-Controlled, Double-Blind Study of Community-Dwelling Older Adults. *Br. J. Nutr.* **2016**, *115*, 2106–2113. [CrossRef] [PubMed]
184. Sharma, R.A.; Steward, W.P.; Gescher, A.J. Pharmacokinetics and Pharmacodynamics of Curcumin. *Adv. Exp. Med. Biol.* **2007**, *595*, 453–470. [PubMed]
185. Wang, Y.-J.; Pan, M.-H.; Cheng, A.-L.; Lin, L.-I.; Ho, Y.-S.; Hsieh, C.-Y.; Lin, J.-K. Stability of Curcumin in Buffer Solutions and Characterization of Its Degradation Products. *J. Pharm. Biomed. Anal.* **1997**, *15*, 1867–1876. [CrossRef] [PubMed]
186. Anand, P.; Kunnumakkara, A.B.; Newman, R.A.; Aggarwal, B.B. Bioavailability of Curcumin: Problems and Promises. *Mol. Pharm.* **2007**, *4*, 807–818. [CrossRef]
187. Siviero, A.; Gallo, E.; Maggini, V.; Gori, L.; Mugelli, A.; Firenzuoli, F.; Vannacci, A. Curcumin, a Golden Spice with a Low Bioavailability. *J. Herb. Med.* **2015**, *5*, 57–70. [CrossRef]
188. Shoba, G.; Joy, D.; Joseph, T.; Majeed, M.; Rajendran, R.; Srinivas, P. Influence of Piperine on the Pharmacokinetics of Curcumin in Animals and Human Volunteers. *Planta Med.* **1998**, *64*, 353–356. [CrossRef]
189. Prasad, S.; DuBourdieu, D.; Srivastava, A.; Kumar, P.; Lall, R. Metal-Curcumin Complexes in Therapeutics: An Approach to Enhance Pharmacological Effects of Curcumin. *Int. J. Mol. Sci.* **2021**, *22*, 7094. [CrossRef]

190. Baek, J.-S.; Cho, C.-W. Surface Modification of Solid Lipid Nanoparticles for Oral Delivery of Curcumin: Improvement of Bioavailability through Enhanced Cellular Uptake, and Lymphatic Uptake. *Eur. J. Pharm. Biopharm.* **2017**, *117*, 132–140. [CrossRef]
191. Hegde, M.; Girisa, S.; BharathwajChetty, B.; Vishwa, R.; Kunnumakkara, A.B. Curcumin Formulations for Better Bioavailability: What We Learned from Clinical Trials Thus Far? *ACS Omega* **2023**, *8*, 10713–10746. [CrossRef]
192. Li, Z.; Peng, S.; Chen, X.; Zhu, Y.; Zou, L.; Liu, W.; Liu, C. Pluronics Modified Liposomes for Curcumin Encapsulation: Sustained Release, Stability and Bioaccessibility. *Food Res. Int.* **2018**, *108*, 246–253. [CrossRef]
193. Zeng, L.; Yang, T.; Yang, K.; Yu, G.; Li, J.; Xiang, W.; Chen, H. Efficacy and Safety of Curcumin and Curcuma Longa Extract in the Treatment of Arthritis: A Systematic Review and Meta-Analysis of Randomized Controlled Trial. *Front. Immunol.* **2022**, *13*, 891822. [CrossRef] [PubMed]
194. Sharifi-Rad, J.; El Rayess, Y.; Rizk, A.A.; Sadaka, C.; Zgheib, R.; Zam, W.; Sestito, S.; Rapposelli, S.; Zielińska, D.; Setzer, W.N. Turmeric and Its Major Compound Curcumin on Health: Bioactive Effects and Safety Profiles for Food, Pharmaceutical, Biotechnological and Medicinal Applications. *Front. Pharmacol.* **2020**, *11*, 550909. [CrossRef] [PubMed]
195. Sahebkar, A. Are Curcuminoids Effective C-Reactive Protein-Lowering Agents in Clinical Practice? Evidence from a Meta-Analysis. *Phytother. Res.* **2014**, *28*, 633–642. [CrossRef] [PubMed]
196. Vogel, A.; Pelletier, J. Examen Chimique de La Racine de Curcuma. *J. Pharm* **1815**, *1*, 289–300.
197. Gupta, S.C.; Patchva, S.; Koh, W.; Aggarwal, B.B. Discovery of Curcumin, a Component of Golden Spice, and Its Miraculous Biological Activities. *Clin. Exp. Pharmacol. Physiol.* **2012**, *39*, 283–299. [CrossRef]
198. Liju, V.B.; Jeena, K.; Kuttan, R. Acute and Subchronic Toxicity as Well as Mutagenic Evaluation of Essential Oil from Turmeric (*Curcuma Longa* L). *Food Chem. Toxicol.* **2013**, *53*, 52–61. [CrossRef]
199. Kim, D.-C.; Ku, S.-K.; Bae, J.-S. Anticoagulant Activities of Curcumin and Its Derivative. *BMB Rep.* **2012**, *45*, 221–226. [CrossRef]
200. Shah, B.H.; Nawaz, Z.; Pertani, S.A.; Roomi, A.; Mahmood, H.; Saeed, S.A.; Gilani, A.H. Inhibitory Effect of Curcumin, a Food Spice from Turmeric, on Platelet-Activating Factor-and Arachidonic Acid-Mediated Platelet Aggregation through Inhibition of Thromboxane Formation and Ca^{2+} Signaling. *Biochem. Pharmacol.* **1999**, *58*, 1167–1172. [CrossRef]
201. Chaudhari, S.P.; Tam, A.Y.; Barr, J.A. Curcumin: A Contact Allergen. *J. Clin. Aesthet. Dermatol.* **2015**, *8*, 43–48.
202. Sathyabhama, M.; Priya Dharshini, L.C.; Karthikeyan, A.; Kalaiselvi, S.; Min, T. The Credible Role of Curcumin in Oxidative Stress-Mediated Mitochondrial Dysfunction in Mammals. *Biomolecules* **2022**, *12*, 1405. [CrossRef]
203. Barclay, L.R.C.; Vinqvist, M.R.; Mukai, K.; Goto, H.; Hashimoto, Y.; Tokunaga, A.; Uno, H. On the Antioxidant Mechanism of Curcumin: Classical Methods Are Needed to Determine Antioxidant Mechanism and Activity. *Org. Lett.* **2000**, *2*, 2841–2843. [CrossRef] [PubMed]
204. Hussain, T.; Tan, B.; Yin, Y.; Blachier, F.; Tossou, M.C.B.; Rahu, N. Oxidative Stress and Inflammation: What Polyphenols Can Do for Us? *Oxid. Med. Cell. Longev.* **2016**, *2016*, 7432797. [CrossRef] [PubMed]
205. Paulraj, F.; Abas, F.; Lajis, N.H.; Othman, I.; Naidu, R. Molecular Pathways Modulated by Curcumin Analogue, Diarylpentanoids in Cancer. *Biomolecules* **2019**, *9*, 270. [CrossRef] [PubMed]
206. Giordano, A.; Tommonaro, G. Curcumin and Cancer. *Nutrients* **2019**, *11*, 2376. [CrossRef] [PubMed]
207. Zhou, H.; Beevers, C.S.; Huang, S. The Targets of Curcumin. *Curr. Drug Targets* **2011**, *12*, 332–347. [CrossRef]
208. Zhang, F.; Altorki, N.K.; Mestre, J.R.; Subbaramaiah, K.; Dannenberg, A.J. Curcumin Inhibits Cyclooxygenase-2 Transcription in Bile Acid-and Phorbol Ester-Treated Human Gastrointestinal Epithelial Cells. *Carcinogenesis* **1999**, *20*, 445–451. [CrossRef]
209. Setyono, J.; Harini, I.M.; Sarmoko, S.; Rujito, L. Supplementation of Curcuma Domestica Extract Reduces Cox-2 and Inos Expression on Raw 264.7 Cells. *J. Phys. Conf. Ser.* **2019**, *1246*, 12059. [CrossRef]
210. Lee, S.-Y.; Cho, S.-S.; Li, Y.; Bae, C.-S.; Park, K.M.; Park, D.-H. Anti-Inflammatory Effect of Curcuma Longa and Allium Hookeri Co-Treatment via NF-KB and COX-2 Pathways. *Sci. Rep.* **2020**, *10*, 5718. [CrossRef]
211. Sreejayan, X.X.; Rao, M.N.A. Nitric Oxide Scavenging by Curcuminoids. *J. Pharm. Pharmacol.* **1997**, *49*, 105–107. [CrossRef]
212. Sreejayan, N.; Rao, M.N. Free Radical Scavenging Activity of Curcuminoids. *Arzneimittelforschung* **1996**, *46*, 169–171.
213. Carvalho, D.d.M.; Takeuchi, K.P.; Geraldine, R.M.; de Moura, C.J.; Torres, M.C.L. Production, Solubility and Antioxidant Activity of Curcumin Nanosuspension. *Food Sci. Technol.* **2015**, *35*, 115–119. [CrossRef]
214. Priyadarsini, K.I.; Maity, D.K.; Naik, G.H.; Kumar, M.S.; Unnikrishnan, M.K.; Satav, J.G.; Mohan, H. Role of Phenolic O-H and Methylene Hydrogen on the Free Radical Reactions and Antioxidant Activity of Curcumin. *Free Radic. Biol. Med.* **2003**, *35*, 475–484. [CrossRef] [PubMed]
215. Jayaprakasha, G.K.; Rao, L.J.; Sakariah, K.K. Antioxidant Activities of Curcumin, Demethoxycurcumin and Bisdemethoxycurcumin. *Food Chem.* **2006**, *98*, 720–724. [CrossRef]
216. Lin, X.; Bai, D.; Wei, Z.; Zhang, Y.; Huang, Y.; Deng, H.; Huang, X. Curcumin Attenuates Oxidative Stress in RAW264. 7 Cells by Increasing the Activity of Antioxidant Enzymes and Activating the Nrf2-Keap1 Pathway. *PLoS ONE* **2019**, *14*, e0216711.
217. Ren, L.; Zhan, P.; Wang, Q.; Wang, C.; Liu, Y.; Yu, Z.; Zhang, S. Curcumin Upregulates the Nrf2 System by Repressing Inflammatory Signaling-Mediated Keap1 Expression in Insulin-Resistant Conditions. *Biochem. Biophys. Res. Commun.* **2019**, *514*, 691–698. [CrossRef]
218. Liu, F.; Gao, S.; Yang, Y.; Zhao, X.; Fan, Y.; Ma, W.; Yang, D.; Yang, A.; Yu, Y. Antitumor Activity of Curcumin by Modulation of Apoptosis and Autophagy in Human Lung Cancer A549 Cells through Inhibiting PI3K/Akt/MTOR Pathway. *Oncol. Rep.* **2018**, *39*, 1523–1531. [CrossRef]

219. Kuttikrishnan, S.; Siveen, K.S.; Prabhu, K.S.; Khan, A.Q.; Ahmed, E.I.; Akhtar, S.; Ali, T.A.; Merhi, M.; Dermime, S.; Steinhoff, M. Curcumin Induces Apoptotic Cell Death via Inhibition of PI3-Kinase/AKT Pathway in B-Precursor Acute Lymphoblastic Leukemia. *Front. Oncol.* **2019**, *9*, 484. [CrossRef]
220. Panahi, Y.; Rahimnia, A.; Sharafi, M.; Alishiri, G.; Saburi, A.; Sahebkar, A. Curcuminoid Treatment for Knee Osteoarthritis: A Randomized Double-blind Placebo-controlled Trial. *Phyther. Res.* **2014**, *28*, 1625–1631. [CrossRef]
221. Panahi, Y.; Saadat, A.; Beiraghdar, F.; Sahebkar, A. Adjuvant Therapy with Bioavailability-Boosted Curcuminoids Suppresses Systemic Inflammation and Improves Quality of Life in Patients with Solid Tumors: A Randomized Double-Blind Placebo-Controlled Trial. *Phytother. Res.* **2014**, *28*, 1461–1467. [CrossRef]
222. Panahi, Y.; Hosseini, M.S.; Khalili, N.; Naimi, E.; Simental-Mendía, L.E.; Majeed, M.; Sahebkar, A. Effects of Curcumin on Serum Cytokine Concentrations in Subjects with Metabolic Syndrome: A Post-Hoc Analysis of a Randomized Controlled Trial. *Biomed. Pharmacother.* **2016**, *82*, 578–582. [CrossRef]
223. Abe, Y.; Hashimoto, S.H.U.; Horie, T. Curcumin Inhibition of Inflammatory Cytokine Production by Human Peripheral Blood Monocytes and Alveolar Macrophages. *Pharmacol. Res.* **1999**, *39*, 41–47. [CrossRef] [PubMed]
224. Cianciulli, A.; Calvello, R.; Porro, C.; Trotta, T.; Salvatore, R.; Panaro, M.A. PI3k/Akt Signalling Pathway Plays a Crucial Role in the Anti-Inflammatory Effects of Curcumin in LPS-Activated Microglia. *Int. Immunopharmacol.* **2016**, *36*, 282–290. [CrossRef] [PubMed]
225. Yadav, V.S.; Mishra, K.P.; Singh, D.P.; Mehrotra, S.; Singh, V.K. Immunomodulatory Effects of Curcumin. *Immunopharmacol. Immunotoxicol.* **2005**, *27*, 485–497. [CrossRef]
226. Li, W.; Wang, Z.; Xiao, X.; Han, L.; Wu, Z.; Ma, Q.; Cao, L. Curcumin Attenuates Hyperglycemia-Driven EGF-Induced Invasive and Migratory Abilities of Pancreatic Cancer via Suppression of the ERK and AKT Pathways. *Oncol. Rep.* **2019**, *41*, 650–658. [CrossRef]
227. Mohan, R.; Sivak, J.; Ashton, P.; Russo, L.A.; Pham, B.Q.; Kasahara, N.; Raizman, M.B.; Fini, M.E. Curcuminoids Inhibit the Angiogenic Response Stimulated by Fibroblast Growth Factor-2, Including Expression of Matrix Metalloproteinase Gelatinase B. *J. Biol. Chem.* **2000**, *275*, 10405–10412. [CrossRef]
228. El-Azab, M.; Hishe, H.; Moustafa, Y.; El-Awady, E.-S. Anti-Angiogenic Effect of Resveratrol or Curcumin in Ehrlich Ascites Carcinoma-Bearing Mice. *Eur. J. Pharmacol.* **2011**, *652*, 7–14. [CrossRef]
229. Bae, M.-K.; Kim, S.-H.; Jeong, J.-W.; Lee, Y.M.; Kim, H.-S.; Kim, S.-R.; Yun, I.; Bae, S.-K.; Kim, K.-W. Curcumin Inhibits Hypoxia-Induced Angiogenesis via down-Regulation of HIF-1. *Oncol. Rep.* **2006**, *15*, 1557–1562. [CrossRef]
230. Nakamura, K.; Yasunaga, Y.; Segawa, T.; Ko, D.; Moul, J.W.; Srivastava, S.; Rhim, J.S. Curcumin Down-Regulates AR Gene Expression and Activation in Prostate Cancer Cell Lines. *Int. J. Oncol.* **2002**, *21*, 825–830. [CrossRef]
231. Dorai, T.; Gehani, N.; Katz, A. Therapeutic Potential of Curcumin in Human Prostate Cancer—I. Curcumin Induces Apoptosis in Both Androgen-Dependent and Androgen-Independent Prostate Cancer Cells. *Prostate Cancer Prostatic Dis.* **2000**, *3*, 84–93. [CrossRef]
232. Saxena, A.R.; Ilic, Z.; Sripada, V.; Crawford, D.R. Lower Concentrations of Curcumin Inhibit Her2-Akt Pathway Components in Human Breast Cancer Cells, and Other Dietary Botanicals Potentiate This and Lapatinib Inhibition. *Nutr. Res.* **2020**, *78*, 93–104. [CrossRef]
233. Miyazaki, K.; Morine, Y.; Xu, C.; Nakasu, C.; Wada, Y.; Teraoku, H.; Yamada, S.; Saito, Y.; Ikemoto, T.; Shimada, M.; et al. Curcumin-Mediated Resistance to Lenvatinib via EGFR Signaling Pathway in Hepatocellular Carcinoma. *Cells* **2023**, *12*, 612. [CrossRef] [PubMed]
234. Lee, J.-Y.; Lee, Y.-M.; Chang, G.-C.; Yu, S.-L.; Hsieh, W.-Y.; Chen, J.J.W.; Chen, H.-W.; Yang, P.-C. Curcumin Induces EGFR Degradation in Lung Adenocarcinoma and Modulates P38 Activation in Intestine: The Versatile Adjuvant for Gefitinib Therapy. *PLoS ONE* **2011**, *6*, e23756. [CrossRef] [PubMed]
235. Park, Y.-G.; Cho, J.-H.; Choi, J.; Ju, E.-M.; Adam, G.O.; Hwang, D.-I.; Lee, J.-H.; An, S.-Y.; Choi, H.-K.; Park, C.-B. Immunomodulatory Effects of *Curcuma Longa* L. and *Carthamus Tinctorius* L. on RAW 264.7 Macrophages and Cyclophosphamide-Induced Immunosuppression C57BL/6 Mouse Models. *J. Funct. Foods* **2022**, *91*, 105000. [CrossRef]
236. Huang, M.-T.; Lysz, T.; Ferraro, T.; Abidi, T.F.; Laskin, J.D.; Conney, A.H. Inhibitory Effects of Curcumin on in Vitro Lipoxygenase and Cyclooxygenase Activities in Mouse Epidermis. *Cancer Res.* **1991**, *51*, 813–819.
237. Srimal, R.C.; Dhawan, B.N. Pharmacology of Diferuloyl Methane (Curcumin), a Non-steroidal Anti-inflammatory Agent. *J. Pharm. Pharmacol.* **1973**, *25*, 447–452. [CrossRef]
238. Cao, J.; Han, Z.; Tian, L.; Chen, K.; Fan, Y.; Ye, B.; Huang, W.; Wang, C.; Huang, Z. Curcumin Inhibits EMMPRIN and MMP-9 Expression through AMPK-MAPK and PKC Signaling in PMA Induced Macrophages. *J. Transl. Med.* **2014**, *12*, 266. [CrossRef]
239. Youn, G.S.; Kwon, D.-J.; Ju, S.M.; Choi, S.Y.; Park, J. Curcumin Ameliorates TNF-α-Induced ICAM-1 Expression and Subsequent THP-1 Adhesiveness via the Induction of Heme Oxygenase-1 in the HaCaT Cells. *BMB Rep.* **2013**, *46*, 410–415. [CrossRef]
240. Machova Urdzikova, L.; Karova, K.; Ruzicka, J.; Kloudova, A.; Shannon, C.; Dubisova, J.; Murali, R.; Kubinova, S.; Sykova, E.; Jhanwar-Uniyal, M.; et al. The Anti-Inflammatory Compound Curcumin Enhances Locomotor and Sensory Recovery after Spinal Cord Injury in Rats by Immunomodulation. *Int. J. Mol. Sci.* **2015**, *17*, 49. [CrossRef]
241. Binion, D.G.; Heidemann, J.; Li, M.S.; Nelson, V.M.; Otterson, M.F.; Rafiee, P. Vascular Cell Adhesion Molecule-1 Expression in Human Intestinal Microvascular Endothelial Cells Is Regulated by PI 3-Kinase/Akt/MAPK/NF-KappaB: Inhibitory Role of Curcumin. *Am. J. Physiol. Gastrointest. Liver Physiol.* **2009**, *297*, G259–G268. [CrossRef]

242. Wang, J.; Qi, L.; Zheng, S.; Wu, T. Curcumin Induces Apoptosis through the Mitochondria-Mediated Apoptotic Pathway in HT-29 Cells. *J. Zhejiang Univ. Sci. B* **2009**, *10*, 93–102. [CrossRef]
243. Yang, Z.; Li, X.; Peng, Z.; Song, J.; Ren, J. Curcumin Down-Regulates PCNA, Cyclin D1 and Bcl-XL Expression in Human Keratinocyte Cell Lines. *J. Med. Coll. PLA* **2010**, *25*, 321–330.
244. Meena, R.; Kumar, S.; Gaharwar, U.S.; Rajamani, P. PLGA-CTAB Curcumin Nanoparticles: Fabrication, Characterization and Molecular Basis of Anticancer Activity in Triple Negative Breast Cancer Cell Lines (MDA-MB-231 Cells). *Biomed. Pharmacother.* **2017**, *94*, 944–954. [CrossRef] [PubMed]
245. Dhandapani, K.M.; Mahesh, V.B.; Brann, D.W. Curcumin Suppresses Growth and Chemoresistance of Human Glioblastoma Cells via AP-1 and NFkappaB Transcription Factors. *J. Neurochem.* **2007**, *102*, 522–538. [CrossRef] [PubMed]
246. Kliem, C.; Merling, A.; Giaisi, M.; Köhler, R.; Krammer, P.H.; Li-Weber, M. Curcumin Suppresses T Cell Activation by Blocking Ca^{2+} Mobilization and Nuclear Factor of Activated T Cells (NFAT) Activation. *J. Biol. Chem.* **2012**, *287*, 10200–10209. [CrossRef]
247. Jung, E.M.; Lim, J.H.; Lee, T.J.; Park, J.-W.; Choi, K.S.; Kwon, T.K. Curcumin Sensitizes Tumor Necrosis Factor-Related Apoptosis-Inducing Ligand (TRAIL)-Induced Apoptosis through Reactive Oxygen Species-Mediated Upregulation of Death Receptor 5 (DR5). *Carcinogenesis* **2005**, *26*, 1905–1913. [CrossRef]
248. Chen, Y.-R.; Tan, T.-H. Inhibition of the C-Jun N-Terminal Kinase (JNK) Signaling Pathway by Curcumin. *Oncogene* **1998**, *17*, 173–178. [CrossRef]
249. Thulasiraman, P.; McAndrews, D.J.; Mohiudddin, I.Q. Curcumin Restores Sensitivity to Retinoic Acid in Triple Negative Breast Cancer Cells. *BMC Cancer* **2014**, *14*, 724. [CrossRef]
250. Li, Q.; Sun, J.; Mohammadtursun, N.; Wu, J.; Dong, J.; Li, L. Curcumin Inhibits Cigarette Smoke-Induced Inflammation via Modulating the PPARγ-NF-KB Signaling Pathway. *Food Funct.* **2019**, *10*, 7983–7994. [CrossRef]
251. Zhu, T.; Chen, Z.; Chen, G.; Wang, D.; Tang, S.; Deng, H.; Wang, J.; Li, S.; Lan, J.; Tong, J.; et al. Curcumin Attenuates Asthmatic Airway Inflammation and Mucus Hypersecretion Involving a PPARγ-Dependent NF-KB Signaling Pathway in Vivo and in Vitro. *Mediat. Inflamm.* **2019**, *2019*, 4927430. [CrossRef]
252. Bradley, J. TNF-mediated Inflammatory Disease. *J. Pathol.* **2008**, *214*, 149–160. [CrossRef]
253. Anwar, M.J.; Alenezi, S.K.; Alhowail, A.H. Molecular Insights into the Pathogenic Impact of Vitamin D Deficiency in Neurological Disorders. *Biomed. Pharmacother.* **2023**, *162*, 114718. [CrossRef] [PubMed]
254. Jang, D.; Lee, A.-H.; Shin, H.-Y.; Song, H.-R.; Park, J.-H.; Kang, T.-B.; Lee, S.-R.; Yang, S.-H. The Role of Tumor Necrosis Factor Alpha (TNF-α) in Autoimmune Disease and Current TNF-α Inhibitors in Therapeutics. *Int. J. Mol. Sci.* **2021**, *22*, 2719. [CrossRef] [PubMed]
255. Díez, J.J.; Hernanz, A.; Medina, S.; Bayón, C.; Iglesias, P. Serum Concentrations of Tumour Necrosis Factor-alpha (TNF-α) and Soluble TNF-α Receptor P55 in Patients with Hypothyroidism and Hyperthyroidism before and after Normalization of Thyroid Function. *Clin. Endocrinol.* **2002**, *57*, 515–521. [CrossRef] [PubMed]
256. Tzanavari, T.; Giannogonas, P.; Karalis, K.P. TNF-α and Obesity. *TNF Pathophysiol.* **2010**, *11*, 145–156.
257. Olivera, A.; Moore, T.W.; Hu, F.; Brown, A.P.; Sun, A.; Liotta, D.C.; Snyder, J.P.; Yoon, Y.; Shim, H.; Marcus, A.I. Inhibition of the NF-KB Signaling Pathway by the Curcumin Analog, 3, 5-Bis (2-Pyridinylmethylidene)-4-Piperidone (EF31): Anti-Inflammatory and Anti-Cancer Properties. *Int. Immunopharmacol.* **2012**, *12*, 368–377. [CrossRef]
258. Wang, S.L.; Li, Y.; Wen, Y.; Chen, Y.F.; Na, L.X.; Li, S.T.; Sun, C.H. Curcumin, a Potential Inhibitor of up-Regulation of TNF-Alpha and IL-6 Induced by Palmitate in 3T3-L1 Adipocytes through NF-KappaB and JNK Pathway. *Biomed. Environ. Sci.* **2009**, *22*, 32–39. [CrossRef]
259. Panaro, M.A.; Corrado, A.; Benameur, T.; Paolo, C.F.; Cici, D.; Porro, C. The Emerging Role of Curcumin in the Modulation of TLR-4 Signaling Pathway: Focus on Neuroprotective and Anti-Rheumatic Properties. *Int. J. Mol. Sci.* **2020**, *21*, 2299. [CrossRef]
260. Ben, P.; Liu, J.; Lu, C.; Xu, Y.; Xin, Y.; Fu, J.; Huang, H.; Zhang, Z.; Gao, Y.; Luo, L. Curcumin Promotes Degradation of Inducible Nitric Oxide Synthase and Suppresses Its Enzyme Activity in RAW 264.7 Cells. *Int. Immunopharmacol.* **2011**, *11*, 179–186. [CrossRef]
261. Ghafouri-Fard, S.; Shoorei, H.; Bahroudi, Z.; Hussen, B.M.; Talebi, S.F.; Taheri, M.; Ayatollahi, S.A. Nrf2-Related Therapeutic Effects of Curcumin in Different Disorders. *Biomolecules* **2022**, *12*, 82. [CrossRef]
262. Atiaa, A.; Abdullah, A. NQO1 Enzyme and Its Role in Cellular Protection; an Insight. *Iberoam. J. Med.* **2020**, *2*, 306–313. [CrossRef]
263. Battino, M.; Giampieri, F.; Pistollato, F.; Sureda, A.; de Oliveira, M.R.; Pittalà, V.; Fallarino, F.; Nabavi, S.F.; Atanasov, A.G.; Nabavi, S.M. Nrf2 as Regulator of Innate Immunity: A Molecular Swiss Army Knife! *Biotechnol. Adv.* **2018**, *36*, 358–370. [CrossRef] [PubMed]
264. Vomund, S.; Schäfer, A.; Parnham, M.J.; Brüne, B.; Von Knethen, A. Nrf2, the Master Regulator of Anti-Oxidative Responses. *Int. J. Mol. Sci.* **2017**, *18*, 2772. [CrossRef] [PubMed]
265. Ferguson, B.S.; Nam, H.; Morrison, R.F. Curcumin Inhibits 3T3-L1 Preadipocyte Proliferation by Mechanisms Involving Post-Transcriptional P27 Regulation. *Biochem. Biophys. Rep.* **2016**, *5*, 16–21. [CrossRef] [PubMed]
266. Yu, C.; Yang, B.; Najafi, M. Targeting of Cancer Cell Death Mechanisms by Curcumin: Implications to Cancer Therapy. *Basic Clin. Pharmacol. Toxicol.* **2021**, *129*, 397–415. [CrossRef]
267. Shen, Q.; Hang, M.; Shi, Y. Curcumin Boosts Natural Killer Cell-Based Immunotherapy in Impeding Progression of Hepatocellular Carcinoma Through Androgen Receptor/UL16 Binding Protein-2 Signal. *Sci. Adv. Mater.* **2022**, *14*, 188–195. [CrossRef]

268. Bhattacharyya, S.; Md Sakib Hossain, D.; Mohanty, S.; Sankar Sen, G.; Chattopadhyay, S.; Banerjee, S.; Chakraborty, J.; Das, K.; Sarkar, D.; Das, T.; et al. Curcumin Reverses T Cell-Mediated Adaptive Immune Dysfunctions in Tumor-Bearing Hosts. *Cell. Mol. Immunol.* **2010**, *7*, 306–315. [CrossRef]
269. Alinejad, S.; Khademvatan, S.; Amani, S.; Asadi, N.; Tappeh, K.H.; Yousefi, E.; Miandoabi, T. The Effect of Curcumin on the Expression of INFγ, TNF-α, and INOS Genes in PBMCs Infected with Leishmania Major [MRHO/IR/75/ER]. *Infect. Disord. Drug Targets* **2022**, *22*, e040422203031. [CrossRef]
270. Draghiciu, O.; Lubbers, J.; Nijman, H.W.; Daemen, T. Myeloid Derived Suppressor Cells-An Overview of Combat Strategies to Increase Immunotherapy Efficacy. *Oncoimmunology* **2015**, *4*, e954829. [CrossRef]
271. Wang, T.; Wang, J.; Jiang, H.; Ni, M.; Zou, Y.; Chen, Y.; Wu, T.; Ding, D.; Xu, H.; Li, X. Targeted Regulation of Tumor Microenvironment through the Inhibition of MDSCs by Curcumin Loaded Self-Assembled Nano-Filaments. *Mater. Today Bio* **2022**, *15*, 100304. [CrossRef]
272. Ahmad, I.; Hoque, M.; Alam, S.S.M.; Zughaibi, T.A.; Tabrez, S. Curcumin and Plumbagin Synergistically Target the PI3K/Akt/MTOR Pathway: A Prospective Role in Cancer Treatment. *Int. J. Mol. Sci.* **2023**, *24*, 6651. [CrossRef]
273. Song, J.; Choi, B.; Jin, E.-J.; Yoon, Y.; Choi, K.-H. Curcumin Suppresses Streptococcus Mutans Adherence to Human Tooth Surfaces and Extracellular Matrix Proteins. *Eur. J. Clin. Microbiol. Infect. Dis.* **2012**, *31*, 1347–1352. [CrossRef] [PubMed]
274. Rudrappa, T.; Bais, H.P. Curcumin, a Known Phenolic from Curcuma Longa, Attenuates the Virulence of Pseudomonas Aeruginosa PAO1 in Whole Plant and Animal Pathogenicity Models. *J. Agric. Food Chem.* **2008**, *56*, 1955–1962. [CrossRef] [PubMed]
275. Dai, C.; Lin, J.; Li, H.; Shen, Z.; Wang, Y.; Velkov, T.; Shen, J. The Natural Product Curcumin as an Antibacterial Agent: Current Achievements and Problems. *Antioxidants* **2022**, *11*, 459. [CrossRef] [PubMed]
276. Kumbar, V.M.; Peram, M.R.; Kugaji, M.S.; Shah, T.; Patil, S.P.; Muddapur, U.M.; Bhat, K.G. Effect of Curcumin on Growth, Biofilm Formation and Virulence Factor Gene Expression of Porphyromonas Gingivalis. *Odontology* **2021**, *109*, 18–28. [CrossRef]

pharmaceuticals

MDPI

Article

Potential of Newly Synthesized Sea Buckthorn Phytocarriers as Anti-Inflammatory Active Agents

Ionela Daniela Popescu [1,†], Elena Codrici [1,2,†], Sevinci Pop [1], Tudor Emanuel Fertig [1,2], Maria Dudău [1], Iliuta Laurentiu Anghelache [1], Nicoleta Constantin [1], Radu Marian Marinescu [2], Vlad Mihai Voiculescu [2], Georgiana Ileana Badea [3], Mirela Diaconu [3], Monica Elisabeta Maxim [4], Mihaela Scurtu [5], Kliment Zanov [5], Ana-Maria Enciu [1,2,*], Simona Carmen Litescu [3] and Cristiana Tanase [1,6]

1 Victor Babes National Institute of Pathology, 99-101 Splaiul Independentei, Sector 5, 050096 Bucharest, Romania; spop@ivb.ro (S.P.); emanuel.fertig@umfcd.ro (T.E.F.); laurentiu.anghelache@ivb.ro (I.L.A.); cristianatp@yahoo.com (C.T.)
2 Faculty of Medicine, Carol Davila University of Medicine and Pharmacy, 8 Eroilor Sanitari, 050047 Bucharest, Romania; radu.gh.marinescu@stud.umfcd.ro (R.M.M.)
3 Centre of Bioanalysis, National Institute of Research and Development for Biological Sciences, 296 Independenței Bd., District 6, 060031 Bucharest, Romania
4 "Ilie Murgulescu" Institute of Physical Chemistry, Romanian Academy, 202 Splaiul Independentei, 060021 Bucharest, Romania; mmaxim@icf.ro
5 Cromatec Plus SRL Str. Petre Ispirescu nr. 1, Sat Tancabesti, Comuna Snagov, 077167 Ilfov, Romania
6 Cajal Institute, Titu Maiorescu University, 22 Dâmbovnicului, Sector 4, 040441 Bucharest, Romania
* Correspondence: ana.enciu@ivb.ro or ana.enciu@umfcd.ro
† These authors contributed equally to this work.

Abstract: Background: Phytocarriers are advanced drug delivery systems that use biocompatible and biodegradable materials to enhance the efficacy, stability, and bioavailability of natural products. The sea buckthorn (*Hippophae rhamnoides* L.) berry extract is rich in essential fatty acids and antioxidants, including vitamin C, vitamin E, and anthocyanins, which contribute to its wide-ranging health benefits. In this study, we assessed the morphology, intracellular delivery, and anti-inflammatory effect of sodium cholate (NaC) and sodium deoxycholate (NaDC)-based phytocarriers loaded with ethanolic extract from sea buckthorn berries (sea buckthorn carrier nanostructures, further defined as phytocarriers). **Methods:** Negative and electron cryo-microscopy were used to analyze hollow and loaded nanocarriers. The cyto-compatibility of nanocarriers was assessed by endpoint (LDH and MTS) and real-time cell assays, on both human fibroblasts (HS27) and human normal monocytes (SC). The anti-inflammatory effect of hollow and loaded nanocarriers was tested by multiplexing. **Results:** The negative and electron cryo-microscopy analyses showed that NaC-based phytocarriers were spherical, whilst NaDC-based phytocarriers were predominantly polymorphic. Moreover, the NaDC-based phytocarriers frequently formed large lipid networks or "plaques". Although 24 h cytotoxicity testing showed both types of nanocarriers are biocompatible with human fibroblasts and monocytes, based on a long-term real-time assay, NaDC delayed fibroblast proliferation. NaC sea buckthorn phytocarriers did not impair fibroblast proliferation in the long term and they were uptaken by cells, as shown by hyperspectral microscopy. NaC nanocarriers and NaC sea buckthorn phytocarriers induced an anti-inflammatory effect, lowering IL-8 cytokine production in normal human monocytes as soon as 4 h of treatment lapsed. **Conclusions:** NaC-derived phytocarriers loaded with sea buckthorn alcoholic extract are a cell-compatible delivery system with anti-inflammatory properties.

https://doi.org/10.3390/ph18020212

Keywords: sea buckthorn ethanolic extract; nanocarriers; phytocarriers; anti-inflammatory effect; IL-8

1. Introduction

Phytocarriers are advanced drug delivery systems that use biocompatible and biodegradable materials to enhance the efficacy, stability, and bioavailability of natural products [1]. Depending on the structure and formulation method, nanocarriers are classified into several categories, whose number increases with technological development. Most are organic, such as the widely used lipid-based nanocarriers (liposomes, microemulsion drug delivery systems, nanostructured lipid carriers, solid lipid nanoparticles, transferomes, and ethosomes), but also polymeric nanocarriers (in the nanoparticles, micelles, and dendrimers). There are also inorganic and hybrid nanocarriers. Some novel nanocarriers are niosomes, liquid crystals, and nanotubes [2].

One natural product benefiting from nanocarrier delivery is the sea buckthorn extract, derived from the berries, seeds, and leaves of the *Hippophae rhamnoides* plant. The berry extract contains a significant variety of essential fatty acids and antioxidants, including vitamin C, vitamin E, and polyphenols, which contribute to its wide-ranging health benefits and applications [3].

Phytocarriers (the structure formed between the natural compound extract and its nanocarrier) offer several benefits over conventional drug delivery methods as follows: 1. enhanced bioavailability; 2. controlled release, providing a steady therapeutic effect over a longer period [4]; 3. targeted delivery, as phytocarriers can be engineered to deliver the sea buckthorn extract specifically to the desired site of action, thereby reducing side effects and increasing efficacy; and 4. improved stability, protecting the extract from environmental factors such as light, heat, and oxygen [5]. Studies have demonstrated that these nanocarriers enhance the bioavailability of the extract's active components, making it more effective in treating conditions such as arthritis, skin disorders, and even certain types of cancer [6,7]. Additionally, the antioxidant and antimicrobial properties of the encapsulated extract enhance its value as a food supplement, nutraceutical, and cosmeceutical, further broadening its applicability [8].

Several types of nanocarriers have been developed for the delivery of sea buckthorn extracts, each with specific advantages. Liposomes are spherical vesicles consisting of lipid bilayers capable of entrapping both lipophilic and hydrophilic compounds. They are recognized for their safety profile and have been used to enhance the delivery of sea buckthorn extract by protecting its active components and ensuring controlled release [7]. Nanostructured lipid carriers (NLCs) are an advanced type of lipid-based carrier with improved stability and controlled release properties. The encapsulation of sea buckthorn extract into NLCs has been shown to enhance its antioxidant and antimicrobial properties, making it a promising candidate for therapeutic applications [8]. Polymeric nanoparticles, synthesized from biodegradable polymers, have been used to encapsulate various natural products, including sea buckthorn extract. These carriers offer the benefits of high drug loading capacity, controlled release, and targeted delivery, which are crucial for improving the therapeutic outcomes of encapsulated bioactive compounds [5]. Solid lipid nanoparticles (SLNs) are another lipid-based carrier system known for their stability and ability to encapsulate both lipophilic and hydrophilic substances. They have been employed to enhance the bioavailability of sea buckthorn extract and to protect its sensitive compounds from degradation [9]. The long-term safety and regulatory approval of these nanocarrier systems are still under examination, requiring more comprehensive research and clinical trials [5,9].

Despite these advancements, several issues remain to be solved. Unlike small molecule drugs, phytocarriers presents different challenges related to cytotoxicity testing due to their large size and polarity. Distinct from conventional drugs, some nanocarriers are unable to diffuse through the cell membrane and instead enter cells via endocytosis [9]. There is still a limited understanding of the mechanisms of action and potential toxicity of these drug delivery systems, which requires supplementary studies. Additionally, long-term safety profiles of these nanocarriers need comprehensive evaluation to ensure their viability for clinical use [10]. Recent research efforts are increasingly focusing on the synthesis of nanocarriers through environmentally safe chemical reactions, incorporating plant extracts [11]. As this field advances, it will be crucial to address these challenges to improve the translational value of current nanomedicine research and to fully realize the therapeutic potential of sea buckthorn extract-loaded nanocarriers.

The aim of this study is to produce evidence that nanocarriers, loaded with sea buckthorn extract originating from Romania, are suitable for further potential development as food supplements with health/therapeutic benefits.

2. Results

In order to assess the utility of sodium cholate (NaC) and sodium deoxycholate (NaDC) edge activator nanocarriers for the nanodelivery method, morphological analysis, cytotoxicity and proliferation assays, as well as cellular uptake were investigated. Both nanocarriers, hollow spherical structures loadable with the cargo of choice (further referred to as "hollow nanocarriers") and nanocarriers loaded with sea buckthorn extract (further referred to as "phytocarriers"), were used in the analysis, and the anti-inflammatory effect of the sea buckthorn ethanolic extract was determined by multiplexing.

2.1. *NaC-Derived Phytocarriers Are Spherical, Loadable, and More Homogeneous than NaDC Phytocarriers*

The morphology of both hollow and loaded nanostructures was assessed using NS-TEM and cryo-TEM.

NaC-based nanostructures were relatively homogenous, with diameters ranging from 20 to 35 nm and averages of 28.6 nm in NS-TEM specimens (n = 50, Figure 1a) and 25.8 nm in cryo-EM (n = 40, Figure 1b). Particles larger than 50 nm were absent from the samples analyzed. While, in NS-TEM, particles frequently presented a "cup-shape" morphology with a collapsed center (Figure 1a), in cryo-EM, they appeared spherical due to their frozen-hydrated state (Figure 1b). By contrast, NaDC nanocarriers were frequently polymorphic in NS-TEM and only rare spherical particles were observed (Figure 1c). As these nanostructures appeared as isolated spheres in cryo-EM (Figure 1d), the polymorphism seen in NS-TEM was likely due to increased aggregation and/or fusion during sample dehydration. As compared to NaC nanostructures, NaDC particles were larger, ranging from 29 to 54 nm (average 44.5 nm, n = 40). In cryo-TEM, NaDC nanocarriers appeared more electron-dense (darker) than NaC nanocarriers, suggesting they have a different structural lipid organization.

Similarly to NaC hollow nanocarriers, in cryo-TEM, NaC phytocarriers appeared relatively homogenous in terms of size, with an average diameter of 26.9 nm (min 19, max 41, n = 40) and most particles ranging between 22 and 25 nm. The second most abundant class of particles had diameters below 20 nm. In NS-TEM, occasional larger phytocarriers could be observed (40 to max 240 nm). The absence of these larger particles in cryo-EM preparations can be explained by the differences in particle surface charges, which would favor the deposition of larger phytocarriers to the carbon surface of the grid rather than the holes with vitreous ice. Regardless of size, NaC phytocarriers were spherical in both NS-TEM (Figure 1e) and cryo-TEM (Figure 1f). By contrast, NaDC phytocarriers were predominantly polymorphic in NS-TEM, frequently forming large lipid networks or "plaques" (Figure 1g). In cryo-TEM, NaDC phytocarriers appeared as individual spheres, but with a very broad size distribution, from 17 to 85 nm (average 33.2 nm, n = 40). Some vesicles appeared electron-dense and larger vesicles presented smaller vesicles within, probably as a result of fusion events (Figure 1h).

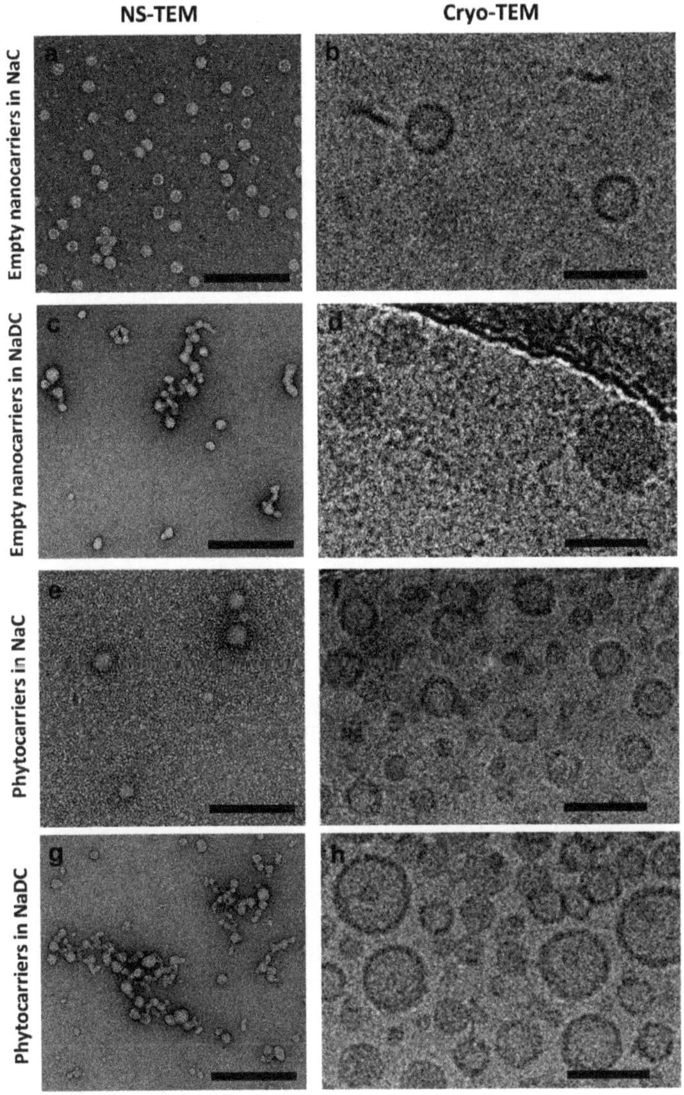

Figure 1. TEM analysis of phytocarriers. NaC hollow nanocarriers were relatively small and highly homogenous in size and shape in both NS-TEM (**a**) and cryo-TEM (**b**). By contrast, NaDC hollow nanocarriers were frequently aggregated and appeared polymorphic in NS-TEM (**c**), whereas individual particles were more electron-dense (darker) and with a comparatively broader size distribution in cryo-TEM (**d**). NaC phytocarriers were also smaller and more homogenous in both size and shape (**e**,**f**), compared to their NaDC counterparts (**g**,**h**). The scale bar is 200 nm for all NS-TEM images and 50 nm for all cryo-TEM images.

The TEM morphological analysis therefore suggests that NaC phytocarriers and hollow nanocarriers are preferable to their NaDC equivalents due to their smaller size and homogeneity, which would facilitate cellular phagocytosis.

The obtained phytocarriers, either hollow or loaded, were assessed by Dynamic Light Scattering, zeta potential, and polydispersity index, as presented in Table 1.

Table 1. Zeta potential and polydispersity index of phytocarriers.

Nanocarriers	Zeta Potential (mV)	Polydispersity Index (PdI)
NaC hollow	−32 ± 6.7	0.283
NaC loaded	−23.9 ± 5.36	0.300
NaDC hollow	−38 ± 6.90	0.253
NaDC loaded	−36 ± 3.19	0.334

Next, we analyzed the biocompatibility of the NaC and NaDC hollow nanocarriers and phytocarriers on the following two cell lines: human fibroblasts and human normal monocytes.

2.2. Biocompatibility Testing of Hollow Nanocarriers and Loaded Nanocarriers/Phytocarriers

Before cytotoxicity testing, the chemical composition of the extract was determined (Table 2). It should be mentioned that, to ensure easier traceability, the extract was normalized to epicatechin and rutin when the encapsulation efficiency was assessed.

Table 2. Composition profile of the sea buckthorn extract.

Composition	Concentration μg/mL
Gallic acid	17.93
Catechin	28.61
Epicatechin	45.77
Syringic acid	4.02
Coumaric acid	1.01
Rutin	46.25
Ellagic acid	7.65
Quercetin	6.38
Isorhamnetin	29.87

The encapsulation efficiency was further assessed, as a percentage of the encapsulated compound reported to the total amount and was determined to be 75.62% for rutin and 82.44% for epicatechin.

The biocompatibility of the nanocarriers was assessed by endpoint cytotoxicity (LDH release) and cell viability assays (MTS), as well as by a real-time cellular proliferation assay.

The effect of two dilutions (1/50, 1/100) of NaC or NaDC loaded and hollow nanocarriers on cell viability and the possible induced cytotoxicity were tested by endpoint assays. Two types of cells were tested as follows: normal human fibroblasts, a generally accepted model for toxicity assays; and human normal monocytes, for the assessment of non-toxic concentrations for the subsequent inflammation-related assays (Figure 2a). After 24 h of treatment, the LDH release for fibroblasts was below 25% at all tested dilutions, which correlated with the percentage of viable cells (over 80%) for all analyzed samples. Similar results were obtained for the treated monocytes, where LDH release was below 20% at all tested dilutions, correlating with the cell viability results which were close to 100% for phytocarriers (loaded with extract) and over 80% for hollow nanostructures. None of the tested samples induced a significant increase in cell proliferation, as determined by endpoint assays for 24 h of treatment.

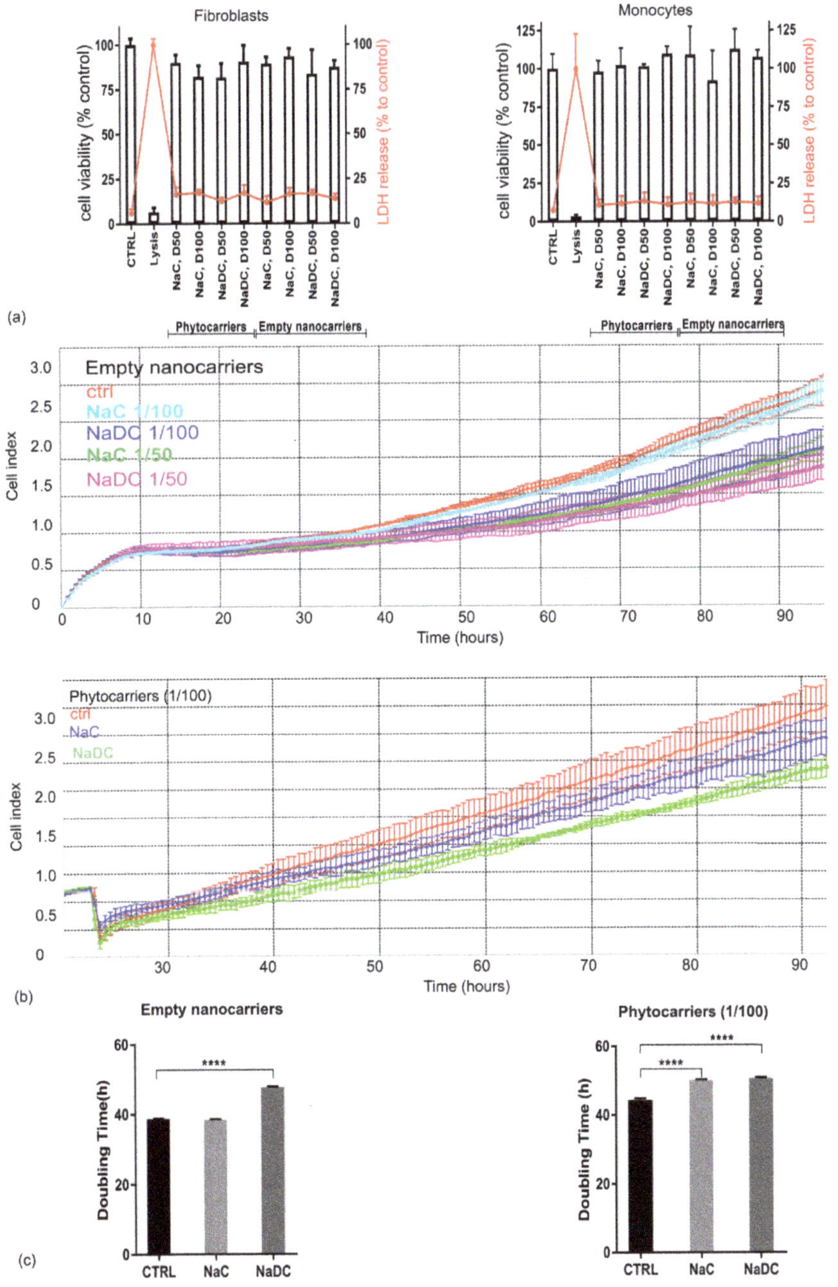

Figure 2. Viability and proliferation rates of cells treated with NaC and NaDC nanocarriers and phytosomes, assessed by endpoint assay (**upper panel**) and real-time assay (**lower panel**). (**a**) MTS bars and LDH points represent the average of triplicates ± S.D. (**b**) Real-time impedance graph points represent the average of triplicates ± S.D. Points were registered every 15 min. (**c**) Doubling times were calculated for 1/100 dilution, and the bars represent the average of triplicates ± S.D. One-way ANOVA, with Dunnet post hoc analysis, was used for the statistical analysis. **** $p < 0.0001$).

The endpoint cell proliferation assay was complemented by a real-time assay for cells adhesion and proliferation, where incubation time was increased, and data collection at intermediate times allowed for the calculation of the doubling times of treated cells.

Regarding NaC and NaDC hollow nanocarriers, no significant difference was observed between treated and non-treated fibroblasts in the first 48 h, consistent with the MTS analysis (Figure 2b). Extending the testing interval to 96 h revealed alterations in the cellular response profiles for both NaC and NaDC hollow nanocarriers at all concentrations, except for the NaC nanocarriers at a 1/100 dilution. Notably, a decrease in cellular index values was observed for NaDC nanocarriers at both dilutions and NaC nanocarriers at a 1/50 dilution. A 1/100 dilution of NaC nanocarrier-treated cells showed a similar proliferation curve as the untreated control for the whole period of time (96 h). A subsequent analysis of doubling time confirmed that NaC nanostructures at a 1/100 dilution do not modify the proliferation rate of normal human fibroblasts. Instead, for NaDC hollow nanocarriers at 1/50 and 1/100 dilutions and NaC at a 1/50 dilution, a stable and statistically significant increase in the doubling times of normal human fibroblasts, visible in real-time after approximately 50 h of incubation, can be observed (Figure 2b, right panel).

Regarding NaC and NaDC phytocarriers, we tested the response of fibroblasts in real time for up to 96 h. To analyze whether phytocarriers can modulate the cellular proliferation process and to avoid any confounding effects of different phytocarriers on initial cell attachment, the fibroblasts were allowed to adhere for 24 h before exposing them to the treatments. The results obtained for cells incubated with phytocarriers at a 1/50 dilution confirmed that human fibroblasts proliferate at lower rates than untreated control cells, an effect that is visible after approximately 24 h of treatment. The same is observed for the 1/100 dilution (Figure 2c, left panel). The decrease in proliferation rate can be observed after at least 24 h of incubation, and this is maintained throughout the entire experimental time. The doubling time analysis showed that, although the effect induced by the NaC phytocarriers is smaller than that induced by NaDC, it is still statistically significant when compared to the control (Figure 2c, right panel).

To conclude, NaC edge activator hollow nanocarriers do not modify fibroblast proliferation in either short or long term, confirming their effectiveness as biocompatible delivery vehicles, as opposed to NaDC-based nanocarriers. Interestingly, the sea buckthorn extract phytocarriers based on either NaC edge activator or NaDC edge activator, diluted 100-fold, induced an anti-proliferative effect on fibroblast cells when treated for longer periods of time.

2.3. NaC Nanocarriers and Sea Buckthorn-Loaded Phytocarriers Are Uptaken by Cells, Making Them Useful Vectors for Active Compounds Delivery

To answer the question of whether these carriers (hollow or loaded) were internalized by cells, hyperspectral imaging (HSI) libraries were acquired. These libraries were used to characterize the spectral signatures of the carriers and the cell background. By comparing these spectra, the intracellular presence of the carriers could be determined.

Both NaC and NaDC carriers were characterized using hyperspectral microscopy, but the cell-based analysis focused on the NaC nanocarriers. This decision was based on previous real-time data, as well as electron microscopy images, which demonstrated that NaC nanocarriers are superior in terms of morphologic homogeneity as well as biocompatibility to NaDC nanocarriers.

Hyperspectral data of hollow and loaded nanocarriers (phytocarriers) were measured in terms of the spectral mean (Figure 3a). No significant difference was noticed between hollow nanocarriers, while loading them with sea buckthorn extract induced a spectral shift to the right of the NaC-based phytocarriers (a maximum between 650 and 675 nm, compared to 610–630 nm). This spectral shift was used to identify the intracellular presence of a specific nanocarrier.

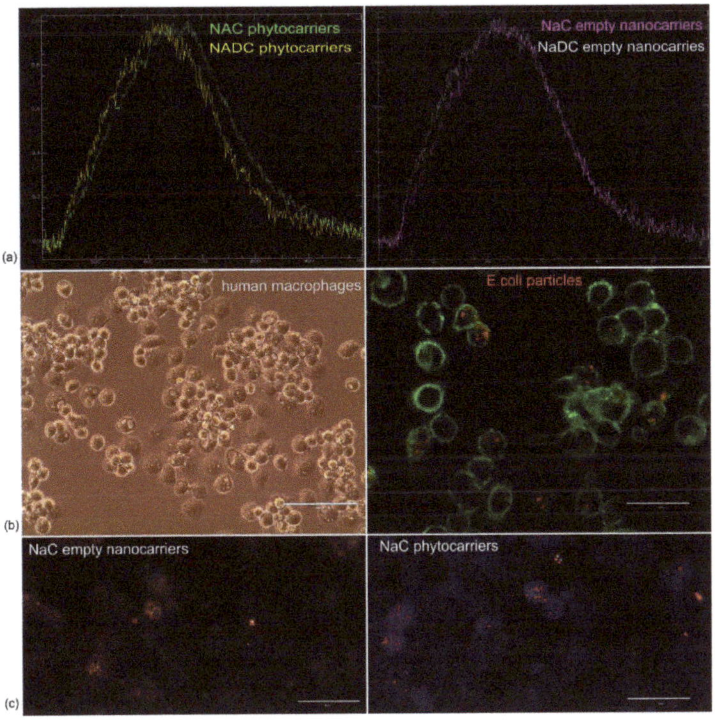

Figure 3. Phase-contrast and dark-field fluorescence hyperspectral imaging of phytocarriers. (**a**) Mean spectral analysis of phytocarriers obtained via hyperspectral analysis; (**b**) phagocytosis abilities of normal human macrophages investigated by phase-contrast microscopy (left, 40×) and fluorescence microscopy (60×), using fluorescently labeled E coli particles; (**c**) digitally highlighted overlayed HSI libraries of NaC phytocarriers and nanocarriers onto macrophage cell cultures (60×), which demonstrated their presence inside the cells. The focal plane was chosen based on the nucleus focal plane.

Fluorescence images were used to assess the uptake of NaC hollow nanocarriers and phytocarriers by macrophages. The phagocytic ability of macrophages was demonstrated using *E. coli* particles, which become fluorescent in an acidic environment (e.g., lysosomes) (Figure 3b). The NaC hollow nanocarriers and phytocarriers were uptaken by cells and were detectable after 24 h incubation (Figure 3c). The presence of hollow carriers and phytocarriers in treated macrophages was demonstrated by overlaying the hyperspectral data of each library over the microscopy images of phagocytosing cells.

To conclude, using hyperspectral microscopy, we demonstrated that both hollow and loaded NaC nanocarriers are uptaken by cells, hence their utility as intracellular delivery vehicles.

2.4. Pro-Inflammatory Cytokines Decreased in a Dose-Dependent Pattern After Nanocarrier Treatment

Next, the biological response of cells to selected hollow and loaded nanocarriers was tested from the following two points of view: whether the nanocarriers, loaded or not with sea buckthorn extract, induced inflammation themselves and, secondly, whether they can protect against inflammation. For the latter, cells were challenged with LPS and then treated with phytocarriers and hollow nanostructures. Dexamethasone treatment was used as a positive anti-inflammatory effect.

To assess whether the tested nanostructures induced a response from the exposed cells, normal human monocytes were incubated for 20 h and supernatant was harvested at 4 h (for early response) and 20 h (late response). Several pro- and anti-inflammatory cytokines were tested (IL-1beta, IL-2, IL-4, IL-6, IL-8, IL-10, IL-12p70, TNFa, TNFb, and INFg), but only IL-6 and IL-8 were detectable during 20 h of treatment. The early response was significant only for IL-8 expression, whereas IL-6 was detectable only at 20 h. Neither hollow nor loaded nanostructures induced, by themselves, an inflammatory response, highlighting their use as biocompatible carriers. In addition, when cells were challenged with LPS, both tested nanostructures induced a time-dependent anti-inflammatory response (Figure 4).

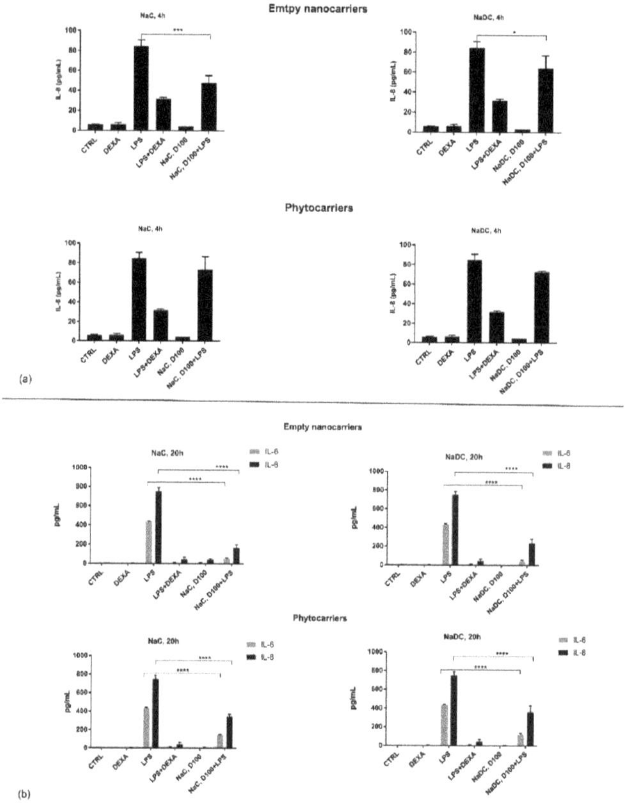

Figure 4. Dose-dependent pattern inhibition of IL-8 at 4 h (**a**) and of IL-6 and IL-8 at 20 h (**b**). One-way ANOVA, Dunnett's post hoc analysis; * $p < 0.05$, *** $p < 0.001$, and **** $p < 0.0001$.

Treating cells for 20 h with LPS and 1/100 of NaC phytosomes led to significant decreases in IL-6 levels by 66% (ratio 0.34, $p < 0.0001$) and IL-8 by 54% (ratio 0.46, $p < 0.0001$). Additionally, treating cells with LPS and 1/100 concentrations of NaDC phytocarriers significantly reduced the levels of IL-6 (by 88.4% and 73%, respectively; $p < 0.0001$) and IL-8 (by 70% and 52%, respectively; $p < 0.0001$) (Figure 4). Similar results were also found when examining cells treated with hollow nanostructures and LPS compared to the LPS control group. Both IL-6 and IL-8 levels were significantly different between these groups ($p < 0.0001$).

3. Discussions

Incorporation of sea buckthorn extracts in lipid nanoparticles was previously described to successfully preserve the biological activity of the natural compounds [12,13]. Soy lecithin lipid nanoparticles were shown to be well tolerated by fibroblasts and monocytes after short-term incubation (24 h) [14]. Their proven lack of toxicity in the short term might account for why, in many studies, the cell viability was usually compared between the extract and the liposome-encapsulated extract at 24 h [15] or 48 h of treatment [16], while the nanocarrier was no longer tested. Our study also showed that, at 24 h, the hollow soy lecithin nanocarriers, as well as the sea buckthorn loaded nanocarriers, are well tolerated by human fibroblasts and monocytes.

One particular finding of this study is that, when assessed in real time for longer periods of time (96 h), both hollow nanocarriers, as well as sea buckthorn loaded nanocarriers, without being cytotoxic, decreased fibroblast proliferation. The effect was persistent for NaDC nanocarriers, even with increased dilution. In contrast, NaC nanocarrier-treated fibroblasts at a 1/100 dilution behaved similarly to the control. However, when loaded with sea buckthorn extract, even at a 1/100 dilution, the loaded NaC nanocarriers also decreased the proliferation of the fibroblasts. The ethanolic extract of sea buckthorn was previously reported to impair cell proliferation in reports mostly addressing tumor cells [17,18]. Sadowska et al. [19] noted an impaired fibroblast migration in the presence of non-polar components of the extract, while the phenolic component did not induce significant changes.

It has been previously shown that NaC and NaDC act differently in terms of micelle formation [20], which potentially impacts cellular uptake. Our study confirmed, through electron microscopy, that the type of edge activator used to generate nanocarriers influences their morphology and size. NaC-based nanoformulation performed better in the generation of spherical, possibly hollow nanocarriers, as assessed by electron microscopy. NaDC nanocarriers yielded elongated and ramified structures, which can potentially explain the inhibitory effect on cell proliferation observed in long-term real-time analysis. DLS data, the obtained negative zeta potential values, support the assertion that the obtained nanostructures are less subjected to aggregation in biological samples.

In terms of anti-inflammatory activity, the aqueous berry extract of sea buckthorn was shown to decrease the secretion of IL-6 and IL-8 in immune cells [21] and various epithelial cell models ($CaCo_2$ [21], HaCaT [22]). For TNFα, the response depends on the cell model used—PMA-induced macrophages [23] respond differently than PBMC [21]. In animal models, the anti-inflammatory properties of sea buckthorn were exploited, especially in dermal applications [24] and intestinal pathologies [25]. Increasing the bioavailability of the active components found in sea buckthorn extracts can potentially bring additional benefits in pathologies characterized by systemic low-grade inflammation. This study also demonstrated the dose-dependent anti-inflammatory activity of both tested nanostructures, hollow or loaded, but the effect on cell proliferation should be taken into consideration. Correlated with the lack of toxicity of the 1/100 diluted nanocarriers, this study provided evidence for the delivery and anti-inflammatory effect of NaC nanocarriers and phytocarriers. Notably, NaC nanocarriers, by themselves, showed an anti-inflammatory effect, possibly attributable to phosphatidylcholine, a natural phospholipid known to have an anti-inflammatory effect, by the inhibition of the NF-kB pathway [26], including following LPS stimulation [27].

4. Materials and Method

4.1. Phytocarriers Preparation and Encapsulation

4.1.1. Phytocarriers Preparation

Solutions of 24 mg of lecithin in 3 mL of 96% ethanol (8 mg/mL) were used to prepare hollow carrier nanostructures, further defined as hollow nanocarriers. Solutions of 24 mg lecithin in 3 mL sea buckthorn hydro-alcoholic extract (obtained by accelerated solvent extraction, ASE, in 96% alcohol and purified) were used to prepare nanostructures loaded with extract (further defined as phytocarriers). For the formation of the composite nano-architecture of phytocarriers, the minimum reaction time was 12 h under continuous stirring. This optimized time was used both for phytocarriers formation and for hollow nanocarriers preparations. After the 12 h, the high-pressure micro-homogenization of the nude lecithin and lecithin-phytoactive compound solution was performed, using 3 cycles of passage through Microfluidics LM20 at 20 kPa. Following this step, the homogenized solution was injected in very small volumes (smaller than 3 μL) of aqueous surfactant solution with edge activators (0.5% sodium cholate—NaC—or sodium deoxycholate—NaDC—and 0.5% Tween 80). In this case, the homogenized solution was either an alcoholic solution of lecithin or a lecithin solution with sea buckthorn extract in 96% alcohol. The injection of small volumes was performed under continuous stirring, at a ratio of 1:10 (v:v, 3 mL phospholipid-phytoactive compound solution to 30 mL aqueous solution with surfactants and edge activators). Finally, the 3 passages through Microfluidics LM20 at 20 kPa were repeated, resulting in nanostructures of lecithin in the composite nano-architectures (phytocarriers).

4.1.2. Composition of Initial Sea Buckthorn Extract and Encapsulation Efficacy

The profile composition of the initial sea buckthorn extract was obtained by high performance liquid chromatography with diode array detection using a method previously developed by our group [28].

4.2. Cell Cultures and Treatments

Normal human fibroblasts Hs27 (ATCC CRL-1634™) were grown in Dulbecco's Modified Eagle Medium (DMEM) with 4.5 g/L glucose, supplemented with 10% fetal bovine serum. Fibroblast cultures were grown and propagated in T-75 flasks, at 37 °C and 5% CO_2 atmosphere. The cell culture medium was changed every 3 days. The cells at 80% confluence were passed 1/3. The tested solutions were diluted in the culture medium before the treatment. Untreated cells (control sample) refer to the normal cell medium supplemented with the vehicle in a corresponding concentration to the samples.

SC normal human monocytes (ATCC 9855) were routinely maintained in culture using IMDM medium, supplemented with 1% HT supplement and 0.1% 2-mercaptoethanol, according to the manufacturer's protocol. To induce the macrophage phenotype, 25 ng/mL phorbol 12-myristate 13-acetate (PMA) treatment for 48 h was used, according to a previously published protocol [29]. The inflammation model was obtained by treatment with LPS (50 ng/mL) and dexamethasone (40 ng/mL) was used as an anti-inflammatory positive control.

4.3. Macrophage Phagocytosis Assay

The phagocytosis assay was performed on PMA-induced macrophages using fluorescently labeled *E. coli* particles (Invitrogen P35360), adhered on 8-well glass slides as described above (Nunc Lab-Tek #154526PK, ThermoFisher Scientific, Waltham, MA, USA). To test for liposome and phytosome phagocytosis, hyperspectral images associated with each type of carrier were plotted against live cell imaging. For ease of interpretation, a digital mask was applied to highlight the intracellular presence of particles.

4.4. Cytotoxicity and Viability Assay

4.4.1. Cell Viability

Cell viability was measured after the cells' exposure to hollow nanocarrier and phytocarrier suspensions by MTS tetrazolium compound [3-(4,5-dimethylthiazol-2-yl)-5-(3-carboxymethoxyphenyl)-2-(4-sulfophenyl)-2H-tetrazolium, inner salt] spectrophotometric test. A total of 15,000 cells/well were seeded in 96-well plates and treated for 24 h with two dilutions (1/50 and 1/100)) of NaC and NaDC phytocarriers. Following this timeframe, 20 µL of CellTiter 96® AQueous One Solution Reagent (CellTiter 96® Aqueous One Solution Cell Proliferation Assay, G3580, Promega, Madison, WI, USA) were subsequently added to each well, each of which contained 100 µL of fresh culture medium. Incubation was carried out at 37 °C for a duration of 3 h, in a humidified atmosphere containing 5% CO_2. Cell metabolic activity, assessed by MTS reduction and formazan formation, was quantified by measuring absorbance at 490 nm on a Microplate Multimode Detector Zenyth 3100 (Anthos Labtec Instruments GmbH, Salzburg, Austria). Cell viability was determined as follows: viability (%) = 100 × [(experimental OD490) − (background mean OD490)]/mean absorbance at 490 nm of untreated cells.

4.4.2. Cytotoxicity Assay

Cell membrane integrity was assessed by quantifying LDH (lactate dehydrogenase) release into the culture medium using the CytoTox 96® assay (G1780, G1782, Promega). A maximum LDH release control was generated using lysis solution, in accordance with the manufacturer's instructions. Following a 45 min incubation with lysis solution, plates were centrifuged at 600 rpm for 5 min. Subsequently, 50 µL of culture supernatant from each well was transferred to a new 96-well flat-bottom, clear plate, followed by the addition of 50 µL of CytoTox 96® Reagent. Plates were incubated in the dark for 30 min, at room temperature. Subsequently, the reaction was stopped by adding 50 µL of stop solution. The absorbance was then measured at 490 nm using a Zenyth 3100 Microplate Multimode Detector (Anthos Labtec Instruments GmbH, Salzburg, Austria). We calculated cytotoxicity using the following formula: cytotoxicity (%) = 100 × [experimental LDH release (OD490) − background mean LDH release (OD490))/mean of maximum LDH release (OD490)].

4.4.3. Real-Time Proliferation Assay

Normal fibroblasts HS27 cell adherence and proliferation were assessed using RTCA-DP xCelligence platform (Agilent). The cell adherence assay in the presence of the investigated nanostructures, hollow or loaded, in solvent solution of NaC and NaDC were performed at two dilutions as follows: 1/50 and 1/100. A number of 10,000 Hs27 cells were resuspended in cell culture media supplemented with carrier solutions, seeded in triplicates for each experimental condition, and monitored for 96 h. The experiments were repeated three times. The phytocarriers' effect on cell proliferation was tested on cells which were left to adhere on E-plates for 24 h prior to cell treatment. After 24 h, the culture medium in each well was replaced by culture medium containing the NaC and NaDC phytocarrier solutions at the appropriate dilutions. Doubling times were calculated using RTCA software (Version 2.0).

4.5. Inflammatory Model in Monocytes/Macrophages

To assess the anti-inflammatory effects of the obtained nanostructures, phytocarrier 1×10^5 monocytes were seeded per well in 24-well plates, pre-treated with 50 ng/mL LPS for 1 h, and then incubated with two dilutions (1/50, 1/100) of NaC and NaDC phytocarriers for 4 and 20 h. As part of the evaluation, we included a positive pro-inflammatory control (50 ng/mL LPS; L4391; Sigma Aldrich, Saint Louis, MO, USA; Merck KGaA, Darmstadt, Germany), a negative inflammation control (40 ng/mL dexamethasone sodium phosphate; E.I.P.I. Co., Tenth of Ramadan City, Egypt), and a combination of 50 ng/mL LPS with 40 ng/mL dexamethasone as a positive control for the anti-inflammatory effect. The cell culture supernatants were collected and stored at −80 °C until analysis.

4.6. *In Vitro Quantification of Anti-Inflammatory Activity Using xMAP Technology*

The analysis of the cell culture supernatants was performed using a multiplex bead-based assay (HCYTOMAG Milliplex MAP 10-plex, Millipore, Billerica, MA, USA) as per the manufacturer's instructions. The beads (IL-1beta, IL-2, IL-4, IL-6, IL-8, IL-10, IL-12p70, TNFa, TNFb, and INFg) provided within the kit were incubated with buffer, cytokine standards, or samples in a 96-well plate at 4 °C, with 800 rpm orbital shaking o/n. Subsequent incubations with detection antibodies and Streptavidin Phycoerythrin Conjugate (SAPE) were performed in the dark with orbital shaking (800 rpm) and at room temperature. The Luminex 200 platform (Luminex Corp., Austin, TX, USA) was used for multiplex data acquisition, followed by data analysis with xPONENT 4.2 software. A 5-parameter logistic fit was used to generate calibration curves for each analyte. For each sample, duplicate analyses were performed, and the mean concentration was used for statistical analysis.

4.7. *Transmission Electron Microscopy*

Negative stain transmission electron microscopy (NS-TEM) and electron cryo-microscopy (cryo-TEM) were performed for the morphology assessment of isolated particles from samples of interest, following previously published methods [30]. Briefly, copper grids specific to each application (AGS160-3H, Agar Scientific, Rotherham, UK and R2/2, Quantifoil MicroTools, Großlöbichau, Germany, respectively) were glow-discharged before 3.5 μL of each suspension were deposited on the carbon-coated surface. Then, the grids were stained with 2.5% uranyl acetate for NS-TEM, or frozen for cryo-EM by rapid plunging in liquid ethane using a Leica EM GP system (Leica Microsystems, Wetzlar, Germany). For both sample preparation methods, image acquisition was carried out on a 200 kV Talos F200C, equipped with a Ceta 4k × 4k CMOS camera (Thermo Fisher Scientific, Waltham, MA, USA).

4.8. *Fluorescence and Dark-Field Hyperspectral Microscopy*

The acquisition of fluorescence and hyperspectral images (HSIs) was performed using Cytoviva Hyperspectral Imaging System equipped with a dual mode fluorescence (DMF) module (CytoViva, Auburn, AL, USA). Hyperspectral images were obtained from 20 μL of the phytocarriers suspension and a HSI acquisition with a 60× oil immersion objective. The HSIs were stored and analyzed using ENVI v.4.8 software (Harris Geospatial Solutions, Boulder, CO, USA). Phytocarriers' spectral signature was collected using automatic particle filtration with an intensity ranging from 400 to 2000 units in order to remove unwanted spectra and save the selected ones in a spectral library. The identification of phytocarriers in samples containing cells was performed by the classification of the HSI to the saved spectral library using the spectral angle mapper. The spectral comparison of the phytocarriers (hollow or loaded) was performed after the normalization of the intensity and the calculation of the mean spectral analysis. The fluorescence images were acquired using the DMF module and QCapture Pro 7 software (QImaging, Surrey, BC, Canada).

4.9. Dynamic Light Scattering

Dynamic light scattering measurements were performed using a Zetasizer Nano ZS instrument (Malvern Instruments, Worcestershire, UK) with a detection angle of 173°. The surface charge (measured as Zeta potential) and polydispersity index were determined using the light scattering technique, according to the Smoluchowski model (in aqueous medium). All measurements were made at a temperature of 25 °C. The Zetasizer Nano software v3 was used for data processing.

4.10. Statistical Analysis

Statistical analysis was performed using GraphPad v7 data analysis software. One-way ANOVA test was used, with Dunnett's multiple comparison post hoc analysis (* $p < 0.05$, ** $p < 0.01$, *** $p < 0.001$, and **** $p < 0.0001$.).

5. Conclusions

This study explored the use of liposomes as a delivery system for sea buckthorn extract to enhance intracellular uptake with potential therapeutic benefits. Two types of edge activators (sodium cholate—NaC—or sodium deoxycholate—NaDC) were used to generate nanocarriers. Both had an impact on their morphology and influenced cell behavior. NaC nanocarriers formed small and homogenous nanovesicles, with an average diameter of 25.8 nm in cryo-EM and with no cytotoxicity or impairment of fibroblast proliferation when studied in real time for up to 96 h. NaC- diluted hollow nanocarriers and phytocarriers (nanocarriers loaded with sea buckthorn extract) are uptaken by cells and induce an anti-inflammatory response in the presence of a low concentration of LPS (50 ng/mL). In conclusion, cell-compatible, therapeutically effective phytocarriers for sea buckthorn extract delivery were obtained and can be further tested in in vivo models.

Author Contributions: Conceptualization, V.M.V., S.C.L. and C.T.; methodology, I.D.P., E.C., S.P., T.E.F., M.D. (Maria Dudău), I.L.A., N.C., R.M.M., G.I.B., M.D. (Mirela Diaconu), M.E.M., M.S., K.Z. and A.-M.E.; formal analysis, T.E.F., G.I.B., M.D. (Mirela Diaconu), A.-M.E. and S.C.L.; investigation, I.D.P., E.C., S.P., M.D. (Maria Dudău), I.L.A., R.M.M., G.I.B., M.D. (Mirela Diaconu), M.E.M. and A.-M.E.; writing—original draft preparation, E.C., S.P., T.E.F., I.L.A., A.-M.E. and S.C.L.; writing—review and editing, E.C., T.E.F., M.E.M., A.-M.E., S.C.L. and C.T.; supervision, S.C.L. and C.T.; project administration, S.C.L. and C.T.; funding acquisition, S.C.L. and C.T. All authors have read and agreed to the published version of the manuscript.

Funding: This research was supported by the POC/1033/1/3/, PTI 2022, SMIS code 156316 and the Core Program within the National Research, Development and Innovation Plan, 2022–2027, with the support of MCID, project no. 10N/01.01.2023, PN 23.16.02.03.

Data Availability Statement: The original contributions presented in this study are included in the article. Further inquiries can be directed to the corresponding author.

Acknowledgments: Data gathering for the Section 1 used STORM—a writing system for the synthesis of topic outlines through retrieval and multi-perspective question asking [31]. After using this tool, the authors reviewed and edited the content as needed and take full responsibility for the content of the published article.

Conflicts of Interest: The authors declare no conflict of interest.

References

1. Vilas-Franquesa, A.; Saldo, J.; Juan, B. Potential of Sea Buckthorn-Based Ingredients for the Food and Feed Industry—A Review. *Food Prod. Process Nutr.* **2020**, *2*, 17. [CrossRef]
2. Stan, D.; Enciu, A.-M.; Mateescu, A.L.; Ion, A.C.; Brezeanu, A.C.; Stan, D.; Tanase, C. Natural Compounds With Antimicrobial and Antiviral Effect and Nanocarriers Used for Their Transportation. *Front. Pharmacol.* **2021**, *12*, 723233. [CrossRef]

3. Wang, Z.; Zhao, F.; Wei, P.; Chai, X.; Hou, G.; Meng, Q. Phytochemistry, Health Benefits, and Food Applications of Sea Buckthorn (*Hippophae rhamnoides* L.): A Comprehensive Review. *Front. Nutr.* **2022**, *9*, 1036295. [CrossRef] [PubMed]
4. Kodel, H.D.A.C.; Alizadeh, P.; Ebrahimi, S.N.; Machado, T.O.X.; Oliveira, M.B.P.P.; Fathi, F.; Souto, E.B. Liposomes and Niosomes: New Trends and Applications in the Delivery of Bioactive Agents for Cancer Therapy. *Int. J. Pharm.* **2025**, *668*, 124994. [CrossRef] [PubMed]
5. Patra, J.K.; Das, G.; Fraceto, L.F.; Campos, E.V.R.; Rodriguez-Torres, M.D.P.; Acosta-Torres, L.S.; Diaz-Torres, L.A.; Grillo, R.; Swamy, M.K.; Sharma, S.; et al. Nano Based Drug Delivery Systems: Recent Developments and Future Prospects. *J. Nanobiotechnol.* **2018**, *16*, 71. [CrossRef] [PubMed]
6. Enkhtaivan, G.; Maria John, K.M.; Pandurangan, M.; Hur, J.H.; Leutou, A.S.; Kim, D.H. Extreme Effects of Seabuckthorn Extracts on Influenza Viruses and Human Cancer Cells and Correlation Between Flavonol Glycosides and Biological Activities of Extracts. *Saudi J. Biol. Sci.* **2017**, *24*, 1646–1656. [CrossRef] [PubMed]
7. Su, S.; Kang, P.M. Recent Advances in Nanocarrier-Assisted Therapeutics Delivery Systems. *Pharmaceutics* **2020**, *12*, 837. [CrossRef] [PubMed]
8. Manea, A.-M.; Ungureanu, C.; Meghea, A. Effect of Vegetable Oils on Obtaining Lipid Nanocarriers for Sea Buckthorn Extract Encapsulation. *Comptes Rendus. Chim.* **2014**, *17*, 934–943. [CrossRef]
9. Alshawwa, S.Z.; Kassem, A.A.; Farid, R.M.; Mostafa, S.K.; Labib, G.S. Nanocarrier Drug Delivery Systems: Characterization, Limitations, Future Perspectives and Implementation of Artificial Intelligence. *Pharmaceutics* **2022**, *14*, 883. [CrossRef] [PubMed]
10. Tehrani, S.F.; Garcia Ac, A.; Minani Tuyaga, M.A.; Rode Garcia, T.; Banquy, X.; Roullin, V.G. Critical Assessment of Purification Processes for the Robust Production of Polymeric Nanomedicine. *Int. J. Pharm.* **2025**, *668*, 124975. [CrossRef]
11. Kalinova, R.; Grancharov, G.; Doumanov, J.; Mladenova, K.; Petrova, S.; Dimitrov, I. Green Synthesis and the Evaluation of a Functional Amphiphilic Block Copolymer as a Micellar Curcumin Delivery System. *Int. J. Mol. Sci.* **2023**, *24*, 10588. [CrossRef] [PubMed]
12. Manea-Saghin, A.-M.; Marin, C.A. Sea Buckthorn Extract Loaded into Solid Lipid Nanoparticles. *Mol. Cryst. Liq. Cryst.* **2019**, *695*, 85–98. [CrossRef]
13. Popovici, V.; Boldianu, A.-B.; Pintea, A.; Caraus, V.; Ghendov-Mosanu, A.; Subotin, I.; Druta, R.; Sturza, R. In Vitro Antioxidant Activity of Liposomal Formulations of Sea Buckthorn and Grape Pomace. *Foods* **2024**, *13*, 2478. [CrossRef] [PubMed]
14. Asprea, M.; Tatini, F.; Piazzini, V.; Rossi, F.; Bergonzi, M.C.; Bilia, A.R. Stable, Monodisperse, and Highly Cell-Permeating Nanocochleates from Natural Soy Lecithin Liposomes. *Pharmaceutics* **2019**, *11*, 34. [CrossRef]
15. Jung, W.H.; Song, J.; You, G.; Lee, J.H.; Lee, S.W.; Ahn, J.-H.; Mok, H. Protection of Skin Fibroblasts from Infrared-A-Induced Photo-Damage Using Ginsenoside Rg3(S)-Incorporated Soybean Lecithin Liposomes. *J. Microbiol. Biotechnol.* **2023**, *33*, 135–141. [CrossRef] [PubMed]
16. Allaw, M.; Manconi, M.; Caboni, P.; Bacchetta, G.; Escribano-Ferrer, E.; Peris, J.E.; Nacher, A.; Diez-Sales, O.; Manca, M.L. Formulation of Liposomes Loading Lentisk Oil to Ameliorate Topical Delivery, Attenuate Oxidative Stress Damage and Improve Cell Migration in Scratch Assay. *Biomed. Pharmacother.* **2021**, *144*, 112351. [CrossRef] [PubMed]
17. Visan, S.; Soritau, O.; Tatomir, C.; Baldasici, O.; Balacescu, L.; Balacescu, O.; Muntean, P.; Gherasim, C.; Pintea, A. The Bioactive Properties of Carotenoids from Lipophilic Sea Buckthorn Extract (*Hippophae rhamnoides* L.) in Breast Cancer Cell Lines. *Molecules* **2023**, *28*, 4486. [CrossRef] [PubMed]
18. Dienaitė, L.; Pukalskas, A.; Pukalskienė, M.; Pereira, C.V.; Matias, A.A.; Venskutonis, P.R. Phytochemical Composition, Antioxidant and Antiproliferative Activities of Defatted Sea Buckthorn (*Hippophaë rhamnoides* L.) Berry Pomace Fractions Consecutively Recovered by Pressurized Ethanol and Water. *Antioxidants* **2020**, *9*, 274. [CrossRef] [PubMed]
19. Sadowska, B.; Rywaniak, J.; Cichocka, A.; Cichocka, K.; Żuchowski, J.; Wójcik-Bojek, U.; Więckowska-Szakiel, M.; Różalska, B. Phenolic and Non-Polar Fractions of the Extracts from Fruits, Leaves, and Twigs of *Elaeagnus rhamnoides* (L.) A. Nelson—The Implications for Human Barrier Cells. *Molecules* **2020**, *25*, 2238. [CrossRef]
20. Kumar, K.; Patial, B.S.; Chauhan, S. Conductivity and Fluorescence Studies on the Micellization Properties of Sodium Cholate and Sodium Deoxycholate in Aqueous Medium at Different Temperatures: Effect of Selected Amino Acids. *J. Chem. Thermodyn.* **2015**, *82*, 25–33. [CrossRef]
21. Laskowska, A.K.; Wilczak, A.; Skowrońska, W.; Michel, P.; Melzig, M.F.; Czerwińska, M.E. Fruits of Hippophaë Rhamnoides in Human Leukocytes and Caco-2 Cell Monolayer Models-A Question About Their Preventive Role in Lipopolysaccharide Leakage and Cytokine Secretion in Endotoxemia. *Front. Pharmacol.* **2022**, *13*, 981874. [CrossRef]
22. Gu, Y.; Wang, X.; Liu, F.; Zhang, J.; Zhang, X.; Liu, J.; Li, S.; Wang, D.; Guan, H.; Hou, D. Total Flavonoids of Sea Buckthorn (*Hippophae rhamnoides* L.) Improve MC903-Induced Atopic Dermatitis-like Lesions. *J. Ethnopharmacol.* **2022**, *292*, 115195. [CrossRef]
23. Pap, N.; Reshamwala, D.; Korpinen, R.; Kilpeläinen, P.; Fidelis, M.; Furtado, M.M.; Sant'Ana, A.S.; Wen, M.; Zhang, L.; Hellström, J.; et al. Toxicological and Bioactivity Evaluation of Blackcurrant Press Cake, Sea Buckthorn Leaves and Bark from Scots Pine and Norway Spruce Extracts under a Green Integrated Approach. *Food Chem. Toxicol.* **2021**, *153*, 112284. [CrossRef] [PubMed]

24. Sajeeda, A.; Bhat, A.M.; Gorke, S.; Wani, I.A.; Sidiqui, A.; Ahmed, Z.; Sheikh, T.A. Naringenin, a Flavanone Constituent from Sea Buckthorn Pulp Extract, Prevents Ultraviolet (UV)-B Radiation-Induced Skin Damage via Alleviation of Impaired Mitochondrial Dynamics Mediated Inflammation in Human Dermal Fibroblasts and Balb/c Mice Models. *J. Photochem. Photobiol. B Biol.* **2024**, *256*, 112944. [CrossRef]
25. Zhao, L.; Geng, T.; Sun, K.; Su, S.; Zhao, Y.; Bao, N.; Pan, L.; Sun, H.; Li, M. Proteomic Analysis Reveals the Molecular Mechanism of Hippophae Rhamnoides Polysaccharide Intervention in LPS-Induced Inflammation of IPEC-J2 Cells in Piglets. *Int. J. Biol. Macromol.* **2020**, *164*, 3294–3304. [CrossRef] [PubMed]
26. Treede, I.; Braun, A.; Sparla, R.; Kühnel, M.; Giese, T.; Turner, J.R.; Anes, E.; Kulaksiz, H.; Füllekrug, J.; Stremmel, W.; et al. Anti-Inflammatory Effects of Phosphatidylcholine. *J. Biol. Chem.* **2007**, *282*, 27155–27164. [CrossRef] [PubMed]
27. Chen, M.; Pan, H.; Dai, Y.; Zhang, J.; Tong, Y.; Huang, Y.; Wang, M.; Huang, H. Phosphatidylcholine Regulates NF-κB Activation in Attenuation of LPS-Induced Inflammation: Evidence from in Vitro Study. *Anim. Cells Syst.* **2018**, *22*, 7–14. [CrossRef]
28. Cosmulescu, S.; Vijan, L.; Mazilu, I.C.; Badea, G. Bioactive Compounds in the Residue Obtained from Fruits of Some Cultivars of Lonicera Caerulea. *Horticulturae* **2024**, *10*, 211. [CrossRef]
29. Marinescu, R.M.; Mickael, M.E.; Enciu, A.M. Normal Human Monocytic Cell Line CRL9855 Can Be Transformed into Macrophages with Very Low Concentrations of Phorbol 12-Myristate 13-Acetate. *JCI* **2022**, *1*, 5–12. [CrossRef]
30. Sorop, A.; Iacob, R.; Iacob, S.; Constantinescu, D.; Chitoiu, L.; Fertig, T.E.; Dinischiotu, A.; Chivu-Economescu, M.; Bacalbasa, N.; Savu, L.; et al. Plasma Small Extracellular Vesicles Derived miR-21-5p and miR-92a-3p as Potential Biomarkers for Hepatocellular Carcinoma Screening. *Front. Genet.* **2020**, *11*, 712. [CrossRef] [PubMed]
31. Shao, Y.; Jiang, Y.; Kanell, T.A.; Xu, P.; Khattab, O.; Lam, M.S. Assisting in Writing Wikipedia-like Articles from Scratch with Large Language Models. 2024. Available online: https://aclanthology.org/2024.naacl-long.347/ (accessed on 27 September 2024).

pharmaceuticals

MDPI

Article

Protective Effects of Phycobiliproteins from *Arthrospira maxima* (Spirulina) Against Cyclophosphamide-Induced Embryotoxicity and Genotoxicity in Pregnant CD1 Mice

Yuliana García-Martínez [1], Amparo Celene Razo-Estrada [1], Ricardo Pérez-Pastén-Borja [1], Candelaria Galván-Colorado [1], Germán Chamorro-Cevallos [1], José Jorge Chanona-Pérez [2], Oscar Alberto López-Canales [3], Hariz Islas-Flores [4], Salud Pérez-Gutiérrez [5], Joaquín Cordero-Martínez [6,*] and José Melesio Cristóbal-Luna [1,*]

[1] Departamento de Farmacia, Escuela Nacional de Ciencias Biológicas, Instituto Politécnico Nacional, Av. Wilfrido Massieu 399, Mexico City C.P. 07738, Mexico; ygarciamart@hotmail.com (Y.G.-M.); arazoe@ipn.mx (A.C.R.-E.); rpastenb@ipn.mx (R.P.-P.-B.); cgalvanc2001@alumno.ipn.mx (C.G.-C.); gchamcev@yahoo.com.mx (G.C.-C.)

[2] Laboratorio de Micro y Nanobiotecnología, Departamento de Ingeniería Bioquímica, Escuela Nacional de Ciencias Biológicas, Instituto Politécnico Nacional, Av. Wilfrido Massieu 399, Mexico City C.P. 07738, Mexico; jchanona@ipn.mx

[3] Departamento de Fisiología, Facultad de Medicina, Universidad Nacional Autónoma de México, Mexico City C.P. 04510, Mexico; oscaralberto_123@hotmail.com

[4] Laboratorio de Toxicología Ambiental, Facultad de Química, Universidad Autónoma del Estado de México, Paseo Colón Intersección Paseo Tollocan, Colonia Residencial Colón, Toluca C.P. 50120, Mexico; hislasf@uaemex.mx

[5] Departamento de Sistemas Biológicos, Universidad Autónoma Metropolitana-Xochimilco, Calzada del Hueso 1100, Del. Coyoacán, Mexico City C.P. 04960, Mexico; msperez@correo.xoc.uam.mx

[6] Laboratorio de Bioquímica Farmacológica, Departamento de Bioquímica, Escuela Nacional de Ciencias Biológicas, Instituto Politécnico Nacional, Mexico City C.P. 11340, Mexico

* Correspondence: jcorderom@ipn.mx (J.C.-M.); jcristoball@ipn.mx (J.M.C.-L.); Tel.: +52-5513782861 (J.C.-M.); +52-5520670441 (J.M.C.-L.)

Abstract: Background/Objectives: In recent years the global incidence of cancer during pregnancy is rising, occurring in 1 out of every 1000 pregnancies. In this regard, the most used chemotherapy drugs to treat cancer are alkylating agents such as cyclophosphamide (Cp). Despite its great efficacy, has been associated with the production of oxidative stress and DNA damage, leading to embryotoxicity, genotoxicity, and teratogenicity in the developing *conceptus*. Therefore, this study aimed to investigate the protective role of phycobiliproteins (PBP) derived from *Arthrospira maxima* (spirulina) in reducing Cp-induced embryotoxicity and genotoxicity in pregnant CD1 mice. **Methods**: Pregnant CD1 mice were divided into five groups: control, Cp 20 mg/kg, and three doses of PBP (50, 100, and 200 mg/kg) + Cp co-treatment. PBP were administered orally from day 6 to 10.5 *dpc*, followed by a single intraperitoneal dose of Cp on 10.5 *dpc*. Embryos were collected at 12.5 *dpc* to assess morphological development and vascular alterations, while maternal DNA damage was evaluated using micronucleus assays and antioxidant enzyme activity in maternal plasma. **Results**: PBP exhibited a dose-dependent protective effect against Cp-induced damage. The 200 mg/kg PBP dose significantly reduced developmental abnormalities, micronucleated polychromatic erythrocytes, and oxidative stress, (as evidenced by increased SOD and GPx activity). **Conclusions**: Phycobiliproteins from *Arthrospira maxima* (spirulina) effectively reduced Cp-induced morphological and vascular alterations in embryos and genotoxicity in pregnant mice. These findings highlight their potential as a complementary therapy to mitigate teratogenic risks during chemotherapy. Further research is needed to optimize dosing and explore clinical applications.

https://doi.org/10.3390/ph18010101

Keywords: phycobiliproteins; cyclophosphamide; teratogenesis; genotoxicity; oxidative stress; antioxidant therapy; pregnant mice; chemotherapy-induced damage; complementary cancer therapy

1. Introduction

Pregnancy is a multifaceted biological and physiological state that supports the development of a fertilized egg into a fetus within a woman's uterus, beginning at conception and lasting around 266 days until childbirth [1]. Unlike polyparous species such as mice, who can have multiple offspring in a single litter and have a gestation period of only 19 to 21 days, humans usually experience singleton pregnancies. Not to mention that mice do not experience spontaneous abortion; instead, they reabsorb non-viable embryos [2]. Understanding these and other unique aspects of gestation in mice is the basis for the study of alterations like embryotoxicity and genotoxicity in humans through murine models. During pregnancy, the mother's body undergoes significant physiological changes that affect all organ systems and the developing fetus. So, it is crucial for healthcare providers to recognize these physiological changes to offer optimal care for the mother and the fetus [3]. Common diseases that may arise during pregnancy include infections, heart disease, gestational diabetes, and cancer, the latter being particularly concerning due to its prevalence and complexity of treatment during pregnancy [4].

Cancer is a disease characterized by the uncontrolled proliferation of transformed cells [5]. One of its most recent definitions states that "cancer is a disease of uncontrolled proliferation by transformed cells subject to evolution by natural selection" [6]. According to data from the International Agency for Research on Cancer (IARC), in 2022 nearly 20 million new cancer cases were reported worldwide, with approximately 9.7 million cancer-related deaths. The most diagnosed cancers were lung cancer (12.4%), breast cancer (11.6%), colorectal cancer (9.6%), prostate cancer (7.3%), and stomach cancer (4.9%) [7]. Although previously rare, the incidence of cancer in pregnant women has increased due to improved diagnostic methods and rising maternal age at conception. It is estimated that cancer affects 1 in 1000 pregnancies [8]. In Mexico, it is estimated that around 2000 to 3000 cases of cancer are diagnosed in pregnant women each year [9]. The most common malignancies diagnosed during pregnancy include breast cancer, cervical cancer, ovarian cancer, melanoma, lymphoma, and thyroid cancer. Similarly, systemic lupus erythematosus [10], Crohn's disease [11], and sclerosis [12] affects women predominantly in their reproductive years, posing significant risks to both maternal and fetal health.

Pregnancy associated with cancers and autoimmune disease can lead to adverse birth outcomes such as preterm birth, low birth weight, growth restrictions, and a wide range of birth defects affecting the central nervous system [13]. This highlights the necessity of aggressive anticancer treatments like nitrosoureas, antimetabolites, mitosis inhibitors, and alkylating agents like cyclophosphamide (Cp) [14]. As a prodrug, Cp is particularly effective in treating various types of cancers by interfering with DNA replication and cell division [15]. Additionally, Cp is employed to suppress the immune system, making it a versatile and essential medication in modern medical practice [16].

Once in the body, Cp is activated in the liver via cytochrome P450-mediated 4-hydroxylation, producing 4-hydroxycyclophosphamide (4-OHCP) [17]. 4-OHCP rapidly equilibrates with aldophosphamide, which undergoes β-elimination to form the phosphoramide mustard (PM), the DNA-crosslinking therapeutic agent [18] (Figure 1). This bioactivation process also generates acrolein (Acr), a toxic aldehyde associated with bladder damage and hemorrhagic cystitis [15].

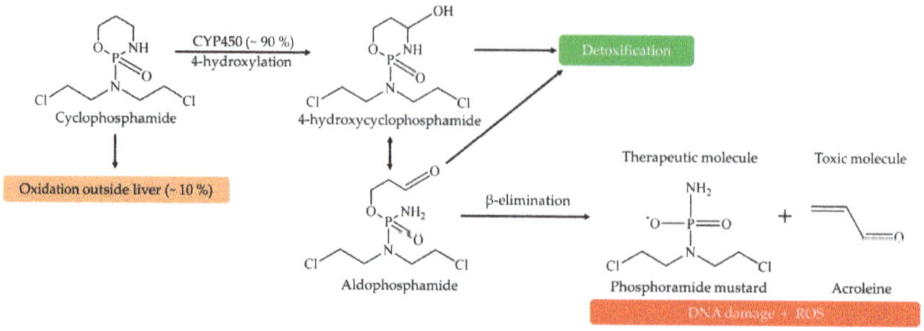

Figure 1. Schematic representation of the hepatic biotransformation of cyclophosphamide. Metabolic activation leads to the formation of the phosphoramide mustard and acrolein.

Despite its beneficial biological properties, Cp causes adverse effects in pregnant women and fetuses; nausea, hair loss, bone marrow suppression, hepatotoxicity [19], cardiotoxicity, neurotoxicity, immunosuppression [20], and birth defects [13]. The latter is of particular interest to this study, although Cp-induced teratogenesis involves complex mechanisms such as caspases activation or NF-kappaB suppression, the main mechanisms responsible are associated with DNA damage by bioactivation of toxic metabolites and induction of oxidative stress. PM forms covalent bonds with DNA, causing crosslinking, replication errors, and double-strand breaks, while Acr reacts with cellular components, forming Acr-deoxyguanosine adducts that inhibit DNA repair and induce damage through replication interference, mutagenesis, and apoptosis [21–23]. If the damage is extensive and cannot be repaired, it can trigger apoptosis or propagation of genetic defects, disrupting embryonic development and causing malformations [23].

On the other hand, Cp induces oxidative stress through reactive oxygen species (ROS) generated during its bioactivation and via angiotensin II overproduction [24]. At same time, Acr exacerbates this by depleting cellular antioxidants like glutathione, leading to mitochondrial dysfunction and increased DNA damage [25]. This oxidative stress activates pro-inflammatory pathways, disrupting embryonic growth and differentiation. Combined with DNA damage, it results in teratogenic effects, including growth restriction, craniofacial and skeletal malformations, and soft tissue defects like hydrocephalus and aphakia [13,26,27].

Projections based on demographic trends suggest that the number of new cancer cases could reach 35 million by 2050 [7]. As a result, the risk that many pregnant women or women of reproductive age are at is palpable. Therefore, it is essential to investigate alternatives that can help prevent or reduce the unwanted effects of Cp. In this context, *Arthrospira maxima*, spirulina (Am), a photosynthetic cyanobacterium that is widely consumed as a nutraceutical is particularly notable for its substantial protein content, 50–70% of its dry weight [28]. This blue-green alga is also rich in micronutrients (thiamine, riboflavin, niacin, cobalamin, folic acid, and A, E, and K vitamins), which are considered valuable tools to counteract the action of free radicals in cells [29]. Additionally, Am contains a variety of essential minerals and bioactive compounds, essential fatty acids and antioxidants like flavonoids, terpenes, phenolic compounds, and pigments such as carotenoids, chlorophylls, and phycobiliproteins (PBP) [30]. Research has shown that Am offers numerous health benefits, including antioxidant, immunostimulatory, antineoplastic, and antiviral properties, as well as a significant detoxifying effect against pollutants like chemicals and heavy metals [31]. Although Am contains a wide variety of bioactive compounds and pigments, multiple studies have demonstrated that one of its most crucial components responsible for its biological effects are the PBP. These protein complexes, in addition to serving as photopigments, have shown significant protective effects against oxidative damage and a low acute toxicity in mice (LD_{50} > 2000 mg/kg) [32].

In this sense, the investigation of antioxidant agents is promising in the context of cancer treatment during pregnancy, especially due to the adverse effects of alkylating drugs such as Cp, which, although effective, generate ROS which subsequently causes oxidative stress. Since this oxidative damage is closely related to embryotoxicity and DNA damage, it is necessary to explore alternative antioxidants capable of mitigating the oxidative stress and toxic effects derived from the use of Cp. Therefore, the ability of PBP to reduce oxidative stress suggests that its inclusion in treatment regimens could offer a complementary approach to protect both mothers and their developing fetuses from damage derived from Cp therapy. Therefore, this study aimed to investigate the protective effect of PBP, protein pigments with broad antioxidant capacity, isolated from Am against Cp-induced damage during the embryonic development of CD1 mice, as well as their antigenotoxic effect in the mothers.

2. Results

2.1. *Phycobiliproteins Extraction and Characterization*

The extraction of PBP from Am using thermal shock cryofracturing, centrifugation, and lyophilization had a yield of 23.41%. In addition, the major component extracted was C-PC, APC and in minor amount PE. With a relative purity of 0.88 ± 0.03, 0.39 ± 0.01, and 0.40 ± 0.01, respectively (Table 1).

Table 1. PBP extraction, concentration, and relative purity.

PBP	Ratio Biomass (g): Solvent (mL)	Concentration (mg/mL)	Relative Purity
C-PC		1.77 ± 0.067	0.88 ± 0.03
APC	1:4	0.66 ± 0.027	0.39 ± 0.01
PE		0.07 ± 0.001	0.40 ± 0.01

The concentration and relative purity with which the PBP were obtained from the aqueous ex-tract of Am are shown. Data are expressed as mean ± SEM. PBP, phycobiliproteins; C-PC, c-phycocyanin; APC, allophycocyanin; PE, phycoerythrin.

2.2. *Results of Teratogenic Test*

The administration of the treatments did not result in significant alterations in the weight gain of pregnant females between gestational days 6.5 and 10.5, with all treated groups showing consistent weight increases (Figure 2). During this period, no post-treatment signs of toxicity were observed in females that received PBP as regards its physical appearance and behavior. However, it is important to note that following the administration of Cp at 10.5 *dpc* lethargy, reduced motor activity, and occasional diarrhea were observed in pregnant females. On gestational day 12.5, a weight reduction of nearly 3 g was observed in the group treated solely with Cp at 20 mg/kg (30.94 ± 0.23 g) compared to the control group (33.87 ± 0.28 g). Conversely, the groups pretreated with PBP exhibited a dose-dependent attenuation of weight loss, with the 200 mg/kg dose of PBP maintaining weight gain at levels comparable to the control, and the 50 mg/kg dose resulting in a weight similar to the group Cp 20 mg/kg (34.47 ± 0.26 g and 31.08 ± 0.31 g, respectively).

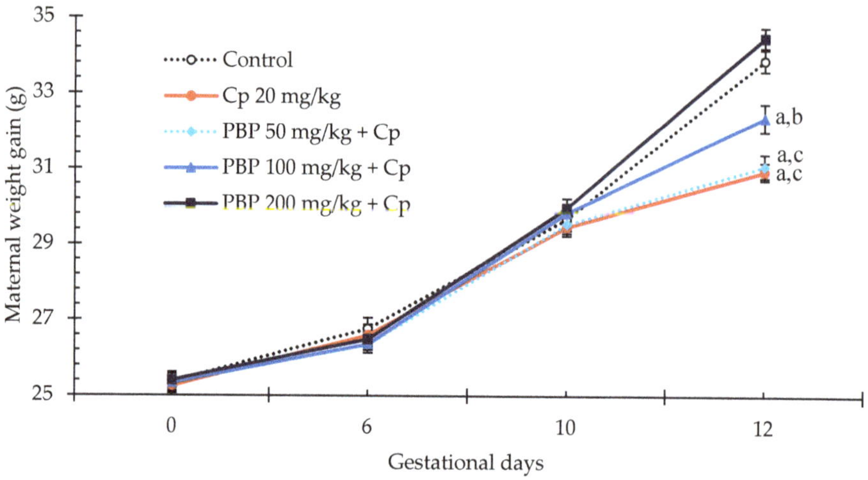

Figure 2. Weight gain of pregnant females from 0.5 to 12.5 *dpc*. Each point represents the mean ± SEM ($n = 15$). PBP, phycobiliproteins; Cp, cyclophosphamide. Two-way ANOVA for repeated measures *post hoc* Student–Newman–Keuls revealed significant differences ($p \leq 0.05$) vs. [a] Control, [b] Cp 20 mg/kg, and [c] PBP 200 mg/kg on 12.5 *dpc*.

In addition to the remarkable irregularities in the weight gain of pregnant females, the administration of Cp resulted in notable damage in embryonic development. At 12.5 *dpc*, the embryos of the control group showed a normal development characterized by a prominent cephalocaudal curvature, in which the head is bent towards the trunk. The semi-transparent skin allows the visualization of some internal organs such as the liver and heart, which are well developed. As well as the underlying blood vessels, which are well defined and developed at the cephalic level. And in parallel, we can see that the brain has been divided into three main vesicles (forebrain, midbrain, and hindbrain). Externally, the well-defined optic and otic vesicles are clearly visible; the formation of the face has begun showing outlines of the jaws and well-defined branchial arches. In the trunk, the forelimbs and hindlimbs are not rounded but have developed digital outlines (fingers). And the limbs show a clear segmentation in arms, forearms, thighs, and legs (long bones are present), without vascular alterations or hemorrhages (Figure 3a).

In contrast, embryos treated only with Cp 20 mg/kg show poor embryonic development evidenced by a significantly smaller and less developed body than the control embryos. They were also severe alterations in the cephalic vascular network showing dilatation, disorganization, poor development, and possible punctate hemorrhages. In parallel, although the three main cerebral vesicles are observed, they are poorly developed and differentiated. On the other hand, optic and otic vesicles, although well defined, present vascular alterations and hemorrhages in their periphery. Something similar is observed in the embryonic trunk and in the upper and lower limbs; where in addition to less structural development, the vascular patterns are observed disordered and with hemorrhages in the somites or in the periphery of the plates of the upper and lower limbs. Finally, mandibular outlines and facial development, in general, are severely altered (Figure 3b).

For their part, embryos exposed to PBP show a clear dose-dependent protective effect against Cp damage. At doses of 50 mg/kg of PBP, the embryonic alterations are practically the same as in the group that only received Cp (Figure 3c), showing no protection against Cp. While at doses of 100 and 200 mg/kg of PBP, an improvement in the parameters described above is observed (Figure 3d,e). At the highest dose of PBP, the cephalocaudal length and the development of facial structures and upper and lower limbs were practically the same (or with similar development) as those observed in the control group. The most remarkable feature of this analysis is the clear improvement in the vascular network in embryos exposed to 200 mg/kg of PBP, which is very similar to that of the control group, with slight dilatations and microbleeds that can still be seen at the cephalic level or in the periphery of the plates of the upper and lower limbs. The same as compared to Cp 20 mg/kg group are minimal.

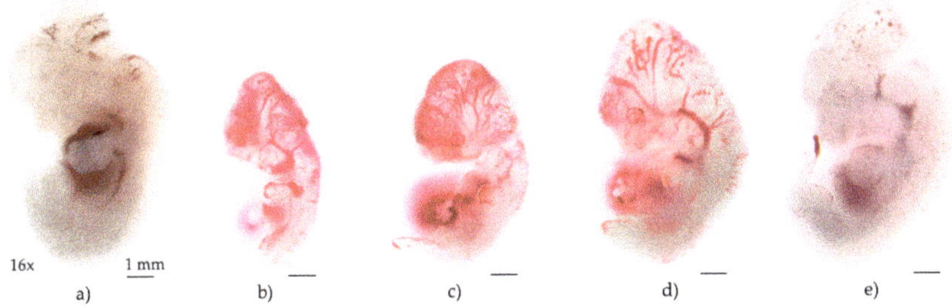

Figure 3. Dose-dependent protective effects of PBP against Cp-induced teratogenicity in CD1 mouse embryos at 12.5 *dpc*. All images were taken on a Wild Heerbrugg M7S stereo microscope at 16x magnification, black bars represent 1 mm. (**a**) Control embryo shows normal development of facial structures, upper and lower limbs, and blood vessels; (**b**) embryos exposed to Cp 20 mg/kg are small, they show delayed embryonic development, disordered somites (lumbar, sacral, and coccygeal), as well as dilatation and disorganization of the blood vessels (mainly at the level of the brain, eyes and limbs); (**c**) embryos treated with PBP 50 mg/kg + Cp show the similar type and severity of developmental and vasculature alterations as those shown by embryos exposed to Cp alone; (**d**) embryos treated with PBP 100 mg/kg + Cp show better embryonic development, the upper and lower limbs have less vascular alterations and better development. Although dilatation of the encephalic blood vessels is still observed, it is more organized (probably due to the more advanced development of the embryo). In parallel, although the somites show a better organization, they present alterations in their vasculature; (**e**) embryos treated with PBP 200 mg/kg + Cp show a practically normal embryonic development, with slight blood vessels alterations at the encephalic level in the form of small dilatations. The somites are perfectly organized and there are no vascular alterations.

Table 2 displays the effects of PBP at different doses on various parameters of embryonic development that include vascular network of the yolk sac, cephalo-caudal length, number of somites, and several morphological and functional markers. It is observed that Cp treatment caused significant alterations in embryonic development compared to the control group. The vascular network of the yolk sac, embryo rotation, caudal extension, and cephalo-caudal length were all notably reduced in the Cp-treated group, resulting in a decrease in cephalo-caudal length decrease from 9.11 mm (control) to 6.27 mm (Cp-treated). The number of somites also dropped drastically from 51.13 in the control group to 37.63, indicating a developmental delay. These negative effects were also observed in the primitive brain, heart development, and pharyngeal arches, showing significant disruptions. Conversely, co-treatment with PBP showed a protective effect, mitigating the teratogenic effects of Cp in a dose-dependent manner. The highest dose of PBP (200 mg/kg) demonstrated near-complete recovery in most developmental parameters evaluated. For example, the cephalo-caudal length in the PBP 200 mg/kg + Cp group (9.18 mm) almost matched that of the control group (9.11 mm). Similarly, the number of somites in the PBP 200 mg/kg group (51.81) was comparable to the control (51.13), while lower doses (50 and 100 mg/kg) showed a gradual improvement in somite numbers (38.93 and 42.12, respectively), though still below control values. The heart rate measured in beats per minute also reflected the protective effects of PBP, where the Cp group showed a decrease to 137.19 beats/min compared to the control (147.38 beats/min). Treatment with PBP improved this parameter, with the 100 mg/kg group reaching 148.45 beats/min. In summary, PBP co-treatment at 200 mg/kg, effectively mitigated the adverse effects induced by Cp on embryonic development. The data suggest a dose-dependent protective effect, with higher doses of PBP providing the most significant recovery in embryo morphology and function, approaching normal developmental conditions observed in the control group.

Table 2. Development score of embryos at 12.5 *dpc*, exposed to PBP and Cp.

	Dosis (mg/kg)				
Embryonic Development	**Control**	**Cp 20**	**PBP 50 + Cp**	**PBP 100 + Cp**	**PBP 200 + Cp**
n	**202**	**191**	**208**	**211**	**199**
Vascular network of the yolk sac	4.91 ± 0.04	4.78 ± 0.07	4.83 ± 0.06	4.88 ± 0.02	4.94 ± 0.05
Caudal extension	4.97 ± 0.03	4.51 ± 0.09 [a,c]	4.71 ± 0.06 [a]	4.81 ± 0.11 [a,b]	4.95 ± 0.03 [b]
Cephalo-caudal length (mm)	9.11 ± 0.20	6.27 ± 0.19 [a,c]	6.81 ± 0.18 [a]	8.01 ± 0.11 [a,b,c]	9.18 ± 0.09 [b]
Number of somites	51.13 ± 0.78	37.63 ± 0.93 [a,c]	38.93 ± 0.98 [a,c]	42.12 ± 0.74 [a,b,c]	51.81 ± 0.97 [b]
Primitive brain	5.00 ± 0.00	3.72 ± 0.12 [a,c]	3.78 ± 0.13 [a]	4.66 ± 0.07 [a,b]	4.91 ± 0.15 [b]
Heart	5.00 ± 0.00	4.07 ± 0.11 [a,c]	4.11 ± 0.15 [a]	4.68 ± 0.08 [a,b]	4.97 ± 0.05 [b]
Pharyngeal arches	4.98 ± 0.01	4.21 ± 0.05 [a,c]	4.11 ± 0.09 [a]	4.72 ± 0.03 [a,b]	4.93 ± 0.03 [b]
Facial morphology	4.98 ± 0.02	3.41 ± 0.14 [a,c]	3.50 ± 0.11 [a]	4.56 ± 0.15 [a,b]	4.77 ± 0.09 [b]
Beats/min	112.38 ± 8.36	117.19 ± 6.93	123.44 ± 9.89 [a]	118.45 ± 7.67	112.95 ± 8.41
Maldevelopment (%)	6.4	78.59 [a,c]	75.34 [a]	51.18 [a,b,c]	9.8 [b]

Data on the development score of embryos exposed to different treatments, 15 litters per group, are shown. The values are based on a dysmorphology scoring system (0–5). Data are expressed as mean ± SEM, and percentage. PBP, phycobiliproteins; Cp, cyclophosphamide; *dpc*, *day post coitum*. ANOVA on ranks (Kruskal–Wallis test) and Chi-square test followed by Fisher's exact test (for maldevelopment), revealed significant differences ($p \leq 0.05$) vs. [a] Control, [b] Cp 20 mg/kg, and [c] PBP 200 mg/kg on 12.5 *dpc*.

2.3. Micronucleus Test

2.3.1. Cytotoxicity and Genotoxic Effects

In the micronucleus test, the polychromatic erythrocytes (PCE) and micronucleated PCE (MN-PCE) frequency in the peripheral blood of pregnant mice exposed to Cp was determined as a measure of cytotoxicity and genotoxicity. Our determinations revealed significant cytotoxic effects induced by Cp on bone marrow cells. As shown in Figure 4, a significant decrease in the number of PCE was observed in the Cp 20 mg/kg group, starting from a baseline level at 0 h of exposure (63 ± 2.93) and progressively decreasing at 24 h (39.2 ± 2.87) until reaching its lowest number at 48 h (26.1 ± 2.06) following its administration. Compared to the control group, which maintained a constant number of PCE at the three sampling times (61.1 ± 3.05, 60.3 ± 3.08, and 60.8 ± 3.04, respectively), these results indicate that Cp significantly impaired the proliferation and/or survival of bone marrow cells, a hallmark of cytotoxicity. Interestingly, co-treatment with PBP demonstrated a protective effect against Cp-induced cytotoxicity. The 200 mg/kg dose maintained PCE numbers with minor reductions at all sampling times (62.6 ± 2.79, 56.1 ± 2.99, and 46 ± 2.55), compared to the control group. In contrast, the 50 mg/kg dose showed no protective effect, with values at the three sampling times similar to those of the group that received only Cp (63.5 ± 3.00, 39.5 ± 2.66, 26.2 ± 1.96).

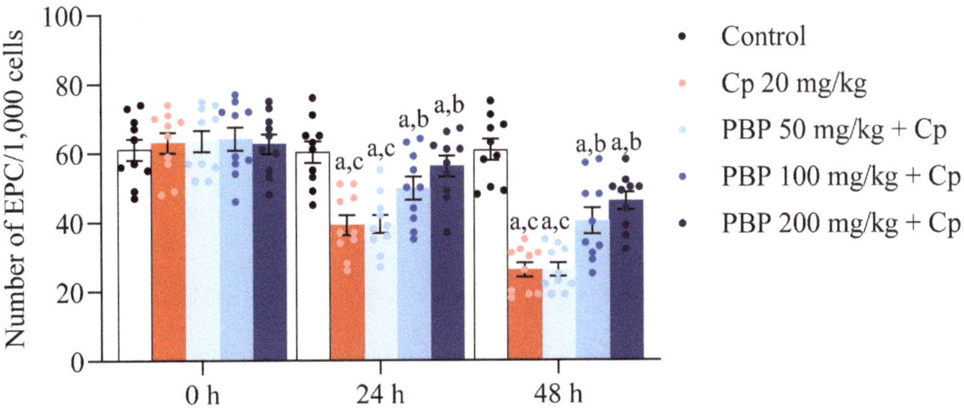

Figure 4. Number of polychromatic erythrocytes found in the peripheral blood of pregnant treated mice. Each bar represents the mean ± SEM of PCE in 1000 cells per mouse (n = 10) in 10.5 (0 h), 11.5 (24 h) and 12.5 (48 h) *dpc*. In addition, points in each bar represent the dispersion of the individual data. Polychromatic erythrocytes, PCE; cyclophosphamide, Cp; phycobiliproteins, PBP. ANOVA on ranks for repeated measures *post hoc* Student–Newman–Keuls revealed significant differences ($p \leq 0.05$) vs. [a] Control, [b] Cp 20 mg/kg, and [c] PBP 200 mg/kg.

2.3.2. Genotoxic Effect

Parallel to cytotoxicity the micronucleus assay revealed significant genotoxic effects induced by Cp on bone marrow cells. As shown in Figure 5, treatment with Cp resulted in a significant increase in micronucleus frequency compared to the control group, starting from a baseline level at 0 h of exposure (3.5 ± 0.40), increasing at 24 h (35.8 ± 3.00), and reaching its highest frequency of micronuclei at 48 h post-treatment (43.2 ± 3.18). In contrast, the control group maintained a constant micronucleus frequency at all sampling times (3.7 ± 0.60, 3.4 ± 0.39, 3.2 ± 0.60, respectively). These findings indicate Cp-induced DNA damage and chromosomal instability in bone marrow cells. Co-treatment with PBP significantly reduced the frequency of micronuclei induced by Cp, suggesting a protective effect against Cp-induced genotoxicity. The decrease in micronucleus frequency was dose-dependent, with the highest dose of PBP (200 mg/kg) providing greater protection at 24 and 48 h post-treatment by reducing the increase in MN frequency to 9.1 ± 1.16 and 17.2 ± 1.09, respectively. The time-dependent increase in micronucleus frequency in the Cp-treated groups highlights the progressive nature of the genotoxic damage. The initial genotoxic effects were most pronounced at 24 h, and the persistent increase at 48 h suggests continued DNA damage or impaired repair mechanisms.

Table 3 illustrates the percentage of damage reduction (% DR) in cytotoxicity and genotoxicity induced by Cp and mitigated by pre-treatment with PBP at doses of 50, 100, and 200 mg/kg. The results are shown for two time points: 24 h (T2) and 48 h (T3) post-treatment. PBP co-treatment demonstrated a dose-dependent protective effect against both cytotoxic and genotoxic damage. At 24 h post-treatment, the group receiving 200 mg/kg of PBP exhibited the highest reduction in cytotoxic damage, achieving an 80.09% reduction in PCE per 1000 cells, followed by 100 (50.23%) and 50 mg/kg PBP (1.42%). This trend continued at 48 h, where the 200 mg/kg dose again showed the greatest protective effect (57.34%), compared to 100 mg/kg (40.92%), and 50 mg/kg (0.28%).

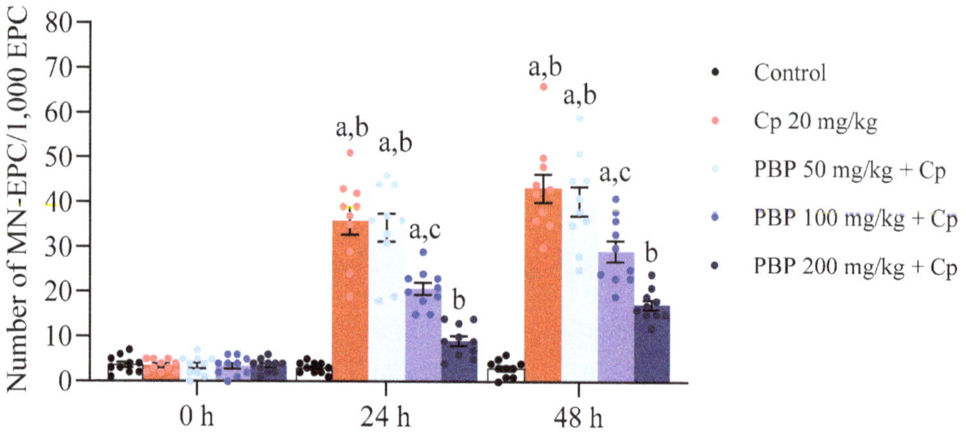

Figure 5. Number of micronucleated polychromatic erythrocytes found in the peripheral blood of pregnant treated mice. Each bar represents the mean ± SEM of MN-PCE in 1000 PCE per mouse (n = 10) in 10.5 (0 h), 11.5 (24 h) and 12.5 (48 h) *dpc*. In addition, points in each bar represent the dispersion of the individual data. Micronucleated polychromatic erythrocytes, MN-PCE; polychromatic erythrocytes, PCE; cyclophosphamide, Cp; phycobiliproteins, PBP. ANOVA on ranks for repeated measures *post hoc* Student–Newman–Keuls revealed significant differences ($p \leq 0.05$) vs. [a] Control, [b] Cp 20 mg/kg, and [c] PBP 200 mg/kg.

Table 3. Reduction in cytotoxic and genotoxic damage in the micronucleus test.

	PCE/1000 Cells (% DR)			MN-PCE/1000 PCE (% DR)		
Treatments	**T0 (0 h)**	**T2 (24 h)**	**T3 (48 h)**	**T0 (0 h)**	**T2 (24 h)**	**T3 (48 h)**
Control	-	-	-	-	-	-
Cp 20 mg/kg	-	-	-	-	-	-
PBP 50 mg/kg + Cp	0	1.42	0.28	0	4.26	7.21
PBP 100 mg/kg + Cp	0	50.23	40.92	0	46.03	34.82
PBP 200 mg/kg + Cp	0	80.09	57.34	0	81.40	64.67

%DR, damage reduction; PCE, polychromatic erythrocytes; MN-PCE, micronucleated polychromatic erythrocytes; PBP, phycobiliproteins; Cp, cyclophosphamide.

For genotoxicity, measured as the reduction in MN-PCE per 1000 PCE, a similar dose-dependent pattern was observed. At 24 h, the highest reduction in genotoxic damage was observed in the 200 mg/kg PBP group (81.40%), followed by 100 (46.03%) and 50 mg/kg (4.26%). At 48 h, the 200 mg/kg dose maintained the most significant reduction (64.67%), followed by 100 (34.82%) and 50 mg/kg (7.21%). In summary, the 200 mg/kg PBP dose consistently provided the greatest protection against both cytotoxic and genotoxic damage at 24 and 48 h, confirming a dose-dependent protective effect.

2.4. Results of Antioxidant Enzymatic Activity

Results shown in Table 4 display the activity of SOD and GPx in the plasma of pregnant CD1 mice subjected to different treatments. The control group exhibited high SOD activity (4.16 ± 0.041 U/mg protein) and correspondingly high GPx activity (416.33 ± 24.11 U/mL). Cyclophosphamide treatment (Cp 20) significantly reduced the activity of both enzymes, with SOD dropping to 1.88 ± 0.044 U/mg protein and GPx to 197.13 ± 28.24 U/mL, indicating oxidative stress induced by the drug. The pretreatment with PBP at different doses mitigated the oxidative damage caused by Cp. At the lowest dose of PBP (50 mg/kg), there was a slightly increased SOD and GPx activity. A more pronounced recovery was observed with 100 mg/kg PBP, where SOD rose to 3.13 ± 0.055 U/mg protein and GPx to 348.55 ± 19.99 U/mL. The highest dose of PBP (200 mg/kg) restored the enzyme activities to levels comparable to or slightly higher than the control group, with SOD at 4.30 ± 0.031 U/mg protein and GPx at 434.81 ± 23.41 U/mL. These results suggest that phycobiliproteins offer a dose-dependent protective effect against cyclophosphamide-induced oxidative damage in pregnant mice, as evidenced by the restoration of SOD and GPx activities.

Table 4. Antioxidant enzyme activity in plasma of pregnant CD1 mice treated with cyclophosphamide and phycobiliproteins.

Treatments (mg/kg)	SOD (U/mg Protein)	GPx (U/mg/mL)
Control	4.16 ± 0.041	416.33 ± 24.11
Cp 20	1.88 ± 0.044 ^{a,c}	197.13 ± 28.24 ^{a,c}
PBP 50 + Cp 20	2.03 ± 0.053 ^{a,c}	224.09 ± 17.4 ^{a,c}
PBP 100 + Cp 20	3.13 ± 0.055 ^{a,b}	348.55 ± 19.99 ^{a,b}
PBP 200 + Cp 20	4.30 ± 0.031 ^{b}	434.81 ± 23.41 ^{b}

Cp treatment significantly reduced antioxidant enzyme activities, whereas co-administration of PBP restored SOD and GPx activities in a dose-dependent manner. SOD activity is expressed as units per mg of protein (U/mg protein), and GPx activity is expressed as units per mL (U/mL). Data are presented as mean ± SEM (n = 15). All experiments were performed in triplicate. SOD, superoxide dismutase; GPx, glutathione peroxidase; Cp, cyclophosphamide; PBP, phycobiliproteins. One-way ANOVA *post hoc* Student–Newman–Keuls revealed significant differences ($p \leq 0.05$) vs. ^{a} Control, ^{b} Cp 20 mg/kg, and ^{c} PBP 200 mg/kg on 12.5 *dpc*.

3. Discussion

This year a study reported that 1 in every 1000 pregnant women worldwide has been diagnosed with some form of cancer, and the number appears to be increasing [8]. Such situations present pregnant women diagnosed with cancer with a challenging dilemma: to undergo treatments to improve their health such as chemotherapy, which can harm the developing fetus, or to prioritize the health of the baby by delaying their treatments and putting their health at risk. In addition, considering that chemotherapy options have become more diverse and complex in recent years, the decision-making process in these cases has become more challenging. This fact has brought increased attention to the concept of shared decision-making (SDM), which is gaining popularity within the medical community as a collaborative approach to addressing these difficult choices [33]. Thus, the present study investigated PBP as an alternative or complementary therapy to help decrease Cp-induced embryotoxicity and genotoxicity during gestation. Our results demonstrated that PBP co-treatment mitigated the negative effects of Cp in a dose-dependent manner, with the highest dose (200 mg/kg) showing the greatest protective effects. These findings could serve as a foundation for developing new complementary cancer therapies.

In our study, pregnant mice exposed to PBP did not show signs of toxicity until 10.5 *dpc* when Cp administration produced lethargy. At 12.5 *dpc*, weight loss was observed in the Cp-exposed groups, mainly in those who received the lowest dose of PBP. Although it was observed that the administration of Cp caused lethargy in pregnant females and some episodes of diarrhea, as well as discomfort that could have been reduced the food consumption, our results indicate that the decrease in weight gain was due to a delay in embryonic development observed in the *conceptus*. The consequences of prenatal exposure to Cp-induced embryopathy are characterized by intrauterine growth restriction, developmental delays, a wide range of congenital malformations, and intrauterine death through oxidative stress and DNA damage [13,34]. Notably, PBP co-treatment effectively preserved maternal weight gain and prevented embryonic malformations, reduced cephalo-caudal length, decreased the number of somites and neural tube defects, among others, which results in a normal embryonic development similar to that of the control group. These findings are supported by research that highlights the antioxidant properties of PBP in reducing oxidative stress and preventing damage to developing tissues [35,36].

In accordance with the literature, the protective effects of PBP against Cp-induced embryotoxicity are attributed to four main mechanisms: neutralization of free radicals, reduction in oxidative stress, cell protection, and to a lesser extent, modulation of immune response. The strong ability of PBP to inhibit free radicals is of great interest because they can neutralize and sequester a wide variety of ROS and reactive nitrogen species (NRS) due to its chemical structures like phycobilins (linear tetrapyrrole chromophores) and α and β subunits [37]. Such neutralization is complemented by the chelating properties of PBP, which allow them to trap ferrous ions and reduce oxidative stress more efficiently [38]. Some authors have shown that another way in which PBP can reduce oxidative stress is decreasing the production of ROS [39], and at the same time increasing the activity of antioxidant enzymes such as SOD, CAT, or GPx, that play a vital role in neutralizing the ROS generated [36]. In the same way, it has been reported that PBP protects against cell damage thanks to its ability to delay or inhibit protein oxidation, lipid peroxidation, and DNA degradation [40]. In addition, some reports have shown that PBP can modulate the immune response, acting on pathways such as NF-κB, TLR, PI3K/Akt/mTOR and Nrf2 to inhibit inflammation [41].

In terms of the protective effects on embryonic development, the improvement observed in PBP-treated groups aligns with the well-established role of antioxidants in protecting against teratogenicity [42]. PBP administration promoted normal development by neutralizing ROS and RNS and enhancing the activity of internal antioxidant defenses, which together helped to maintain a balance between oxidative stress and the organism's antioxidant capacity, thus protecting both maternal tissues and developing embryos from oxidative damage. Not to mention that PBP can modulate inflammatory processes that could impair embryonic development, and at the same time protects against DNA damage. The latter aspect is of particular importance given the fragility of embryonic processes considering the high rate of DNA replication and cell division required during embryogenesis—DNA replication in embryonic stages occurs 20 to 60 times faster than in somatic cells [43]. It is important to note that the protective response of PBP, in which higher doses show greater protection against Cp-induced damage, is consistent with the literature on antioxidants as they often show greater efficacy at higher concentrations [44].

In addition to their antioxidant, anti-inflammatory, and immunomodulatory properties, PBP offers a unique advantage in embryonic development that not all antioxidant compounds possess: their ability to restore vascular contractility [45]. This effect is of special interest for our research, since functional assays using mesenteric arteries from Cp-treated mice have demonstrated a significant decrease in vascular contractility associated with vascular lipoperoxidation, indicating that Cp causes significant vascular damage [46,47]. As observed when analyzing the main structures of the embryos exposed to Cp, the blood system was one of the most affected. The CNS, somites, eyes, and upper and lower limbs showed severe damage in their blood vessels such as dilatation, microbleeds, and alterations in the pattern of vascular development. Our results indicate that Cp significantly alters embryonic vascular development, thereby impairing normal embryonic growth and maternal health. Consequently, we can infer that the improvement in embryonic development observed in the PBP-treated group is not solely attributable to the reduction in ROS and protection against genetic damage. In contrast, PBP have the ability to protect not only against vascular lipoperoxidation, but can also restore vascular contractility, which is a crucial factor contributing to their antiteratogenic effect against Cp at the CNS level. This aspect warrants further investigation to fully understand its implications and action mechanisms.

In a complementary manner, the results of the micronucleus assay support the protective effect of PBP against Cp, as the frequency of MN-PCE decreased significantly in the PBP-treated groups. Such findings suggest that PBP mitigates the DNA damage caused by Cp, which is known to induce double-strand breaks and chromosomal instability via its active metabolites, PM and Acr [21]. The protective effect of PBP on MN-PCE frequency is likely linked to its ability to reduce oxidative stress, which plays a key role in DNA damage [22]. In the same way, the observed reduction in cytotoxicity, as indicated by the preservation of PCE frequency, further supports the role of PBP in maintaining cellular integrity against Cp-induced damage, possibly through antioxidant mechanisms or by modulating cellular signaling pathways involved in cell death. The observed decrease in the number of PCE as a function of time highlights the dynamic nature of the cytotoxic response. While cytotoxic effects were visible from the first 24 h, the persistent decline at 48 h suggests ongoing cell damage or poor recovery. Overall, these results provide convincing evidence that CP induces cytotoxicity in bone marrow cells, as evidenced by the significant reduction in the number of PCE [48]. And at the same time, co-treatment with PBP appears to alleviate these cytotoxic effects, indicating a protective role of PBP against Cp-induced cytotoxicity.

The dose-dependent antigenotoxic and anticytotoxic capacity in the presence of Cp was previously reported by Oliveira et al. [49], whose research demonstrates that antioxidant compounds such as β-glucan can reduce Cp-induced bone marrow suppression by protecting hematopoietic cells from oxidative damage (significantly reducing MN-PCE frequency and preventing PCE loss) in Cp-treated pregnant females. Our data are consistent with previous research that highlights the ability of antioxidants such as melatonin, β-caryophyllene, carvedilol, L-carnitine, quercetin, etc., to reduce Cp-induced malformations and DNA damage by neutralizing ROS and enhancing cellular repair mechanisms [25,26,50–52].

The results of this study suggest that PBP could be a promising candidate for adjuvant therapy in pregnant women undergoing treatment with Cp, either for cancer, autoimmune diseases, nephrotic syndrome, or any other disease for which the treatment includes alkylating agents such as Cp. The ability of PBP to reduce embryotoxicity and genotoxicity resulting from Cp treatment is particularly noteworthy, as it opens the possibility of reducing the teratogenic risks associated with alkylating agent chemotherapy. It also allows the patient to continue with her treatment without endangering the integrity of her developing baby. However, further research is needed to demonstrate that PBP, in addition to reducing the toxic effects of Cp, does not compromise the efficacy of cancer treatment.

Despite these promising findings, it is important to acknowledge certain limitations: the mouse model does not fully replicate human physiological responses to PBP and Cp; although we explored different doses of PBP the optimal dosing regimen for maximizing protective effects while minimizing potential toxicity remains to be fully established; PBP were shown to reduce the toxic effects of Cp, but we do not know whether PBP interfere with the therapeutic capacity of this alkylating agent. Therefore, future studies should also investigate the long-term developmental outcomes in offspring exposed to PBP and Cp during gestation, as well as the optimal dosing regimen for balancing protective effects with potential toxicity. Molecular studies focusing on the specific pathways involved in PBP-mediated protection could provide valuable insights into its therapeutic potential. Among these, it would be interesting to explore its ability to restore vascular contractility, and to determine whether PBP interferes with the therapeutic effects of Cp.

The present study reinforces the notion that PBP, potent natural antioxidant, has a great potential to be utilized as a complementary strategy alongside existing chemotherapy regimens. By mitigating oxidative stress and enhancing cellular protection, PBP could improve treatment outcomes and reduce the adverse effects associated with conventional chemotherapeutic agents.

4. Materials and Methods

4.1. Aqueous Extract of Arthrospira Maxima (Spirulina)

A total of 5 g of Am powder (generously donated by Alimentos Esenciales para la Humanidad S.A. de C.V., Ciudad de México, Mexico) were suspended in 20 mL of phosphate-buffered saline (PBS) (20 mmol, pH 7.4). The suspension underwent two cycles of freezing (−70 °C for 2 h) and thawing (37 °C for 30 min), followed by centrifugation at 13,000 rpm × 30 min using a JA-17 rotor in a Beckman Coulter centrifuge (Beckman Coulter, Inc., California, CA, USA) for two cycles to ensure the purity of the PBP by separating the characteristic dark blue, PBP-rich supernatant from the cell precipitate. The aqueous extract was analyzed spectrophotometrically to assess its purity and subsequently lyophilized (FreeZone 4.5, Labconco, Kansas City, MO, USA) at −50 °C and 0.0133 mBar for 36 h until a fine light blue powder was obtained under dark conditions. The lyophilized extract was then stored at −70 °C, protected from light until its use [53].

The optical densities (O.D.) of the aqueous extract rich in PBP were measured at specific wavelengths (615, 652, and 562 nm) using a Shimadzu BioSpec-mini DNA/RNA/Protein UV-Visible Spectrophotometer (Shimadzu Corporation, Kyoto, Japan), in order to determine the absorbance of C-phycocyanin (C-PC, λ_{max} = 610–620 nm), allophycocyanin (APC, λ_{max} = 650–655 nm), and phycoerythrin (PE, λ_{max} = 540–570 nm), respectively [54]. The concentration of three PBP were calculated following the method described by Bennett and Bogorad [55], with the following equations:

$$\text{C-PC}\left(\frac{\text{mg}}{\text{mL}}\right) = \frac{A_{615} - 0.474(A_{652})}{5.34}$$

$$\text{APC}\left(\frac{\text{mg}}{\text{mL}}\right) = \frac{A_{652} - 0.208(A_{615})}{5.09}$$

$$\text{PE}\left(\frac{\text{mg}}{\text{mL}}\right) = \frac{A_{562} - 2.41[\text{C-PC}] - 0.849[\text{APC}]}{9.62}$$

The relative purity was estimated using the method described by Boussiba and Richmond [53,54,56] with the following equations:

$$\text{C-PC purity} = \left(\frac{A_{615}}{A_{280}}\right), \quad \text{APC} = \left(\frac{A_{652}}{A_{280}}\right), \quad \text{PE} = \left(\frac{A_{562}}{A_{280}}\right)$$

The extraction of the PBP was estimated following the equation proposed by Silveira et al. [57], where C-PC, APC, and PE are expressed as mg/mL, V is the solvent volume (mL), and DB is the dry biomass (g):

$$\text{PBP Yield}\left(\frac{\text{mg}}{\text{g}}\right) = \frac{(\text{C-PC} + \text{ACP} + \text{PE})(\text{V})}{\text{DB}}$$

4.2. Teratogenic Test

4.2.1. Animals and Housing Conditions

A total of 10 sexually mature male and 75 nulliparous female CD1 mice aged 8 weeks were obtained from the breeding colony of the Laboratory Animal Production and Experimentation Unit (UPEAL) of the Universidad Autónoma Metropolitana (UAM) Xochimilco, located in Mexico City, Mexico. All animals were housed in polycarbonate cages with sterile pinewood shavings as bedding in an air-conditioned room under controlled conditions; 23 ± 2 °C, 55–60% relative humidity, and a 12 h light/dark cycle (lights on at 10:00 h). They received a standard diet (Rodent Lab Chow 5001, Purina, St. Luis, MO, USA) and access to purified water *ad libitum*, and were acclimatized for 2 weeks prior to the initiation of the experiment. Approval for the study was obtained from the Research Ethics Committee of the Escuela Nacional de Ciencias Biológicas (CEI-ENCB) under protocol number 09-CEI-002-20190327. All procedures and animal handling were conducted in strict adherence to the Mexican Official Standard "NOM-062-ZOO-1999" concerning technical statements for production, care, and use of experimental laboratory animals [58].

4.2.2. Study Design and Treatment Administration

Females were housed three per cage and males housed individually, after 2 weeks of acclimatization animals were coupled during the last 3 h of the dark phase of their light/dark cycle. This was performed with the aim of having better control over the moment of fertilization. At the end of the dark phase, the vaginal cavity of each female was examined, the presence of a vaginal plug was taken as evidence that mating had occurred, and that day was designated as *day post coitum* 0.5 (0.5 *dpc*), also referred to by some researchers as gestation day 0 (GD0).

Each mated female was assigned a unique identification number through coat staining and randomly allocated to one of five groups ($n = 15$): control (vehicle, purified water), Cp 20 mg/kg, and three different doses of PBP: 50, 100, and 200 mg/kg. Similarly, Cp doses were selected based on data in the literature that ensured the induction of malformations in developing embryos of mice [59]. All solutions were freshly prepared before its administration; all treatments, except for Cp, were administered by gavage in a constant volume of 10 mL/kg from 6.5 to 10.5 *dpc*, at the same time once a day. On the other hand, Cp was administered as a single intraperitoneal (IP) dose only on 10.5 *dpc* in the same constant volume. On 12.5 *dpc*, pregnant females were euthanized by cervical dislocation and the uterine horns were removed through a transverse abdominal incision. The position of every embryo on the uterine horns was registered, and the embryos were dissected and analyzed for external morphological alterations, modifications in the embryonic vasculature, and antioxidant enzyme activity.

4.2.3. Embryonic Morphological Analysis

Embryos were carefully extracted and placed in cold PBS, pH = 7.4, to measure crown-rump length and develop a morphological and structural analysis of alterations using a Wild Heerbrugg M7S stereo microscope (Leica Microsystems, Heerbrugg, Switzerland). A descriptive value was assigned based on the dysmorphology scoring system proposed by Zhang et al. [60].

4.2.4. Statistical Analysis

Maternal body weight was analyzed using two-way ANOVA for repeated measures *post hoc* Student–Newman–Keuls test. Somatometric variables were analyzed using one-way ANOVA followed by a *post hoc* Student–Newman–Keuls test. Implantation and embryonic parameters (live or dead embryos, heartbeats, number of somites, development scoring, etc.) were evaluated using ANOVA on ranks (Kruskal–Wallis test), and maldevelopment was evaluated using a Chi-square test followed by Fisher's exact test. All data were processed using the statistical software SigmaPlot 15.0, with statistical significance set at $p \leq 0.05$.

4.3. *Micronuclei Assay*

Micronuclei evaluation was performed on peripheral blood reticulocytes from pregnant females of the previously described five groups (in the teratogenic test), from which 10 were randomly selected for each group of 15 females ($n = 10$). Peripheral blood samples were collected from the tail of each mouse (5 μL approximately) prior to Cp administration at 10.5 *dpc* (0 h). After Cp administration, the remaining samples were collected every 24 h for the next 48 h. The last blood sample was collected at 12.5 *dpc*, prior to euthanasia. To prepare each smear, a drop of blood was placed at the end of each clean slide and extended (two smears of each sampling time per mouse). Next, cells were fixed in 96% methanol for 3 min, briefly rinsed under running water, dried, and stained with 5% Giemsa (Sigma-Aldrich, St. Louis, MO, USA) in PBS for 10 min [61]. The stained and coded slides were examined under a Zeiss light microscope (Carl Zeiss Microscopy GmbH, Jena, Germany) using a 100× objective to count the number of young PCE and mature normochromatic erythrocytes (NCE) within 1000 cells per mouse at each sampling time, to determine the PCE/NCE ratio as an indicator of the cytotoxicity of the treatments. Additionally, the frequency of MN-PCE was quantified within 1000 PCE per mouse at each sampling time, as a measure of the genotoxic effects of the treatments. Finally, to assess the chemopreventive capacity of PBP against Cp in the micronuclei test, the percentage of damage reduction (%DR) was calculated with the equation proposed by Manoharan and Beneriee [62,63]:

$$\%DR = \left(\frac{MN_{\text{positive control}} - MN_{\text{treated group}}}{MN_{\text{positive control}} - MN_{\text{negative control}}} \right)(100).$$

Statistical Analysis of Micronuclei Assay

The data corresponding to the PCE and MN-PCE were analyzed using an ANOVA on ranks for repeated measures followed by a *post hoc* Student–Newman–Keuls test. All statistical analyses were performed using the statistical software SigmaPlot 15.0, with significance set at $p \leq 0.05$.

4.4. Antioxidant Enzymatic Activity

At 12.5 *dpc*, peripheral blood samples were collected from pregnant females via retro-orbital puncture using heparinized capillary tubes to prevent coagulation. The blood samples were immediately transferred into EDTA-treated Eppendorf tubes to prevent clotting. The samples were centrifuged at 2000× *g* for 10–15 min at 4 °C to separate plasma from the cellular components. Plasma, rather than serum, is ideal for enzymatic antioxidant assays as it preserves the integrity of enzymes like superoxide dismutase (SOD) and glutathione peroxidase (GPx). The plasma was carefully aliquoted to avoid contamination from cellular components and stored at −70 °C until further analysis. The total protein concentration and the activity of antioxidant enzymes SOD and GPx were determined using validated spectrophotometric assays.

The activities of SOD and GPx were determined in collected plasma using commercial kits (RANSOD SD125 and RANSEL RS504, Randox Laboratories Ltd., Crumlin, Co., Antrim, UK). The assays were performed according to the manufacturer's instructions, with absorbance measured at 505 nm for SOD and 340 nm for GPx. The SOD assay utilizes xanthine and xanthine oxidase to generate superoxide radicals, which react with 2-(4-iodophenyl)-3-(4-nitrophenol)-5-phenyltetrazolium chloride (INT) to form a red formazan dye. SOD inhibits this reaction by dismutating superoxide radicals. SOD activity was expressed as units per mg of protein [64]. The GPx assay is based on the oxidation of glutathione (GSH) by cumene hydroperoxide, catalyzed by GPx. The oxidized glutathione (GSSG) is then reduced by glutathione reductase (GR) in the presence of NADPH, which is oxidized to NADP+. The decrease in absorbance at 340 nm was monitored, and GPx activity was expressed as units per mg of protein [65]. Total protein concentration was measured using the Randox Total Protein Kit (TP245, Randox Laboratories Ltd., Crumlin, Antrim, UK). The assay is based on the Biuret method, in which proteins form a

violet-colored complex with copper ions in an alkaline solution. The determination was performed according to the manufacturer's protocol, with absorbance measured at 546 nm using a spectrophotometer. Bovine serum albumin (BSA) was used as the calibration of the standard for protein quantification [66].

Statistical Analysis

Enzymatic activity data were analyzed with a one-way ANOVA *post hoc* Student–Newman–Keuls. All statistical analyses were performed using the statistical software SigmaPlot 15.0, with significance set at $p \leq 0.05$.

5. Conclusions

Cp administration significantly reduced SOD and GPx activities, indicating increased oxidative stress in pregnant CD1 mice. PBP from Am effectively mitigated the embryotoxic and genotoxic effects of Cp in a dose-dependent manner. The highest dose of PBP tested (200 mg/kg) was THE most effective in reducing developmental abnormalities and DNA damage, likely through the enhancement of antioxidant enzyme activity to counter oxidative stress. While multiple mechanisms are involved, one of the most intriguing mechanisms through which PBP appears to prevent Cp-induced embryonic damage is through their protective effects against vascular injury. This mechanism merits additional exploration in future studies.

These findings suggest that PBP could be considered a potential adjunct therapy for pregnant women undergoing chemotherapy, providing embryofetal protection without compromising maternal cancer treatment. Further research is needed to ensure that PBP does not interfere with the therapeutic effect of Cp and to establish optimal dosing, safety, and efficacy in clinical settings.

Author Contributions: Formal analysis and writing—original draft preparation, Y.G.-M.; methodology and research, A.C.R.-E.; data curation, R.P.-P.-B.; software, J.J.C.-P.; validation, H.I.-F.; Conceptualization, S.P.-G.; investigation, G.C.-C.; resources, C.G.-C.; visualization, O.A.L.-C.; supervision, project administration, J.C.-M.; writing—review and editing, funding acquisition, J.M.C.-L. All authors have read and agreed to the published version of the manuscript.

Funding: This research was funded by the Secretaría de Investigación y Posgrado del Instituto Politécnico Nacional, grant number 20241423.

Institutional Review Board Statement: The animal study protocol was approved by the Research Ethics Committee of the Escuela Nacional de Ciencias Biológicas del Instituto Politécnico Nacional, Mexico City (protocol code 09-CEI-002-20190327).

Informed Consent Statement: Not applicable.

Data Availability Statement: The data presented in this study are available upon request from the corresponding author due to privacy considerations.

Acknowledgments: I would like to take a moment to acknowledge the profound impact that Germán Chamorro-Cevallos had on my academic journey and personal growth. His steadfast support, profound wisdom, and unyielding thirst for knowledge shaped not only my journey but also the lives of countless others in our field. Dr. Chamorro was far more than a mentor; he was a trusted colleague and a cherished friend. His absence is a wound deeply felt—a stark reminder of life's fleeting nature and the indelible legacies we leave behind. Though he is no longer with us, his contributions will echo through every effort in our research, and his spirit will remain an eternal beacon of inspiration. With profound sorrow and endless gratitude, I dedicate this work to his memory; for men like him do not fade into oblivion, they become timeless guides for those of us left behind.

Requiescat in pace, magister et amicus dilectus; cum magno dolore, sed etiam cum gratitudine profunda, te meminimus.

Conflicts of Interest: The authors declare no conflicts of interest.

References

1. Davis, E.P.; Narayan, A.J. Pregnancy as a period of risk, adaptation, and resilience for mothers and infants. *Dev. Psychopathol.* **2020**, *32*, 1625–1639. [CrossRef]
2. Crocker, K.; Calder, M.D.; Edwards, N.A.; Betts, D.H.; Watson, A.J. CD-1 mouse fertility rapidly declines and is accompanied with early pregnancy loss under conventional housing conditions. *Theriogenology* **2018**, *108*, 245–254. [CrossRef] [PubMed]
3. Vinnars, M.T.; Bixo, M.; Damdimopoulou, P. Pregnancy-related maternal physiological adaptations and fetal chemical exposure. *Mol. Cell. Endocrinol.* **2023**, *578*, 112064. [CrossRef] [PubMed]
4. Jin, X.; Wang, G.; Xu, X.; Bai, Y.; An, R.; Jiang, D. Coexistence of Crohn's disease and systemic lupus erythematosus: A case report and literature review. *Eur. J. Gastroenterol. Hepatol.* **2020**, *32*, 1256–1262. [CrossRef] [PubMed]
5. Hausman, D.M. What Is Cancer? *Perspect. Biol. Med.* **2019**, *62*, 778–784. [CrossRef]
6. Brown, J.S.; Amend, S.R.; Austin, R.H.; Gatenby, R.A.; Hammarlund, E.U.; Pienta, K.J. Updating the Definition of Cancer. *Mol. Cancer Res.* **2023**, *21*, 1142–1147. [CrossRef] [PubMed]
7. Bray, F.; Laversanne, M.; Sung, H.; Ferlay, J.; Siegel, R.L.; Soerjomataram, I.; Jemal, A. Global cancer statistics 2022: GLOBOCAN estimates of incidence and mortality worldwide for 36 cancers in 185 countries. *CA Cancer J. Clin.* **2024**, *74*, 229–263. [CrossRef]
8. Heimovaara, J.H.; van Calsteren, K.; Lok, C.A.R.; Evens, A.M.; Hoegl, J.; Ferber, A.; Fernandes, A.; Vriens, I.; van Zuylen, L.; Amant, F. Results of an international survey on the current organization of care for pregnant women with cancer. *Acta Obstet. Gynecol. Scand.* **2024**, *103*, 751–756. [CrossRef] [PubMed]
9. Heraldo de México. Available online: https://heraldodemexico.com.mx/nacional/2023/1/30/en-mexico-fundacion-padma-les-da-una-oportunidad-las-mujeres-embarazadas-con-cancer-477254.html (accessed on 22 August 2024).
10. Dao, K.H.; Bermas, B.L. Systemic Lupus Erythematosus Management in Pregnancy. *Int. J. Womens Health* **2022**, *14*, 199–211. [CrossRef]
11. Cushing, K.; Higgins, P.D.R. Management of Crohn Disease: A Review. *JAMA* **2021**, *325*, 69–80. [CrossRef] [PubMed]
12. Villaverde-González, R. Updated Perspectives on the Challenges of Managing Multiple Sclerosis During Pregnancy. *Degener. Neurol. Neuromuscul. Dis.* **2022**, *12*, 1–21. [CrossRef] [PubMed]
13. Rengasamy, P. Congenital Malformations Attributed to Prenatal Exposure to Cyclophosphamide. *Anticancer Agents Med. Chem.* **2017**, *17*, 1211–1227. [CrossRef]
14. Miyamoto, S.; Yamada, M.; Kasai, Y.; Miyauchi, A.; Andoh, K. Anticancer drugs during pregnancy. *Jpn. J. Clin. Oncol.* **2016**, *46*, 795–804. [CrossRef] [PubMed]
15. Dabbish, E.; Scoditti, S.; Shehata, M.N.I.; Ritacco, I.; Ibrahim, M.A.A.; Shoeib, T.; Sicilia, E. Insights on cyclophosphamide metabolism and anticancer mechanism of action: A computational study. *J. Comput. Chem.* **2024**, *45*, 663–670. [CrossRef]
16. Liu, B.; Zhou, H.; Tan, L.; Siu, K.T.H.; Guan, X.Y. Exploring treatment options in cancer: Tumor treatment strategies. *Signal Transduct. Target. Ther.* **2024**, *9*, 175. [CrossRef] [PubMed]
17. Helsby, N.; Yong, M.; Burns, K.; Findlay, M.; Porter, D. Cyclophosphamide bioactivation pharmacogenetics in breast cancer patients. *Cancer Chemother. Pharmacol.* **2021**, *88*, 533–542. [CrossRef] [PubMed]
18. Stork, C.M.; Schreffler, S.M. Cyclophosphamide. In *Encyclopedia of Toxicology*, 4th ed.; Wexler, P., Ed.; Academic Press: London, UK, 2024; Volume 3, pp. 417–421.
19. Bhat, N.; Kalthur, S.G.; Padmashali, S.; Monappa, V. Toxic Effects of Different Doses of Cyclophosphamide on Liver and Kidney Tissue in Swiss Albino Mice: A Histopathological Study. *Ethiop. J. Health Sci.* **2018**, *28*, 711–716. [CrossRef]
20. Caruso, G.; Privitera, A.; Antunes, B.M.; Lazzarino, G.; Lunte, S.M.; Aldini, G.; Caraci, F. The Therapeutic Potential of Carnosine as an Antidote against Drug-Induced Cardiotoxicity and Neurotoxicity: Focus on Nrf2 Pathway. *Molecules* **2022**, *27*, 4452. [CrossRef] [PubMed]
21. Singh, R.K.; Kumar, S.; Prasad, D.N.; Bhardwaj, T.R. Therapeutic journey of nitrogen mustard as alkylating anticancer agents: Historic to future perspectives. *Eur. J. Med. Chem.* **2018**, *151*, 401–433. [CrossRef] [PubMed]
22. Tang, M.S.; Wang, H.T.; Hu, Y.; Chen, W.S.; Akao, M.; Feng, Z.; Hu, W. Acrolein induced DNA damage, mutagenicity and effect on DNA repair. *Mol. Nutr. Food Res.* **2011**, *55*, 1291–1300. [CrossRef]
23. Ibrahim, K.M.; Darwish, S.F.; Mantawy, E.M.; El-Demerdash, E. Molecular mechanisms underlying cyclophosphamide-induced cognitive impairment and strategies for neuroprotection in preclinical models. *Mol. Cell. Biochem.* **2024**, *479*, 1873–1893. [CrossRef] [PubMed]
24. Akomolafe, S.F.; Olasehinde, T.A.; Oyeleye, S.I.; Aluko, T.B.; Adewale, O.O.; Ijomone, O.M. Curcumin Administration Mitigates Cyclophosphamide-Induced Oxidative Damage and Restores Alteration of Enzymes Associated with Cognitive Function in Rats' Brain. *Neurotox. Res.* **2020**, *38*, 199–210. [CrossRef]

25. Wang, H.T.; Lin, J.H.; Yang, C.H.; Haung, C.H.; Weng, C.W.; Maan-Yuh Lin, A.; Lo, Y.L.; Chen, W.S.; Tang, M.S. Acrolein induces mtDNA damages, mitochondrial fission and mitophagy in human lung cells. *Oncotarget* **2017**, *8*, 70406–70421. [CrossRef] [PubMed]
26. Mahabady, K.M.; Varzi, N.H.; Jahromi, Z.S. L-Carnitine Protect against Cyclophosphamide Induced Skeletal and Neural Tube Malformations in Rat Fetuses. *Acta Med. Iran.* **2015**, *53*, 703–710.
27. Metwally, E.; Hefny, B.; Safwat, M.; Biram, D. The teratogenic effect of cyclophosphamide on the embryos of albino rats and the protective effect of folic acid: Morphologic study. *Zagazig Univ. Med. J.* **2022**, *28*, 1312–1331. [CrossRef]
28. Jung, F.; Krüger-Genge, A.; Waldeck, P.; Küpper, J.H. Spirulina platensis, a super food? *J. Cell. Biotechnol.* **2019**, *5*, 43–54. [CrossRef]
29. Grosshagauer, S.; Kraemer, K.; Somoza, V. The True Value of Spirulina. *J. Agric. Food Chem.* **2020**, *68*, 4109–4115. [CrossRef]
30. Martí-Quijal, F.J.; Ramon-Mascarell, F.; Pallarés, N.; Ferrer, E.; Berrada, H.; Phimolsiripol, Y.; Barba, F.J. Extraction of Antioxidant Compounds and Pigments from Spirulina (*Arthrospira platensis*) Assisted by Pulsed Electric Fields and the Binary Mixture of Organic Solvents and Water. *Appl. Sci.* **2021**, *11*, 7629. [CrossRef]
31. Pérez-Alvarez, I.; Islas-Flores, H.; Sánchez-Aceves, L.M.; Gómez-Olivan, L.M.; Chamorro-Cevallos, G. Spirulina (*Arthrospira maxima*) mitigates the toxicity induced by a mixture of metal and NSAID in *Xenopus laevis*. *Reprod. Toxicol.* **2023**, *120*, 108422. [CrossRef] [PubMed]
32. Grover, P.; Bhatnagar, A.; Kumari, N.; Narayan, B.A.; Kumar, N.D.; Purkayastha, J. C-Phycocyanin-a novel protein from Spirulina platensis- In vivo toxicity, antioxidant and immunomodulatory studies. *Saudi J. Biol. Sci.* **2021**, *28*, 1853–1859. [CrossRef]
33. Hori, R.; Suzuki, S. Shared Decision-Making Support Process for Healthcare Professionals for Pregnant Cancer Patients and Their Families. *APJON* **2021**, *8*, 304–313. [CrossRef] [PubMed]
34. Xu, J.; Fang, H.; Chong, Y.; Lin, L.; Xie, T.; Ji, J.; Shen, C.; Shi, C.; Shan, J. Cyclophosphamide Induces Lipid and Metabolite Perturbation in Amniotic Fluid during Rat Embryonic Development. *Metabolites* **2022**, *12*, 1105. [CrossRef] [PubMed]
35. Bae, H.K.; Hwang, I.S.; Kim, J.Y.; Lee, S.Y.; Park, C.K.; Yang, B.K.; Cheong, H.T. Antioxidant treatment during manipulation procedures prevents mitochondrial and DNA damage and enhances nuclear reprogramming of bovine somatic cell nuclear transfer embryos. *Reprod. Fertil. Dev.* **2015**, *27*, 1088–1096. [CrossRef] [PubMed]
36. Guzmán-Gómez, O.; García-Rodríguez, R.V.; Pérez-Gutierrez, S.; Rivero-Ramírez, N.L.; García-Martínez, Y.; Pablo-Pérez, S.S.; Pérez-Pastén-Borja, R.; Cristóbal-Luna, J.M.; Chamorro-Cevallos, G. Protective Effect of the Phycobiliproteins from *Arthrospira maxima* on Indomethacin-Induced Gastric Ulcer in a Rat Model. *Plants* **2023**, *12*, 1586. [CrossRef] [PubMed]
37. Jha, S.; Singh, V.K.; Singh, A.P.; Gupta, A.; Rana, P.; Sinha, R.P. The Radiant World of Cyanobacterial Phycobiliproteins: Examining Their Structure, Functions, and Biomedical Potentials. *Targets* **2024**, *2*, 32–51. [CrossRef]
38. Peña-Medina, R.L.; Fimbres-Olivarría, D.; Enríquez-Ocaña, L.F.; Martínez-Córdova, L.R.; Del-Toro-Sánchez, C.L.; López-Elías, J.A.; González-Vega, R.I. Erythroprotective Potential of Phycobiliproteins Extracted from Porphyridium cruentum. *Metabolites* **2023**, *13*, 366. [CrossRef] [PubMed]
39. Li, Y. The Bioactivities of Phycocyanobilin from Spirulina. *J. Immunol. Res.* **2022**, *2022*, 4008991. [CrossRef] [PubMed]
40. Sharifi-Rad, M.; Anil Kumar, N.V.; Zucca, P.; Varoni, E.M.; Dini, L.; Panzarini, E.; Rajkovic, J.; Tsouh Fokou, P.V.; Azzini, E.; Peluso, I.; et al. Lifestyle, Oxidative Stress, and Antioxidants: Back and Forth in the Pathophysiology of Chronic Diseases. *Front. Physiol.* **2020**, *11*, 694. [CrossRef]
41. Liu, R.; Qin, S.; Li, W. Phycocyanin: Anti-inflammatory effect and mechanism. *Biomed. Pharmacother.* **2022**, *153*, 113362. [CrossRef] [PubMed]
42. Ornoy, A. Embryonic oxidative stress as a mechanism of teratogenesis with special emphasis on diabetic embryopathy. *Reprod. Toxicol.* **2007**, *24*, 31–41. [CrossRef]
43. Kermi, C.; Lo Furno, E.; Maiorano, D. Regulation of DNA Replication in Early Embryonic Cleavages. *Genes* **2017**, *8*, 42. [CrossRef] [PubMed]
44. Schmidt, H.H.; Stocker, R.; Vollbracht, C.; Paulsen, G.; Riley, D.; Daiber, A.; Cuadrado, A. Antioxidants in Translational Medicine. *ARS* **2015**, *23*, 1130–1143. [CrossRef] [PubMed]
45. Castro-García, S.Z.; Chamorro-Cevallos, G.; Quevedo-Corona, L.; McCarty, M.F.; Bobadilla-Lugo, R.A. Beneficial effects of phycobiliproteins from Spirulina maxima in a preeclampsia model. *Life Sci.* **2018**, *211*, 17–24. [CrossRef]
46. Ayza, M.A.; Zewdie, K.A.; Tesfaye, B.A.; Wondafrash, D.Z.; Berhe, A.H. The Role of Antioxidants in Ameliorating Cyclophosphamide-Induced Cardiotoxicity. *Oxidative Med. Cell. Longev.* **2020**, *2020*, 4965171. [CrossRef]
47. Pimenta, G.F.; Awata, W.M.C.; Orlandin, G.G.; Silva-Neto, J.A.; Assis, V.O.; da Costa, R.M.; Bruder-Nascimento, T.; Tostes, R.C.; Tirapelli, C.R. Melatonin prevents overproduction of reactive oxygen species and vascular dysfunction induced by cyclophosphamide. *Life Sci.* **2024**, *338*, 122361. [CrossRef]
48. Yadav, V.; Krishnan, A.; Zahiruddin, S.; Ahmad, S.; Vohora, D. Amelioration of cyclophosphamide-induced DNA damage, oxidative stress, and hepato- and neurotoxicity by Piper longum extract in rats: The role of γH2AX and 8-OHdG. *Front. Pharmacol.* **2023**, *14*, 1147823. [CrossRef] [PubMed]

49. Oliveira, R.J.; Salles, M.J.; da Silva, A.F.; Kanno, T.Y.; Lourenço, A.C.; Freiria, G.A.; Matiazi, H.J.; Ribeiro, L.R.; Mantovani, M.S. Effects of the polysaccharide beta-glucan on clastogenicity and teratogenicity caused by acute exposure to cyclophosphamide in mice. *RTP* **2009**, *53*, 164–173. [PubMed]
50. Khaksary Mahabady, M.; Najafzadeh Varzi, H.; Bakhtiari, E. The effects of cyclophosphamide, melatonin and carvedilol on neural tube and skeletal system of mice fetuses in prenatal period. *Ann. Anat.* **2011**, *193*, 459–465. [CrossRef] [PubMed]
51. Lourenço, A.; Baroneza, J.; Ramos, S.; Miguel, L.; Juliani, L.; Pic-Taylor, A.; Salles, M. Effects of Copaiba Oil on Cyclophosphamide-Induced Teratogenesis in Mice. *Am. J. Plant Sci.* **2014**, *5*, 3464–3473. [CrossRef]
52. Khaksary Mahabady, M.; Gholami, M.R.; Najafzadeh Varzi, H.; Zendedel, A.; Doostizadeh, M. Protective effect of quercetin on skeletal and neural tube teratogenicity induced by cyclophosphamide in rat fetuses. *Vet. Res. Forum* **2016**, *7*, 133–138.
53. Guzmán-Gómez, O.; García-Rodríguez, R.V.; Quevedo-Corona, L.; Pérez-Pastén-Borja, R.; Rivero-Ramírez, N.L.; Ríos-Castro, E.; Pérez-Gutiérrez, S.; Pérez-Ramos, J.; Chamorro-Cevallos, G.A. Amelioration of Ethanol-Induced Gastric Ulcers in Rats Pretreated with Phycobiliproteins of *Arthrospira (Spirulina) Maxima*. *Nutrients* **2018**, *10*, 763. [CrossRef] [PubMed]
54. Patel, H.M.; Rastogi, R.P.; Trivedi, U.; Madamwar, D. Structural characterization and antioxidant potential of phycocyanin from the cyanobacterium *Geitlerinema* sp. H8DM. *Algal Res.* **2018**, *32*, 372–383. [CrossRef]
55. Bennett, A.; Bogorad, L. Complementary chromatic adaptation in a filamentous blue-green alga. *J. Cell Biol.* **1973**, *58*, 419–435. [CrossRef]
56. Boussiba, S.; Richmond, A.E. Isolation and characterization of phycocyanins from the blue-green alga Spirulina platensis. *Arch. Microbiol.* **1979**, *120*, 155–159. [CrossRef]
57. Silveira, S.T.; Burkert, J.F.; Costa, J.A.; Burkert, C.A.; Kalil, S.J. Optimization of phycocyanin extraction from Spirulina platensis using factorial design. *Bioresour. Technol.* **2007**, *98*, 1629–1634. [CrossRef]
58. *NOM-062-ZOO-1999*; Animales de Laboratorio y la Norma Oficial Mexicana. Norma Oficial Mexicana: Ciudad de México, México, 1999.
59. Vega-Navarro, A.C.; Moreno-Vázquez, S.E.; Hernández-Delgado, N.C.; Cristóbal-Luna, J.M.; García Martínez, Y.; Gutiérrez-Salmeán, G.; Chamorro-Cevallos, G.A. Spirulina (*Arthrospira maxima*), protects from cyclophosphamide teratogenicity in mice. *Vet. Méx. OA* **2022**, *9*. [CrossRef]
60. Zhang, C.; Panzica-Kelly, J.; Augustine-Rauch, K. The rat whole embryo culture assay using the Dysmorphology Score system. *Methods Mol. Biol.* **2013**, *947*, 423–450.
61. Cristóbal-Luna, J.M.; Paniagua-Castro, N.; Escalona-Cardoso, G.N.; Pérez-Gutiérrez, M.S.; Álvarez-González, I.; Madrigal-Bujaidar, E.; Chamorro-Cevallos, G. Evaluation of teratogenicity and genotoxicity induced by kramecyne (KACY). *Saudi Pharm. J.* **2018**, *26*, 829–838. [CrossRef] [PubMed]
62. Manoharan, K.; Banerjee, M.R. Beta-Carotene reduces sister chromatid exchanges induced by chemical carcinogens in mouse mammary cells in organ culture. *Cell Biol. Int. Rep.* **1985**, *9*, 783–789. [CrossRef]
63. Sánchez-De-La-Rosa, S.V.; Lazalde-Ramos, B.P.; Morales-Velazquez, G.; Zúñiga-González, G.M.; Gómez-Meda, B.C.; Sánchez-Rivera, S.O.; Ortiz-García, Y.M.; Guerrero-Velazquez, C.; Zamora-Perez, A.L. Evaluation of Genotoxic Effect and Antigenotoxic Potential against DNA Damage of the Aqueous and Ethanolic Leaf Extracts of Annona muricata Using an In Vivo Erythrocyte Rodent Micronucleus Assay. *BioMed Res. Int.* **2022**, *16*, 9554011. [CrossRef]
64. Zheng, M.; Liu, Y.; Zhang, G.; Yang, Z.; Xu, W.; Chen, Q. The Applications and Mechanisms of Superoxide Dismutase in Medicine, Food, and Cosmetics. *Antioxidants* **2023**, *12*, 1675. [CrossRef] [PubMed]
65. Ahmed, A.Y.; Aowda, S.A.; Hadwan, M.H. A validated method to assess glutathione peroxidase enzyme activity. *Chem. Pap.* **2021**, *75*, 6625–6637. [CrossRef]
66. Zheng, K.; Wu, L.; He, Z.; Yang, B.; Yang, Y. Measurement of the total protein in serum by biuret method with uncertainty evaluation. *Measurement* **2017**, *112*, 16–21. [CrossRef]

pharmaceuticals

MDPI

Article

Antinociceptive and Anti-Inflammatory Activities of Acetonic Extract from *Bougainvillea x buttiana* (var. Rose)

Gabriela Castañeda-Corral, Mayra Cedillo-Cortezano, Magdalena Aviles-Flores, Misael López-Castillo, Juan José Acevedo-Fernández and Vera L. Petricevich *

Facultad de Medicina, Universidad Autónoma del Estado de Morelos, Calle Iztaccihuatl Esq. Leñeros, Col. Volcanes, Cuernavaca 62350, Morelos, Mexico; gabriela.castaneda@uaem.mx (G.C.-C.); mayra.cedillo@uaem.edu.mx (M.C.-C.); magda.aviles0711@gmail.com (M.A.-F.); misael.pez@gmail.com (M.L.-C.); juan.acevedo@uaem.mx (J.J.A.-F.)
* Correspondence: vera.petricevich@uaem.mx

Abstract: Background: *Bougainvillea x buttiana* is an ornamental plant with antioxidant, anti-inflammatory, and cytotoxic activities, which has been traditionally used to treat respiratory diseases. This study aimed to investigate whether the acetonic extract of *Bougainvillea x buttiana* var. Rose (BxbRAE-100%) has analgesic and anti-inflammatory properties and its potential action mechanisms. **Methods:** Analgesic and anti-inflammatory activities were evaluated using three murine pain models and two acute inflammation models. In vitro, the ability of the extract to inhibit proteolytic activity and the activities of the enzymes phospholipase A2 (PLA2) and cyclooxygenase (COX) were evaluated. In silico analysis was performed to predict the physicochemical and Absorption, distribution, metabolism, and excretion (ADME) profiles of the compounds previously identified in BxbRAE-100%. **Results:** In vivo BxbRAE-100% decreased the nociceptive behaviors in the writhing model, the tail immersion, and the formalin test, suggesting that the extract has the potential to relieve pain at peripheral and central levels. Additionally, topical or oral BxbRAE-100% treatment reduced dose-dependent 12-*O*-Tetradecanoylphorbol-13-acetate (TPA)-induced ear inflammation and carrageenan-induced paw edema, respectively. In vitro, BxbRAE-100% significantly inhibited proteolytic activity and PLA2, COX-1 and COX-2 activities. In silico, the compounds previously identified in BxbRAE-100% met Lipinski's rule of five and showed adequate ADME properties. **Conclusions:** These results support the use of *B. x buttiana* in Traditional Mexican Medicine and highlight its potential for the development of new treatments for pain and inflammation.

Keywords: acetonic extract *Bougainvillea x buttiana*; anti-nociceptive activity; anti-inflammatory activity; COX- and PLA2 inhibition; in silico analysis

1. Introduction

Inflammation is the response of the human body to a wound or infection. It is a fundamental mechanism for the clearance of the infectious agent and repairing the affected tissues. The goals of the inflammatory process are the complete recovery of health and return to homeostasis through cellular and molecular processes [1]. However, inflammation is also associated with both pain and multiple conditions, such as autoimmune diseases like arthritis and osteoarthritis, sports injuries, headaches, and musculoskeletal pain [2–4]. Pain is defined as an unpleasant sensory and emotional experience associated with, or resembling that associated with, actual or potential tissue damage [5]. Acute pain is a symptom that acts as a warning signal for the body to protect it from possible damage or injury and, thus, avoid harmful consequences. Therefore, it has an adaptive role. However, when pain becomes chronic, it can have detrimental effects on individuals' health and quality of life, and sometimes, more than a symptom, it can be a disease by itself [6].

Standard anti-inflammatory and analgesic treatments include nonsteroidal anti-inflammatory drugs (NSAIDs) and glucocorticoids. However, these medications are associated with several side effects that affect the gastrointestinal and cardiovascular systems, kidneys, and liver, among other organs [7]. Furthermore, an insufficient response to treatment is frequently observed. As a result, the scientific community is seeking novel drugs and therapeutic agents for inflammation and pain management, particularly those of natural origin [8].

It is worth noting that medicinal plants are important sources of compounds with high therapeutic value. Examples include the approved drugs morphine, quinine, and acetyl-salicylic acid [9]. The discovery of these drugs has significantly contributed to the development of knowledge about chemical structures and mechanisms of action [10]. Furthermore, there are numerous reports in the literature about the presence of a wide variety of bioactive compounds found in medicinal plants, which exhibit beneficial biological activities such as analgesic, antibacterial, anti-inflammatory, antipyretic, antispasmodic, and antitumor activities [11]. Therefore, pure compounds or standardized extracts provide more opportunities to develop new medications. The World Health Organization aims to ensure the quality of plants for medicinal use. In this sense, the techniques to obtain extracts have been standardized because extraction, separation, and identification are critical steps that can potentially modify the type and number of bioactive compounds present in an extract [12].

Bougainvillea is a genus consisting of at least 18 species of ornamental and horticultural plants with colorful flowers belonging to the Nyctaginaceae family. It is endemic to Brazil and other South American regions. It was introduced pantropically and distributed in warm regions of Mexico, Asia, Australia, the Caribbean, South Africa, and the United States [13]. In Mexico, several species of *Bougainvillea* exist, including *B. spectabilis*, *B. glabra*, and *B. x buttiana*. *Bougainvillea* bracts, which are commonly confused with flower petals, are the most used part in traditional Mexican medicine to treat respiratory conditions such as cough, asthma, flu, and bronchitis. It has also been reported to be useful in treating gastrointestinal problems such as diarrhea and dysentery, as well as people suffering from lung pain, whooping cough, drowning, nausea, and wound cleaning [14]. It is commonly used in traditional medicine as an infusion of flowers and bracts that are administered orally [15].

The antinociceptive and anti-inflammatory properties of the ethanolic extract of *B. x buttiana* (var. Orange) were described for the first time by Alvarez Perez Gil et al., 2012 [16]. Subsequent studies found that the extract has significant antioxidant and immunomodulatory activities [17,18]. In our previous report, several extracts of *B. x buttiana* (var. Rose) of different polarities demonstrated cytotoxic and antioxidant activities. The phytochemical analysis showed that the polarity of the solvent influenced the composition of the extracts. In this sense, the main compounds identified in the extracts of *B. x buttiana* (var. Rose) include flavonoids (e.g., rutin and quercetin), carbohydrates (e.g., 3-*O*-Methyl-d-glucose), saturated fatty acids (e.g., *n*-Hexadecanoic acid) and polyunsaturated (e.g., 9,12-octadecadienoic (Z,Z)-), fatty alcohols (e.g., 1-Dotriacontanol), and phytosterols (e.g., Stigmasta-5,22-dien-3-ol and Stig-mast-7-en-3-ol, (3β,5α)) [19,20]. However, the antinociceptive and anti-inflammatory activities and mechanism of action of extracts made from flowers and bracts of plants of different colors have not yet been established.

This study aims to investigate the in vivo and in vitro anti-inflammatory activity of the acetonic extract of *Bougainvillea x buttiana* (var. Rose) (BxbRAE) as well as its peripheral and central analgesic actions. Finally, an in silico analysis of the physicochemical and ADME profiles of the bioactive compounds previously identified in the extract was performed.

2. Results

2.1. Extraction and Yields

In this study, the extraction process was conducted with 8.38 g of flowers and bracts, in acetone (100%), and the yield obtained was 2.37%. The solid residue obtained was resuspended in 5% Tween 20 in saline solution and orally administered at different concentrations. The extraction yield was used as an indicator of the effects of extraction conditions. Under the test conditions used in this study, no mouse mortality or macroscopic changes in the skin, eyes, or fur were observed.

2.2. Analgesic Activity

In this study, the antinociceptive properties of the acetonic extract from *Bougainvillea x buttiana* var. Rose (BxbRAE-100%) were evaluated using three different murine models: the acetic acid-induced writhing model, the tail immersion test, and the formalin test. Figure 1 shows the results obtained in the writhing model. It was observed that the groups of animals treated orally with BxbRAE 100% in the dose range between 0.4 and 400 mg/kg showed a statistically significant decrease in the percentage of pain (% pain) compared to the group treated with the vehicle. The doses of 40, 100, and 400 mg/kg showed the most significant reduction in % pain and were more effective than aspirin (1 mg/kg), dexamethasone (1 mg/kg), and diclofenac (10 mg/kg; Figure 1A). The dose-response curve analysis showed that the antinociceptive effect of BxbRAE 100% was dose-dependent, with a calculated ED_{50} of 10.14 mg/kg and an average maximum effect of 86 ± 2.0% (Figure 1B).

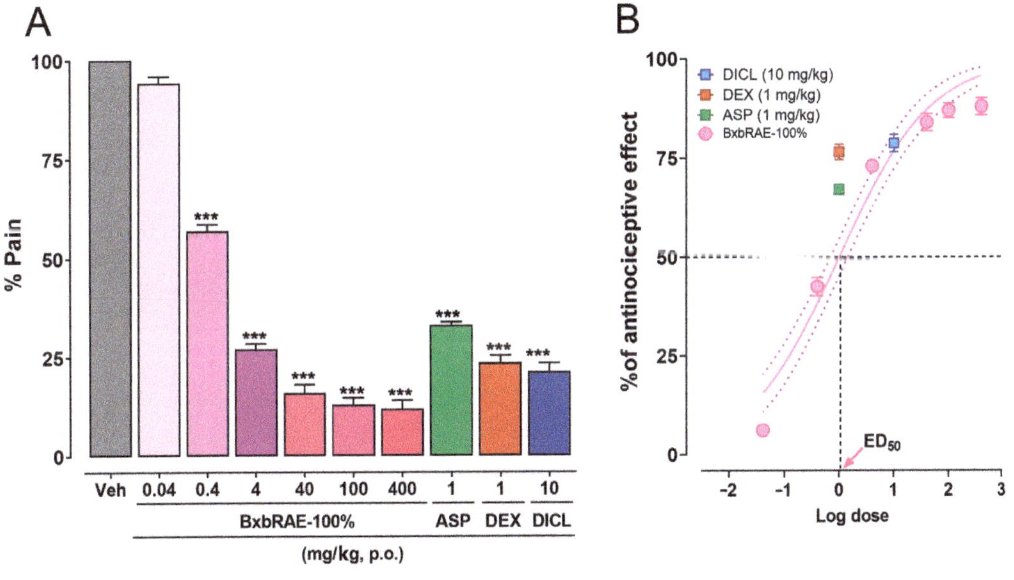

Figure 1. BxbRAE decreased in a dose-dependent manner acetic acid-induced pain in mice. (**A**) Bar graph showing the effect of BxbRAE 100% in the % of pain. (**B**) Dose–response curve (DRC) of the anti-nociceptive effect. In (**B**), the dashed lines represent the dose that achieves 50% of the anti-nociceptive effect (ED_{50}). Aspirin (ASP), dexamethasone (DEX), and diclofenac (DICL) were used as positive controls. Data are shown as the mean ± SD (n = 4). *** $p < 0.001$ vs. the Veh group through one-way ANOVA followed by Dunnett's test.

The pain experimental design included the evaluation of the effect of the extract on pain induced by a thermal noxious stimulus using the tail immersion test. The pain percentages obtained from the tail immersion assay are presented in Figure 2. The results showed that all doses of the extract used in this study significantly reduced the pain percentage compared to the results of the group treated with the vehicle ($p < 0.001$). This reduction in the percentage of pain was observed from the first 30 min to 120 min of the test. The pain percentages in the BxbRAE-100%-treated groups were equal to those observed in the aspirin-treated group. In contrast, the pain percentages of the dexamethasone-treated group at 60 and 120 min were significantly higher than those of the BxbRAE-100% and aspirin.

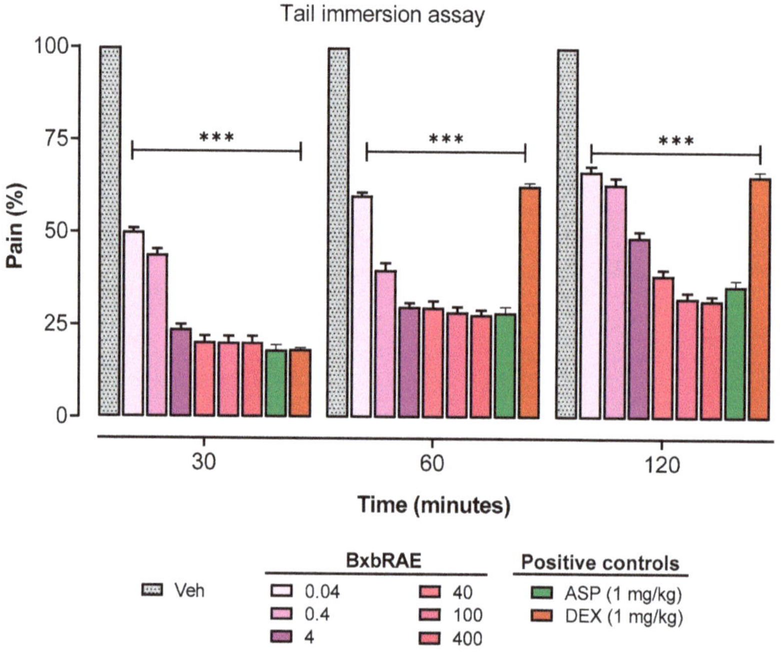

Figure 2. Effect of BxbRAE-100% in the tail immersion assay in mice. Aspirin (ASP) and dexamethasone (DEX) were used as positive controls. Data are shown as the mean ± SD ($n = 4$). *** $p < 0.001$ vs. the Veh group through one-way ANOVA followed by the Dunnett's test.

Formalin-induced pain behaviors is a model used to determine the central and peripheral activity of substances with analgesic properties, such as BxbRAE-100%. This test involves two phases: the early phase (0 to 5 min post-formalin injection) and the late phase (15 to 30 min post-formalin injection). In the present study, the results showed that the pretreatment of BxbRAE-100% at the doses between 0.04 and 400 mg/ kg significantly reduced pain percentages in a dose-dependent manner in both the early (Figure 3A) and the late phase (Figure 3B) of the formalin test. In both phases, the groups treated with the doses of 40, 100, and 400 mg/kg displayed the lowest pain percentages and were akin to those observed in the dexamethasone- or aspirin-treated groups in the early or late phases, respectively.

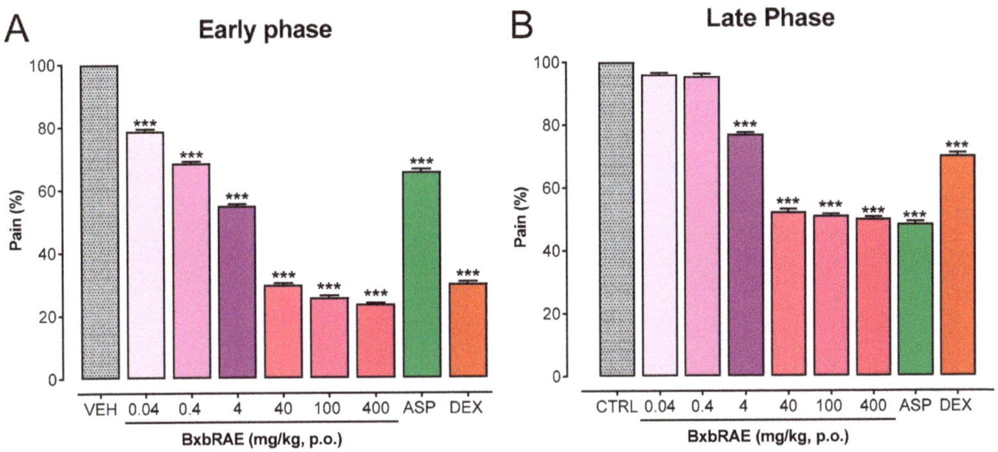

Figure 3. BxbRAE-100% decreased in a dose-dependent manner formalin-induced pain behaviors. Aspirin (ASP; 1 mg/kg) and dexamethasone (DEX; 1 mg/kg) were used as positive controls. Data are shown as the mean ± SD ($n = 4$). *** $p < 0.001$ vs. the Veh group through one-way ANOVA followed by the Dunnet's test.

2.3. *In Vivo Anti-Inflammatory Activity*

To determine the anti-inflammatory activity of BxbRAE-100% two murine models of inflammation were used. First, the topical anti-inflammatory activity of the extract was determined using the TPA (12-*O*-Tetradecanoylphorbol-13-acetate)-induced ear edema. Thus, increasing doses of BxbRAE-100% (0.1–0.57 mg/ear) or the positive controls indomethacin (0.25–1.25 mg/ear) were applied topically into the ear 5 min after TPA. The results of the present study demonstrate that topical BxbRAE-100% strongly inhibited TPA-induced inflammation in a dose-dependent fashion (Figure 4A). The maximum anti-inflammatory effect of the extract (68.2 ± 5.3%) was observed at the dose of 5.7 mg/ear, with an ED_{50} of 1.45 mg/ear. However, indomethacin displayed higher efficacy (89.3 ± 0.9%) and potency than the extract (0.54 mg/ear, Figure 4B).

In the same way the carrageenan-induced paw edema model in mice, a well-validated acute inflammatory model was used to determine the anti-inflammatory activity of BxbRAE-100%. Figure 4C shows that the BxbRAE-100% administrated orally reduced paw edema in a dose-dependent manner at 1, 2, 3, 4, 5, and 6 h after the carrageenan injection in the dose range from 4–400 mg/kg. The groups treated with 0.04 and 0.4 mg/kg of BxbRAE-100% did not show significant changes in paw volume compared to the control group. The reduction of paw edema was observed from the first hour after carrageenan injection, which lasted at least six hours. The maximal reduction in paw edema was observed between 4 and 6 h post carrageenan injection. The analysis of the inhibition of paw edema showed that the oral treatment with BxbRAE-100% inhibited paw edema in a range between 41.75 and 83.16%. The dose of 400 mg/kg most effectively reduced carrageenan-induced paw edema. However, its anti-inflammatory effect was not greater than that of the positive control, indomethacin (Figure 4D). These results showed that BxbRAE-100% produces anti-inflammatory effects whether administered topically or orally.

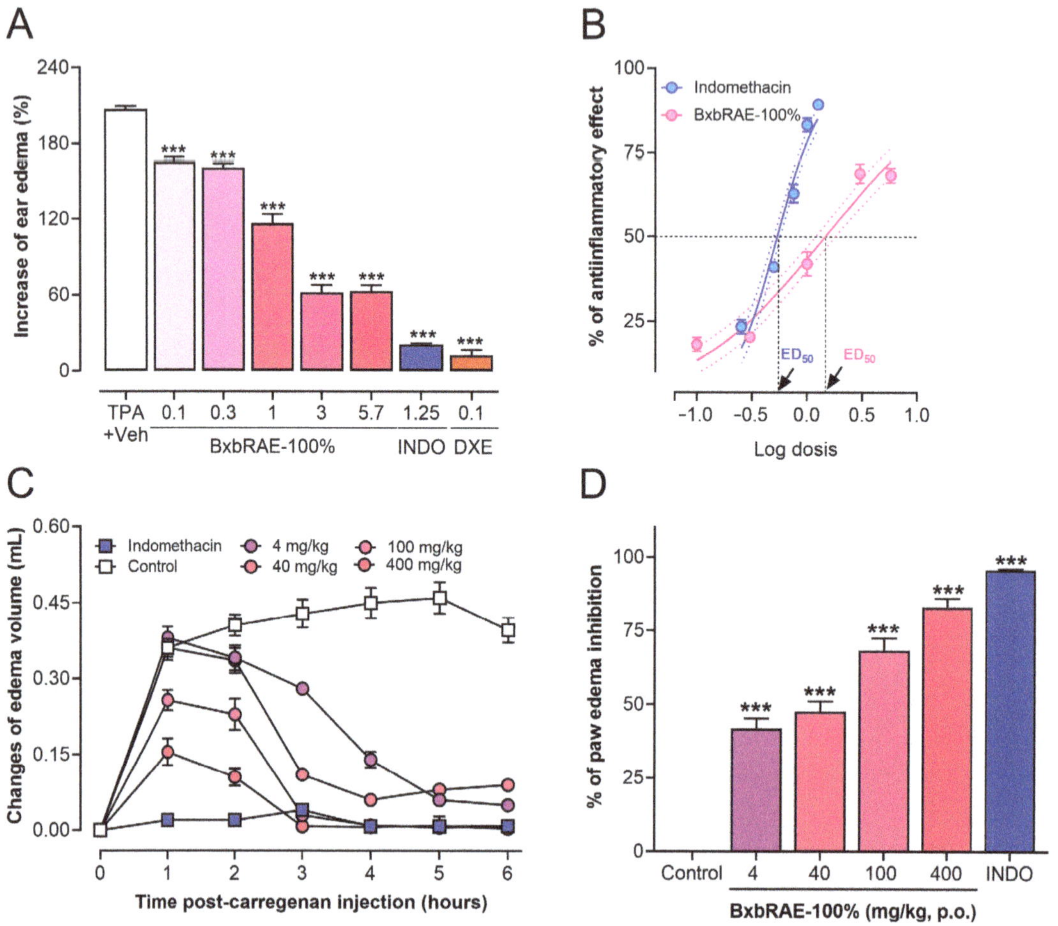

Figure 4. BxbRAE-100% reduced ear and paw edema in mice. (**A**) Effect of the topical treatment with the extract in the TPA-induced ear edema model. (**B**) Dose–response curve (DRC) of the anti-inflammatory effect of BxbRAE-100% vs. the positive control indomethacin (INDO). The dashed lines represent the dose that achieves a 50% anti-inflammatory effect (ED_{50}). (**C**) Effect of BxbRAE-100% on the time course of carrageenan-induced paw edema. (**D**) Data are presented as the % of paw edema inhibition. Each point or bar represents the average ± SD. *** $p < 0.001$ vs. the Veh + TPA group or control group through one-way ANOVA followed by Dunnett's test.

2.4. Inhibition of Proteolytic Activity of BxbRAE-100%

To determine the anti-inflammatory effect of BxbRAE-100%, the inhibition of proteolytic activity was evaluated using azocasein as a substrate. Figure 5 shows that BxbRAE-100% decreased the proteolytic activity percentage in a concentration- and time-dependent manner. The relative activity percentages induced by the extract after a 30 min incubation period at 40, 100, and 400 mg/mL concentrations were 59%, 12%, and 0%, respectively.

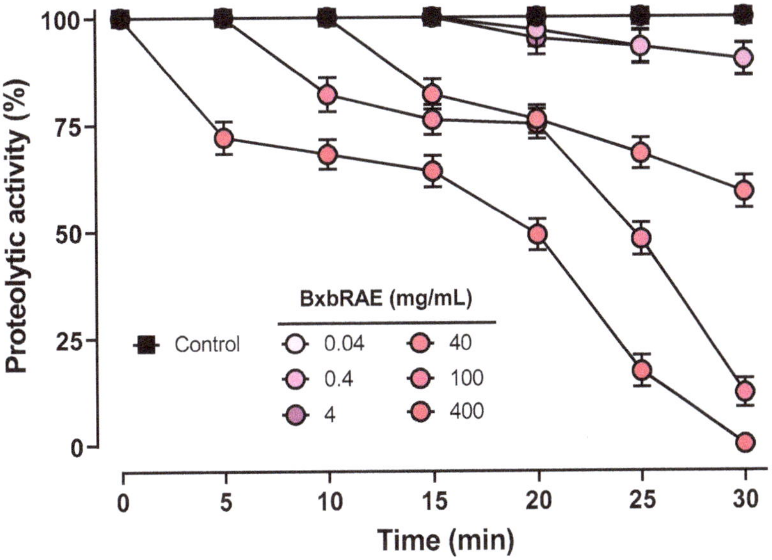

Figure 5. BxbRAE-100% inhibited proteolytic activity in vitro. Each point corresponds to the results of three different preparations.

2.5. *Effect of BxbRAE-100% on the Activity of the Phospholipase A2 and Cyclooxygenase Enzymes*

Secretory phospholipase A2 (PLA2) is the first enzyme in the arachidonic acid pathway. This enzyme catalyzes the hydrolysis of membrane phospholipids, releasing arachidonic acid and a lysophospholipid. Subsequently, cyclooxygenase (COX) can oxidize free arachidonic acid to produce prostaglandins, considered important pro-inflammatory mediators [21]. In this study, to preliminarily explore the possible mechanism of action of BxbRAE-100%, the effect of the extract on the activity of sPLA2 and COX enzymes was evaluated.

2.5.1. Anti-Phospholipase Activity of BxbRAE-100%

The extract was assessed for its inhibitory effect toward the two Human group IIA secreted phospholipase A2 (hG-IIA) and Porcine group IB phospholipase A2 (pG-IB) at a range concentration between 0.04 and 400 mg/mL. hG-IIA participates in the inflammatory process, while pG-IB is responsible for the hydrolysis of dietary phospholipids. We hypothesized that the extract could selectively inhibit group IIA pro-inflammatory phospholipase A2, with little or no inhibitory effect on group IB digestive phospholipase A2. The results showed that the extract inhibited in a concentration-dependent manner the activity of hG-IIA. It is important to highlight that the greatest inhibitory activities (72.4 ± 2.9%, and 81.5 ± 3.3%) were observed at the concentrations of 100 and 400 mg/mL. The calculated concentration that inhibits the 50% of hG-IIA activity (IC_{50}) was 25.94 mg/mL. On the other hand, the same doses of BxbRAE-100% inhibited pG-IB activity by less than 38% (Figure 6A). These results suggest that inhibition of PLA2 is one of the mechanisms underlying the antinociceptive and anti-inflammatory activities of *B. x buttiana*.

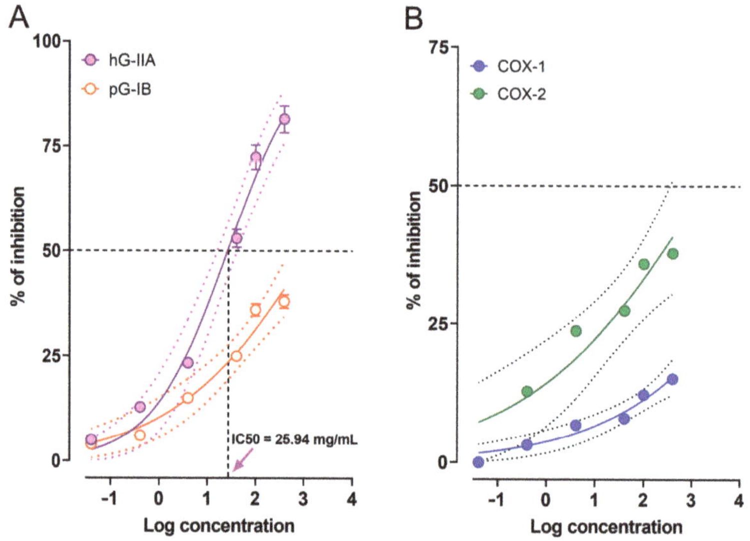

Figure 6. BxbRAE 100% inhibits the activity of sPLA2 and COX isoforms 1 and 2. (**A**) Inhibitory effect of the extract on human group IIA secreted phospholipase A2 (hG-IIA) and porcine group IB phospholipase A2 (pG-IB) activities. (**B**) Inhibitory effect of the extract on the activity of COX-1 and COX-2. The dashed lines represent the concentration that produces 50% inhibition of enzymatic activity (IC_{50}). Values represent the average of triplicate measurements.

2.5.2. Cyclooxygenase Inhibitory Activity of BxbRAE-100%

In order to evaluate the effect of BxbRAE-100% on the activity of COX-1 and COX-2 isoforms, different concentrations (0.4–400 mg/mL) of BxbRAE-100% were assessed. It was observed that BxbRAE-100% inhibited in a concentration-dependent manner the activity of COX-I and COX-2. The effect was moderate since the highest inhibitory activity was 15.15% and 37.76% for COX-1 and COX-2, respectively. However, as observed, the extract showed higher selectivity for COX-2 than for COX-1 (Figure 6B). Thus, these results suggest that COX inhibition is partially responsible for *B. x buttiana* activities.

2.6. Compounds Identified in BxbRAE 100%

In our previous study, BxbRAE-100% was analyzed via gas chromatography-mass spectrometry (GC-MS). Acetone was used since it allowed for the extraction of secondary plant metabolites of intermediate polarity. Accordingly, the next compounds were identified in the extract: 3-*O*-Methyl-d-glucose, *n*-Hexadecanoic acid, 9,12-Octadecadienoic (Z,Z), 1-Dotriacontanol, Stigmasta-5,22-dien-3-ol and Stigmast-7-en-3-ol, (3β,5α) [19]. Their structure and bioactivities are detailed in Table 1.

Table 1. Compounds identified in BxbRAE-100% and their reported bioactivities.

Compound Name and Structure	Activity	Reference
	Carbohydrates	
3-*O*-Methyl-d-glucose 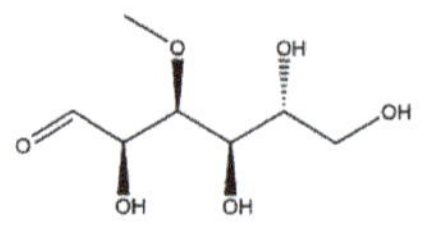	Increased the rate of hexose transport into myotubes by increasing glucose transporter type 4 (GLUT-4) activity	[22,23]

Table 1. *Cont.*

Compound Name and Structure	Activity	Reference
Saturated Fatty Acids		
n-Hexadecanoic acid 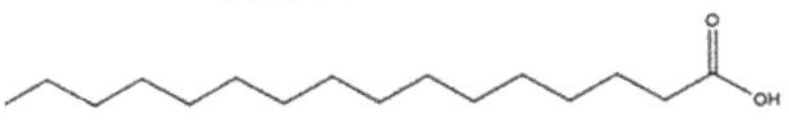	Antioxidant, anti-inflammatory, antinociceptive, hypocholesterolemic, nematicide, hemolytic, anti-androgenic, 5-alfa reductase inhibitor and immunomodulator	[22–25]
Polyunsaturated Fatty Acids		
9,12-Octadecadienoic(Z,Z)- 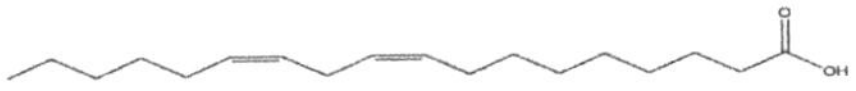	Antioxidant, antibacterial, anti-inflammatory neuroprotective, hypocholesterolemic, cancer preventive, hepatoprotector, antihistaminic, and antieczemic	[26–30]
Fatty Alcohol		
1-Dotriacontanol 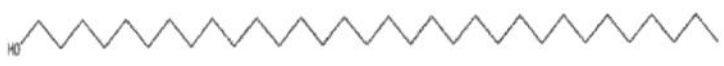	Antimicrobial, and antioxidant	[31,32]
Phytosterols		
Stigmasta-5,22-dien-3-ol 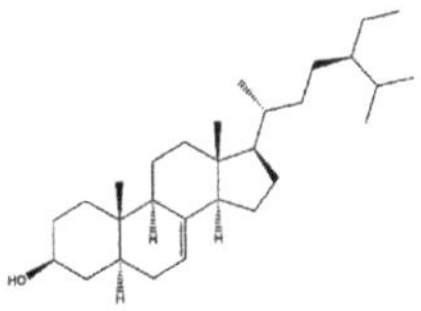	Antioxidant, anti-inflammatory, antibacterial, cytotoxic, anti-hepatotoxic, antiviral, and hypercholesteremic	[33–35]
Stigmast-7-en-3-ol, (3β,5α) 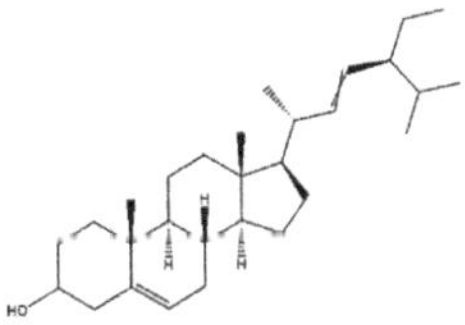	Anti-cancer, antidiabetic, and anti-inflammatory	[36,37]

2.7. In Silico Analysis of the Physicochemical Profile and ADME Properties of BxbRAE-100% Metabolites

At this point, we do not know if just one metabolite or a group of them is responsible for the observed activities of *B. x buttiana*. However, since at least 6 metabolites have been identified in the extract, it is possible to infer that they could be responsible for the observed biological activities. To preliminarily determine whether the compounds found in the acetonic extract of *B. x buttiana* have drug-like properties, an in silico analysis was performed to determine their physicochemical profile and ADME properties using the online free software swissADME, pre-ADME, and pcKSM. The molecular descriptors were calculated according to Lipinski's rule of five (Ro5), an experimental method to estimate water and lipid solubility, membrane permeability, and pharmacological effectiveness in drug discovery [34]. We found that all six compounds have a molecular weight of less than 500, fewer than five hydrogen bond donors (HBD), and fewer than six hydrogen bond acceptors (HBA). However, they showed, with the exception of 3-*O*-Methyl-d-glucose, a partition coefficient between *n*-octanol and water (log P) greater than five due to their high lipophilicity. These results suggested that the compounds in BxbRAE-100% meet Lipinski's Ro5 criteria.

Furthermore, the six compounds showed topological polar surface area (TPSA) values lower than 140 Å^2. Five of them have very small values (37.3 and 23.3), indicating that they can easily cross the cell membrane (Table 2). However, three of the six compounds showed more than 10 rotatable bonds, indicating that they are highly flexible molecules. Altogether, these results suggest that the bioactive compounds present in BxbRAE-100% are highly likely to be absorbed orally and have good cell membrane permeability.

Table 2. Physicochemical profiles of compounds found in BxbRAE-100% according to Lipinski's Ro5.

Compound	MW	nHBD	nHBA	Log P	N_{Vio}	Meet Lipinski RO5 Criteria	TPSA (Å^2)	nRotB
	<500	<5	<10	≤5	<1	Yes/No	<140	<10
3-*O*-Methyl-d-glucose	194.18	4	6	−2.25	0	Yes	107.22	6
n-Hexadecanoic acid	256.43	1	2	7.06	1	Yes	37.30	14
9,12-Octadecadienoic(Z,Z)-	280.45	1	2	6.86	1	Yes	37.30	13
1-Dotriacontanol	466.88	1	1	10.11	1	Yes	20.23	30
Stigmasta-5,22-dien-3-ol	414.72	1	1	8.62	1	Yes	20.23	6
Stigmast-7-en-3-ol, (3β,5α)	414.72	1	1	8.05	1	Yes	20.23	5

MW: molecular weight; nHBD: number of hydrogen-bond donors; nHBA: number of hydrogen bond acceptors; Log P: logarithm of partition coefficient of the compound between *n*-octanol and water; N_{Vio}: number of RO5 violated; TPSA: topological polar surface area; nRotB: Num. rotatable bonds.

The ADME properties, solubility (log S), human intestinal absorption (HIA), skin penetration (log Kp), and the ability to be a P-glycoprotein substrate (P-gp) were calculated to predict absorption. The results showed that 3-*O*-methyl-d-glucose is highly soluble in water but showed very low HIA and low skin penetration. These properties could affect its bioavailability after oral administration. In contrast, the remaining five compounds were moderately to poorly soluble in water, but their predicted HIA values were greater than 90%. None of them, except 1-Dotriacontanol, are P-gp substrates. Together, these results suggest that the metabolites found in BxbRAE-100% will have moderate to good absorption. For distribution, we predicted descriptors such as plasma protein binding (PPB), brain–blood barrier penetration (BBB), and volume of distribution (Vd). It was found that five of the six compounds showed PPB values very close to 100%, which is consistent with their high log P values, that is, with their lipophilicity.

Furthermore, it was determined that only *n*-Hexadecanoic acid and 9,12-Octadecadienoic acid(Z,Z)- could cross the BBB. All compounds showed Vd values between 0.04–20 L/kg, which are considered optimal values. Finally, 3-*O*-Methyl-d-glucose, *n*-Hexadecanoic acid, 9,12-Octadecadienoic(Z,Z)- and 1-Dotriacontanol showed Cl values < 5 mL/min/kg, indicating low clearance. In contrast, Stigmasta-5,22-dien-3-ol and Stigmast-7-en-3-ol, (3β,5α) showed CL values between 5 and 15 mL/min/kg; suggesting moderate clearance. None of the compounds was a substrate for renal OCT2, suggesting no renal excretion (Table 3).

Drug metabolism is a process that helps to prevent xenobiotics, like drugs, from reaching toxic concentrations and producing toxic side effects. The human cytochrome P450 (CYP) superfamily of enzymes metabolizes both endogenous and exogenous compounds such as drugs, cellular metabolites, and toxins [38]. CYP1A2, 2C9, 2C19, 2D6, and 3A4 isoforms mainly metabolize commercially available drugs. In this study, the metabolism of the compounds present in BxbRAE-100% was analyzed using free online software. The in-silico analysis showed that the six compounds were not CYP1A2, 2C19, 2C9, or 2D6 substrates. Moreover, CYP enzymes also play an essential role in drug–drug and herb–drug interactions. The inhibition of CYP enzymes is strongly associated with adverse drug reactions encompassing metabolic failures and induced side effects. Here we found that *n*-Hexadecanoic acid and 9,12-Octadecadienoic(Z,Z)- are potential inhibitors of CYP1A2. Moreover, *n*-Hexadecanoic acid could also be a CYP2D6 inhibitor. However, it is important to note that most of the compounds did not have the potential of being CYP inhibitors (Table 4). The in-silico results showed that each compound had a unique ADME profile, but, these predictions could help to better understand whether the extract or its metabolites had suitable ADME properties. However, these results need to be rigorously verified through in vitro and in vivo experiments to establish their clinical significance.

Table 3. ADME properties of the bioactive compounds identified on BxbRAE-100%.

Compound	Absorption				Distribution			Excretion	
	Log S	HIA	Log Kp	P-gp	PPB%	BBB	Vd	Cl_{tot}	Renal OCT2 Substrate
3-*O*-Methyl-d-glucose	1.17 Highly soluble	27.2	−9.54	No	29.67	No	0.43	1.84	No
n-Hexadecanoic acid	−5.02 Moderately soluble	91.9	−2.77	No	98.95	Yes	0.61	2.38	No
9,12-Octadecadienoic (Z,Z)-	−4.67 Moderately soluble	90.4	−3.37	No	98.95	Yes	0.61	2.37	No
1-Dotriacontanol	−10.7 Insoluble	84.3	−2.06	Yes	100	No	5.1	4.73	No
Stigmasta-5,22-dien-3-ol	−7.74 Poorly soluble	95.9	−2.38	No	95.04	No	1.27	7.35	No
Stigmast-7-en-3-ol, (3β,5α)	−7.99 Poorly soluble	97.8	−2.17	No	95.17	No	1.46	11.31	No

Water solubility: Log S (mol/L); human intestinal absorption: HIA (%); human skin permeability: Log Kp (cm/h); plasma protein binding: PPB (%); blood–brain barrier permeability: BBB (Log BB); volume of distribution: Vd; total clearance: Cl_{tot} (Log mL/min/kg); organic cation transporter 2: OCT2.

Table 4. Metabolism profile predicted in silico.

Compound	Metabolism									
	CYP1A2		CYP2C9		CYP2C19		CYP2D6		CYP3A4	
	S	I	S	I	S	I	S	I	S	I
3-*O*-Methyl-d-glucose	No	No	No	No	No	No	No	No	No	No
n-Hexadecanoic acid	No	**Yes**	No	No	No	No	No	**Yes**	**Yes**	No
9,12-Octadecadienoic(Z,Z)-	No	**Yes**	No	**Yes**	No	No	No	No	**Yes**	No
1-Dotriacontanol	No	No	No	No	No	No	No	No	**Yes**	No
Stigmasta-5,22-dien-3-ol	No	No	No	No	No	No	No	No	**Yes**	No
Stigmast-7-en-3-ol, (3β,5α)	No	No	No	No	No	No	No	No	**Yes**	No

S: substrate; I: inhibitor.

3. Discussion

In this study, we aimed to expand the knowledge of the biological properties of *Bougainvillea* by evaluating the antinociceptive and anti-inflammatory activities of the acetonic extract of *B. x buttiana* (var. Rose). Our findings showed that BxbRAE-100% significantly reduced nociception in three well-validated murine models of acute pain by acting at peripheral and central levels.

The acetic acid-induced abdominal constriction model allows the evaluation of the potential analgesic properties of test compounds at the peripheral level since acetic acid stimulates the endings of the primary afferent nerve fibers and produced a localized inflammatory response [39–41]. In this model, oral treatment with BxbRAE-100% dose-dependently (0.4 to 400 mg/kg) reduced pain percentages. The groups treated with 40, 100, and 400 mg/kg were more effective in reducing pain than the groups treated with the control drugs aspirin (1 mg/kg), dexamethasone (1 mg/kg), and diclofenac (10 mg/kg). These results suggest that BxbRAE-100% produces analgesic activity at the peripheral level.

Similarly, in the tail immersion test, BxbRAE-100% significantly reduced the pain percentages at 30, 60, and 120 min after oral administration. The efficacy of BxbRAE-100% was comparable to that of the reference drug aspirin but significantly lower than that of dexamethasone. In this test, the opioid drugs, which produce their effects in the central nervous system, show greater sensitivity [41]. Then, our findings suggest an analgesic central action of the extract.

The formalin test is widely used for assessing central and peripheral analgesic activities. This pain model is characterized by a distinctive biphasic nociceptive response. In mice, the early or neurogenic phase occurs between 0 and 5 min after formalin injection into the paw. It is caused by the direct chemical activation of primary nociceptive afferents. The late or inflammatory phase occurs between 15 and 30 min after formalin injection and results from various mechanisms, including inflammation of peripheral tissues and central sensitization [42–44]. Our findings showed that BxbRAE-100% reduced, in a dose-dependent manner, the pain percentage in both phases of the formalin test. The most significant effect of BxbRAE-100% was observed at 40, 100, and 400 mg/kg. These doses decreased the percentages of pain in the early and late phases by 70% and 50%, respectively. It is well established that centrally acting drugs, such as opioids, inhibit equally the early and late phases [44], while peripheral acting drugs, such as nonsteroidal anti-inflammatory drugs (NSAIDs; e.g., aspirin) or corticosteroids (e.g., dexamethasone), mainly inhibit the late phase [41]. Thus, our results suggest that BxbRAE-100% has central and peripheral antinociceptive activity in the formalin test.

The peripheral and central analgesic activity of BxbRAE-100% is consistent with the results of a previous study, which demonstrated that the ethanolic extract of *B. x buttiana* (var. Orange) also produces analgesia in the acetic acid-induced writhing model and the formalin test [16].

Several studies have demonstrated the role of inflammation in the development of various health conditions. Inflammation is the body's response to injury and involves a series of events, including the inflammatory reaction, a sensory response perceived as pain, and the repair process. Infection, tissue injury caused by external noxious stimuli, or immunological injuries are the main causes of the inflammatory response [1,2]. In this study, the anti-inflammatory properties of BxbRAE-100% were determined using both in vivo and in vitro approaches. In vivo, the anti-inflammatory activity was determined with two well-validated models to identify compounds with potential anti-inflammatory activity [45,46].

This is the first time the TPA model has been used to test the topically anti-inflammatory properties of *B. x buttiana*. TPA rapidly promotes edema development, peaking 4 to 6 h after topical application and lasting at least 24 h. Our findings show that BxbRAE-100% significantly decreased, in a dose-dependent manner, 4 h post TPA application. The extract achieved its maximum anti-inflammatory effect (68.2 $\pm$ 5.3%) with a 5.7 mg/ear dose, and the calculated ED50 was 1.45 mg/ear. However, indomethacin and dexamethasone displayed higher efficacy and potency than the extract. These results confirm the anti-inflammatory effect of BxbRAE-100% and suggest that the topical route could be an alternative to its administration.

The carrageenan-induced paw edema model in rodents is biphasic. The first phase begins immediately after carrageenan injection and decreases within two hours, while the second phase starts at the end of the first phase and remains at least six hours [47]. The mice treated with 4 to 400 mg/kg BxbRAE-100% showed a statistically significant ($p < 0.001$) reduction of carrageenan-induced paw edema in the second phase (between 2 and 6 h) of the inflammatory response. The 400 mg/kg dose produced the maximum edema inhibition (83%). These results were similar to those obtained in the group treated with indomethacin. The second phase in this model is characterized by PGs and bradykinin production, the release of proteases, and the infiltration of neutrophils [47]. Then, the results suggest that the extract produced its anti-inflammatory properties by modulating some of these events.

It is important to highlight that our findings agree with a previous study that showed the anti-inflammatory properties in vivo and in vitro of *B. x buttiana* (var. Orange) [16–18].

Conventional anti-inflammatory treatment includes NSAIDs and corticosteroids, drugs that work by inhibiting elements of inflammatory pathways [7,48]. Corticosteroids have structural similarities to steroid hormones, and one of their mechanisms of action is the inhibition of the pro-inflammatory enzyme phospholipase A2 (PLA2). NSAIDs are structurally diverse drugs that share analgesic, anti-inflammatory, and antipyretic activity. These drugs are classified based on their mechanism of action as non-selective inhibitors or selective COX-2 inhibitors [21,48].

In this study, BxbRAE-100% showed activity in two models of inflammatory pain, and in two models of acute inflammation, which are highly sensitive to conventional analgesic and anti-inflammatory treatments. Therefore, we can infer that the pharmacological activities of BxbRAE-100% can be attributed, at least in part, to the inhibition of enzymes involved in the production of pro-inflammatory and pronociceptive mediators. Therefore, to preliminarily explore its mode of action, we evaluated its effect on the activity of PLA2 and COX enzymes.

Until now, ten mammalian subtypes of sPLA2 have been identified: groups IB, IIA, IIC, IID, IIE, IIF, III, V, X, and XII. The second secretory PLA2 (sPLA2), or group II PLA2, is stored in immune cell secretory granules and markedly induced by inflammatory stimuli. Meanwhile, pancreatic sPLA2 IB (pG-IB) mainly participates in the digestion of dietary phospholipids [49]. sPLA2 releases arachidonic acid from membranes, which is the precursor to eicosanoids known for their potent pro-inflammatory actions. In the next step, the rate-limiting reaction enzyme prostaglandin H synthase (PGHS), the peroxidase activity of COX, catalyzes the formation of PGs. The constitutive isoform of COX-1 produces PGs that protect the stomach and kidneys from damage, while the COX-2 isoform is induced during inflammation and produces PGs that play an essential role in pain and inflammation [50]. Therefore, the arachidonic acid pathway has been a target for developing anti-inflammatory treatments.

In this work, our findings showed that the extract inhibited the activity of group IIA PLA2 by 81% with an IC_{50} of 25.94 mg/mL. However, low inhibitory activity was observed for pG-IB. Similarly, we observed that BxbRAE-100% moderately inhibited the activity of COX-1 and COX-2, with a slightly greater selectivity for COX-2. These results suggest that BxbRAE-100% exerts its biological effects by modulating the metabolism of arachidonic acid by reducing the activities of PLA2 and COX enzymes, which decreases the production of pro-inflammatory mediators.

Protease enzymes found in all living organisms catalyze the cleavage of peptide bonds in other proteins. Human proteases are divided into five mechanistic classes according to the catalytic mechanism of hydrolysis: aspartate, cysteine, metalloproteinases, serine, and threonine proteases [51]. Protease signaling pathways are strictly regulated, and the dysregulation of protease activity can lead to pathologies such as cardiovascular and inflammatory diseases and neurological disorders [52]. In inflammation, rapid protease activity is a key component of the innate immune system that contributes to the microenvironment and regulates the expression and activity of different pro-inflammatory cytokines and for tissue remodeling [53]. Therefore, they are attractive biological target-identifying molecules that can modulate their activity. In this study, BxbRAE-100% significantly decreased the percentage of proteolytic activity in a concentration- and time-dependent manner, reinforcing the evidence of its anti-inflammatory activity.

Numerous studies have shown the anti-inflammatory activity in plant extracts through in vitro and in vitro studies as well as the identification and characterization of the bioactive compounds involved in their anti-inflammatory action [48,54,55]. This study showed that BxbRAE-100% significantly inhibited edema formation and reduced pain. Therefore, we can infer that the active compounds present in BxbRAE-100%, alone or synergically, are responsible for their anti-inflammatory and analgesic properties. In our previous study, we identified that BxbRAE-100% is composed of the carbohydrate *O*-3-methyl-d-glucose (16.80%); the saturated fatty acid *n*-Hexadecanoic acid (23.10%), the polyunsaturated acid (9-Z,12-Z),-9,12 octadecanoic acid (19.90%), the fatty alcohol 1-Dotriacontanol (19.90%) and the phytosterols (3β,22E)-stigmata-5,22-dien-3-ol (10.60%) and (3β,5α)-stigmast-7-en-3 (9.62%) [19]. These bioactive compounds have been studied and found to produce several pharmacological activities that support their role in the anti-inflammatory properties of *B. x buttiana* var. Rose (see Table 1).

Fatty acids, known for their metabolic role, have now been identified as important regulators of immune function. Among them, *n*-Hexadecanoic acid, also known as Palmitic acid (PA), stands out with its unique properties. This saturated-free fatty acid exhibits antibacterial and antifungal properties [25]. Moreover, this fatty acid also inhibits PLA2, modulates cytokine production, and reprograms the innate immune cell response to secondary inflammatory stimuli in vitro and in vivo [24].

Polyunsaturated fatty acids, essential components in the architecture and function of cell membranes, play a key role in several biological processes, such as metabolic precursors of prostaglandins and leukotrienes [25]. 9,12-Octadecadienoic (Z,Z)-or Linoleic Acid (LA) is the most abundant ω-6 polyunsaturated fatty acid (PUFA) and is essential in the human diet with several functions in health and disease. Several studies have demonstrated that high dietary intake or high plasma concentrations of LA do not appear to result in increased tissue arachidonic acid or in increased in vivo or ex vivo concentrations of inflammatory markers in humans. Moreover, a recent study reported their in vivo and in vitro anti-inflammatory and neuroprotective actions in Parkinson's disease models [26,27].

Plant-derived sterols, phytosterols, are abundant in lipid-rich plant materials. These compounds are well known for their serum cholesterol-lowering and anti-inflammatory activities [33]. Previous studies found Stigmasta-5,22-dien-3-ol, also called Stigmasterol, in the acetonic extracts of *Sideritis foetens* and the hexane extract of *Eryngium foetidum.* Oral or topical treatment with *Sideritis foetens* extract reduced carrageenan-induced paw edema and inhibited TPA-induced ear edema, respectively. Similarly, the extract of *Eryngium foetidum* inhibited TPA-induced ear inflammation [34,35]. Furthermore, an in vitro study showed that Stigmasterol downregulated PGE2 and MMP-3 in IL-1β-treated cells without affecting IL-6 levels, suggesting that Stigmasterol inhibited the NF-κB pathway [56]. Similarly, in vitro studies showed that Stigmast-7-en-3-ol (3β,5α) inhibited nitric oxide production in macrophages activated by LPS, suggesting potent anti-inflammatory properties [57].

The evidence cited shows that most bioactive compounds reported in BxbRAE-100% exhibit anti-inflammatory activity, suggesting that they could act alone or synergistically to produce the observed analgesic and antinociceptive effects. To better understand how the compounds contribute to the biological activities of the extract, an in silico study was performed to determine the physicochemical profile and ADME properties, as well as the drug-likeness of each compound.

Lipinski's RO5 was designed to estimate the probability of malabsorption or membrane permeability. If the analysis of a molecule showed that two of the following parameters are out of range, "poor absorption or permeability is possible": (1) molecular weight greater than 500, (2) more than five hydrogen bond donors, (3) more than 10 hydrogen bond acceptors, and (4) octanol–water partition coefficient (log P) greater than five [58]. The physicochemical properties of all compounds found on BxbRAE-100% met Lipinski´s RO5, suggesting that they will have high oral bioavailability despite their high log P value. These results are consistent with the absorption predictions and the fact that the extract showed efficacy when administered orally. Furthermore, the extract was also active topically, which is consistent with the high lipophilicity of the compounds. The topical activity of BxbRAE-100% opens up the option to investigate different routes of administration that maintain efficacy but limit side effects.

Regarding drug metabolism, we found that five out of six compounds were substrates of CYP3A4. This finding was expected because CYP3A4 is the main isoform involved in more than 50% of the commercially available drugs [59]. Moreover, it was also observed that most of the compounds, except *n*-Hexadecanoic acid and 9,12-Octadecadienoic(Z,Z)-, did not have the potential to be CYP inhibitors. Since inhibition or induction of CYP enzymes may modify the bioavailability or other pharmacokinetic parameters of drugs, which can lead to therapeutic failure and/or toxic effects [60], these results suggest that the BxbRAE-100% had a low potential for herb–drug interactions. While the in silico analysis results are promising, it is crucial that they are rigorously verified through in vitro and in vivo experiments to establish their clinical significance. However, these predictions could significantly enhance our understanding of the ADME properties of the extract or its metabolites.

4. Materials and Methods

4.1. Chemicals, Drugs and Solvents

Pentobarbital sodium (Lot 20104) was purchased from Laboratorios Aranda S.A de C.V, Querétaro, Mexico. Acetonitrile, azocasein, dexamethasone acetate (Lot LRAC8664), indomethacin (Lot 0000118216), oleic acid, 2-*O*-tetradecanoylphorbol 13-acetate (TPA; Lot MKCL1143), Carrageenan (Lot 095K1394), and bovine pancreas phospholipase A2 were purchased from Sigma-Aldrich Chemical Co. (St. Louis, MO, USA). The COX inhibitor detection assay kit (ovine/human), hG-IIA, and pG-IB phospholipases were purchased from Cayman Chemical Co. (Ann Arbor, MI, USA). Diclofenac was donated by Arroli Organics (Mumbai, India). For the TPA model, the indomethacin, TPA, and the different doses of the extract were dissolved in acetone and applied topically to the ear. For the anti-inflammatory and antinociceptive evaluation, the extract was dissolved in 5% Tween 20 in sterile saline solution and prepared for administration on the day of the experiment.

4.2. Animals

In the present study, female mice of the BALB/c strain weighing between 20 and 25 g acquired from the biotherium of the National Institute of Public Health (Cuernavaca-Morelos, Mexico) were used. Before conducting the experiments, the mice were allowed an adaptation period of 7 to 10 days to our laboratory conditions. All experimental procedures followed the Mexican Official Norm of Animal Care and Handling and the International Association for the Study of Pain guidelines. Moreover, the protocol was validated (002/2016) by the Care and Use of Animals of the Faculty of Medicine, UAEM (CCUAL-FM-UAEM). At the end of the experiments, the mice were sacrificed via asphyxiation with CO_2. All efforts were made to minimize animal suffering and reduce the number of animals used.

4.3. Extraction of Plant Material

The flowers and bracts of *Bougainvillea x buttiana* were collected in Cuernavaca, Morelos, Mexico. A voucher specimen of *Bougainvillea x buttiana* Holttum & Standl was cataloged with the number 33872 for reference and subsequent consultation in the HUMO Herbarium, CIByC (UAEM A mixture of 200 g of flowers and bracts was air-dried for 14 days at 25 °C and ground into powder to obtain the acetonic extract. Nearly 5 g of air-dried powder was poured into 100 mL of 100% acetone (1:20 ratio). This preparation was stored and stirred continuously for 72 h and filtered through Whatman No. 1 filter paper. The residue was subjected to the same procedure three more times. The filtrates obtained on each occasion were mixed and then concentrated at 50 °C, using a rotary evaporator at reduced pressure to produce a dry crude extract. The crude extract was allowed to dry for approximately 72 h at room temperature to determine the percentage yield of the extracts. The extract obtained was called crude acetonic extract of *Bougainvillea x buttiana* (var. Rose) (BxbRAE-100%) and was kept at −20 °C until the experiments were carried out. The BxbRAE-100% performance percentage was calculated using the following formula:

$$\%\ \text{yield} = \left(\frac{\text{Weigh of extract material}}{\text{Weigh of original plant material used}}\right) \times 100$$

4.4. Analgesic Activity

The peripheral antinociceptive activity of BxbRAE-100% was evaluated using the acetic acid-induced writhing model, while the central action was determined using the formalin test and the tail immersion assay.

4.4.1. Acetic Acid-Induced Writhing Model

This test was performed according to the Koster method [61]. Briefly, to evaluate the antinociceptive activity of BxbRAE-100%, 11 independent groups of 4 mice were orally administered with the following treatments: Group 1,vehicle (sterile saline solution 0.9%); Groups 2–7, the BxbRAE-100% at the doses of 0.04, 0.4, 4, 40, 100 and 400 mg/kg, respectively; and Group 8–10 the reference drugs aspirin (1 mg/Kg), diclofenac (10 mg/Kg), and dexamethasone (1 mg/Kg), respectively. Immediately after treatment administration, each mouse was placed in a transparent acrylic box. Sixty minutes later, the mice were injected intraperitoneally with a 0.7% acetic acid solution (0.1 mL/10 g body weight). Then, the number of writhes (contraction of the abdominal muscle together with a stretch of the hind limbs or rotation of the trunk) was immediately quantified 20 min after the intraperitoneal injection of acetic acid [62]. The sum of the number of writhes was used to calculate the percentage of pain (%P) and the % of antinociceptive effect using the following formulas:

$$\%\ \text{Pain} = \frac{\text{number of writhes of the treated group}}{\text{number of writhes of the vehicle group}} \times 100$$

$$\%\ \text{Antinociceptive effect} = 100 - \%\ \text{Pain}$$

4.4.2. Tail Immersion Assay

This test was carried out following the method described by [63]. This method consists of dipping the lower portion (approximately 4 cm) of the tail of a mouse in hot water (51 ± 1 °C) contained in a one-liter beaker and studying, before and after administration of a potential bioactive substance, the time taken by the animal to remove its tail (latency of tail withdrawal). To determine the antinociceptive effect of the extract, the mice were randomly selected and divided into nine groups of 4 mice each and administered orally, with one of the following treatments: vehicle (physiological saline solution), increasing doses of BxbRAE-100% (0.04, 0.4, 4, 40, 100 and 400 mg/kg) and the positive controls aspirin and dexamethasone (1 mg/kg). Subsequently, the tail withdrawal latency was measured at 0, 30, 60, and 120 min post treatment administration. If the mouse did not withdraw its tail, a cutting time of 10 s was set to avoid tissue damage. The results were expressed as a percentage of pain calculated with the following formula:

$$\%\ \text{Pain} = (\text{Ttcg}/\text{Tttg}) \times 100$$

where: Tttg = tail withdrawal latency of the treated group and Ttcg = tail withdrawal latency of the vehicle group.

4.4.3. Formalin Test

To determine the antinociceptive effect of the extract, formalin, a model of inflammatory pain, was used following the method described by Rosland et al., 1990 [64]. To apply this model, different groups of 5 mice were treated orally with the following doses of BxbRAE-100% 0.04, 0.4, 4, 40, 100, and 400 mg/kg, the vehicle. Aspirin was used as a positive control (4 mg/kg). Immediately, each mouse was placed in a transparent acrylic cylinder 30 cm in diameter and 30 cm high, surrounded by 30 cm × 30 cm mirrors to observe the mouse throughout the test. One hour after treatment administration, the mouse was removed from the cylinder for subcutaneous injection of 20 μL of 1% formalin into the dorsum of the right hind paw. Immediately thereafter, the mouse was returned to the cylinder, and quantification of nociceptive licking/biting and shuddering behaviors was assessed in two phases. The early phase was evaluated between 0 and 5 min, and the late phase was evaluated between 15 and 30 min after formalin injection.

4.5. *In Vivo Anti-Inflammatory Activity*

4.5.1. TPA-Induced Ear Edema

The mouse model of phorbol 12-myristate 13-acetate (TPA)-induced ear edema was used to determine the topical anti-inflammatory effect of BxbRAE-100% [65]. Briefly, under general anesthesia induced with pentobarbital (63 mg/kg; i.p.), TPA dissolved in ethanol (0.25 µg/µL) was applied to the inner and outer surfaces of the mouse's ear. Subsequently, the vehicle, increasing doses of the BxbRAE-100% (var. Rosa) (0.1, 0.3, 1, 3, and 5.7 mg/ear) or the positive controls indomethacin (0.25, 0.5, 0.75, 1 and 1.25 mg/ear) and dexamethasone (0.1 mg/ear) were applied in the same way as TPA. Four hours after TPA application, the mice were euthanized via CO_2 asphyxiation, and a 6-mm ear biopsy was obtained and weighed. The % anti-inflammatory effect was calculated by comparing the biopsies of the TPA groups and the treatments with the TPA + vehicle group. The % anti-inflammatory effect was used to construct the dose–response curve (DRC). Maximum efficacy (maximum anti-inflammatory effect), potency (effective dose 50, ED_{50}), and relative potency compared to indomethacin were obtained from the DRC.

4.5.2. Carrageenan-Induced Paw Edema

The carrageenan edema method was carried out according to the method described by Sugishita et al., 1981 [66]. The animals were randomly divided into 8 groups of 5 animals. Six groups were administered orally with different doses of the acetonic extract (0.04, 0.4, 4, 40, 100, and 400 mg/kg); a negative control group did not receive treatment, and the positive control group was treated with 1% indomethacin. One hour after treatment administration, each mouse received an intraplantar injection of 0.1 mL of 1% carrageenan into the right hind paw and into the left paw an equal volume of 0.1% saline solution. The edema produced by carrageenan was measured by using a plethysmograph at different time intervals, and the increase in volume was determined by subtracting the value obtained in the left paw. Next, the area under the curve (AUC) of the time courses was calculated using the trapezoidal rule. The AUC was used to estimate the % Inhibition with the following formula:

$$\% \text{ of inhibition} = 100 - \left(\frac{\text{AUC of treated mice}}{\text{UC of control mice}} \times 100 \right)$$

4.6. *In Vitro Anti-Inflammatory Activity*

4.6.1. Inhibitory Proteolytic Activity of BxbRAE-100%

The activity of BxbRAE-100% was assessed using the colorimetric method previously described by Adulyatham and Owusu-Apenten, 2005 [67] with slight modification. Briefly, 1.0 mg/mL of azocasein as substrate was prepared in 100 mM Potassium phosphate buffer (pH 7). One milliliter of this substrate solution was transferred to an Eppendorf tube containing 0.6 mL of buffer solution and 0.1 mL of different concentrations of BxbRAE-100% (0.04, 0.4, 4, 40, 100, 400 mg/mL). This mixture was then incubated at 60 °C for 20 min. The reaction was stopped by adding 0.3 mL of 10% (w/v) of trichloroacetic acid solution, followed by centrifugation at 9000× g for 10 min at room temperature. The supernatants were collected and mixed with 0.5 mL of 2 M NaOH for 10 min at room temperature. The blank was prepared in the same way as the test samples but with the enzyme previously inactivated in a boiling water bath for 5 min. The final solutions were analyzed spectrophotometrically at an absorbance of 450 nm, and the results were expressed as the percentage of relative activity. All tests were conducted in triplicate (n = 3).

4.6.2. Inhibition of Secretory Phospholipase A2 (sPLA2)

The effect of BxbRAE-100% on sPLA2 activity was measured according to the protocol described by de Araújo and Radvanyi, 1987 [68] using inhibitors of group IIA sPLA2, including hG-IIA and pG-IB forms. Briefly, the substrate buffer was prepared with 3.5 mM lecithin solubilized in 100 mM NaCl, 3 mM sodium taurodeoxycholate, 10 mM $CaCl_2$, and

0.055 mM phenol red at pH 7.6. Ten microliters of BxbRAE-100% at concentrations of 0.04, 0.4, 4, 40, 100, and 400 mg/mL were mixed with 10 μL of PLA2-GIB and incubated for 20 min at 25 °C. Subsequently, 1 mL of the PLA2 substrate was added to each tube, and the kinetics of hydrolysis were monitored over 5 min by measuring the absorbance at 558 nm. The inhibition percentage was calculated by comparing the residual activity to that of the negative control (absence of BxbRAE-100%). The IC_{50} values were determined from the resulting inhibition curves.

4.6.3. Cyclooxygenase Inhibitory Activity

The in vitro COX-1/2 inhibitory activity of BxbRAE-100% was evaluated using a COX (Ovine/Human) inhibitor screening kit with 96-well plates purchased from Cayman Chemical (Ann Arbor, MI, USA). The assay was performed according to the manufacturer´s instructions. This screening measures PGF2 produced by $SnCl_2$ reduction of COX-derived PGH2. Initial COX-2 activity was measured using 105 μL of reaction buffer and 10 μL of COX-1/2 enzymes. Similarly, COX-1/2 inhibitor tubes were prepared by adding 20 μL of each concentration of BxbRAE in each tube in addition to the above ingredients. The background tubes correspond to inactivated COX-1/2 enzymes by boiling water for 3 min. For the initial reactions, 10 μL of arachidonic acid was added to each tube and quenched with 50 μL of 1 M HCl. The PGH2 formed was reduced to PGF2 a by adding 100 μL $SnCl_2$ and reading the plate at 405 nm. The results were expressed as the percentage of inhibition.

4.7. *In Silico Analysis of Compounds Present in BxbRAE-100%*

The molecular descriptors and drug likeliness of the compounds identified in BxbRAE-100% were analyzed according to Lipinski's RO5 (Table 5). The parameters to predict the properties of Absorption, Distribution, Metabolism, and Elimination (ADME) (Table 5) were calculated with the three widely used online free software: SwissADME (http://www.swissadme.ch/ accessed on 31 May 2024), PreADMET 2.0 (https://preadmet.webservice.bmdrc.org/ accessed on 31 May 2024), and pkCSM (https://biosig.lab.uq.edu.au/pkcsm/prediction accessed on 31 May 2024) [69,70]. In all the cases, the descriptors calculation was conducted by uploading the standard smile files on the web servers.

Table 5. Molecular descriptors calculated in silico.

Physicochemical profile	Lipinski's RO5 descriptors	• Molecular weight (MW) • Number of hydrogen bond donors (nHBD) • Number of hydrogen bond acceptors (nHBA) • Partition coefficient of the compound between *n*-octanol and water (log P) • Topological polar surface area (TPSA) • Num. of rotatable bonds (nRotB)
ADME properties	Absorption	• Aqueous solubility in mol/L (Log S) • Human intestinal absorption (%HIA) • Skin permeation coefficient (LogKp) • P-glycoprotein substrate(P-gp)
	Distribution	• Plasma protein binding (%PPB) • Blood–Brain Barrier permeability (BBB) • Volume of distribution (Vd)

Table 5. *Cont.*

ADME properties	Metabolism	• Phase I of drug metabolism: • Cytochrome P450 isoenzyme: • CYP1A2 • CYP2C9; CYP2C19, CYP2D6 • CYP3A4
	Excretion	• Total body clearance (Cltot) • Renal organic cation transporter 2 (OCT2) Substrate

4.8. Statistical Analysis

Data are expressed as the mean ± SD. Statistical analysis was conducted using GraphPad Prism 8 (GraphPad Software, Inc., San Diego, CA, USA). One-way ANOVA followed by a post hoc test of Dunnet was used to determine statistical significance between more than three experimental groups. The significance level was set at $p < 0.05$.

5. Conclusions

BxbRAE showed significant antinociceptive and anti-inflammatory activities in vivo and in vitro, at least in part through the inhibition of PLA2 and COX. These activities can be attributed to the unique or synergistic action of the bioactive compounds present in the extract. These compounds meet the Lipinski Ro5 criteria, suggesting good bioavailability for oral administration. These findings support the use of *Bougainvillea x buttiana* in traditional Mexican medicine. Furthermore, they highlight the potential of *B. x buttiana* extracts to continue studying them in order to develop new phytomedicines for pain and inflammation treatment.

Author Contributions: Conceptualization, V.L.P. and G.C.-C.; methodology, M.C.-C., M.A.-F. and M.L.-C.; software, M.A.-F. and M.L.-C.; formal analysis, V.L.P., J.J.A.-F. and G.C.-C.; investigation, G.C.-C. and J.J.A.-F.; writing—original draft preparation, V.L.P. and G.C.-C.; writing—review and editing, V.L.P.; visualization, G.C.-C.; supervision, V.L.P.; project administration, V.L.P. All authors have read and agreed to the published version of the manuscript.

Funding: This research was partially funded by Secretaria de Educación Pública (México) and Consejo Nacional de Humanidades, Ciencia y Tecnología (CONAHCyT; Grant number 140607).

Institutional Review Board Statement: All experimental procedures followed the Mexican Official Norm of Animal Care and Handling [71] and the international Association for the Study of Pain guidelines. The protocol was validated (002/2016) by the Care and Use of Animals of the Faculty of Medicine, UAEM (CCUAL-FM-UAEM).

Informed Consent Statement: Not applicable.

Data Availability Statement: The original contributions presented in the study are included in the article, further inquiries can be directed to the corresponding author.

Conflicts of Interest: The authors declare no conflicts of interest.

References

1. Medzhitov, R. Inflammation 2010: New adventures of an old flame. *Cell* **2010**, *140*, 771–776. [CrossRef]
2. Fioranelli, M.; Roccia, M.G.; Flavin, D.; Cota, L. Regulation of Inflammatory Reaction in Health and Disease. *Int. J. Mol. Sci.* **2021**, *22*, 5277. [CrossRef]
3. Sánchez-Flórez, J.C.; Seija-Butnaru, D.; Valero, E.G.; Acosta, C.; Amaya, S. Pain Management Strategies in Rheumatoid Arthritis: A Narrative Review. *J. Pain Palliat. Care Pharmacother.* **2021**, *35*, 291–299. [CrossRef]
4. VanderPluym, J. Indomethacin-responsive headaches. *Curr. Neurol. Neurosci. Rep.* **2015**, *15*, 516. [CrossRef]
5. Raja, S.N.; Carr, D.B.; Cohen, M.; Finnerup, N.B.; Flor, H.; Gibson, S.; Keefe, F.J.; Mogil, J.S.; Ringkamp, M.; Sluka, K.A.; et al. The revised International Association for the Study of Pain definition of pain: Concepts, challenges, and compromises. *Pain* **2020**, *161*, 1976–1982. [CrossRef] [PubMed]

6. Treede, R.D.; Rief, W.; Barke, A.; Aziz, Q.; Bennett, M.I.; Benoliel, R.; Cohen, M.; Evers, S.; Finnerup, N.B.; First, M.B.; et al. Chronic pain as a symptom or a disease: The IASP Classification of Chronic Pain for the International Classification of Diseases (ICD-11). *Pain* **2019**, *160*, 19–27. [CrossRef] [PubMed]
7. Cascorbi, I. Inflammation: Treatment Progress and Limitations. *Clin. Pharmacol. Ther.* **2017**, *102*, 564–567. [CrossRef]
8. Calixto, J.B.; Beirith, A.; Ferreira, J.; Santos, A.R.; Filho, V.C.; Yunes, R.A. Naturally occurring antinociceptive substances from plants. *Phytother. Res.* **2000**, *14*, 401–418. [CrossRef]
9. Mathur, S.; Hoskins, C. Drug development: Lessons from nature (Review). *Biomed. Rep.* **2017**, *6*, 612–614. [CrossRef] [PubMed]
10. Cos, P.; Vlietinck, A.J.; Berghe, D.V.; Maes, L. Anti-infective potential of natural products: How to develop a stronger in vitro 'proof-of-concept'. *J. Ethnopharmacol.* **2006**, *106*, 290–302. [CrossRef]
11. Duraipandiyan, V.; Ignacimuthu, S. Antibacterial and antifungal activity of *Cassia fistula* L.: An ethnomedicinal plant. *J. Ethnopharmacol.* **2007**, *112*, 590–594. [CrossRef]
12. Ye, M.; Han, J.; Chen, H.; Zheng, J.; Guo, D. Analysis of phenolic compounds in rhubarbs using liquid chromatography coupled with electrospray ionization mass spectrometry. *J. Am. Soc. Mass Spectrom.* **2007**, *18*, 82–91. [CrossRef] [PubMed]
13. Ornelas García, I.G.; Guerrero Barrera, A.L.; Avelar González, F.J.; Chávez Vela, N.A.; Gutiérrez Montiel, D. Bougainvillea glabra Choisy (Nyctinaginacea): Review of phytochemistry and antimicrobial potential. *Front. Chem.* **2023**, *11*, 1276514. [CrossRef] [PubMed]
14. Schalepfer, L.; Bernarda, G.O. *Las Flores de Casa Libertad*; UACM, Ed.; UACM: Mexico City, Mexico, 2017.
15. Poswal, F.S.; Russell, G.; Mackonochie, M.; MacLennan, E.; Adukwu, E.C.; Rolfe, V. Herbal Teas and their Health Benefits: A Scoping Review. *Plant Foods Hum. Nutr.* **2019**, *74*, 266–276. [CrossRef]
16. Alvarez Perez Gil, A.L.; Barbosa Navarro, L.; Patipo Vera, M.; Petricevich, V.L. Anti-inflammatory and antinociceptive activities of the ethanolic extract of Bougainvillea xbuttiana. *J. Ethnopharmacol.* **2012**, *144*, 712–719. [CrossRef] [PubMed]
17. Arteaga Figueroa, L.; Abarca-Vargas, R.; García Alanis, C.; Petricevich, V.L. Comparison between Peritoneal Macrophage Activation by *Bougainvillea × buttiana* Extract and LPS and/or Interleukins. *BioMed Res. Int.* **2017**, *2017*, 4602952. [CrossRef]
18. Arteaga Figueroa, L.; Barbosa Navarro, L.; Patiño Vera, M.; Petricevich, V.L. Preliminary Studies of the Immunomodulator Effect of the *Bougainvillea × buttiana* Extract in a Mouse Model. *Evid.-Based Complement. Altern. Med.* **2015**, *2015*, 479412. [CrossRef] [PubMed]
19. Abarca-Vargas, R.; Peña Malacara, C.F.; Petricevich, V.L. Characterization of Chemical Compounds with Antioxidant and Cytotoxic Activities in *Bougainvillea × buttiana* Holttum and Standl, (var. Rose) Extracts. *Antioxidants* **2016**, *5*, 45. [CrossRef]
20. Abarca-Vargas, R.; Zamilpa, A.; Petricevich, V.L. Development and Validation of Conditions for Extracting Flavonoids Content and Evaluation of Antioxidant and Cytoprotective Activities from *Bougainvillea × buttiana* Bracteas (var. Rose). *Antioxidants* **2019**, *8*, 264. [CrossRef]
21. Yeung, Y.T.; Aziz, F.; Guerrero-Castilla, A.; Arguelles, S. Signaling Pathways in Inflammation and Anti-inflammatory Therapies. *Curr. Pharm. Des.* **2018**, *24*, 1449–1484. [CrossRef]
22. Figueroa, L.A.; Navarro, L.B.; Vera, M.P.; Petricevich, V.L. Antioxidant activity, total phenolic and flavonoid contents, and cytotoxicity evaluation of *Bougainvillea × buttiana*. *Int. J. Pharm. Pharm. Sci.* **2014**, *6*, 497–502.
23. Shamni, O.; Cohen, G.; Gruzman, A.; Zaid, H.; Klip, A.; Cerasi, E.; Sasson, S. Regulation of GLUT4 activity in myotubes by 3-*O*-methyl-D-glucose. *Biochim. Biophys. Acta (BBA) Biomembr.* **2017**, *1859*, 1900–1910. [CrossRef] [PubMed]
24. Seufert, A.L.; Napier, B.A. A new frontier for fat: Dietary palmitic acid induces innate immune memory. *Immunometabolism* **2023**, *5*, e00021. [CrossRef] [PubMed]
25. Chapkin, R.S.; McMurray, D.N.; Davidson, L.A.; Patil, B.S.; Fan, Y.Y.; Lupton, J.R. Bioactive dietary long-chain fatty acids: Emerging mechanisms of action. *Br. J. Nutr.* **2008**, *100*, 1152–1157. [CrossRef] [PubMed]
26. Belury, M.A. Dietary conjugated linoleic acid in health: Physiological effects and mechanisms of action. *Annu. Rev. Nutr.* **2002**, *22*, 505–531. [CrossRef] [PubMed]
27. Alarcon-Gil, J.; Sierra-Magro, A.; Morales-Garcia, J.A.; Sanz-SanCristobal, M.; Alonso-Gil, S.; Cortes-Canteli, M.; Niso-Santano, M.; Martínez-Chacón, G.; Fuentes, J.M.; Santos, A.; et al. Neuroprotective and Anti-Inflammatory Effects of Linoleic Acid in Models of Parkinson's Disease: The Implication of Lipid Droplets and Lipophagy. *Cells* **2022**, *11*, 2297. [CrossRef]
28. Odiase-Omoighe, J.; Agoreyo, B. Identification of Bioactive Compounds in Sclerotia Extracts from *Pleurotus tuber-regium* (Fr.) Sing. using Gas Chromatograph–Mass Spectrometer (GC-MS). *Niger. J. Biotechnol.* **2022**, *38*, 39–50. [CrossRef]
29. Nava Lauson, C.B.; Tiberti, S.; Corsetto, P.A.; Conte, F.; Tyagi, P.; Machwirth, M.; Ebert, S.; Loffreda, A.; Scheller, L.; Sheta, D.; et al. *Linoleic acid* potentiates CD8(+) T cell metabolic fitness and antitumor immunity. *Cell Metab.* **2023**, *35*, 633–650.e9. [CrossRef] [PubMed]
30. Hagr, T.; Ali, K.; Satti, A.; Omer, S. GC-MS analysis, phytochemical, and antimicrobial activity of sudanese *Nigella sativa* (L) oil. *Eur. J. Biomed. Pharmaceut. Sci.* **2018**, *5*, 23–29.
31. Alrumman, S.; Mostafa, Y.; Al-Qahtani, S.; Sahlabji, T.; Taha, T. Antimicrobial Activity and GC-MS Analysis of Bioactive Constituents of Thermophilic Bacteria Isolated from Saudi Hot Springs. *Arab. J. Sci. Eng.* **2018**, *44*, 75–85. [CrossRef]
32. Oluyori, A.P.; Nwonuma, C.; Akpo, T.; Inyinbor, A.A.; Dada, O.A.; Oladeji, O.S.; Ogunnupebi, T.A. In Vivo Antiplasmodial Potential of the Leaf, Mesocarp, and Epicarp of the *Raphia hookeri* Plant in Mice Infected with *Plasmodium berghei* NK65. *Evid.-Based Complement. Altern. Med.* **2022**, *2022*, 4129045. [CrossRef]

33. Dash, R.; Mitra, S.; Ali, M.C.; Oktaviani, D.F.; Hannan, M.A.; Choi, S.M.; Moon, I.S. Phytosterols: Targeting Neuroinflammation in Neurodegeneration. *Curr. Pharm. Des.* **2021**, *27*, 383–401. [CrossRef]
34. García, M.D.; Sáenz, M.T.; Gómez, M.A.; Fernández, M.A. Topical antiinflammatory activity of phytosterols isolated from *Eryngium foetidum* on chronic and acute inflammation models. *Phytother. Res.* **1999**, *13*, 78–80. [CrossRef]
35. Navarro, A.; De las Heras, B.; Villar, A. Anti-inflammatory and immunomodulating properties of a sterol fraction from Sideritis foetens Clem. *Biol. Pharm. Bull.* **2001**, *24*, 470–473. [CrossRef]
36. Tan, D.C.; Kassim, N.K.; Ismail, I.S.; Hamid, M.; Ahamad Bustamam, M.S. Identification of Antidiabetic Metabolites from *Paederia foetida* L. Twigs by Gas Chromatography-Mass Spectrometry-Based Metabolomics and Molecular Docking Study. *BioMed Res. Int.* **2019**, *2019*, 7603125. [CrossRef]
37. Wikarta, J.; Kim, S.M. Anti-Inflammatory Activity and Cytotoxicity of the Starfish Extracts on Cancer Cells in Culture. *Med. Chem.* **2016**, *6*, 331–338. [CrossRef]
38. Hakkola, J.; Hukkanen, J.; Turpeinen, M.; Pelkonen, O. Inhibition and induction of CYP enzymes in humans: An update. *Arch. Toxicol.* **2020**, *94*, 3671–3722. [CrossRef]
39. Adebayo, A.; John-Africa, L.; Chike-Ekwughe, A.; Omotosho, O.; Mosaku, T. Anti-nociceptive and anti-inflammatory activities of extract of *Anchomanes difformis* in rats. *Pak. J. Pharm. Sci.* **2014**, *27*, 265–270.
40. Afify, E.; Alkreathy, H.; Ali, A.; Alfaifi, H.; Khan, L. Characterization of the Antinociceptive Mechanisms of Khat Extract (*Catha edulis*) in Mice. *Front. Neurol.* **2017**, *8*, 69. [CrossRef]
41. Aziz, M.A. Qualitative phytochemical screening and evaluation of anti-inflammatory, analgesic and antipyretic activities of Microcos paniculata barks and fruits. *J. Integr. Med.* **2015**, *13*, 173–184. [CrossRef]
42. Le Bars, D.; Gozariu, M.; Cadden, S.W. Animal models of nociception. *Pharmacol. Rev.* **2001**, *53*, 597–652.
43. Costa, E.A.; Lino, R.C.; Gomes, M.N.; Nascimento, M.V.; Florentino, I.F.; Galdino, P.M.; Andrade, C.H.; Rezende, K.R.; Magalhães, L.O.; Menegatti, R. Anti-inflammatory and antinociceptive activities of LQFM002—A 4-nerolidylcatechol derivative. *Life Sci.* **2013**, *92*, 237–244. [CrossRef]
44. Shibata, M.; Ohkubo, T.; Takahashi, H.; Inoki, R. Modified formalin test: Characteristic biphasic pain response. *Pain* **1989**, *38*, 347–352. [CrossRef]
45. Carlson, R.P.; O'Neill-Davis, L.; Chang, J.; Lewis, A.J. Modulation of mouse ear edema by cyclooxygenase and lipoxygenase inhibitors and other pharmacologic agents. *Agents Actions* **1985**, *17*, 197–204. [CrossRef]
46. Morris, C.J. Carrageenan-induced paw edema in the rat and mouse. *Inflamm. Protoc.* **2003**, *225*, 115–121.
47. Chatpalliwar, V.; Joharapurkar, A.; Wanjari, M.; Chakraborty, R.; Kharkar, V. Anti-inflammatory activity of *Martynia diandra* glox. *Indian Drugs* **2002**, *39*, 543–545.
48. Yatoo, M.I.; Gopalakrishnan, A.; Saxena, A.; Parray, O.R.; Tufani, N.A.; Chakraborty, S.; Tiwari, R.; Dhama, K.; Iqbal, H.M.N. Anti-Inflammatory Drugs and Herbs with Special Emphasis on Herbal Medicines for Countering Inflammatory Diseases and Disorders—A Review. *Recent Pat. Inflamm. Allergy Drug Discov.* **2018**, *12*, 39–58. [CrossRef]
49. Murakami, M.; Kudo, I. Phospholipase A2. *J. Biochem.* **2002**, *131*, 285–292. [CrossRef]
50. Vane, J.R.; Bakhle, Y.S.; Botting, R.M. Cyclooxygenases 1 and 2. *Annu. Rev. Pharmacol. Toxicol.* **1998**, *38*, 97–120. [CrossRef]
51. Rawlings, N.D.; Barrett, A.J. Evolutionary families of peptidases. *Biochem. J.* **1993**, *290 Pt 1*, 205–218. [CrossRef]
52. Turk, B. Targeting proteases: Successes, failures and future prospects. *Nat. Rev. Drug Discov.* **2006**, *5*, 785–799. [CrossRef]
53. Demir, F.; Troldborg, A.; Thiel, S.; Lassé, M.; Huesgen, P.F.; Tomas, N.M.; Wiech, T.; Rinschen, M.M. Proteolysis and inflammation of the kidney glomerulus. *Cell Tissue Res.* **2021**, *385*, 489–500. [CrossRef]
54. Khumalo, G.P.; Van Wyk, B.E.; Feng, Y.; Cock, I.E. A review of the traditional use of southern African medicinal plants for the treatment of inflammation and inflammatory pain. *J. Ethnopharmacol.* **2022**, *283*, 114436. [CrossRef]
55. Kaabi, Y.A. Potential Roles of Anti-Inflammatory Plant-Derived Bioactive Compounds Targeting Inflammation in Microvascular Complications of Diabetes. *Molecules* **2022**, *27*, 7352. [CrossRef]
56. Gabay, O.; Sanchez, C.; Salvat, C.; Chevy, F.; Breton, M.; Nourissat, G.; Wolf, C.; Jacques, C.; Berenbaum, F. Stigmasterol: A phytosterol with potential anti-osteoarthritic properties. *Osteoarthr. Cartil.* **2010**, *18*, 106–116. [CrossRef]
57. Innes, J.K.; Calder, P.C. Omega-6 fatty acids and inflammation. *Prostaglandins Leukot. Essent. Fat. Acids* **2018**, *132*, 41–48. [CrossRef]
58. Lipinski, C.A.; Lombardo, F.; Dominy, B.W.; Feeney, P.J. Experimental and computational approaches to estimate solubility and permeability in drug discovery and development settings. *Adv. Drug Deliv. Rev.* **2001**, *46*, 3–26. [CrossRef]
59. Guengerich, F.P. Cytochrome P-450 3A4: Regulation and role in drug metabolism. *Annu. Rev. Pharmacol. Toxicol.* **1999**, *39*, 1–17. [CrossRef]
60. Feltrin, C.; Farias, I.V.; Sandjo, L.P.; Reginatto, F.H.; Simões, C.M.O. Effects of Standardized Medicinal Plant Extracts on Drug Metabolism Mediated by CYP3A4 and CYP2D6 Enzymes. *Chem. Res. Toxicol.* **2020**, *33*, 2408–2419. [CrossRef]
61. Koster, R.; Anderson, W.; De Beer, E. Acetic acid for analgesic screening. *Fed. Proc.* **1959**, *18*, 412–417.
62. Siegmund, E.; Cadmus, R.; Lu, G. A method for evaluating both non-narcotic and narcotic analgesics. *Proc. Soc. Exp. Biol. Med.* **1957**, *4*, 729–731. [CrossRef]
63. Parimaladevi, B.; Boominathan, R.; Mandal, S.C. Studies on analgesic activity of *Cleome viscosa* in mice. *Fitoterapia* **2003**, *74*, 262–266. [CrossRef]
64. Rosland, J.H.; Tjølsen, A.; Mæhle, B.; Hole, K. The formalin test in mice: Effect of formalin concentration. *Pain* **1990**, *42*, 235–242. [CrossRef]

65. Romero-Estudillo, I.; Viveros-Ceballos, J.L.; Cazares-Carreño, O.; González-Morales, A.; de Jesús, B.F.; López-Castillo, M.; Razo-Hernández, R.S.; Castañeda-Corral, G.; Ordóñez, M. 000Synthesis of new α-aminophosphonates: Evaluation as anti-inflammatory agents and QSAR studies. *Bioorg. Med. Chem.* **2019**, *27*, 2376–2386. [CrossRef]
66. Sugishita, E.; Amagaya, S.; Ogihara, Y. Anti-inflammatory testing methods: Comparative evaluation of mice and rats. *J. Pharmacobio-Dyn.* **1981**, *4*, 565–575. [CrossRef]
67. Adulyatham, P.; Owusu-Apenten, R. Stabilization and partial purification of a protease from ginger rhizome (*Zingiber offinale* Roscoe). *J. Food Sci.* **2005**, *70*, C231–C234. [CrossRef]
68. de Araújo, A.L.; Radvanyi, F. Determination of phospholipase A2 activity by a colorimetric assay using a pH indicator. *Toxicon* **1987**, *25*, 1181–1188. [CrossRef]
69. Daina, A.; Michielin, O.; Zoete, V. SwissADME: A free web tool to evaluate pharmacokinetics, drug-likeness and medicinal chemistry friendliness of small molecules. *Sci. Rep.* **2017**, *7*, 42717. [CrossRef]
70. Pires, D.E.; Blundell, T.L.; Ascher, D.B. pkCSM: Predicting Small-Molecule Pharmacokinetic and Toxicity Properties Using Graph-Based Signatures. *J. Med. Chem.* **2015**, *58*, 4066–4072. [CrossRef]
71. NORMA Oficial Mexicana NOM-062-ZOO-1999, Especificaciones Técnicas para la Producción, Cuidado y Uso de los Animales de Laboratorio. Diario Oficial de la Federación, 1999. pp. 107–165. Available online: https://dof.gob.mx/nota_detalle.php?codigo=764738&fecha=18/06/2001#gsc.tab=0 (accessed on 20 January 2024).

pharmaceuticals

MDPI

Article

Analgesic and Anti-Arthritic Potential of Methanolic Extract and Palmatine Obtained from *Annona squamosa* Leaves

Caren Naomi Aguero Ito [1], Elisangela dos Santos Procopio [1], Natália de Matos Balsalobre [1], Lucas Luiz Machado [2], Saulo Euclides Silva-Filho [2,*], Taíse Fonseca Pedroso [3], Caroline Caramano de Lourenço [3], Rodrigo Juliano Oliveira [4], Arielle Cristina Arena [5], Marcos José Salvador [3] and Cândida Aparecida Leite Kassuya [1,*]

1 Health Sciences College, Federal University of Grande Dourados (UFGD), Dourados 79804-970, MS, Brazil; itonaomi@live.com (C.N.A.I.); elisangelaprocopiosan@gmail.com (E.d.S.P.); nataliabalsalobre@hotmail.com (N.d.M.B.)

2 Pharmaceutical Sciences, Food and Nutrition College, Federal University of Mato Grosso do Sul (UFMS), Campo Grande 79070-900, MS, Brazil; lucaslmachado11@gmail.com

3 Institute of Biology, Department of Plant Biology, University of Campinas (UNICAMP), Campinas 13083-862, SP, Brazil; taisefpedroso@gmail.com (T.F.P.); ca_jau@hotmail.com (C.C.d.L.); marcosjs@unicamp.br (M.J.S.)

4 Stem Cell, Cell Therapy and Toxicological Genetics Research Centre (CeTroGen), Medical School, Federal University of Mato Grosso do Sul (UFMS), Campo Grande 79070-900, MS, Brazil; rodrigo.oliveira@ufms.br

5 Institute of Biosciences of Botucatu, Department of Structural and Functional Biology, São Paulo State University (UNESP), Botucatu 18618-970, SP, Brazil; arielle.arena@unesp.br

* Correspondence: saulo.e@ufms.br (S.E.S.-F.); candida2005@gmail.com (C.A.L.K.)

Abstract: Background/Objectives: *Annona squamosa* is used in folk medicine to treat pain and arthritis. Palmatine is an alkaloid isolated from several plants, including *A. squamosa* leaves. The aim of the present study was to investigate the analgesic, anti-arthritic, and anti-inflammatory potential of the methanolic extract of *A. squamosa* (EMAS) and palmatine. **Methods**: The chemical profile of EMAS was evaluated by ultra high-performance liquid chromatography with electrospray ionization coupled to mass spectrometry (UHPLC-ESI/MS). EMAS and palmatine were evaluated in carrageenan-induced pleurisy, zymosan-induced joint inflammation, formalin-induced nociception, and tumor necrosis factor (TNF)-induced mechanical hyperalgesia in experimental models in mice. A cytotoxicity test of EMAS and palmatine was performed using a methylthiazolidiphenyl-tetrazolium (MTT) bromide assay. **Results**: The analysis of the chemical profile of the extract showed the presence of palmatine, liriodenine, and anonaine. Oral administration of EMAS and palmatine significantly reduced leukocyte migration and oxide nitric production in the carrageenan-induced pleurisy model. EMAS and palmatine reduced mechanical hyperalgesia, leukocyte migration, and edema formation in the joint inflammation induced by zymosan. In the formalin test, palmatine was effective against the second-phase nociceptive response, mechanical hyperalgesia, and cold allodynia. In addition, palmatine reduced mechanical hyperalgesia induced by TNF. EMAS and palmatine did not demonstrate cytotoxicity. **Conclusions**: The present study showed that *A. squamosa* and palmatine are analgesic and anti-inflammatory agents, and that the anti-hyperalgesic properties of palmatine may involve the TNF pathway. Palmatine may be one of the compounds responsible for the anti-hyperalgesic and/or anti-arthritic properties of this medicinal plant.

Keywords: *Annona*; alkaloids; anti-hyperalgesic; arthritis; efficiency; inflammation

1. Introduction

Inflammation is a complex process involving multiple signaling pathways that, if unsolved, can lead to a chronic inflammatory process [1]. Neutrophils are normally the first responders (among others) to acute inflammation, and they contribute to the release of inflammatory (prostaglandins (PGs), leukotrienes, cytokines, chemokines) and pro-resolving mediators [2]. When this process is not healed, the subacute phase can occur. In this phase, neutrophils release lysosomal enzymes, which increase capillary permeability and cause tissue destruction, and monocytes (macrophages) act as cellular defense cells. Failure to resolve inflammatory processes can lead to increased cells and several inflammatory mediators, resulting in chronic inflammation [2,3]. In chronic inflammation, pain, edema, and loss of tissue function are three of the five cardinal signs that [4] may be present [5].

The main pharmacological treatments of pain are opioid analgesics and nonsteroidal anti-inflammatory drugs (NSAIDs), whose long-term use can cause various side effects. These adverse effects include opioid-induced dependence, NSAID-induced ulcers (non-selective NSAIDS), and/or cardiovascular thrombotic events (selective cyclooxygenase(COX)-2 inhibitors) [6,7]. The main drugs used to treat inflammation are NSAIDs and glucocorticoids analogs. Chronic treatment with the latter can lead to adrenal insufficiency, insulin resistance, and other health problems [8,9]. Considering the need for new anti-inflammatory and analgesic drugs, analysis of the biological activities of medicinal plants and their isolated compounds is important for the development and discovery of new drugs.

Annona squamosa L. (Annonaceae) is an exotic tree, known as "fruta-do-conde" (Brazil) [10] or Seetha pazham [11], popularly used by oral route for urinary disorders (Philippines) [12], hair growth (India) [13], inflammation, and cancer, among others [11,14,15]. In the Philippines, it is popularly used topically for headache and mumps, cuts, and wounds [12,16]. *A. squamosa* can be found in various tropical and subtropical regions of the world, especially in the American continent [17]. Several states in Brazil cultivate this plant, which is known for its fruit. The trees grow from 3 m to 8 m high, with large branches, brownish bark, and thin leaves [18].

The juice of the whole plant or the powder of the leaves are used for body aches [13,19] and arthritis [20]. The decoction of the leaves is widely used in folk medicine in China to treat lymphadenopathy [14] and in Brazil, after preparation by maceration, infusion, or decoction, the leaves are used to treat hemorrhoids, labyrinthitis, digestive, and rheumatic disorders [17,21,22]. In scientific studies, the ethanolic extract obtained from the leaves of *A. squamosa* have shown efficacy in the acetic acid-induced nociception model and in the hot plate test [23]. In addition, an ethanolic extract of the leaves and seeds of *A. squamosa* reduced carrageenan-induced paw edema [23,24]. Caryophyllene oxide was isolated from petroleum ether extract of the bark of *A. squamosa*, and it seems to be the compound responsible for several biological properties [25]. Palmatine has several pharmacological properties such as hypolipidemic action [26], antiproliferative [27], gastroprotective [28], neuroprotective [29], antidepressant [30], chondroprotective [31], anti-inflammatory [32], antibacterial, antiviral, and hepatoprotective activities [33,34], and alleviating lung injury [35], among others. In addition, palmatine showed anti-hyperalgesic effects against diabetic neuropathy (mechanical and thermal hyperalgesia) [30] and trigeminal neuralgia models (mechanical hyperalgesia) in rats [36]. No studies have shown the anti-nociceptive action of palmatine.

In view of this, the present research evaluated the presence of alkaloids and the chemical profile of the methanolic extract of *A. squamosa* leaves (EMAS). The biological properties (anti-inflammatory, anti-nociceptive, and anti-hyperalgesic) of EMAS and its isolated compound (palmatine) were analyzed in models of nociception (formalin), paw (carrageenan), and articular (zymosan) inflammation as well as its cytotoxic activity. The mechanisms of action of palmatine were also investigated in relation to the tumor necrosis factor (TNF) pathway. This work is relevant since the involvement of palmatine in the analgesic and anti-arthritic responses of *A. squamosa* has not been fully elucidated.

2. Results

2.1. Chemical Analysis of EMAS and Isolation and Structure Elucidation of Palmatine

The results of ESI-MS and UHPLC-MS-MS analysis of EMAS allowed for the identification of the alkaloids anonaine, liriodenine, and palmatine (Table 1 and Figure 1). These data are in agreement with the chemical profile presented by the Annona genera and the Annonaceae family. As the main constituents of the *Annona* leaves are alkaloids, for further purification, an acid–basic extraction was performed with EMAS, resulting in the alkaloidal fraction. Fractionation of the alkaloidal fraction resulted in the isolation of palmatine alkaloid. The purity and identification of this substance were confirmed using spectroscopic (UV, IR, 1D, and 2D NMR) and mass spectrometric (ESI-MS) methods, and by comparison with the literature data [37]. The elucidation of the structure of palmatine, with the interpretation of carbon and proton NMR data and a reference article which helped to confirm the structure, is shown in the Supplementary Materials.

Table 1. UHPLC-MS analysis of the alkaloids (confirmed by a comparison with a standard sample) in the methanolic extract of *A. squamosa* leaves (EMAS).

Analyzed Compounds [a]	Masses Calculated	Positive Ion Mode $[M + H]^+$ (m/z)	Retention Time (min)	EMAS
Anonaine	265	266	2.86	+
Asimilobine	267	268	2.19	-
Liriodenine	275	276	3.00	+
Lysicamine	291	292	3.63	-
Isomoschatoline	307	308	4.01	-
O-methyl-isomoschatoline	321	322	4.45	-
Coreximine	327	328	1.36	-
Isocoreximine	327	328	1.36	-
Reticuline	329	330	1.61	-
9-Methoxy-isomoscatoline	337	338	4.18	-
Palmatine	352	353	2.44	+

+: compound detected; -: compound not detected. [a] Standard sample.

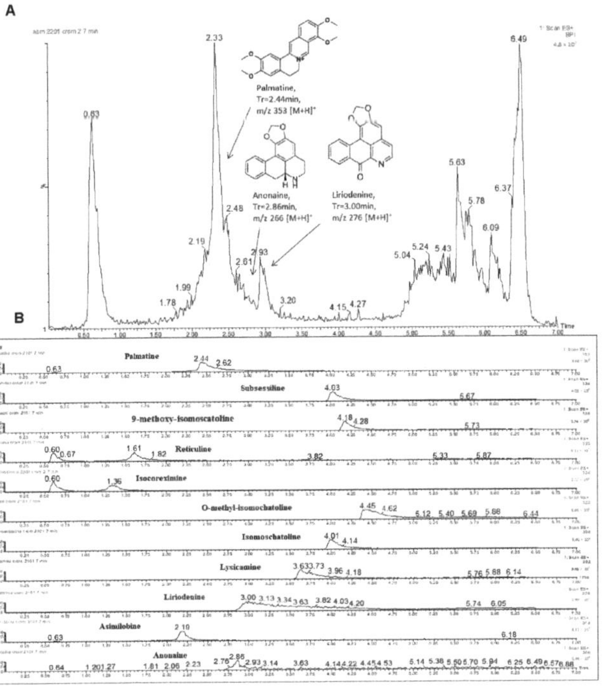

Figure 1. UHPLC-MS chromatograms. (**A**) From the methanolic extract of the leaves of *A. squamosa* (EMAS) with some identified alkaloids. (**B**) From the standard samples of alkaloids used as a standard.

2.2. *Effects of EMAS and Palmatine on Carrageenan-Induced Pleurisy*

Evaluation of pleurisy induced by carrageenan showed a reduction in leukocyte migration of 74% for a dose of 100 mg/kg of EMAS, 81% for a dose of 300 mg/kg of EMAS, 50% for a dose of 1 mg/kg of palmatine, and 75% for a dose of 3 mg/kg of palmatine (Figure 2A,B), when compared to the control group of mice. The oral administration of 30 mg/kg of EMAS and 0.3 mg/kg of palmatine did not interfere with leukocyte migration to the mouse pleural cavity. Furthermore, the groups treated with EMAS (100 and 300 mg/kg) did not differ statistically from the groups treated with the reference drug (prednisolone) or those from the naïve group.

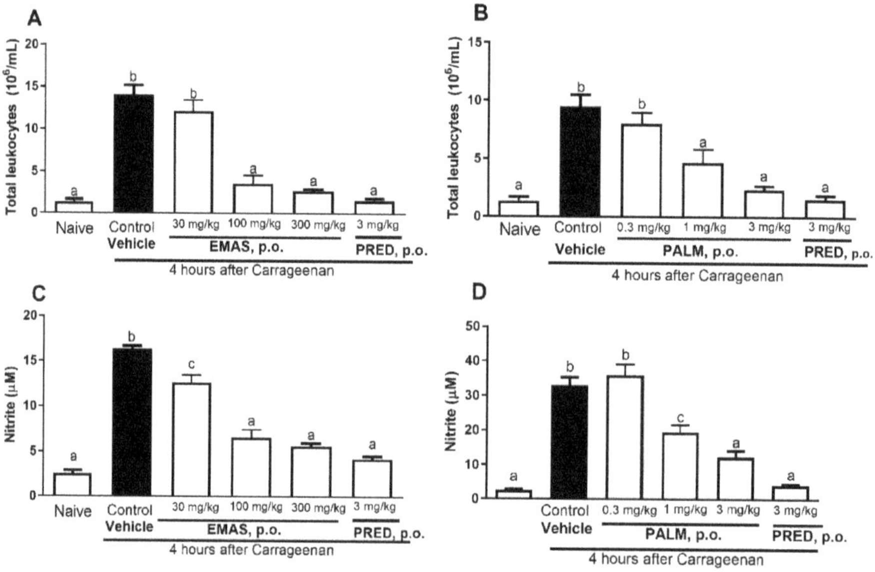

Figure 2. Effects of oral administration of EMAS and palmatine on leukocyte migration (**A**,**B**) and nitric oxide production (**C**,**D**) in pleurisy model induced by carrageenan. Animals received, by gavage, EMAS (30, 100, 300 mg/kg), palmatine (0.3, 1, 3 mg/kg), vehicle (naïve and control groups), or prednisolone (PRED, 3 mg/kg), and, after 1 h, intrathoracic injection of carrageenan was given to groups, except naïve. Each bar represents mean ± SEM of 6 animals. Letters a, b and c indicate significant differences among groups according to Tukey's multiple comparison test.

Evaluation of pleurisy induced by carrageenan showed a reduction in leukocyte migration of 22.64% for a dose of 30 mg/kg of EMAS, 59.85% for a dose of 100 mg/kg of EMAS, 65.48% for a dose of 300 mg/kg of EMAS, 40.61% for a dose of 1 mg/kg of palmatine, and 62.42% for a dose of 3 mg/kg of palmatine (Figure 2C,D), when compared to the control group of mice. The oral administration of 0.3 mg/kg of palmatine did not interfere with nitrite production in the pleural cavity. Oral administration of EMAS (Figure 2C) and palmatine (Figure 2D) did not differ statistically from the groups treated with prednisolone or those from the naïve group, when compared to the control group. Moreover, the analysis demonstrated that palmatine could act in a dose-dependent manner.

2.3. *Effects of EMAS and Palmatine on Zymosan-Induced Joint Inflammation*

After 4 h of zymosan administration in the knee, oral exposure to a dose of 100 mg/kg of EMAS, 1 mg/kg of palmatine, and prednisolone (PRED) significantly inhibited mechanical hyperalgesia in 68, 70, and 70%, respectively. After 6 h of zymosan administration in the knee, the inhibition of mechanical hyperalgesia induced by EMAS was 70% for 100 mg/kg, while for palmatine it was 73%, and for prednisolone (PRED) it was 77% (Figure 3A,B).

The results of palmatine- and EMAS-treated groups showed no statistical difference from those treated with prednisolone; however, all these groups differed from the control group (Figure 3A,B).

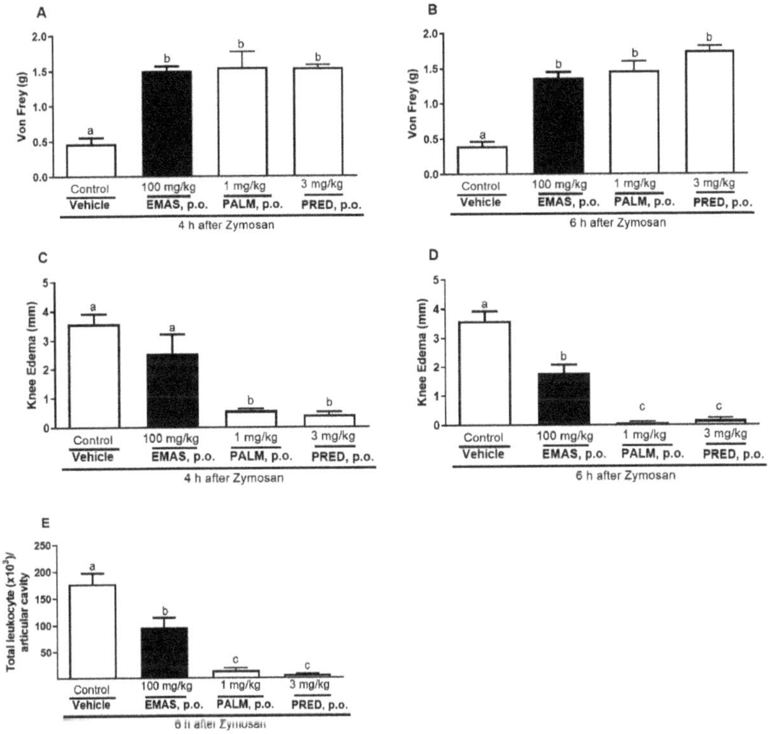

Figure 3. Effects of oral administration of EMAS and palmatine on mechanical hyperalgesia (**A**,**B**), knee edema (**C**,**D**), and on leukocyte migration (**E**) caused by zymosan-induced joint inflammation in female mice. Animals received, by gavage, EMAS (100 mg/kg), palmatine (1 mg/kg), saline solution (control group), or the reference drug prednisolone (PRED, 3 mg/kg) and, after 1 h, 200 μg of zymosan was injected into left knee. After induction of inflammation, mechanical hyperalgesia and edema were measured four (**A**,**C**) and six (**B**,**D**) hours later, respectively. After that, animals were euthanized and joint exudate was used to assess leukocyte migration (**E**). Each bar represents mean ± SEM of 6 animals. Letters a, b, and c indicate significant differences among groups according to Tukey's multiple comparison test.

After 4 h of zymosan administration in the knee, oral exposure to a dose of 1 mg/kg of palmatine, and of prednisolone (PRED) significantly inhibited edema in 84 and 88%, respectively. EMAS did not interfere with the edema at this point. After 6 h of zymosan administration in the knee, oral exposure to a dose of 100 mg/kg of EMAS, 1 mg/kg of palmatine, and of prednisolone (PRED) significantly inhibited edema in 51%, 98%, and 96%, respectively. The results of the palmatine- and prednisolone-treated groups showed no statistical difference between themselves; however, both groups differed from the control group and EMAS-treated group (Figure 3C,D).

Six hours after the induction of joint inflammation by zymosan (Figure 3E), leukocyte recruitment was reduced by the treatment with EMAS (51%), palmatine (91%), and prednisolone (96%). Regarding leukocyte recruitment, the results of the groups treated with palmatine and prednisolone showed no statistical difference between themselves; however, both groups differed from the control group and EMAS-treated group (Figure 3E).

2.4. Effects of EMAS and Palmatine on Formalin-Induced Nociception

Formalin-induced nociception and paw edema were not reduced by EMAS (100 mg/kg) and palmatine (1 mg/kg) in the first phase (Figure 4A,E). In the second phase (inflammatory phase) (Figure 4B), treatment with palmatine significantly reduced the time the animals bit or licked the paw (83%), when compared to the control group.

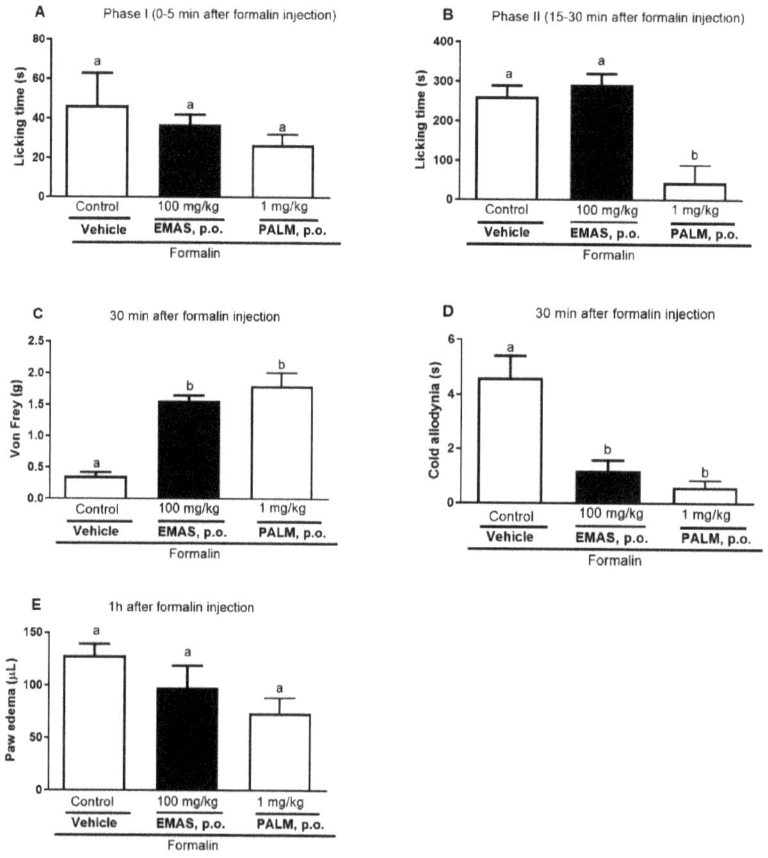

Figure 4. Effects of oral administration of EMAS and palmatine on formalin test. One hour before applying 30 μL of 1% formalin, animals were orally treated with EMAS (100 mg/kg), palmatine (PALM 1 mg/kg), or vehicle (control group). First phase represents neurogenic phase (**A**), while second phase is inflammatory phase (**B**). Paw withdrawal threshold (Von Frey test) (**C**) and cold sensitivity (**D**) were performed immediately after formalin test. Formalin-induced edema was measured one hour after formalin application (**E**). Each bar represents mean ± SEM of 5 animals. Letters a and b indicate significant differences between groups according to Tukey's multiple comparison test.

Furthermore, EMAS (77%) and palmatine (80%) decreased mechanical hyperalgesia (Figure 4C) and reduced cold sensitivity (Figure 4D) by 74% and 87%, respectively, when compared to the control group.

2.5. Effect of Palmatine on TNF-Induced Hyperalgesia

Intraplantar treatment of 3 μg/paw (73% and 71%) and 30 μg/paw (71% and 81%) of palmatine prevented mechanical hyperalgesia 3 and 4 h after TNF compared to the control group (Figure 5). Furthermore, these two doses (3 and 30 μg/paw) of oral palmatine administration, 3 and 4 h after TNF injection, differed from the control group and did not statistically differ from baseline. The baseline values of the three groups were not statistically different.

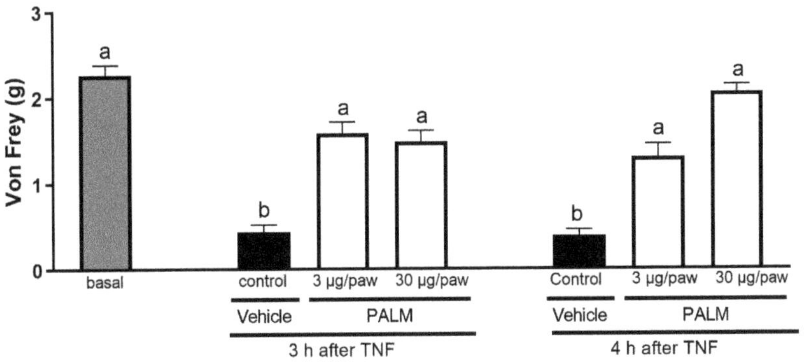

Figure 5. The effects of the intraplantar administration of palmatine on TNF-induced mechanical hyperalgesia. One hour before the injection of 20 μL of TNF into the right hind paw, the animals were intraplantar treated with saline solution or palmatine (PALM 3 and 30 μg/paw) in the same region as the inducing agent. Three and four hours after the TNF injection, mechanical hyperalgesia (Von Frey test) was analyzed. In addition, the basal response to mechanical stimulus was performed before treating the animals. Each bar represents the mean ± SEM of 5 animals. The letters a and b indicate significant differences among groups according to Tukey's multiple comparison test.

2.6. Effect of EMAS and Palmatine on Leukocyte Viability by MTT

EMAS and palmatine showed no cytotoxicity in vitro. The cell viability of EMAS (96, 93, and 84%) and palmatine (72.89, and 88%) at concentrations of 10, 30, and 90 μg/mL did not induce cytotoxicity (results not shown).

3. Discussion

The present research showed the anti-nociceptive and anti-arthritic properties of EMAS and palmatine in experimental models. The anti-inflammatory effects of *A. squamosa* leaves have been extensively explored in the literature [23,38,39]; however, available studies of analgesic [23] and anti-arthritic properties with this plant are scarce. The leaves of *A. squamosa* are used by the population to treat body pain [13,19] and rheumatic disorders [17,20]. To our knowledge, this is the first study to demonstrate that EMAS is effective against painful and inflammatory parameters in zymosan and formalin models. No cytotoxicity was found for EMAS and palmatine in the tests performed in this study, corroborating the studies showing that palmatine is not cytotoxic. Palmatine was isolated from EMAS and the purity of the substance was demonstrated (Supplementary Materials). Palmatine is an alkaloid, with a wide spectrum of its pharmacological effects already described in the literature; however, its anti-nociceptive and anti-arthritic effects have not been totally explored. In the present work, the analgesic and anti-arthritic activities of EMAS seem to be induced by palmatine, and the mechanisms of action could be related to the TNF pathway.

Different parts of *A. squamosa* (bark, leaves, fruit, seeds) have shown substances with pharmacological, nutraceutical, and biological potential [18,40,41]. The peel of its fruit (epicarp), for example, has mostly shown spathulenol, a substance with anti-inflammatory, anti-nociceptive, antimicrobial, and antiproliferative potential [42,43]. In the ethanolic extract of the leaves, sesquiterpenes such as *trans*-caryophyllene have been identified [44]. *Trans*-caryophyllene, for example, reduced mechanical hyperalgesia and thermal nociception in a chronic model of neurogenic pain (sciatic nerve constriction) [45]. *Trans*-caryophyllene reduced mechanical hyperalgesia and IL-6 and IL-1 β levels in a model of chronic diabetic neuropathy induced by streptozotocin [46]. This substance reduced paw inflammation induced by several inflammatory agents [47]. In another study, *trans*-caryophyllene reduced capsaicin-induced nociception [48]. In addition to these, other substances with anti-inflammatory and anti-nociceptive potential present in the leaves of *A. squamosa* have also been identified, such as trans-caryophyllene, phytol, and humulene. *Trans*-caryophyllene (23.0%) and β-elemene were isolated from the essential oil of *A. squamosa* [44,49]. Phytol and trans-caryophyllene have shown thermal (hot plate test) and chemical (formalin, acetic acid) anti-nociceptive effects in acute nociception models [45,50].

The carrageenan-induced pleurisy model in mice is a relevant model to study the anti-inflammatory effects of new drugs in vivo [51]. Pure palmatine and EMAS have been tested in a pleurisy model and the analysis demonstrated that doses of 100 and 300 mg/kg, but not the dose of 30 mg/kg, of EMAS, and that doses of 1 and 3 mg/kg, but not the dose of 0.3 mg/kg, of palmatine are effective, which could indicate that palmatine induced a dose-dependent inhibition (Figure 2A,B). In relation to nitrite production, all the tested doses of EMAS inhibited this parameter, indicating a possible action in oxide nitric production. Doses of 1 and 3 mg/kg, but not a dose of 0.3 mg/kg, of palmatine inhibited nitrite production in pleural exudate, corroborating the findings of Yan et al. [28] that showed the inhibition of the oxide nitric pathway (in vitro) by palmatine. The ethanolic extract obtained from *A. squamosa* leaves also showed an anti-inflammatory property in carrageenan-induced paw edema [23], while palmatine, in an in vitro study, reduced the production of pro-inflammatory mediators (TNF-α, IL-1β, IL-6, and NO) and increased the production of IL-10 [32]. These new results indicate that EMAS and palmatine had anti-inflammatory action in the pleurisy model and showed that palmatine could act in a dose-dependent manner.

Several scientists have classified zymosan-induced joint inflammation in rodents as an arthritis experimental model for drug discovery [52,53]. Zymosan is derived from *Saccharomyces cerevisiae* and is classified as an immunogenic and inflammatory agent. When zymosan is injected into the knee cavity, it can induce hyperalgesia, joint edema, and neutrophil recruitment [53], which can characterize acute inflammatory processes in the knee. In previous studies, palmatine demonstrated chondroprotective effects in an osteoarthritis model [31]. The 100 mg/kg dose of EMAS and the 1 mg/kg dose of palmatine were effective in inhibiting mechanical hyperalgesia, leukocyte migration, and edema in zymosan joint inflammation. These results show that EMAS and palmatine have anti-arthritic potential, which may explain, at least in part, the popular use of *A. squamosa* for the treatment of arthritis.

The formalin test is a nociceptive model used to evaluate new products with analgesic activity in the two phases of pain: neurogenic pain, related to direct stimulation of nociceptor fibers, and inflammatory pain, related to inflammatory mediators [54]. Previous studies have shown that extracts of *A. squamosa* leaves exhibited anti-nociceptive effects in acetic acid (peripheral action) and the hot plate test (central action) [23], while seed extract showed anti-edematogenic effect in a carrageenan-induced paw edema model [23,24]. Palmatine showed anti-hyperalgesic effects against diabetic neuropathy (mechanical and thermal hyperalgesia) [30] and trigeminal neuralgia models (mechanical hyperalgesia) in rats. Our results showed that EMAS (100 mg/kg) and palmatine (1 mg/kg) had no activity in the first phase (Figure 4A), but in the second phase (inflammatory phase) (Figure 4B), nociception was antagonized by palmatine. Furthermore, EMAS and palmatine prevented mechanical hyperalgesia (Figure 4C) and cold sensitivity (Figure 4D). The present study was the first to demonstrate palmatine anti-nociceptive properties in the formalin model, which could partially explain the popular analgesic use of *A. squamosa*.

The extract was chemically analyzed and revealed the presence of palmatine, lirio-denine, and anonaine. Palmatine is an alkaloid present in several medicinal plants and has a wide range of pharmacological activities already described in the literature [34], including anti-cancer [23,38,55], antioxidant [56,57], anti-inflammatory [31,32], neuroprotective [29,56,58], antibacterial [59,60], antiviral [59,61], and hypolipidemic properties [26,62]. Previous studies have demonstrated the anti-inflammatory activity of liriodenine. Liriodenine reduced NO production by macrophages obtained from lipopolysaccharide (LPS)-induced peritonitis in rats [63], interacted with the COX-2 binding site and inhibited COX-2 in silico [64], decreased cell proliferation in the rat synovial cavity, and reduced splenocyte proliferation in vitro [63]. Anonaine has not been evaluated for inflammatory or analgesic effects. The effective dose of EMAS was 100 mg/kg, and the dose of 1 mg/kg of palmatine was selected to be tested in zymosan and formalin models, since palmatine comprises approximately 1% of EMAS (performed by validated quantitative HPLC-ESI method). Both EMAS (100 mg/kg) and palmatine (1 mg/kg) had efficacy in all the models tested in the present work. The present study was the first to show that palmatine is the main compound found in EMAS, responsible for anti-nociceptive and anti-arthritic effects.

Given the effects of palmatine on pain and inflammation, this study evaluated the involvement of the TNF pathway in the anti-hyperalgesic effect of this substance. TNF is a potent pro-inflammatory cytokine that plays an important role in pathological spinal pain [65,66]. This cytokine acts as a neuromodulator in the dorsal horn of the spinal cord [65] and regulates both inflammatory and neuropathic pain [66–68]. In this study, palmatine was observed to inhibit TNF-induced mechanical hyperalgesia, which is consistent with previous studies showing that palmatine antagonized TNF-α and IL-1β in neuropathy models [30,36]. The anti-hyperalgesic effect of palmatine was associated with the up-regulation of calcitonin gene-related peptide (CGRP) expression, a neurotransmitter with an important role in pain transmission [36]. In diabetic neuropathy, palmatine decreased phosphorylation of the ERK1/2 pathway, which contributed to a reduction in the expression of P2X7, a receptor with an important role in the development of pain and depression [30]. Palmatine showed efficacy in the TNF model, but the result of this test does not exclude that palmatine antagonizes other inflammatory/nociceptive pathways.

Considering the role of leukocytes in the regulation of inflammation and, consequently, inflammatory pain, the viability of leukocytes treated with palmatine and EMAS was evaluated by the in vitro MTT test. Although no significant cytotoxicity was observed, it is interesting to note that studies have been published linking palmatine to the induction of DNA modification [34]. In addition, palmatine has a complex effect on metabolic enzymes in the liver, with glucuronidation and sulfation being the main metabolic pathways [34]. In in vitro tests, palmatine showed cytotoxic potential in A431 cells (a human skin epithelial carcinoma cell line) [69], while in cardiomyocyte cell culture, this substance showed cardiotoxic potential [70]. In human hepatoma cells and in normal liver cells, this substance did not induce cytotoxic cells [71]. In addition to palmatine, the aqueous extract of the leaves of *A. squamosa* showed no signs of toxicity at a dose of 2000 mg/kg. There were, however, signs of intoxication such as salivation, convulsion, excitation, and motility 48 h after administration of the extract at a dose of 5000 mg/kg [72].

This study has some limitations, for example, palmatine and EMAS were not evaluated in toxicity models. Another limitation is the use of only mice and a few doses of EMAS and palmatine in the experimental models, but the ethics of the use of animal experimentation limits the use of animals.

4. Materials and Methods

4.1. Plant Material, EMAS Acquisition, and Isolation/Chemical Analysis of Palmatine

The leaves of *A. squamosa* were collected from a specimen grown at the Biology Institute of Unicamp (22°49′10.1″ S 47°04′16.3″ W) and registered in the National System for the Management of Genetic Heritage and Associated Traditional Knowledge (Access Register No. A709776). The collected plant raw material was stabilized and dried in a circulating air oven at 40 °C (up to seven days) and then pulverized in a knife mill. In the present work, a methanolic extract of *A. squamosa* leaves was prepared due to the selectivity of the methanol solvent for the extraction of protoberberine alkaloids, the focus of this study, such as palmatine. The obtained powder (1000 g) was successively extracted (maceration) with n-hexane, followed by MeOH, in the ration 1:20 (powder/extracting liquid, *v/v*). The extraction was performed first with hexane (clean up), and then the same material, after treatment with hexane, underwent the extraction with MeOH to extract the alkaloids. After evaporation of the extracted liquid in an evaporator under reduced pressure, the crude hexane (121.5 g) and methanol (EMAS, 72.3 g) extracts were obtained. TLC (thin layer chromatography) and UHPLC-ESI-MS (ultra high-performance liquid chromatography–electrospray ionization tandem mass spectrometry) investigations indicated the presence of alkaloids in the EMAS extract. An aliquot of EMAS (2.0 g) was initially subjected to acid–base extraction according to COSTA et al. (2010) [37] for the isolation of alkaloid constituents, and to give the CH_2Cl_2 alkaloid fraction (0.25 g) and the CH_2Cl_2 neutral fraction (1.75 g). The alkaloid fraction (0.20 g) was subjected to 10% $NaHCO_3$-treated silica gel column chromatography eluted with the following gradient systems: petroleum ether–CH_2Cl_2 from 100:0 to 10:90, followed by CH_2Cl_2-EtOAc from 100:0 to 10:90, and EtOAc-MeOH from 100:0 to 50:50. The eluted fractions (35 fractions of 30 mL each) were evaluated and pooled according to TLC analysis to afford 15 fractions. Fraction 12 (25.0 mg) was purified by preparative TLC eluted with CH_2Cl_2-MeOH (96:04) to give the alkaloid palmatine (20.0 mg). All solvents used in these procedures were rota-evaporated, aiming to ensure their full removal from the product. The isolated protoberberine alkaloid palmatine was identified using spectroscopic (UV, IR, 1D, and 2D NMR) and mass spectrometric (ESI-MS) methods. For the identification analysis by UHPLC-ESI-MS/MS of the dried crude extract (EMAS), the fractions obtained from the chromatographic columns and the standard compounds isolated by our research group were dissolved in methanol (at 1.0 mg/mL) and filtered (0.22 μm) to proceed with the analysis. The chemical profile and analysis of the presence of alkaloids in the extracts was performed by ESI-MS/MS with the crude extracts and fractions. The confirmation of the presence of alkaloids in the samples was performed by direct injection into the Quadrupolar Mass Spectrometer—Micromass (Acquity model from Micromass/Waters) by electrospray in positive mode. The constituents were identified by comparing their ESI-MS/MS fragmentation spectra with the spectra of the standard compound previously isolated by our research group and with data from the literature. All chromatographic analysis of the samples was performed was performed using an Acquity UHPLC chromatograph coupled to an Acquity TQD mass spectrometer (Micromass-Waters, Manchester, UK), with ESI source, using a Waters Acquity C_{18} BEH column (2.1 mm × 50 mm × 1.7 μm particle size). The analysis conditions were as follows: solvent A (Milli-Q water and formic acid 0.1%) and solvent B (methanol). The flow rate was 0.2 mL/min for the entire run time of 7.0 min, with an elution gradient that started with 20% methanol and went up to 100% at minute 5, 100% from 5.01 to 5.50 min, and finally returning to the initial situation. The detection was performed in positive mode ionization under 3.00 kV of capillary voltage, 30.00 V at cone, 130 °C source temperature, 250 °C desolvation temperature, and an injection volume of 5 μL. The analyzed masses were in the range of 100 to 800 *m/z*. Finally, the constituents were identified by UHPLC-MS/MS analysis, comparing the mass spectra, the retention time, and the fragmentation profile (MS/MS) of the standard compound spectra previously isolated by our research group with the fragmentation spectra of the crude extract and fractions. Collision-Induced Dissociation (CID) was performed to identify the ions, and the MS/MS spectra were compared with the fragmentation pattern of the substances annonaine, asimilobine, liriodenine, lysicamine, isomoschatoline, o-methylisomoschatoline, coreximine, isocoreximine, reticuline, 9-methoxy-isomoschatoline, and palmatine, and with data found in the literature (collision energy 30 V). For the quantification of palmatine in the EMAS extract, the palmatine standard (Sigma-Aldrich, St. Louis, MA, USA) at concentrations of 0.010 to 1.0 mg/mL was prepared and analyzed with the HPLC-ESI-MS method described before. An accurately weighed amount of EMAS was dissolved in methanol and analyzed with the same chromatographic conditions as used for palmatine. After chromatographic analysis by UPLC-MS (n = 3), the regression line was obtained by plotting the concentrations of alkaloid on the abscissa axis and the sample area on the ordinate axis. Calibration graphs were plotted, showing a linear relationship between concentrations versus peak areas for the palmatine reference compound. The regression equation curve obtained for the palmatine was y = 138,151,203x − 112,281, R^2 = 0.9887. The attribution of the chromatographic peak was based on the retention time of the single compound and confirmed by analysis in comparison with the isolated standard. Under our working conditions, the mean retention time for palmatine was 2.44 min. The concentration was calculated from the experimental peak area by analytical interpolation in standard calibration line. The limit of quantification (LOQ) for palmatine was 0.010 μg/mL. The relative standard deviation (%RSD) was 0.15%, calculated as the mean of the three replications

4.2. Reagents

Zymosan, carrageenan, Bradford solution, methylthiazolidiphenyl-tetrazolium bromide, and RPMI medium were purchased from Sigma-Aldrich (Saint Louis, MO, USA). Tumor necrosis factor was obtained from Abcam (Cambridge, UK). Phosphate-buffered saline, ethylene diamine tetra acetic acid, acetone, and dimethyl sulfoxide were acquired from Vetec (Rio de Janeir, Brazil). Turk's solution was purchased from Newprov (Pinhais, Brazil). Ketamine and xylazine were obtained from Syntec (Santana de Paraíba, Brazil). Formalin was acquired from Proquimicos (Rio de Janeiro, Brazil). All reagents used for this work have a high analytical grade.

4.3. Animals, Dissolution of EMAS and Palmatine, and Description of the Doses Used in the In Vivo and In Vitro Models

Female and male Swiss mice (28–32 g) were provided by the central biotherium of the Federal University of Grande Dourados (UFGD). Animals were housed in polypropylene boxes in the biotherium of the Health Sciences College under the following conditions: 22 °C, in the presence of a 12-hour light/dark cycle, with food and water ad libitum. The experiments were conducted at the UFGD. The experiments were performed after approval by the UFGD Animal Use Ethics Committee (13.2020).

EMAS and palmatine were dissolved in saline solution (0.9%), which was the vehicle used to treat the animals, and the dose was calculated according to the weight of the animals.

The oral inhibitory effect of EMAS (30, 100 and 300 mg/kg) and palmatine (0.3, 1, or 3 mg/kg) was investigated to evaluate if there was change in the response at different doses in the carrageenan-induced pleurisy model.

The effectives doses of EMAS were 100 and 300 mg/kg, and of palmatine were 1 and 3 mg/kg of palmatine, and a dose of 100 mg of extract and 1 mg/kg of the pure substance were selected to test in the zymosan and formalin models. As mentioned before, the yield of palmatine in EMAS was 1%, and the dose of 100 mg/kg of EMAS was equivalent to 1 mg/kg of palmatine. In addition, prednisolone (3 mg/kg, orally) was used as a positive control drug.

4.4. EMAS and Palmatine Test in Carrageenan-Induced Pleurisy

Female Swiss mice were divided into groups (9 groups with n = 5) and treated orally with vehicle (naive and control groups), EMAS (30, 100 or 300 mg/kg), palmatine (0.3, 1, or 3 mg/kg), and prednisolone (3 mg/kg).

Inflammation in the pleural cavity was induced by a 100 μL injection of carrageenan solution (1% diluted in sterile saline) one hour after previous oral administration [73]. Animals in the naive group received similar volume injections of 0.9% saline. Four hours after the induction of pleurisy, animals were submitted to a euthanasia protocol (ketamine—300 mg/kg, intraperitoneal (i.p.) + xylazine—30 mg/kg, i.p.). The thoracic cavity was opened, and the exudate was collected by washing the cavity in 1000 μL of phosphate-buffered saline/ethylene diamine tetra acetic acid (PBS/EDTA) solution. Part of the obtained sample was diluted in Turk's fluid for leukocyte count using a Neubauer chamber, while another part was used for nitrite dosage (a final product of the nitric oxide oxidation pathway) by the Griess method.

4.5. EMAS and Palmatine Test on Zymosan-Induced Joint Inflammation

Female Swiss mice were divided into four groups and treated with vehicle (control), palmatine (1 mg/kg), EMAS (100 mg/kg), or prednisolone (3 mg/kg—positive control drug). One hour later, inflammation was induced by an intra-articular (i.a.) injection of zymosan (200 µg/cavity in 10 µL sterile saline solution) into the left knee junction through the suprapatellar ligament [74]. Edema (digital micrometer) and mechanical hyperalgesia (electronic Von Frey) were measured 4 and 6 h after zymosan injection. Six hours after the induction of inflammation, the animals were euthanized (with a dose of 300 mg/kg of ketamine and 30 mg/kg of xylazine, by intraperitoneal route (i.p.). The inflamed joint was surgically exposed and washed with 10 µL of PBS containing EDTA (10 mM). Subsequently, 40 µL of this solution of PBS/EDTA was added to the collected exudate. Part of the sample was diluted in Turk's solution for leukocyte count in a Neubauer chamber.

4.6. EMAS and Palmatine Test on Formalin-Induced Nociception

Male Swiss mice were distributed into 3 groups (n = 5) and treated orally with vehicle (control), palmatine (1 mg/kg), or EMAS (100 mg/kg). One hour after administration, 1% formalin (30 µL/animal) was injected into the right hind paw of the animals (intraplantar route). The mice were placed individually in glass funnels and observed for nociceptive behavior (licking and biting) during two phases (0–5 min initially and a second phase at 15–30 min) [54,75].

Subsequently, 30 µL of acetone was applied to the surface of the injected paw, and the times the animal lifted its paw in the first 20 s were counted. In addition, mechanical hyperalgesia was analyzed using the electronic Von Frey, and the edema volume was measured using a digital plethysmometer.

4.7. Palmatine Test on TNF-Induced Hyperalgesia

The TNF-induced hyperalgesia test was performed according to Aquino et al. (2015) [76] to verify whether palmatine has a direct effect on mechanical hyperalgesia. Prior to the intraplantar administration of palmatine, the baseline mechanical score of the right hind paw of all animals was determined using a digital Von Frey algesimeter.

The animals were then distributed into 3 groups (n = 5) and intraplantarly received 30 µL of the following solutions (right hind paw): vehicle (control) and palmatine solution (3 and 30 µg/paw). After 30 min, an intraplantar injection of 20 µL of TNF (100 pg) was made into the same previously treated paw. Three and four hours after the induction of inflammation by TNF, the mechanical hyperalgesia of the right hind paw was measured by the digital Von Frey algesimeter and the animals were euthanized with dose of 300 mg/kg of ketamine and 30 mg/kg of xylazine (i.p.) after the last measurement of mechanical hyperalgesia.

4.8. Analysis of EMAS and Palmatine on Leukocyte Viability by Methylthiazolidiphenyl-Tetrazolium (MTT) Bromide Test

The MTT assay is based on applying the mitochondrial enzyme reduction in tetrazolium dye to detect and determine cell viability. This assay was performed as previously described by Silva-Filho et al. [77]. The leukocytes were obtained from the peritoneal cavity of male Swiss mice 4 h after an intraperitoneal injection of zymosan (1 mg/cavity). The cells numbers were plated at 5×10^5 cells/well in 100 µL RPMI medium (supplemented with 10% of fetal bovine serum and penicillin 100 U/mL + streptomycin 100 µg/mL) into 96-well plates. The cells were exposed to EMAS or palmatine at concentrations of 10, 30, 90 µg/mL, or vehicle, and incubated by 90 min (37 °C/5% CO_2). Then, 10 µL of MTT solution (5 mg/mL) was added to each well. After 2 h of incubation (37 °C/5% CO_2), the supernatant was removed, and 100 µL of dimethyl sulfoxide was added to each well. The plate was incubated for another 10 min and the reading was performed by an ELISA reader at 540 nm. The values of the blank wells were subtracted from each well of the treated and control cells. The percentage of feasibility was determined by the following formula:

$$\%\text{Viable cells} = \frac{(\text{absorbance of the treates cells} - \text{Absorbance of the blank})}{(\text{Absorbance of the control} - \text{Abosorbance of the blank})} \times 100$$

4.9. Statistical Analysis

Data are presented as the mean ± standard error (SEM). Determination of significant differences among groups was performed using a one-way analysis of variance (ANOVA) followed by a Tukey post hoc test (GraphPad Prism Software). The percentage of inhibition was calculated from the control group. Differences were considered significant when $p < 0.05$.

5. Conclusions

This study demonstrated the presence of palmatine and other compounds in the leaves of *A. squamosa*. The analgesic, anti-inflammatory, and anti-arthritic potential effects of EMAS and palmatine were demonstrated in inflammation, arthritis, and nociception experimental models. Taken together, the data suggest that EMAS and palmatine may have therapeutic potential in arthritis and pain disorders. One of the mechanisms of action of palmatine may be the TNF pathway.

Supplementary Materials: The following supporting information can be downloaded at https://www.mdpi.com/article/10.3390/ph17101331/s1, Table S1. Palmatine ^{1}H and ^{13}C-NMR and gHMBC data. Figure S1: Palmatine molecular structure. Figure S2: ^{1}H NMR spectra of palmatine (400 MHz, $CDCl_3$); Figure S3: ^{1}H-^{13}C correlation map from HSQC NMR experiment of palmatine (400 MHz for ^{1}H e 100 MHz for ^{13}C, $CDCl_3$); Figure S4: ^{1}H-^{13}C long-range correlation map from HMBC NMR experiment of palmatine (400 MHz for ^{1}H e 100 MHz for ^{13}C, $CDCl_3$); Figure S5: ESI(+)-MS/MS. Fragmentation of the alkaloid palmatine (m/z 352).

Author Contributions: Conceptualization, C.A.L.K. and C.N.A.I.; methodology, C.N.A.I., E.d.S.P., N.d.M.B., L.L.M. and S.E.S.-F.; validation, T.F.P., C.C.d.L. and A.C.A.; investigation, C.A.L.K., A.C.A. and M.J.S.; resources, S.E.S.-F., A.C.A., R.J.O. and C.A.L.K.; writing—original draft preparation, C.N.A.I.; writing—review and editing, C.A.L.K., S.E.S.-F., R.J.O. and A.C.A.; supervision, C.A.L.K.; funding acquisition, C.A.L.K. and S.E.S.-F. All authors have read and agreed to the published version of the manuscript.

Funding: This study was financed in part by the Coordenação de Aperfeiçoamento de Pessoal de Nível Superior—CAPES—Brazil (Finance Code 001), Conselho Nacional de Desenvolvimento Científico e Tecnológico—CNPq, Fundação de Apoio ao Desenvolvimento do Ensino, Ciência e Tecnologia do Estado de Mato Grosso do Sul—FUNDECT, Universidade Federal da Grande Dourados—UFGD, Universidade Federal de Mato Grosso do Sul—UFMS (Edital PROPP/UFMS N° 57/2024), Fundação de Amparo à Pesquisa do Estado de São Paulo—FAPESP (grant numbers 2009/05992-6, 2014/17436-9, 2015/03726-8, 2016/06407-3, and 2021/09693-5).

Institutional Review Board Statement: The animal study protocol was approved by the Ethical Committee in Animal Experimentation of the Federal University of Grande Dourados, Brazil (protocol number: 13/2020).

Informed Consent Statement: Not applicable.

Data Availability Statement: All data are available in this publication.

Conflicts of Interest: The authors declare no conflicts of interest.

References

1. Furman, D.; Campisi, J.; Verdin, E.; Carrera-Bastos, P.; Targ, S.; Franceschi, C.; Ferrucci, L.; Gilroy, D.W.; Fasano, A.; Miller, G.W.; et al. Chronic Inflammation in the Etiology of Disease across the Life Span. *Nat. Med.* **2019**, *25*, 1822–1832. [CrossRef] [PubMed]
2. Serhan, C.N. Pro-Resolving Lipid Mediators Are Leads for Resolution Physiology. *Nature* **2014**, *510*, 92–101. [CrossRef] [PubMed]
3. Herrero-Cervera, A.; Soehnlein, O.; Kenne, E. Neutrophils in Chronic Inflammatory Diseases. *Cell Mol. Immunol.* **2022**, *19*, 177–191. [CrossRef] [PubMed]

4. Ronchetti, S.; Migliorati, G.; Delfino, D.V. Association of Inflammatory Mediators with Pain Perception. *Biomed. Pharmacother.* **2017**, *96*, 1445–1452. [CrossRef]
5. Baral, P.; Udit, S.; Chiu, I.M. Pain and Immunity: Implications for Host Defence. *Nat. Rev. Immunol.* **2019**, *19*, 433–447. [CrossRef] [PubMed]
6. Arthur, J.; Bruera, E. Balancing Opioid Analgesia with the Risk of Nonmedical Opioid Use in Patients with Cancer. *Nat. Rev. Clin. Oncol.* **2019**, *16*, 213–226. [CrossRef]
7. Bertin, C.; Delage, N.; Rolland, B.; Pennel, L.; Fatseas, M.; Trouvin, A.-P.; Delorme, J.; Chenaf, C.; Authier, N. Analgesic Opioid Use Disorders in Patients with Chronic Non-Cancer Pain: A Holistic Approach for Tailored Management. *Neurosci. Biobehav. Rev.* **2021**, *121*, 160–174. [CrossRef]
8. Barnes, P.J.; Adcock, I.M. Glucocorticoid Resistance in Inflammatory Diseases. *Lancet* **2009**, *373*, 1905–1917. [CrossRef]
9. Quatrini, L.; Ugolini, S. New Insights into the Cell- and Tissue-Specificity of Glucocorticoid Actions. *Cell Mol. Immunol.* **2020**, *18*, 269–278. [CrossRef]
10. Gonçalves, K.G.; Pasa, M.C. The Ethnobotany and Medicinal Plants in Community Sucuri, Cuiabá, MT, Brazil. *Interações* **2015**, *16*, 245–256. [CrossRef]
11. Chinnasamy, P.; Arumugam, R.; Ariyan, S. In Silico Validation of the Indigenous Knowledge of the Herbal Medicines among Tribal Communities in Sathyamangalam Wildlife Sanctuary, India. *J. Tradit. Complement. Med.* **2019**, *9*, 143–155. [CrossRef] [PubMed]
12. Ong, H.G.; Kim, Y.-D. Quantitative Ethnobotanical Study of the Medicinal Plants Used by the Ati Negrito Indigenous Group in Guimaras Island, Philippines. *J. Ethnopharmacol.* **2014**, *157*, 228–242. [CrossRef]
13. Yabesh, J.E.M.; Prabhu, S.; Vijayakumar, S. An Ethnobotanical Study of Medicinal Plants Used by Traditional Healers in Silent Valley of Kerala, India. *J. Ethnopharmacol.* **2014**, *154*, 774–789. [CrossRef]
14. Li, D.; Xing, F. Ethnobotanical Study on Medicinal Plants Used by Local Hoklos People on Hainan Island, China. *J. Ethnopharmacol.* **2016**, *194*, 358–368. [CrossRef] [PubMed]
15. Longuefosse, J.L.; Nossin, E. Medical Ethnobotany Survey in Martinique. *J. Ethnopharmacol.* **1996**, *53*, 117–142. [CrossRef] [PubMed]
16. Abe, R.; Ohtani, K. An Ethnobotanical Study of Medicinal Plants and Traditional Therapies on Batan Island, the Philippines. *J. Ethnopharmacol.* **2013**, *145*, 554–565. [CrossRef]
17. Safira, A.; Widayani, P.; An-Najaaty, D.; Rani, C.A.M.; Septiani, M.; Putra, Y.A.S. A Review of an Important Plants: *Annona squamosa* Leaf. *Pharmacogn. J.* **2022**, *14*, 456–463. [CrossRef]
18. Kumar, M.; Changan, S.; Tomar, M.; Prajapati, U.; Saurabh, V.; Hasan, M.; Sasi, M.; Maheshwari, C.; Singh, S.; Dhumal, S.; et al. Custard Apple (*Annona squamosa* L.) Leaves: Nutritional Composition, Phytochemical Profile, and Health-Promoting Biological Activities. *Biomolecules* **2021**, *11*, 614. [CrossRef]
19. Vijayakumar, S.; Morvin Yabesh, J.E.; Prabhu, S.; Manikandan, R.; Muralidharan, B. Quantitative Ethnomedicinal Study of Plants Used in the Nelliyampathy Hills of Kerala, India. *J. Ethnopharmacol.* **2015**, *161*, 238–254. [CrossRef]
20. Quílez, A.M.; Fernández-Arche, M.A.; García-Giménez, M.D.; De la Puerta, R. Potential Therapeutic Applications of the Genus *Annona*: Local and Traditional Uses and Pharmacology. *J. Ethnopharmacol.* **2018**, *225*, 244–270. [CrossRef]
21. Magalhães, K.d.N.; Guarniz, W.A.S.; Sá, K.M.; Freire, A.B.; Monteiro, M.P.; Nojosa, R.T.; Bieski, I.G.C.; Custódio, J.B.; Balogun, S.O.; Bandeira, M.A.M. Medicinal Plants of the Caatinga, Northeastern Brazil: Ethnopharmacopeia (1980–1990) of the Late Professor Francisco José de Abreu Matos. *J. Ethnopharmacol.* **2019**, *237*, 314–353. [CrossRef] [PubMed]
22. Ribeiro, R.V.; Bieski, I.G.C.; Balogun, S.O.; Martins, D.T.d.O. Ethnobotanical Study of Medicinal Plants Used by Ribeirinhos in the North Araguaia Microregion, Mato Grosso, Brazil. *J. Ethnopharmacol.* **2017**, *205*, 69–102. [CrossRef] [PubMed]
23. Singh, D.; Mishra, B.; Mishra, R. Anti-Nociceptive and Anti-Inflammatory Activity of *Annona squamosa* L. Leaf Extract in Mice and Rats. *Res. J. Pharmacogn. Phytochem.* **2012**, *4*, 182–185.
24. Umamaheshwari, A.; Arunkumar, A.; Vedhahari, B.N.; Suryaprabha, D.; Punitha, S. Phytochemical Evaluation and Antinflammatory Activity of Seed Extract of *Annona squamosa*. *Int. J. Chem. Sci.* **2008**, *6*, 1594–1599.
25. Chavan, M.J.; Wakte, P.S.; Shinde, D.B. Analgesic and Anti-Inflammatory Activity of Caryophyllene Oxide from *Annona squamosa* L. Bark. *Phytomedicine* **2010**, *17*, 149–151. [CrossRef]
26. Ning, N.; He, K.; Wang, Y.; Zou, Z.; Wu, H.; Li, X.; Ye, X. Hypolipidemic Effect and Mechanism of Palmatine from Coptis Chinensis in Hamsters Fed High-Fat Diet. *Phytother. Res.* **2015**, *29*, 668–673. [CrossRef]
27. Hambright, H.G.; Batth, I.S.; Xie, J.; Ghosh, R.; Kumar, A.P. Palmatine Inhibits Growth and Invasion in Prostate Cancer Cell: Potential Role for RpS6/NFκB/FLIP. *Mol. Carcinog.* **2015**, *54*, 1227–1234. [CrossRef]
28. Wang, L.; Wang, X.; Zhang, S.-L.; Zhu, X.-M.; Liu, Y.-Q.; Song, Z.-J.; Du, W.-J.; Ji, J.; Cui, C.-L.; He, X.; et al. Gastroprotective Effect of Palmatine against Acetic Acid-Induced Gastric Ulcers in Rats. *J. Nat. Med.* **2017**, *71*, 257–264. [CrossRef]
29. Haj, E.; Losev, Y.; Guru KrishnaKumar, V.; Pichinuk, E.; Engel, H.; Raveh, A.; Gazit, E.; Segal, D. Integrating in Vitro and in Silico Approaches to Evaluate the "Dual Functionality" of Palmatine Chloride in Inhibiting and Disassembling Tau-Derived VQIVYK Peptide Fibrils. *Biochim. Biophys. Acta Gen. Subj.* **2018**, *1862*, 1565–1575. [CrossRef]
30. Shen, Y.; Guan, S.; Ge, H.; Xiong, W.; He, L.; Liu, L.; Yin, C.; Liu, H.; Li, G.; Xu, C.; et al. Effects of Palmatine on Rats with Comorbidity of Diabetic Neuropathic Pain and Depression. *Brain Res. Bull.* **2018**, *139*, 56–66. [CrossRef]

31. Zhou, X.; Lin, X.; Xiong, Y.; Jiang, L.; Li, W.; Li, J.; Wu, L. Chondroprotective Effects of Palmatine on Osteoarthritis in Vivo and in Vitro: A Possible Mechanism of Inhibiting the Wnt/β-Catenin and Hedgehog Signaling Pathways. *Int. Immunopharmacol.* **2016**, *34*, 129–138. [CrossRef] [PubMed]
32. Yan, B.; Wang, D.; Dong, S.; Cheng, Z.; Na, L.; Sang, M.; Yang, H.; Yang, Z.; Zhang, S.; Yan, Z. Palmatine Inhibits TRIF-Dependent NF-KB Pathway against Inflammation Induced by LPS in Goat Endometrial Epithelial Cells. *Int. Immunopharmacol.* **2017**, *45*, 194–200. [CrossRef]
33. Tarabasz, D.; Kukula-Koch, W. Palmatine: A Review of Pharmacological Properties and Pharmacokinetics. *Phytother. Res.* **2020**, *34*, 33–50. [CrossRef]
34. Long, J.; Song, J.; Zhong, L.; Liao, Y.; Liu, L.; Li, X. Palmatine: A Review of Its Pharmacology, Toxicity and Pharmacokinetics. *Biochimie* **2019**, *162*, 176–184. [CrossRef]
35. Zuo, H.; Zhou, W.; Chen, Y.; Zhou, B.; Wang, Z.; Huang, S.; Alinejad, T.; Chen, C. Palmatine Alleviates Particulate Matter-Induced Acute Lung Injury by Inhibiting Pyroptosis via Activating the Nrf2-Related Pathway. *Inflammation* **2024**. [CrossRef] [PubMed]
36. He, L.; Liu, L.; Guan, S.; Zheng, X.; Ge, H.; Yin, C.; Shen, Y.; Tan, M.; Wang, C.; Gao, Y.; et al. Palmatine Alleviates Hyperalgesia by Inhibiting the Expression of Calcitonin Gene-Related Peptide in the Trigeminal Ganglion of Rats with Chronic Constriction Injury of the Infraorbital Nerve. *Br. J. Oral Maxillofac. Surg.* **2020**, *58*, 443–450. [CrossRef] [PubMed]
37. Costa, E.V.; Pinheiro, M.L.B.; Barison, A.; Campos, F.R.; Salvador, M.J.; Maia, B.H.L.N.S.; Cabral, E.C.; Eberlin, M.N. Alkaloids from the Bark of *Guatteria hispida* and Their Evaluation as Antioxidant and Antimicrobial Agents. *J. Nat. Prod.* **2010**, *73*, 1180–1183. [CrossRef]
38. Hemalatha, K.; Satyanarayana, D. Anti-inflammatory activity of *Annona squamosa* Linn. *Biomed. Pharmacol. J.* **2009**, *2*, 17–20.
39. Singh, T.P.; Singh, R.K.; Malik, P. Analgesic and Anti-Inflammatory Activities of *Annona squamosa* Linn Bark. *J. Sci. Innov. Res.* **2014**, *3*, 60–64. [CrossRef]
40. Chen, Y.-Y.; Li, F.-Q.; Zhu, X.-L.; Chen, J.-W.; Li, X. Chemical Composition and Anti-Hepatoma Effect of *Annona squamosa* L. Pericarp Oil. *Nat. Prod. Res.* **2020**, *36*, 401–404. [CrossRef]
41. Shehata, M.G.; Abu-Serie, M.M.; Abd El-Aziz, N.M.; El-Sohaimy, S.A. Nutritional, Phytochemical, and in Vitro Anticancer Potential of Sugar Apple (*Annona squamosa*) Fruits. *Sci. Rep.* **2021**, *11*, 6224. [CrossRef] [PubMed]
42. do Nascimento, K.F.; Moreira, F.M.F.; Alencar Santos, J.; Kassuya, C.A.L.; Croda, J.H.R.; Cardoso, C.A.L.; Vieira, M.D.C.; Góis Ruiz, A.L.T.; Ann Foglio, M.; de Carvalho, J.E.; et al. Antioxidant, Anti-Inflammatory, Antiproliferative and Antimycobacterial Activities of the Essential Oil of *Psidium guineense* Sw. and Spathulenol. *J. Ethnopharmacol.* **2018**, *210*, 351–358. [CrossRef] [PubMed]
43. Dos Santos, E.; Radai, J.A.S.; do Nascimento, K.F.; Formagio, A.S.N.; de Matos Balsalobre, N.; Ziff, E.B.; Castelon Konkiewitz, E.; Kassuya, C.A.L. Contribution of Spathulenol to the Anti-Nociceptive Effects of Psidium Guineense. *Nutr. Neurosci.* **2022**, *25*, 812–822. [CrossRef] [PubMed]
44. Al-Nemari, R.; Al-Senaidy, A.; Semlali, A.; Ismael, M.; Badjah-Hadj-Ahmed, A.Y.; Ben Bacha, A. GC-MS Profiling and Assessment of Antioxidant, Antibacterial, and Anticancer Properties of Extracts of *Annona Squamosa* L. Leaves. *BMC Complement. Med. Ther.* **2020**, *20*, 296. [CrossRef]
45. Paula-Freire, L.I.G.; Andersen, M.L.; Gama, V.S.; Molska, G.R.; Carlini, E.L.A. The Oral Administration of *Trans*-Caryophyllene Attenuates Acute and Chronic Pain in Mice. *Phytomedicine* **2014**, *21*, 356–362. [CrossRef]
46. Aguilar-Ávila, D.S.; Flores-Soto, M.E.; Tapia-Vázquez, C.; Pastor-Zarandona, O.A.; López-Roa, R.I.; Viveros-Paredes, J.M. β-Caryophyllene, a Natural Sesquiterpene, Attenuates Neuropathic Pain and Depressive-Like Behavior in Experimental Diabetic Mice. *J. Med. Food* **2019**, *22*, 460–468. [CrossRef]
47. Oliveira-Tintino, C.D.d.M.; Pessoa, R.T.; Fernandes, M.N.M.; Alcântara, I.S.; da Silva, B.A.F.; de Oliveira, M.R.C.; Martins, A.O.B.P.B.; da Silva, M.d.S.; Tintino, S.R.; Rodrigues, F.F.G.; et al. Anti-Inflammatory and Anti-Edematogenic Action of the *Croton campestris* A. St.-Hil (Euphorbiaceae) Essential Oil and the Compound β-Caryophyllene in in Vivo Models. *Phytomedicine* **2018**, *41*, 82–95. [CrossRef]
48. Katsuyama, S.; Mizoguchi, H.; Kuwahata, H.; Komatsu, T.; Nagaoka, K.; Nakamura, H.; Bagetta, G.; Sakurada, T.; Sakurada, S. Involvement of Peripheral Cannabinoid and Opioid Receptors in β-Caryophyllene-Induced Antinociception. *Eur. J. Pain* **2013**, *17*, 664–675. [CrossRef]
49. Garg, S.N.; Gupta, D. Composition of the Leaf Oil of *Annona squamosa* L. from the North Indian Plains. *J. Essent. Oil Res.* **2005**, *17*, 257–258. [CrossRef]
50. Santos, C.C.d.M.P.; Salvadori, M.S.; Mota, V.G.; Costa, L.M.; de Almeida, A.A.C.; de Oliveira, G.A.L.; Costa, J.P.; de Sousa, D.P.; de Freitas, R.M.; de Almeida, R.N. Antinociceptive and Antioxidant Activities of Phytol In Vivo and In Vitro Models. *Neurosci. J.* **2013**, *2013*, 949452. [CrossRef]
51. Ahmad, S.F.; Zoheir, K.M.A.; Abdel-Hamied, H.E.; Alrashidi, I.; Attia, S.M.; Bakheet, S.A.; Ashour, A.E.; Abd-Allah, A.R.A. Role of a Histamine 4 Receptor as an Anti-Inflammatory Target in Carrageenan-Induced Pleurisy in Mice. *Immunology* **2014**, *142*, 374–383. [CrossRef] [PubMed]
52. Carlos, F.P.; de Paula Alves da Silva, M.; de Lemos Vasconcelos Silva Melo, E.; Costa, M.S.; Zamuner, S.R. Protective Effect of Low-Level Laser Therapy (LLLT) on Acute Zymosan-Induced Arthritis. *Lasers Med. Sci.* **2014**, *29*, 757–763. [CrossRef] [PubMed]

53. Guazelli, C.F.S.; Staurengo-Ferrari, L.; Zarpelon, A.C.; Pinho-Ribeiro, F.A.; Ruiz-Miyazawa, K.W.; Vicentini, F.T.M.C.; Vignoli, J.A.; Camilios-Neto, D.; Georgetti, S.R.; Baracat, M.M.; et al. Quercetin Attenuates Zymosan-Induced Arthritis in Mice. *Biomed. Pharmacother.* **2018**, *102*, 175–184. [CrossRef] [PubMed]
54. Hunskaar, S.; Hole, K. The Formalin Test in Mice: Dissociation between Inflammatory and Non-Inflammatory Pain. *Pain* **1987**, *30*, 103–114. [CrossRef]
55. Ali, H.; Dixit, S. Extraction Optimization of *Tinospora cordifolia* and Assessment of the Anticancer Activity of Its Alkaloid Palmatine. *ScientificWorldJournal* **2013**, *2013*, 376216. [CrossRef]
56. Chaves, S.K.M.; Afzal, M.I.; Islam, M.T.; Hameed, A.; Da Mata, A.M.O.F.; Da Silva Araújo, L.; Ali, S.W.; Rolim, H.M.L.; De Medeiros, M.d.G.F.; Costa, E.V.; et al. Palmatine Antioxidant and Anti-Acetylcholinesterase Activities: A Pre-Clinical Assessment. *Cell Mol. Biol.* **2020**, *66*, 54–59. [CrossRef] [PubMed]
57. Okechukwu, P.N.; Ekeuku, S.O.; Chan, H.K.; Eluri, K.; Froemming, G.R.A. Palmatine Inhibits Up-Regulation of GRP78 and CALR Protein in an STZ-Induced Diabetic Rat Model. *Curr. Pharm. Biotechnol.* **2021**, *22*, 288–298. [CrossRef]
58. Tang, C.; Hong, J.; Hu, C.; Huang, C.; Gao, J.; Huang, J.; Wang, D.; Geng, Q.; Dong, Y. Palmatine Protects against Cerebral Ischemia/Reperfusion Injury by Activation of the AMPK/Nrf2 Pathway. *Oxid. Med. Cell Longev.* **2021**, *2021*, 6660193. [CrossRef]
59. Kim, J.H.; Ryu, Y.B.; Lee, W.S.; Kim, Y.H. Neuraminidase Inhibitory Activities of Quaternary Isoquinoline Alkaloids from *Corydalis turtschaninovii* Rhizome. *Bioorganic Med. Chem.* **2014**, *22*, 6047–6052. [CrossRef]
60. Zhou, J.-T.; Li, C.-L.; Tan, L.-H.; Xu, Y.-F.; Liu, Y.-H.; Mo, Z.-Z.; Dou, Y.-X.; Su, R.; Su, Z.-R.; Huang, P.; et al. Inhibition of Helicobacter Pylori and Its Associated Urease by Palmatine: Investigation on the Potential Mechanism. *PLoS ONE* **2017**, *12*, e0168944. [CrossRef]
61. Ho, Y.-J.; Lu, J.-W.; Huang, Y.-L.; Lai, Z.-Z. Palmatine Inhibits Zika Virus Infection by Disrupting Virus Binding, Entry, and Stability. *Biochem. Biophys. Res. Commun.* **2019**, *518*, 732–738. [CrossRef]
62. He, K.; Kou, S.; Zou, Z.; Hu, Y.; Feng, M.; Han, B.; Li, X.; Ye, X. Hypolipidemic Effects of Alkaloids from *Rhizoma coptidis* in Diet-Induced Hyperlipidemic Hamsters. *Planta Med.* **2016**, *82*, 690–697. [CrossRef] [PubMed]
63. Yang, N.; Wang, L.; Zhang, Y. Immunological Activities of Components from Leaves of *Liriodendron chinensis*. *Chin. Herbal. Med.* **2015**, *7*, 279–282. [CrossRef]
64. Anita, T.Z.; Mahdi, C.; Beltran, M.A.G.; Aulanni'am, A. Identification and Molecular Docking Analysis Alkaloids *Polyalthia longifolia* Leaves from Indonesia and the Philippines as Anti-Inflammatory. *J. Phys. Conf. Ser.* **2019**, *1374*, 012049. [CrossRef]
65. Liu, Y.-L.; Zhou, L.-J.; Hu, N.-W.; Xu, J.-T.; Wu, C.-Y.; Zhang, T.; Li, Y.-Y.; Liu, X.-G. Tumor Necrosis Factor-Alpha Induces Long-Term Potentiation of C-Fiber Evoked Field Potentials in Spinal Dorsal Horn in Rats with Nerve Injury: The Role of NF-Kappa B, JNK and P38 MAPK. *Neuropharmacology* **2007**, *52*, 708–715. [CrossRef]
66. Schäfers, M.; Svensson, C.I.; Sommer, C.; Sorkin, L.S. Tumor Necrosis Factor-α Induces Mechanical Allodynia after Spinal Nerve Ligation by Activation of P38 MAPK in Primary Sensory Neurons. *J. Neurosci.* **2003**, *23*, 2517–2521. [CrossRef]
67. Park, C.-K.; Lü, N.; Xu, Z.-Z.; Liu, T.; Serhan, C.N.; Ji, R.-R. Resolving TRPV1- and TNF-α-Mediated Spinal Cord Synaptic Plasticity and Inflammatory Pain with Neuroprotectin D1. *J. Neurosci.* **2011**, *31*, 15072–15085. [CrossRef]
68. Xu, J.-T.; Xin, W.-J.; Zang, Y.; Wu, C.-Y.; Liu, X.-G. The Role of Tumor Necrosis Factor-Alpha in the Neuropathic Pain Induced by Lumbar 5 Ventral Root Transection in Rat. *Pain* **2006**, *123*, 306–321. [CrossRef]
69. Ali, D.; Ali, H. Assessment of DNA Damage and Cytotoxicity of Palmatine on Human Skin Epithelial Carcinoma Cells. *Toxicol. Environ. Chem.* **2014**, *96*, 941–950. [CrossRef]
70. Zhang, M.; Yu, Y.; Wang, S.; Zhang, Q.; Wu, H.; Wei, J.; Yang, W.; Li, S.; Yang, H. Cardiotoxicity Evaluation of Nine Alkaloids from Rhizoma Coptis. *Hum. Exp. Toxicol.* **2018**, *37*, 185–195. [CrossRef]
71. Vrba, J.; Havlikova, M.; Gerhardova, D.; Ulrichova, J. Palmatine Activates AhR and Upregulates CYP1A Activity in HepG2 Cells but Not in Human Hepatocytes. *Toxicol. Vitr.* **2014**, *28*, 693–699. [CrossRef] [PubMed]
72. Desai, N.; Burade, K.; Agrawal, R. Evaluation of In Vivo and In Vitro Antiarthritic Potential of Annona Squamosa Leaves. *J. Curr. Pharma Res.* **2021**, *13*, 27–44.
73. Vinegar, R.; Truax, J.F.; Selph, J.L. Some Quantitative Temporal Characteristics of Carrageenin-Induced Pleurisy in the Rat. *Proc. Soc. Exp. Biol. Med.* **1973**, *143*, 711–714. [CrossRef]
74. Penido, C.; Conte, F.P.; Chagas, M.S.S.; Rodrigues, C.a.B.; Pereira, J.F.G.; Henriques, M.G.M.O. Antiinflammatory Effects of Natural Tetranortriterpenoids Isolated from *Carapa guianensis* Aublet on Zymosan-Induced Arthritis in Mice. *Inflamm. Res.* **2006**, *55*, 457–464. [CrossRef] [PubMed]
75. Leitão, M.M.; Radai, J.A.S.; Ferrari, I.C.; Negrão, F.J.; Silva-Filho, S.E.; Oliveira, R.J.; Mota, J.d.S.; Kassuya, C.A.L. Effects of an Ethanolic Extract and Fractions from *Piper glabratum* (Piperaceae) Leaves on Pain and Inflammation. *Regul. Toxicol. Pharmacol.* **2020**, *117*, 104762. [CrossRef]

76. Aquino, D.F.d.S.; Piccinelli, A.C.; Soares, F.L.P.; Arena, A.C.; Salvador, M.J.; Kassuya, C.A.L. Anti-Hyperalgesic and Anti-Inflammatory Activity of *Alternanthera maritima* Extract and 2″-O-α-L-Rhamnopyranosylvitexin in Mice. *Inflammation* **2015**, *38*, 2057–2066. [CrossRef]
77. Silva-Filho, S.E.; Wiirzler, L.A.M.; Cavalcante, H.A.O.; Uchida, N.S.; de Souza Silva-Comar, F.M.; Cardia, G.F.E.; da Silva, E.L.; Aguiar, R.P.; Bersani-Amado, C.A.; Cuman, R.K.N. Effect of Patchouli (*Pogostemon cablin*) Essential Oil on in Vitro and in Vivo Leukocytes Behavior in Acute Inflammatory Response. *Biomed. Pharmacother.* **2016**, *84*, 1697–1704. [CrossRef]

pharmaceuticals

MDPI

Article

Anti-Inflammatory Activity of Two Labdane Enantiomers from *Gymnosperma glutinosum*: An *In Vivo*, *In Vitro*, and *In Silico* Study

Salud Pérez-Gutiérrez [1], Nimsi Campos-Xolalpa [2], Sofía A. Estrada-Barajas [1], Alan Carrasco-Carballo [3], Angel Mendoza [4] and Ernesto Sánchez-Mendoza [1,*]

[1] Departamento de Sistemas Biológicos, Universidad Autónoma Metropolitana-Xochimilco, Calzada del Hueso 1100, Coyoacán, Ciudad de México 04960, Mexico; msperez@correo.xoc.uam.mx (S.P.-G.); sofiiabii11@gmail.com (S.A.E.-B.)

[2] Secretaria de Ciencia, Humanidades, Tecnología e Innovación (SECIHTI), Departamento de Sistemas Biológicos, Universidad Autónoma Metropolitana-Xochimilco, Calzada del Hueso 1100, Coyoacán, Ciudad de México 04960, Mexico; ncampos@correo.xoc.uam.mx

[3] Secretaria de Ciencia, Humanidades, Tecnología e Innovación (SECIHTI), Laboratorio de Elucidación y Síntesis en Química Orgánica, Instituto de Ciencias, Benemérita Universidad Autónoma de Puebla, Blvd. Capitán Carlos Camacho Espíritu, Puebla 72540, Mexico; alan.carrascoc@correo.buap.mx

[4] Centro de Química, Instituto de Ciencias, Benemérita Universidad Autónoma de Puebla, 18 Sur y Av. San Claudio, Col. San Manuel, Puebla 72570, Mexico; angel.mendoza@correo.buap.mx

* Correspondence: esanchez@correo.xoc.uam.mx

Abstract: Background/Objectives: Diseases associated with inflammatory processes continue to grow steadily throughout the world. Unfortunately, prolonged use of drugs induces adverse effects ranging from hypersensitivity reactions to damage to the digestive system. These negative effects open the possibility of continuing the search for anti-inflammatory compounds with less toxicity. The aim of this research was to isolate and evaluate the anti-inflammatory activity of a mixture of two enantiomeric labdanes isolated from *Gymnosperma glutinosum* by *in vivo*, *in vitro*, and *in silico* methods. **Methods**: A brief description of the main methods or treatments applied. This can include any relevant preregistration or specimen information. The structure of the labdanes enantiomers was elucidated by X-ray crystallography and spectroscopies methods. The anti-inflammatory effect was evaluated on a mouse model of ear edema induced with 12-O-tetradecanoyl phorbol-13-acetate; the pro-inflammatory mediators, nitric oxide (NO) and interleukin (IL-6), were quantified on macrophages stimulated with lipopolysaccharide, and the interaction between labdanes and diana was studied by molecular docking. **Results**: We identified the chemical structures of two new labdane enantiomers: *a*-gymglu acid and *b*-*ent*-gymglu acid. The enantiomer mixture, named gymglu acid, diminished ear edema at doses of 1 and 2 mg/ear by 36.07% and 41.99%, respectively. A concentration of 155.16 μM of gymglu acid inhibited the production of NO by 78.06% and IL-6 by 71.04%. The *in silico* results suggest two routes by which these labdanes reduce inflammation: partial agonism toward the corticosteroid receptors and inhibition of nitric oxide synthases. **Conclusions**: These results show that the gymglu acid enantiomers have promising anti-inflammatory activity.

Keywords: enantiomers; molecular docking; cytokines; cell viability; stabilization of membrane

1. Introduction

The incidence of diseases associated with inflammatory processes continues to grow steadily throughout the global population. Conditions such as rheumatoid arthritis, ulcerative colitis, chronic obstructive pulmonary disease, psoriasis, atherosclerosis, and multiple sclerosis, among others, involve inflammatory processes that can become disabling. The treatment of these diseases is based on the prescription of anti-inflammatory drugs and analgesics. Unfortunately, prolonged use of these compounds induces adverse effects ranging from hypersensitivity reactions to digestive system damage. These negative effects have necessitated the continual search for new compounds with anti-inflammatory activity and fewer adverse effects [1].

Inflammation is a natural defense mechanism used by the body to protect itself against infections and injury. It involves cellular and vascular events, including the activation of monocytes, basophils, eosinophils, and macrophages, as well as the overproduction of some inflammatory mediators, such as nitric oxide (NO), tumor necrosis factor-alpha (TNF-α), interleukin (IL-1β), and IL-6 [2]. Dysregulation of these mediators is associated with different diseases, pain, and hyperalgesia.

According to the World Health Organization (WHO), more than 170 countries have reported the use of traditional medicine as an alternative method for the relief and treatment of different diseases. The use of herbal medicines, extracts, infusions, tonics, and even the direct application of plant material is currently a commonly used alternative treatment in the Mexican population for the relief of various diseases. Therefore, there has been a focused scientific effort to isolate and evaluate the biological activity of different plant metabolites and thereby obtain information that can be applied to the development of new drugs. Furthermore, knowledge of the chemical structure of secondary metabolites allows for the prediction of possible mechanisms of action that explain the observed biological effects with the help of bioinformatics. For example, molecular docking revealed that Z-geranial, a compound identified in *Cymbopogon citratus* essential oil, has greater binding energy than does a commercial M1 muscarinic acetylcholine receptor blocker and blocks the M2 receptor, whereas β-pinene and β-myrcene block the M1, M2, and M4 receptors [3]. These actions may positively affect cardiovascular activity, memory, Alzheimer's disease, and schizophrenia.

Gymnosperma glutinosum (Sprengel) Less. is a plant that has been used in traditional Mexican medicine to combat different diseases. Infusions of this species have been used to treat diarrhea, rheumatism, skin infections, ulcers, and abscesses. *G. glutinosum* belongs to the Asteraceae family; it is commonly known as Tatalencho, Escobilla, Jarilla, and Pegajosa. Scientific studies of this plant have demonstrated the presence of essential oil, flavonoids, and diterpenes [4]. Canales et al. found that methanolic extracts of *G. glutinosum* collected from different regions of Mexico presented antimicrobial and antifungal activity [5]. Moreover, for the first time, they isolated two metabolites from these extracts, namely, (−)-17-hydroxy-neo-clerod-3-en-15-oic acid and 5,7-dihydroxy-3,6,8,2,4,5-hexamethoxyflavone. In addition, compounds with other biological activities have been isolated: (−)-13S,14R,15-trihydroxy-7-oxo-ent-labd-8(9)-ene showed cytotoxic activity against the L5178Y-R lymphoma cell line [6], and (+)-8S,13S,14R,15-ent-labdanetetrol exerted antifungal activity [7]. Other diterpenes have also been isolated, including (+)-ent-labd-7-en-13S,14R,15-triol and (−)-17-hydroxy-neo-clerod-3-en-15-oic acid [8] as well as 2-angeloyl ent-dihydrotucumanoic, which exerts moderate *in vitro* anti-inflammatory and *in vivo* antinociceptive effects [9]. Alonso-Castro et al. reported that 2-angeloyl ent-dihydrotucumanoic has anti-inflammatory, antinociceptive, cytotoxic, and antimicrobial effects [10]. In previous studies conducted by our research group, we demonstrated that the dichloromethane extract of this plant had anti-inflammatory activity in auricular edema in mice induced by TPA [11]. Based on this background, we studied the anti-inflammatory effect of methanolic and dichloromethane extracts of *G. glutinosum*. Furthermore, two enantiomeric labdanes were isolated, and their chemical structures were elucidated. *In vivo*, *in vitro*, and *in silico* methods were used to comprehensively evaluate the anti-inflammatory effects of two labdane enantiomers.

2. Results

2.1. Isolation and Structural Analysis of Gymglu Acid

Gymglu acid was isolated from the 60:40 hexane-ethyl acetate fraction from the dichloromethane extract, with a yield of 0.067% and a melting point of 189–190 °C. The spectroscopic data, particularly crystallographic studies, confirmed that the white, needle-shaped crystals of gymglu acid are formed by two diterpenoids of the *ent*-labdane type.

2.1.1. Crystallographic Evaluation

We used the CrysAlisPro software (version 1.171.43) to process the X-ray data and to apply numerical absorption correction [12]. We solved the structures with direct methods via the ShelXT program and refined them with full-matrix least-squares based on F^2 with SHELXL-2019 [13]. We refined the positional and anisotropic atomic displacement parameters for all nonhydrogen atoms. The hydrogen atoms were identified from the Fourier map and included as fixed contributions attached to their parent atoms, with isotropic thermal factors chosen as 1.2 and 1.5 times their respective carrier atoms. We employed the OLEX2 software (version 1.5-alpha) [14] as a graphical interface.

Crystallographic analysis determined that gymglu acid corresponds to a mixture of two enantiomeric labdanes, with the structural elucidation and stereochemical configuration of the carbons determined as follows: (5S,8R,9R,10S)-8-hydroxy-labda-13(Z)-ene-15-oic acid, which we named *a*-gymglu acid, and (5R,8S,9S,10R)-8-hydroxy-labda-13(Z)-ene-15-oic acid, which we named *b-ent*-gymglu acid (Figure 1a–c). *a*-gymglu acid and *b-ent*-gymglu acid crystallize in a monoclinic system with a P21/c space group, and the asymmetric unit corresponds to $C_{20}H_{34}O_3$. The crystallographic parameters are shown in Table S1. The crystal packing shows two hydrogen bonds: one of them is intramolecular, O1—H1···O2, and the other is intermolecular, O3—H3···O1 (Supplementary Material). The crystallographic data for *a*-gymglu acid and *b-ent*-gymglu acid were deposited in the Cambridge Crystallographic Data Center (CCDC numbers 2364580), and Mercury (Version 2022 3.0) [15] was used to represent crystallographic data.

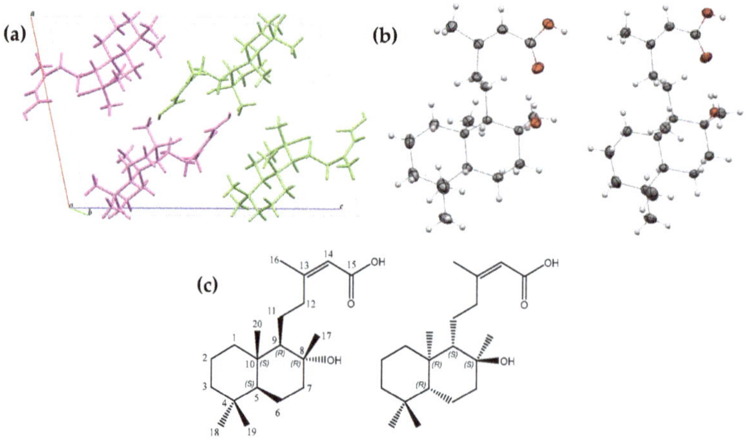

Figure 1. (**a**) Unit cell showing *a*-gymglu acid (violet) and *b-ent*-gymglu acid (green), a, b, and c are the lengths of unit cell edges. (**b**) Molecular structure for each enantiomer showing 30% probability displacement ellipsoids. (**c**) Chemical structure of *a*-gymglu acid and *b-ent*-gymglu acid (IUPAC name in Supplementary Materials).

2.1.2. FT-IR and NMR Evaluation

The FT-IR spectra presented the following peaks: 3408.89 cm^{-1} (OH); 3300.0–2600 cm^{-1} (COOH); 3100 (=C-H); 2923.95, 2889.44, 1458.06, and 1386.37 cm^{-1} (C-H); 1688.88 cm^{-1} (C=O); and 1637.27 cm^{-1} (C=C).

We recorded the ^1H, ^{13}C, gCOSY, TOCSY, gHSQC, and gHMBC NMR spectra in a $CDCl_3$ solution at 299 K (NMR spectra are provided in Supplementary Material). We assigned the correlations between protons and carbons based on an analysis of the gCOSY and gHSQC NMR spectra, and we confirmed the structural position of the quaternary carbon based on the gHMBC NMR correlations (Table 1). The complete NMR assignment included the following:

Table 1. NMR Correlations.

Carbon	HSQC Correlations	HMBC Correlations
1	39.17: 1.96, 0.93	C1, H20
2	18.45: 1.60, 1.43	C2, H3′
3	41.94: 1.37, 1.14	C3, H18; C3, H19
4	33.24	C4, H18; C4, H19
5	55.97: 0.92	C5, H20; C5, H19; C5, H18
6	20.18: 1.64, 1.25	C6, H5; C6, H7′
7	42.96: 1.83, 1.44	C7, H5; C7, H17
8	74.06	C8, H17; C8, H9; C8, H7; C8, H7′; C8, H11
9	61.02: 1.17	C9, H12; C9, H12′; C9, H7; C9, H7′; C9, H17; C9, H20; C9, H5; C9, H11
10	38.73	C10, H5; C10, H20
11	24.23: 1.48	C11, H12; C11, H12′
12	37.27: 2.95, 2.19	C12, H14; C12, H16; C12, H11
13	161.98	C13, H12; C13, H12′; C13, H19; C13, H11; C13, H14
14	115.86: 5.68	C14, H12; C14, H12′; C14, H16
15	168.70	C15, H14
16	25.85: 1.91	C16, H14; C16, H12; C16, H12′
17	24.21: 1.17	C17, H12; C17, H12′; C17, H9; C17, H7; C17, H7′
18	33.34: 0.87	C18, H19; C19, H5; C18, H3′
19	21.44: 0.78	C19, H18; C19, H5; C19, H3′
20	15.48: 0.75	C20, H5; C20, H9

^{13}C NMR (151 MHz, $CDCl_3$) δ (ppm) C1 39.17, C2 18.45, C3 41.94, C4 33.24, C5 55.97, C6 20.18, C7 42.96, C8 74.06, C9 61.02, C10 38.73, C11 24.23, C12 37.27, C13 161.98, C14 115.86, C15 168.70, C16 25.85, C17 24.21, C18 33.34, C19 21.44, and C20 15.48; ^1H NMR (600 MHz, $CDCl_3$ δ (ppm) H1 1.69 (dd, J = 12.7, 3.5 Hz), H1′ 0.93 (m); H2 1.61 (m), H2′ 1.43 (m), H3 1.37 (dd, J = 13.1, 3.4 Hz), H3′ 1.14 (dd, J = 13.1, 4.2 Hz), H5 0.92 (m), H6 1.64 (m), H6′ 1.25 (m), H7 1.83 (dt, J = 12.5, 3.3 Hz), H7′ 1.44 (m), H9 1.17 (m), H11 1.48 (m), H12 2.95 (td, J = 11.3, 5.0 Hz), H12′ 2.19 (td, J = 11.3, 7.1 Hz), H14 5.68 (d, J = 1.5 Hz), H16 1.91 (d, J = 1.5 Hz), H17 1.17 (s), H18 0.87 (s), H19 0.78, and H20 0.75 (s).

2.2. *In Vivo and In Vitro Evaluation of Gymglu Acid*

The mixture of *a*-gymglu acid and *b-ent*-gymglu acid presented a low yield; thus, separating enantiomers was not possible. Therefore, the *in vivo* and *in vitro* analyses were performed only with the mixture, referred to simply as gymglu acid, for these experiments.

2.2.1. Anti-Inflammatory Activity in a Mouse Ear Edema Induced with TPA

Table 2 presents the anti-inflammatory activity of the dichloromethane and methanol extracts of *G. glutinosum* and indomethacin (positive control) in a mouse ear edema induced with TPA. The dichloromethane extract diminished ear edema by 52.83 ± 5.28%, which was better than that of the methanol extract and comparable to that of indomethacin (49.74 ± 4.25%).

Table 2. The anti-inflammatory activity of the *G. glutinosum* extracts and indomethacin on a mouse ear edema induced with 12-O-tetradecanoyl phorbol-13-acetate.

Group	Percent Decrease in Inflammation	Weight Differences (mg)
Methanol extract (2 mg/ear)	41.96 ± 6.5 *	6.14 ± 0.69 #
Dichloromethane extract (2 mg/ear)	52.83 ± 5.28	4.99 ± 0.56 #
Indomethacin (2 mg/ear)	49.74 ± 4.25	5.31 ± 0.48 #
Negative	------	10.58 ± 0.41

The values are the mean ± S.E.M. (n = 8). $p < 0.05$ versus the * Indomethacin group and # Negative group.

Gymglu acid was isolated from the bioactive extract, and its anti-inflammatory activity was evaluated. We tested two doses (1 and 2 mg) of the gymglu acid on the mouse ear edema induced with TPA (Table 3). The results show that 2 mg/ear dose diminished ear edema by 41.99 ± 3.57%, similar to the effect of indomethacin (50.27 ± 4.46%).

Table 3. The anti-inflammatory activity of gymglu acid on a mouse model of ear edema induced with 12-O-tetradecanoyl phorbol-13-acetate.

Group	Percent Decrease in Inflammation	Weight Differences (mg)
Gymglu acid (1 mg/ear)	36.07 ± 0.84 *	7.57 ± 0.19 #
Gymglu acid (2 mg/ear)	41.99 ± 3.57 *	6.7 ± 0.44 #
Indomethacin (2 mg/ear)	50.27 ± 4.46	5.7 ± 0.52 #
Negative	------	11.55 ± 0.36

The values are the mean ± S.E.M. (n = 8). $p < 0.05$ versus the * Indomethacin and # Negative group.

2.2.2. Effect of Gymglu Acid on J774A.1 Macrophages Cell Viability

In accordance with previously described methods, we determined the effect of gymglu acid on the viability of J774A.1 macrophages (Table 4). The results show that the IC_{50} was 390.09 µM. Therefore, in subsequent tests, we used a concentration of 155.04 µM, which did not affect the 70% cell viability.

Table 4. Percentage of the viability of the J774A.1 macrophages treated with gymglu acid.

µM	% Cell Viability
0	100 ± 3.32
3.11	92.93 ± 2.86
15.53	83.79 ± 1.93
31.06	81.92 ± 1.75
77.64	73.33 ± 2.13
155.28	74.27 ± 1.86
232.92	71.24 ± 1.82
310.56	57.03 ± 2.05

The values are the mean ± S.E.M.

2.2.3. Measurement of Proinflammatory Mediator Levels

As mentioned above, we stimulated J774A.1 macrophages with LPS to induce the release of pro-inflammatory mediators such as NO and IL-6. Findings revealed that gymglu acid at a concentration of 155.04 µM inhibited the production of NO by 79.18%, a stronger effect compared with dexamethasone (52.32%) ($p < 0.05$). Moreover, gymglu acid at the same concentration inhibited the production of IL-6 (71.04%), while the reference compound did the same at 83.8% ($p < 0.05$) (Figure 2).

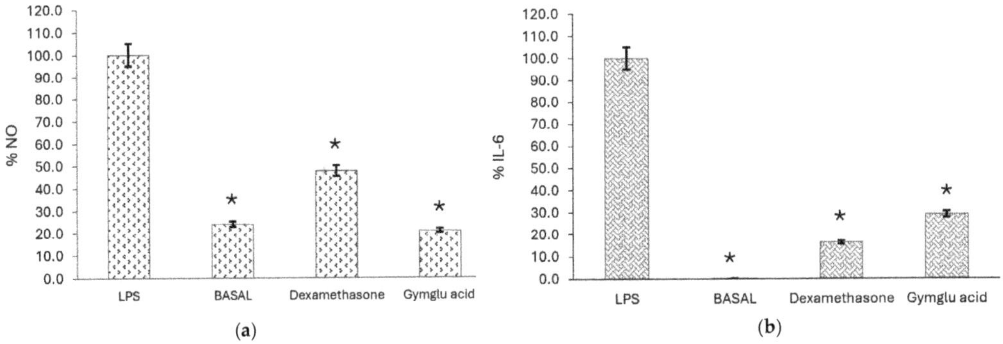

Figure 2. The effect of gymglu acid (155.04 μM) and dexamethasone (12.74 μM) on the release of (**a**) NO and (**b**) IL-6 from J774A.1 macrophages stimulated with LPS. The graph represents the mean ± S.E.M. of three independent experiments (n = 4). * $p < 0.05$ compared with the LPS group.

2.2.4. The Membrane Protective Effect of Gymglu Acid

The membrane protective effect of gymglu acid was evaluated, as presented in Table 5; increasing the gymglu acid concentration increased the percentage of erythrocyte membrane protection. This behavior is similar to that of diclofenac. However, the IC_{50} of diclofenac (38.81 μg/mL) was lower than gymglu acid (94.47 μg/mL).

Table 5. Percentage of the hemolysis of the erythrocyte membrane treated with diclofenac and gymglu acid.

Concentration (μg/mL)	% Erythrocyte Membrane Protection	
	Diclofenac	**Gymglu Acid**
200	63.04 ± 3.98	56.43 ± 0.95
100	61.30 ± 0.54	52.46 ± 0.59
50	51.15 ± 3.05	30.24 ± 0.48
25	45.96 ± 4.81	17.69 ± 1.69
12.5	31.39 ± 5.17	8.57 ± 1.35
0	100.00 ± 0.59	100.00 ± 0.58
IC_{50} (μg/mL)	38.806	94.47

The values are the mean ± S.E.M. (n = 8).

2.3. *In Silico Results*

As the *a*-gymglu acid and *b-ent*-gymglu acid may interact differently with the organism during the inflammatory process, bioinformatics studies were realized with the enantiomeric structures. Based on the chemical structures, we searched for the molecular targets underlying the anti-inflammatory and antioxidant activities of *a*-gymglu acid and *b-ent*-gymglu acid. We performed structural similarity analysis via SwissTargetPrediction in combination with STRING relationship analysis (Figure 3). The second pathway focuses on oxidative stress via PPARA and the downstream response was triggered by this regulation (Figure 3).

We assessed the MR, GR, HSD11B1, PPARA, nNOS, iNOS, and eNOS as molecular targets by molecular docking and MM-GBSA. The results showed the regulation via NOSs based on molecular docking calculations. The results presented in Table 6 indicate that the *b-ent*-gymglu acid has even greater coupling than the reference for the PPARA pathway, suggesting it may be an antagonist of this pathway.

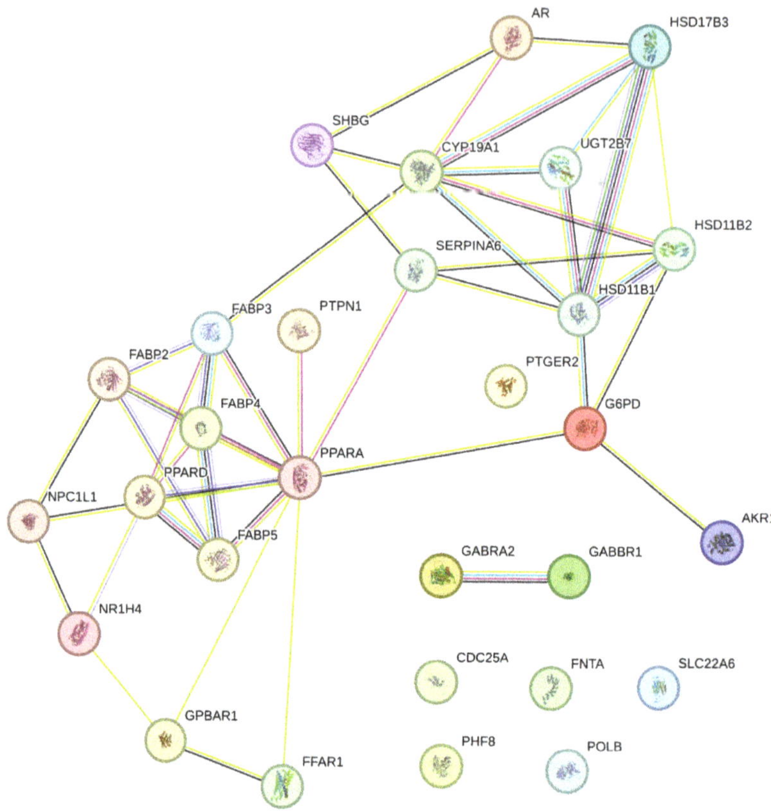

Figure 3. The relationship between the isolated molecules (*a*-gymglu acid and *b-ent*-gymglu acid) and interacting proteins.

Table 6. Docking scores for *a*-gymglu acid and *b-ent*-gymglu acid with select proteins of interest.

Protein	*a*-Gymglu Acid	*b-ent*-Gymglu Acid	Reference
PPARA	NI/NI	−6.229/−55.19	−4.287/−43.56 (thiazolidinediones)
MR	−7.245/−83.98	−6.016/−67.30	−9.324/−93.64 (dexamethasone)
GR	−7.867/−19.98	−7.019/−17.37	−10.258/−31.02 (dexamethasone)
HSD11B1	−6.095/−36.87	−5.064/−39.36	−6.038/−37.26 (glycyrrhizic acid)
iNOS	−4.025/−9.96	−4.318/−12.38	−3.876/−11.38 (L-NMMA)
eNOS	−4.128/−10.12	−3.975/−11.52	−3.957/−11.45 (L-NMMA)
nNOS	−3.017/−9.35	−3.358/−10.98	−3.797/−11.92 (L-NMMA)

NI—no interaction encounter.

In contrast to the corticosteroid route, we observed a partial agonism for the MR and the GR, indicating a direct relationship between the dose and the anti-inflammatory effect. Figure 4 presents the differences in the interactions between the enantiomers and the sites of action. For the MR, the carboxylate of *b-ent*-gymglu acid interacts via Arg817 (Figure 4b), whereas for *a*-gymglu acid, it interacts via Asn770 (Figure 4a), indicating that the three-dimensional arrangement of the enantiomers plays a very important role in the way these molecules couple with their receptors. For example, when coupled with GR, only *a*-gymglu acid hydrogen bonds with Asn564 (Figure 4d); however, both structures maintain an amphipathic environment, characteristic of partial activation of this receptor. In addition, regarding the regulation of corticosteroid production, only *a*-gymglu acid has sufficient energy to overcome cortisol, leading to inhibition of the cortisol to cortisone pathway and resulting in increased cortisol levels. Nevertheless, this action deregulates the system, so the dose is important for regulating the pathway and thus, the cortisol levels.

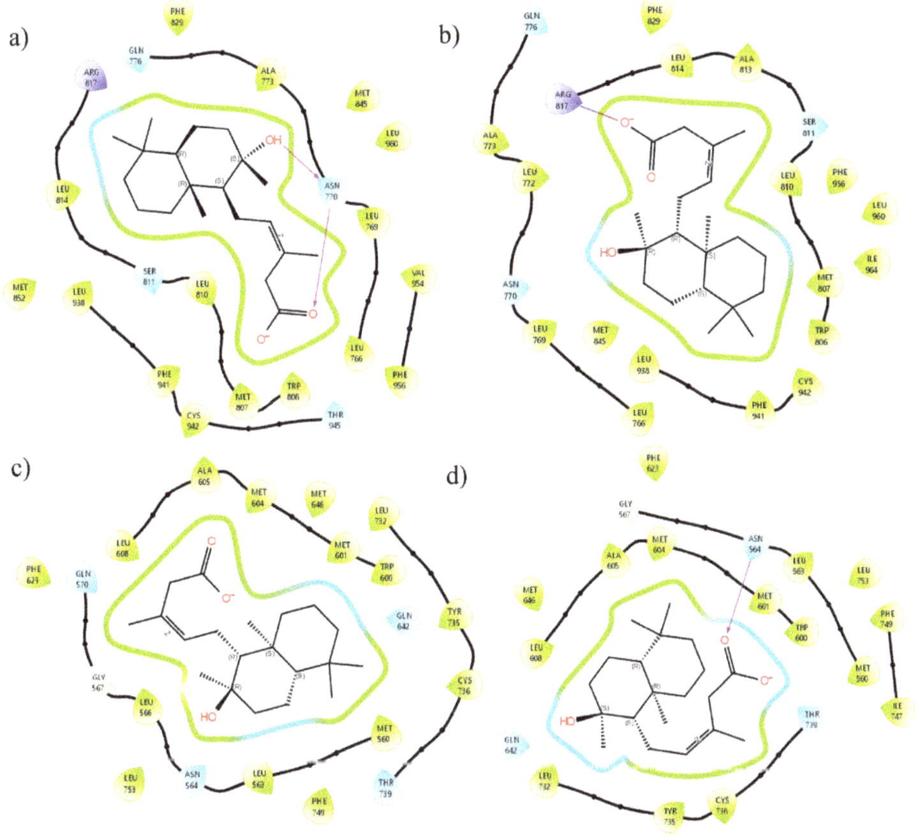

Figure 4. A two-dimensional interaction diagram of (**a**) *b-ent*-gymglu acid with the MR, (**b**) *a*-gymglu acid with the MR, (**c**) *b-ent*-gymglu acid with the GR, and (**d**) *a*-gymglu acid with the GR.

Finally, when analyzing the effects on NOSs, we found a preference for iNOS, followed by eNOS and nNOS (Table 4). These findings indicate a certain specificity for systemic regulation prior to regulation of the central nervous system. This phenomenon explains the decrease in NO levels caused by both compounds. To summarize, the enantiomeric mixture has multitarget activity, starting from partial agonism of the GR and MR, as well as a downregulation of oxidative stress via selective inhibition of NOSs.

3. Discussion

In the present study, for the first time, we obtained a white crystalline solid from the dichloromethane extract of *G. glutinosum*, which we identified as an enantiomeric mixture of labdanes. Many reports suggest that these diterpenoids have a wide variety of bioactivities, including antibacterial, cytotoxic, and anti-inflammatory effects, as well as hepatoprotective and neuroprotective effects. In this work, we found that gymglu acid exhibited anti-inflammatory activity because it inhibited TPA-induced ear edema in mice. TPA leads to edema, erythema, and infiltration of neutrophils and leukocytes and activates protein kinase C [16] and phospholipase A2 [17]. These results suggest that gymglu acid can inhibit the activation of some of these enzymes and inflammatory cells.

NO is involved in physiological functions such as vasodilation and neuronal transmission; it is produced by monocytes, macrophages, and neutrophils as part of the immune response [18]. NO is produced by constitutively expressed NOS isoforms (eNOS and nNOS) as well as by iNOS, which promote the formation of reactive nitrogen species that are involved with tissue damage. NO overexpression promotes the release of inflammatory cytokines, such as IL-1β, TNF-α, and IL-6, among others [19]. IL-6 has pleiotropic activity and plays an important role in the acquired immune response by stimulating the production of antibodies and the development of effector T cells; however, continuous unregulated production of IL-6 leads to the development of different diseases such as those related to inflammation [20]. Therefore, compounds that inhibit the production of NO and IL-6 could be used to treat different inflammatory problems. Our results demonstrated that gymglu acid reduced NO and IL-6 production in LPS-stimulated macrophages. These conclusions are supported by previously published studies that have shown that some diterpene labdanes have anti-inflammatory activity via the inhibition of NF-κB activity, modulation of arachidonic acid metabolism, and reduction of NO production [21].

During the inflammatory response, neutrophils release their lysosomal components, such as proteases and bactericidal enzymes, further increasing inflammation. Lysosomal membrane components are analogous to human erythrocyte membranes [22]. We found that gymglu acid protected the human erythrocyte membrane from hemolysis, with protection increased as the gymglu acid concentration increased.

The *in silico* results suggest two routes by which *a*-gymglu acid and *b-ent*-gymglu acid exert their effects, and biological results are the result of the sum of both. The first mechanism, with a lesser impact, involves partial agonism of the corticosteroid receptors, which can partially explain the ability of *a*-gymglu acid to reduce inflammation. Indeed, GR agonism has been reported to have anti-inflammatory effects. Moreover, partial agonism of the GR and the MR may underlie the positive effects of both enantiomers on hemolysis [23]. The second route is the inhibition of NOSs: *b-ent*-gymglu acid predominately inhibits iNOS, which is directly correlated with its ability to reduce NO production in LPS-stimulated macrophages. However, in further studies, the activity of gymglu on iNOS and GR will be determined.

In summary, the enantiomers studied presented inhibitory inflammatory effects based on the *in silico*, *in vitro*, and *in vivo* results. Therefore, the anti-inflammatory effects of gymglu acid make it a very relevant active ingredient that could be promising to treat acute and chronic inflammation. Therefore, this study suggests that gymglu acid could have the potential to be an alternative anti-inflammatory agent.

4. Materials and Methods

4.1. Materials

Fetal bovine serum (FBS), Dulbecco's Modified Eagle's Medium (DMEM), penicillin-streptomycin antibiotics, indomethacin, 3-(4,5-dimethylthiazol-2-yl)-2,5-diphenyl tetrazolium bromide (MTT), the Griess reagent, dimethyl sulfoxide (DMSO), lipopolysaccharide (LPS), polyvinylpyrrolidone (PVP), and 12-O-tetradecanoylphorbol-13-acetate (TPA) were purchased from Sigma Aldrich (St. Louis, MO, USA). The enzyme-linked immunosorbent assay (ELISA) kits were obtained from TONBO Bioscience (San Diego, CA, USA).

4.2. Plant Material

The plant was gathered through ecological pruning, and aerial parts of *G. glutinosum* were collected on highway 70, San Luis Potosí—Rio Verde, in August 2018. The plant was identified by M.Sc. Gabriel Flores Franco of the Universidad Autónoma del Estado de Morelos (UAEM). A voucher specimen (HUMO35267) was deposited in the herbarium (HUMO) of the UAEM.

4.3. Obtaining Extracts

The aerial parts of *G. glutinosum* were dried in the shade at room temperature. Subsequently, 300 g of previously ground plant was macerated in 2 L of dichloromethane or methanol for 8 days. Then, the mixture was filtered, and the solvent was removed on a rotatory evaporator under reduced pressure. The anti-inflammatory activity of the extracts was evaluated in a mouse ear edema model induced with TPA.

4.4. Isolation of a White Crystalline Solid: Gymglu Acid

The bioactive extract was separated by an open-column chromatography (column height 70 cm; column diameter 3 cm) packed with silica gel (Macherey-Nagel 60, 70–230 mesh ASTM). The mobile phase comprises hexane with increasing amounts of ethyl acetate to increase polarity; 100 mL of each fraction was collected. A white crystalline solid, named gymglu acid, was obtained from the 60:40 hexane–ethyl acetate fraction. The anti-inflammatory activity of this compound was subsequently evaluated in a mouse ear edema model induced with TPA.

4.5. Structural Analysis of the Solid Crystalline

Gymglu acid was analyzed via different spectroscopic techniques: Fourier transform infrared (FTIR) spectra were obtained via a Spectrum Two FT-IR spectrometer (Perkin Elmer, Waltham, MA, USA) with attenuated total reflectance (ATR). Nuclear Magnetic Resonance (NMR) spectra were recorded in a deuterated chloroform ($CDCl_3$) solution at 299 K on a DD2 600 spectrometer (Agilent, Palo Alto, CA, USA). The ^1H and ^{13}C NMR chemical shifts were reported relative to those of TMS and $CDCl_3$, respectively. From a previously reported fraction, suitable crystals of gymglu acid were obtained via slow evaporation. For X-ray diffraction, data were collected with an Oxford Diffraction Gemini-Atlas diffractometer equipped with a charge-coupled device area detector and graphite monochromate Mo-Kα radiation (λ = 0.71073 Å).

4.6. Animals

Male CD1 mice weighing 25–30 g were supplied by the Universidad Autónoma Metropolitana-Xochimilco (UAM-X) bioterium. The animals had free access to water and food and were kept at 20–22 °C under a 12 h photoperiod. The study was conducted according to the Official Mexican Standard (NOM-062-ZOO-1999) [24]. The protocol (number 140) was approved by the Research Bioethics Committee of UAM-X.

4.7. Anti-Inflammatory Activity in Mouse Ear Edema Induced with TPA

Groups were formed with eight mice each and treated as follows: a solution of 2.5 µg of TPA in 20 µL of acetone was topically applied to the right ear of each mouse. After 30 min, one of the following treatments was applied on the right ear by group: 20 µL of vehicle (negative control), 2 mg of indomethacin (positive control), 2 mg of dichloromethane or methanol extract, or 1 or 2 mg of gymglu acid (test groups). All extracts or compounds were dissolved in 20 µL of the vehicle (dichloromethane, acetone or methanol), and in the left ear to all mice, 20 µL of the vehicle was administered. Six hours after the administration of TPA, the mice were euthanized in a CO_2 chamber, and a central 6 mm portion was obtained from both ears of the mice. These portions were weighed to calculate the percentage of edema inhibition according to the following equation [25]:

$$\% \text{ inhibition} = \left(\frac{(\text{Wt} - \text{Wnt})\text{control} - (\text{Wt} - \text{Wnt})\text{treated}}{(\text{Wt} - \text{Wnt})\text{control}} \right) \times 100$$

where Wt is the weight of the treated ear, and Wnt is the weight of the non-treated ear.

4.8. Cell Viability Assay

J774A.1 cells murine macrophage were cultured in 96-well plates (5×10^3 cells per well) with DMEM containing 10% FBS, HEPES/NaOH (20 mM) at pH 7.4, $NaHCO_3$ (2 mM), antibiotics including 100 μg/mL streptomycin and 100 U/mL penicillin at 37 °C, and 5% CO_2. Twenty-four hours later, the cells were treated with 3.10, 15.50, 31.03, 77.52, 155.16, 310.32, or 620.64 μM gymglu acid in phosphate-buffered saline (PBS). Untreated cells served as a negative control. Forty-eight hours after treatment, 10 μL MTT (5 mg/mL) was added, and the plates were incubated for 4 h. Next, the medium was removed, and the formazan crystals were dissolved in 100 μL DMSO. The absorbance was measured at 540 nm via an ELISA plate reader (spectrophotometer, Bio-Rad Laboratories Inc., Hercules, CA, USA). The half-maximal inhibitory concentration (IC_{50}) was calculated via linear regression analysis.

4.9. Determination of NO and IL-6 Levels

Initially, 5×10^5 J774A.1 macrophages were seeded per well in 6-well plates; they were then stimulated with 5 μg/mL LPS. Two hours after treatment with 155.16 μM gymglu acid, 12.74 μM dexamethasone, or PBS, the cells were stimulated with LPS. After 24 h, the supernatants were collected for NO and IL-6 quantification. For NO analysis, 100 μL Griess reagent and 100 μL supernatant were mixed, the mixture was incubated for 30 min at 37 °C, and the absorbance was read at 540 nm with an ELISA plate reader (Bio-Rad spectrophotometer). The percentage of NO production was calculated based on the group treated with only LPS as a reference [26]. To quantify IL-6, a portion of the supernatant was analyzed via a commercial ELISA following the manufacturer's instructions (Promega, Madison, WI, USA). The absorbance was read at 405 nm via a spectrophotometer.

4.10. Membrane Stabilization Assay

Blood samples were collected by the physician of the UAM-X medical service from a healthy volunteer under aseptic conditions. The volunteer signed a letter of consent and declared had not consumed nonsteroidal anti-inflammatory drugs, steroidal anti-inflammatory drugs, or contraceptives 2 weeks prior to collection. The blood samples (10 mL) were washed with an equal volume of Alsever's solution (2% dextrose, 0.8% sodium citrate, 0.05% citric acid, and 0.42% sodium chloride in water) and centrifuged at 3000 rpm for 10 min. Subsequently, a 10% (*v*/*v*) suspension of erythrocytes with isosaline solution (HRBC) was prepared.

Three groups (n = 4) were established; each tube was prepared with 150 μL of HRBC and 550 μL of hyposaline solution (0.036%), and 300 μL of the sample to be evaluated was added. Phosphate buffer was added to the negative control group; diclofenac was added to the positive control group; and gymglu acid was added to the test group at concentrations of 6.25, 12.5, 25, 50, 100, and 200 μg/mL.

All the samples were incubated at 37 °C for 30 min; subsequently, the samples were centrifuged at 3500 rpm for 5 min, and then 100 μL of the supernatant was added to a 96-

well plate. The absorbances were read at 540 nm via a spectrophotometer. The erythrocyte membrane protection percentages were calculated via the following formula [27]:

$$\% \text{ Hemolysis} = \frac{\text{absorbance of test sample}}{\text{Absorbance of control}} \times 100$$

4.11. Statistical Analysis

The results are expressed as the mean ± standard error of the mean (S.E.M.). Statistical analyses were performed with analysis of variance (ANOVA) followed by Tukey's post hoc test, using the statistical program iner-STAT20-a v1.3. In the figures and tables, asterisks (*) indicate statistical significance: * $p < 0.05$.

4.12. Bioinformatics

Based on the structures of the crystals and respecting stereochemistry, the simplified molecular input line entry system (SMILES) was constructed for structural similarity analysis in SwissTargetPrediction (http://www.swisstargetprediction.ch/) [28], together with the main targets previously obtained through STRING [29].

4.12.1. Protein Preparation

The proteins of interest are the mineralocorticoid receptor (MR, 3VHU), the glucocorticoid receptor (GR, 4CSJ), the 11β-hydroxysteroid dehydrogenase type 1 (HSD11B1, 2RBE), the peroxisome proliferator-activated receptor alpha (PPARA, 6GHK), neural nitric oxide synthase (nNOS, 4EUX), inducible nitric oxide synthase (iNOS, 4NOS), and endothelial nitric oxide synthase (eNOS, 3NOS) were prepared in Schrödinger's Protein Preparation Wizard (Version 2023-2) [30], the protonation and tautomeric states of Asp, Glu, Arg, Lys, and His were adjusted to a pH of 7.4. Water molecules inside a sphere of 5 Å in the active site were removed. The orientation of the hydrogen bridge bonds was adjusted around the active site using PROPKA at a pH of 7.4, and water molecules had one or two hydrogen bridges removed. Finally, OPLS4 was used to minimize the complete protein at 0.3 Å root mean square deviation according to the previously reported protocols [31].

4.12.2. Ligand Preparation

The ligation of the crystallized structure was minimized, which led to dissolution conditions and a physiological pH of 7.4 in Macromodel and LigPrep (Schrödinger, Version 2022-1). Water was used as a solvent for minimization, along with the PGRP minimization model with OPLS4 force fields. For LigPrep with OPLS4 force field, all possible protonated centers and ionization states were calculated for scaffolding using an Ionizer at pH 7.4. Stereoisomers were retained according to their original crystal structures, which were limited to 32 isomers for each ligand. Tautomeric states were generated for each group. Conformers with lower energy for each ligand were selected [32].

4.12.3. Molecular Docking

The docking study was carried out in Glide, allowing flexibility at the interaction site and with XP precision. Each grid box was built based on co-crystallized reference ligands or inhibitors; the softening of the nonpolar parts of the receptors was carried out by scaling the van der Waals radii by a 0.08 factor. Atoms were considered nonpolar if they were determined that their absolute partial atomic charge was <0.25. In flexibility, additional ligand rotations were allowed for the hydroxyl groups in Ser, Thr, and Tyr, and the thiol group in Cys residues. Also, the lowest energy binding position of each ligand was maintained. First, docking with the reference molecules of the respective protein targets was performed to validate the docking protocol and select the best coupling by Schrödinger software (2022-1) according to a previously established protocol [32].

4.12.4. MMGBSA Calculations

The binding energy of the selected gymglu acid and references were analyzed using Molecular Mechanics with MM-GBSA of prime Schrödinger molecule [33–35]. The solvation model was set to VSGB (Variable Dielectric Surface Generalized Born) and the force field to OPLS4. Protein residues were delimited 12 Å from the ligand for energy minimization. The binding free energy was calculated by:

$$\Delta G_{Binding} = G_{Complex} - (G_{Protein} - G_{ligand})$$

where $\Delta G_{Binding}$ = binding free energy, $G_{Complex}$ = free energy of the complex, $G_{Protein}$ = free energy of the target protein and G_{ligand}= free energy of the ligand.

Supplementary Materials: The following supporting information can be downloaded at: https://www.mdpi.com/article/10.3390/ph18040516/s1, Table S1. Crystal data and structure refinement for *a*-gymglu acid and *b-ent*-gymglu acid; Table S2. Hydrogen Bonds for *a*-gymglu acid and *b-ent*-gymglu acid; Chemical structure and IUPAC name for *a*-gymglu acid and *b-ent*-gymglu acid; IR spectrum and NMR spectra for gymglu acid.

Author Contributions: S.P.-G.: Conceptualization, methodology, and resources. N.C.-X.: Investigation, methodology, and formal analysis. S.A.E.-B.: Investigation and methodology. A.C.-C.: Software and formal analysis. A.M.: Formal analysis and data curation. E.S.-M.: Formal analysis and writing—original draft preparation. All authors have read and agreed to the published version of the manuscript.

Funding: This work was financially supported by Secretaría de Ciencia, Humanidades, Tecnología e Innovación (SECIHTI) (Grant No. CBF 2023-2024-923), Unidad Autónoma Metropolitana—Xochimilco, UAM-X (Grant No. FI 2024-14). N.C.-X. would like to thank SECIHTI for the fellowship (Project No. 3055040).

Institutional Review Board Statement: The study was conducted according to the Official Mexican Standard (NOM-062-ZOO-1999). The animal study protocol was approved by the Ethics Committee of Unidad de Producción y Experimentación de Animales de Laboratorio UPEAL-bioterio. UAM-Xochimilco (protocol code 140. Approved on 23 July 2015).

Informed Consent Statement: Not applicable.

Data Availability Statement: The research data are contained within the article and Supplementary Materials.

Conflicts of Interest: The authors declare that they have no competing financial interests or personal relationships that could have appeared to influence the work reported in this paper.

Abbreviations

The following abbreviations are used in this manuscript:

ATR	Attenuated total reflectance
$CDCl_3$	Deuterated chloroform
DMEM	Dulbecco's Modified Eagle's Medium
DMSO	Dimethyl sulfoxide
ELISA	Enzyme-linked immunosorbent assay
eNOS, 3NOS	Endothelial nitric oxide synthase
FBS	Fetal bovine serum

FTIR	Fourier-transform infrared
GR, 4CSJ	Glucocorticoid receptor
HRBC	Suspension of erythrocytes with isosaline solution.
HSD11B, 2RBE	Hydroxysteroid 11-beta dehydrogenase 1
IL-1β	Interleukin one beta
IL-6	Interleukin six
IND	Indomethacin
iNOS, 4NOS	Inducible nitric oxide synthase
J774A.1	Cells murine macrophage
MR	Mineralocorticoid receptor
MTT	3-(4,5-dimethylthiazol-2-yl)-2,5-diphenyl tetrazolium bromide
NMR	Nuclear magnetic resonance
nNOS, 4EUX	Neuronal nitric oxide synthase
NO	Nitric oxide
LPS	Lipopolysaccharide
PBS	Phosphate-buffered saline
PPARA, 6GHK	Peroxisome proliferator-activated receptor Alpha
PVP	Polyvinylpyrrolidone
SMILES	Simplified Molecular Input Line Entry System
TNF-α	Tumor Necrosis Factor Alpha
TPA	12-O-tetradecanoyl phorbol-13-acetate
3VHU	Mineralocorticoid receptor ligand-binding domain with spironolactone

References

1. Bindu, S.; Mazumder, S.; Bandyopadhyay, U. Non-Steroidal Anti-Inflammatory Drugs (NSAIDs) and Organ Damage: A Current Perspective. *Biochem. Pharmacol.* **2020**, *180*, 114147. [CrossRef]
2. Koelman, L.; Pivovarova-Ramich, O.; Pfeiffer, A.F.H.; Grune, T.; Aleksandrova, K. Cytokines for Evaluation of Chronic Inflammatory Status in Ageing Research: Reliability and Phenotypic Characterisation. *Immun. Ageing* **2019**, *16*, 11. [CrossRef] [PubMed]
3. Cortes-Torres, A.G.; López-Castillo, G.N.; Marín-Torres, J.L.; Portillo-Reyes, R.; Luna, F.; Baca, B.E.; Sandoval-Ramírez, J.; Carrasco-Carballo, A. Cymbopogon Citratus Essential Oil: Extraction, GC–MS, Phytochemical Analysis, Antioxidant Activity, and In Silico Molecular Docking for Protein Targets Related to CNS. *Curr. Issues Mol. Biol.* **2023**, *45*, 5164–5179. [CrossRef]
4. Domínguez, X.A.; Torre, B. Two Pentamethoxylated Flavonoids from Gymnosperma Glutinosum. *Phytochemistry* **1974**, *13*, 1624–1625. [CrossRef]
5. Canales, M.; Hernández, T.; Serrano, R.; Hernández, L.B.; Duran, A.; Ríos, V.; Sigrist, S.; Hernández, H.L.H.; Garcia, A.M.; Angeles-López, O.; et al. Antimicrobial and General Toxicity Activities of Gymnosperma Glutinosum: A Comparative Study. *J. Ethnopharmacol.* **2007**, *110*, 343–347. [CrossRef] [PubMed]
6. Quintanilla-Licea, R.; Morado-Castillo, R.; Gomez-Flores, R.; Laatsch, H.; Verde-Star, M.J.; Hernández-Martínez, H.; Tamez-Guerra, P.; Tamez-Guerra, R.; Rodríguez-Padilla, C. Bioassay-Guided Isolation and Identification of Cytotoxic Compounds from Gymnosperma Glutinosum Leaves. *Molecules* **2012**, *17*, 11229–11241. [CrossRef]
7. Serrano, R.; Hernández, T.; Canales, M.; García-Bores, A.M.; Romo De Vivar, A.; Céspedes, C.L.; Avila, J.G. Ent-Labdane Type Diterpene with Antifungal Activity from Gymnosperma Glutinosum (Spreng.) Less. (Asteraceae). *Boletín Latinoam. Caribe Plantas Med. Aromáticas* **2009**, *8*, 412–418.
8. Maldonado, E.; Segura-Correa, R.; Ortega, A.; Calderón, J.S.; Fronczek, F.R. Ent-Labdane and Neo-Clerodane Diterpenes from Gymnosperma Glutinosum. *Phytochemistry* **1994**, *35*, 721–724. [CrossRef]
9. González-Chávez, M.M.; Arana-Argáez, V.; Zapata-Morales, J.R.; Ávila-Venegas, A.K.; Alonso-Castro, A.J.; Isiordia-Espinoza, M.; Martínez, R. Pharmacological Evaluation of 2-Angeloyl Ent-Dihydrotucumanoic Acid. *Pharm. Biol.* **2017**, *55*, 873–879. [CrossRef]
10. Alonso-Castro, A.J.; González-Chávez, M.M.; Zapata-Morales, J.R.; Verdinez-Portales, A.K.; Sánchez-Recillas, A.; Ortiz-Andrade, R.; Isiordia-Espinoza, M.; Martínez-Gutiérrez, F.; Ramírez-Morales, M.A.; Domínguez, F.; et al. Antinociceptive Activity of Ent-Dihydrotucumanoic Acid Isolated from Gymnosperma Glutinosum Spreng Less. *Drug Dev. Res.* **2017**, *78*, 340–348. [CrossRef]
11. Salas-Balgañón, K.; Pérez.-Ramos, J.; Serrano-Vega, J.R.; Campos-Xolalpa, N.; Pérez-Gutiérrez, S. Evaluación Antiinflamatoria Del Extracto Metanólico y Clorofórmico de Gymnosperma Glutinosum. In *Proceedings of the 16ª Reunión Internacional de Investigación en Productos Naturales*; Garduño-Ramírez María, L., Rivas-Galindo Verónica, M., Antunez Mojica Mayra, Y., Robles Zepeda Ramón, E., Eds.; AMIPRONAT: Zacatecas, Mexico, 2021; p. 33.

12. *Agilent CrysAlisPro Software System*; Technologies UK Ltd.: Yarnton, UK, 2014; Volume 44.
13. Sheldrick, G.M. Crystal Structure Refinement with SHELXL. *Acta Crystallogr. C Struct. Chem.* **2015**, *71*, 3–8. [CrossRef] [PubMed]
14. Dolomanov, O.V.; Bourhis, L.J.; Gildea, R.J.; Howard, J.A.K.; Puschmann, H. OLEX2: A Complete Structure Solution, Refinement and Analysis Program. *J. Appl. Crystallogr.* **2009**, *42*, 339–341. [CrossRef]
15. Macrae, C.F.; Edgington, P.R.; McCabe, P.; Pidcock, E.; Shields, G.P.; Taylor, R.; Towler, M.; Streek, J.V.D. Mercury: Visualization and analysis of crystal structures. *J. Appl. Crystallogr.* **2006**, *39*, 453–457.
16. Hiraganahalli Bhaskarmurthy, D.; Evan Prince, S. Effect of Baricitinib on TPA-Induced Psoriasis like Skin Inflammation. *Life Sci.* **2021**, *279*, 119655. [CrossRef]
17. Hamaguchi, K.; Kuwata, H.; Yoshihara, K.; Masuda, S.; Shimbara, S.; Oh-Ishi, S.; Murakami, M.; Kudo, I. Induction of Distinct Sets of Secretory Phospholipase A2 in Rodents during Inflammation. *Biochim. Biophys. Acta Mol. Cell Biol. Lipids* **2003**, *1635*, 37–47. [CrossRef]
18. Green, S.J.; Mellouk, S.; Hoffman, S.L.; Meltzer, M.S.; Nacy, C.A. Cellular Mechanisms of Nonspecific Immunity to Intracellular Infection: Cytokine-Induced Synthesis of Toxic Nitrogen Oxides from l-Arginine by Macrophages and Hepatocytes. *Immunol. Lett.* **1990**, *25*, 15–19. [CrossRef]
19. Wu, Z.; Huang, Y.; Hu, W.; Ren, L.; Jiang, P.; Margolskee, R.F.; Wang, H.; Feng, S. Lipopolysaccharide-Induced Inflammation Increases Nitric Oxide Production in Taste Buds. *Brain Behav. Immun.* **2022**, *103*, 145–153. [CrossRef]
20. Jin, J.O.; Han, X.; Yu, Q. Interleukin-6 Induces the Generation of IL-10-Producing Tr1 Cells and Suppresses Autoimmune Tissue Inflammation. *J. Autoimmun.* **2013**, *40*, 28–44. [CrossRef]
21. Tran, Q.T.N.; Wong, W.S.F.; Chai, C.L.L. Labdane Diterpenoids as Potential Anti-Inflammatory Agents. *Pharmacol. Res.* **2017**, *124*, 43–63. [CrossRef]
22. Chetehouna, S.; Derouiche, S.; Boulaares, I.; Réggami, Y. Phytochemical Profile, Anti-Inflammatory Analysis and Cytotoxic Activity of SmE-SeNPs against Breast (MCF-7) Cancer Cells. *Biocatal. Agric. Biotechnol.* **2024**, *57*, 103122. [CrossRef]
23. Obeagu, E.I.; Obeagu, G.U. Exploring the Intersection: Peptic Ulcers and Hemolysis—Unraveling the Complex Relationship. *Medicine* **2024**, *103*, e37565. [CrossRef]
24. Especificaciones Técnicas para la Producción, Cuidado y Uso de los Animales de Laboratorio (NOM-062-ZOO-1999). Available online: https://www.gob.mx/cms/uploads/attachment/file/203498/NOM-062-ZOO-1999_220801.pdf (accessed on 31 March 2025).
25. De Young, L.M.; Kheifets, J.B.; Ballaron, S.J.; Young, J.M. Edema and Cell Infiltration in the Phorbol Ester-Treated Mouse Ear Are Temporally Separate and Can Be Differentially Modulated by Pharmacologic Agents. *Agents Actions* **1989**, *26*, 335–341. [CrossRef] [PubMed]
26. Sun, J.; Zhang, X.; Broderick, M.; Fein, H. Measurement of Nitric Oxide Production in Biological Systems by Using Griess Reaction Assay. *Sensors* **2003**, *3*, 276–284. [CrossRef]
27. Parameswari, P.; Devika, R.; Vijayaraghavan, P. In Vitro Anti-Inflammatory and Antimicrobial Potential of Leaf Extract from Artemisia Nilagirica (Clarke) Pamp. *Saudi J. Biol. Sci.* **2019**, *26*, 460–463. [CrossRef] [PubMed]
28. Gfeller, D.; Grosdidier, A.; Wirth, M.; Daina, A.; Michielin, O.; Zoete, V. SwissTargetPrediction: A Web Server for Target Prediction of Bioactive Small Molecules. *Nucleic Acids Res.* **2014**, *42*, W32–W38. [CrossRef]
29. Szklarczyk, D.; Kirsch, R.; Koutrouli, M.; Nastou, K.; Mehryary, F.; Hachilif, R.; Gable, A.L.; Fang, T.; Doncheva, N.T.; Pyysalo, S.; et al. The STRING Database in 2023: Protein-Protein Association Networks and Functional Enrichment Analyses for Any Sequenced Genome of Interest. *Nucleic Acids Res.* **2023**, *51*, D638–D646. [CrossRef]
30. Schrödinger. *Protein Preparation Wizard*; Version 2023-2; Schrödinger: Cambridge, MA, USA, 2023.
31. Carrasco-Carballo, A.; Mendoza-Lara, D.F.; Rojas-Morales, J.A.; Alatriste, V.; Merino-Montiel, P.; Luna, F.; Sandoval-Ramirez, J. In Silico Study of Coumarins Derivatives With Potential Use in Systemic Diseases. *Biointerface Res. Appl. Chem.* **2023**, *13*, 240. [CrossRef]
32. Schrödinger. *Schrödinger Release 2022-1: Glide*; Schrödinger, LLC: New York, NY, USA, 2022.
33. Lu, C.; Wu, C.; Ghoreishi, D.; Chen, W.; Wang, L.; Damm, W.; Ross, G.A.; Dahlgren, M.K.; Russell, E.; Von Bargen, C.D.; et al. OPLS4: Improving Force Field Accuracy on Challenging Regimes of Chemical Space. *J. Chem. Theory Comput.* **2021**, *17*, 4291–4300. [CrossRef]
34. Rosales-López, A.; López-Castillo, G.; Sandoval-Ramírez, J.; Terán, J.; Carrasco-Carballo, A. Correlation between Molecular Docking and the Stabilizing Interaction of HOMO-LUMO: Spirostans in CHK1 and CHK2, an In Silico Cancer Approach. *Int. J. Mol. Sci.* **2024**, *25*, 8588. [CrossRef]
35. Release Notes: Release 2024-2. Available online: https://www.schrodinger.com/life-science/download/release-notes/release-2024-2/ (accessed on 11 December 2024).

pharmaceuticals

Article

The Anti-Arthritic Potential of the Ethanolic Extract of *Salvia Lachnostachys* Benth. Leaves and Icetexane Dinor-Diterpenoid Fruticuline B

Natália de M. Balsalobre [1,†], Elisangela dos Santos-Procopio [1,†], Cristhian S. Oliveira [2], Silvia C. Neves [3], Maria H. Verdan [4], Saulo E. Silva-Filho [5], Rodrigo J. Oliveira [3], Maria É. A. Stefanello [2] and Cândida A. L. Kassuya [1,*]

1 Faculty of Health Sciences, Federal University of Grande Dourados, Dourados 79804-970, MS, Brazil; nataliabalsalobre@hotmail.com (N.d.M.B.); elisangelaprocopiosan@gmail.com (E.d.S.-P.)
2 Chemistry Department, Federal University of Paraná, Curitiba 81530-900, PR, Brazil; cristhian.so@hotmail.com (C.S.O.); stefanello.elida@gmail.com (M.É.A.S.)
3 Faculty of Health, Federal University of Mato Grosso do Sul, CeTroGen, Campo Grande 79070-900, MS, Brazil; nevessilva@gmail.com (S.C.N.); rjo.rodrigojulianooliveira@gmail.com (R.J.O.)
4 Postgraduate Program in Chemistry, Federal University of Grande Dourados, Dourados 79804-970, MS, Brazil; mhelenaverdan@gmail.com
5 Faculty of Pharmaceutical Sciences, Food and Nutrition, Federal University of Mato Grosso do Sul, Campo Grande 79070-900, MS, Brazil; saulo.e@ufms.br
* Correspondence: candida2005@gmail.com; Tel.: +55-67-3410-2326
† These authors contributed equally to this work.

Abstract: The decoction of *Salvia lachnostachys* Benth. leaves is used in Brazilian folk medicine for anti-spasmodic, antipyretic, and anxiolytic purposes. Some of the biological effects of an *S. lachnostachys* extract have been shown to be anti-inflammatory, anti-cancer, and antidepressant effects. In addition, this medicinal plant produces several compounds including icetexane diterpenoids, such as fruticuline A and fruticuline B. The aim of the present work was to evaluate the anti-hyperalgesic and anti-inflammatory properties of fruticuline B (FRUT B) and the ethanolic extract obtained from the leaves of *S. lachnostachys* (EESL) in experimental mouse models. EESL (30, 100, and 300 mg/kg) and FRUT B (1 mg/kg) were evaluated in articular inflammation-induced models in *Swiss* mice. In articular inflammation induced by Zymosan, EESL (300 mg/kg) and FRUT B (1 mg/kg) significantly reduced mechanical hyperalgesia (83.17% inhibition for EESL and 81.19% for FRUT B); edema (68.75% reduction for EESL and 33.66% for FRUT B); leukocyte migration (81.3% for EESSL and 92.2% for FRUT B), and nitric oxide production (88.3% for EESL and 74.4% for FRUT B). The exposure to fruticuline B significantly inhibited the edema (51.5%), mechanical (88.12%) and cold hyperalgesia (80.8%), and myeloperoxidase (MPO) (63.4%) activity 24 h after CFA injection. In the pleurisy model, FRUT B reduced 89.1% of leukocyte migration and 50.3% in nitric oxide production. Four hours after carrageenan injection, FRUT B (1 mg/kg) diminished 89.11% of mechanical hyperalgesia, 65.8% of paw edema, and 82.12% of the response to cold hyperalgesia. In the MTT test, EESL and fruticuline B caused no cytotoxicity. The present study revealed, for the first time, the anti-arthritic and anti-nociceptive effects of FRUT B, pointing out the therapeutic potential of the species to control inflammation and nociception. Future studies are needed to evaluate other biological properties of fruticuline B and to better understand its mechanism of action.

Keywords: articular inflammation; Lamiaceae; nociception; icetexane diterpenoids

1. Introduction

Inflammation is a defense response of the organism triggered by harmful or infectious agents. The inflammatory process can be acute or chronic, and generally, when not properly solved, it can become persistent, leading to an exaggerated response of the immune system [1]. Inflammation, redness, edema, pain, and joint injury [2] may be present in diseases such as rheumatoid arthritis [3]. These clinical signs can be treated with glucocorticoid analogs and non-steroidal anti-inflammatory drugs (NSAIDs). Most drugs cause adverse effects; thus, drug development and new effective treatment alternatives are still needed [4].

The discovery of bioactive substances extracted from plants has a significant impact on drug development, opening new possibilities for therapeutic treatment. The traditional use of medicinal plants has proven to be an effective option for the treatment of inflammatory diseases [5]. Among Brazilian plant species with potential for new drug development, *Salvia lachnostachys* Benth. (Lamiaceae family), an herbaceous plant native to the southern regions of Brazil and commonly known as "melissa", stands out.

The ethanolic extract of *S. lachnostachys* leaves (EESL) demonstrated an anti-inflammatory effect in pain and inflammation models [6]. Moreover, it has an antitumor and chemopreventive effect against solid Ehrlich carcinoma [7]. Santos Radai and coauthors (2018) demonstrated that the EESL has anti-arthritic activity and no toxic genetic effect, being safe for usage [8]. The EESL additionally exhibited anti-hyperalgesic, antidepressant, and antinociceptive effects [9]. This medicinal plant is used in folk medicine as an antipyretic agent, and non-steroidal anti-inflammatory drugs (NSAIDs) are used to treat fever, pain, and inflammation. In this context, the evaluation of an *S. lachnostachys* extract and fruticuline B (FRUT B) in experimental models of inflammation is relevant.

The EESL has been previously characterized for its chemical constituents [7,10,11]. Phytochemical investigation revealed the predominant presence of unique icetexane *nor*- and *dinor*-diterpenoids, along with ursane and oleanane triterpenoids in fractions of low and medium polarity. Additionally, rosmarinic acid, a phenolic compound commonly found in species of the Lamiaceae family, predominates in the more polar fractions [11,12]. Icetaxenes are biosynthesized from abietanes, featuring a tricyclic 6-7-6 structure (systematic name: 9(10/20)-*abeo*-abietane) and containing a *para*-quinone group [13,14]. In particular, the icetexane FRUT B, a *dinor*-diterpenoid that has a rare tricyclic anthracene-based structure, was initially isolated from *S. fruticulosa* [13]. This represents the second recorded isolation of this diterpenoid. The extraction also yielded one of the main chemical constituents, the icetexane fruticuline A (a *nor*-diterpenoid) (Figure 1). Furthermore, other minor icetexanes were isolated, including isofruticuline A, demethylfruticuline A, demethylfruticuline B, 20-hydroxyfruticuline B, and 6-hydroxyisofruticuline A [10,11].

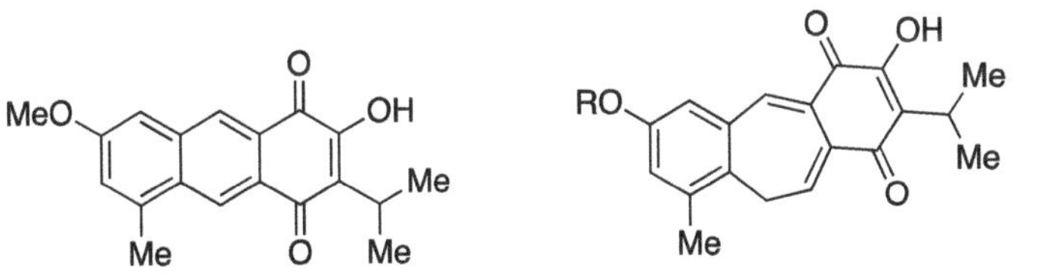

Fruticuline B

R = Me - Fruticuline A
R = H - Demethylfruticuline A

Figure 1. Chemical structures of the icetexane *nor*-diterpenoids fruticuline A and demethylfruticuline A and *dinor*-diterpenoid fruticuline B.

From a pharmacological perspective, fruticuline A has been extensively studied and exhibits significant biological properties, including anti-inflammatory, anti-nociceptive, and antineoplastic activities, as well as antidepressant effects [7,10,13,15]. Similarly, demethylfruticuline A (Figure 1) is known to induce apoptosis [16]. Both fruticuline A and demethylfruticuline A have shown notable binding affinity to CDK-2 compared to known CDK-2 inhibitors [17]. However, FRUT B has been less explored regarding its biological properties, showing only moderate cytotoxic activity (IG_{50} 16.4–116.4 μM) against human tumor cell lines and high antioxidant activity assessed by the ORAC-FL method (1.8 TE) [10,11].

In this perspective, we evaluated the effects of FRUT B in murine models of inflammation, pain, and toxicity, aiming to expand the pharmacological knowledge of these unique chemical skeletons. Additionally, the present study also assessed the effects of the EESL.

2. Results

2.1. Isolation and Identification of FRUT B

Pure FRUT B was isolated using semi-preparative HPLC and its structure was confirmed by NMR (^{1}H, HSQC, and HMBC). The obtained NMR spectra were identical to those previously reported in the literature (Supplementary Figures S1–S3) [10]. The ^{1}H NMR showed the typical signals of FRUT B: an isopropyl group (doublet at δ_H 1.35, six hydrogens; septet at δ_H 3.49, one hydrogen), two tetrasubstituted aromatic rings (two doublets at δ_H 7.14 and δ_H 7.16, one hydrogen each; and two singlets of two unprotected hydrogens at δ_H 8.45 and δ_H 8.69, one hydrogen each), a methoxy group (singlet at δ_H 3.95, three hydrogens), a methyl group (δ_H 2.75, three hydrogens), and a hydroxyl group (broad singlet at δ_H 7.55, one hydrogen). Besides the solvent signal ($CDCl_3$; δ_H 7.26), no other signals were observed, confirming the absence of impurities, such as aliphatic compounds or other aromatic diterpenes, like fruticuline A.

2.2. The Oral Exposure to EESL and FRUT B Reduced Zymosan-Induced Knee Inflammation

After 4 h of Zymosan administration in the knee, oral exposure of female mice to a dose of 100 or 300 mg/kg of EESL, FRUT B, and prednisolone (PRED) significantly inhibited mechanical hyperalgesia in 68.19, 75.17, 81.19, and 91.17%, respectively (Figure 2A). The inhibition of mechanical hyperalgesia induced by EESL was 80.21% for 100 mg/kg and 83.17% for 300 mg/kg, while for FRUT B, it was 81.19, and for prednisolone (PRED), it was 85.15% (Figure 1), after 6 h of Zymosan administration in the knee. The dose of 30 mg/kg of EESL did not interfere with mechanical hyperalgesia (Figures 1 and 2A). After 4 h of Zymosan administration in the knee, no doses of EESL, FRUT B, and prednisolone (PRED) groups interfered statistically with knee edema when compared with the control group (Figure 2C). After 6 h of Zymosan administration in the knee, the oral administration of 100 mg/kg of EESL prevented the knee edema in 66.25% while the dose of 300 mg/kg prevented it in 68.75%, FRUT B in 33.66%, and prednisolone (PRED) in 97.3% (Figure 2D).

In relation to the total migration of leukocyte cells to the knee, the doses of 100 and 300 mg/kg of EESL inhibited 67.2 and 81.3% while FRUT B inhibited 92.2% and prednisolone (PRED) inhibited 89.1% (Figure 2E). Regarding nitric oxide production in the knee, 100 and 300 mg/kg doses of EESL inhibited 68.6 and 88.3%, while FRUT B inhibited 74.4%, and prednisolone (PRED) inhibited 85.1% (Figure 2F).

The oral exposure to the doses of 100 and 300 mg/kg of EESL for mechanical hyperalgesia evaluation did not differ between themselves; however, they differed from the control group and from the dose of 30 mg/kg of EESL. The results suggested that EESL acts in a dose-dependent manner since different doses induced distinct responses (Figure 2A,B).

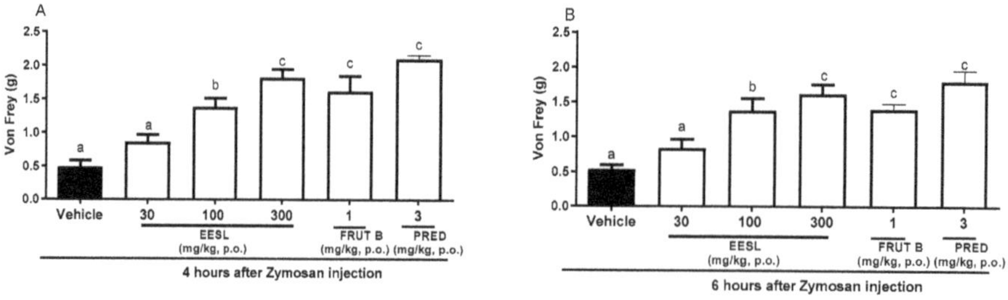

Figure 2. *Cont.*

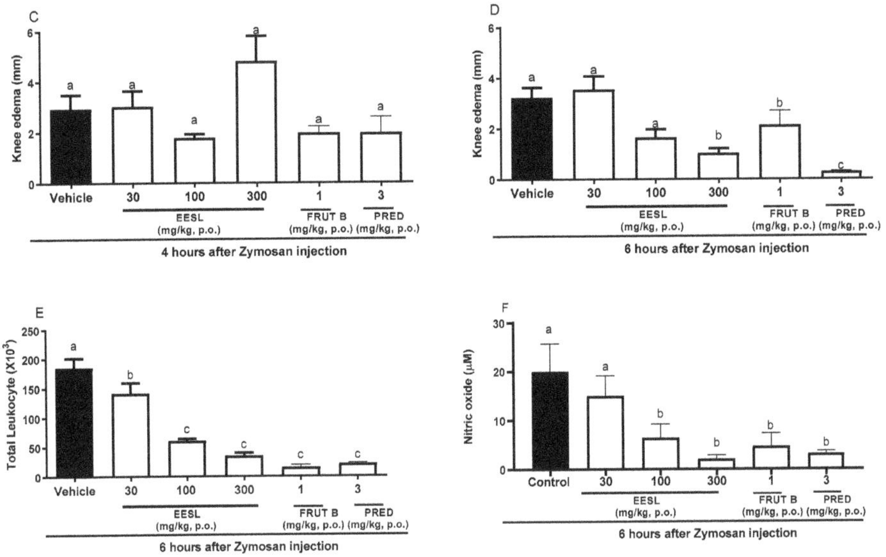

Figure 2. The effect of oral administration of EESL and FRUT B on the Zymosan-induced knee edema, mechanical hyperalgesia, leukocyte migration, and nitric oxide in synovial exudate in mice. The animals received EESL (30, 100, and 300 mg/kg, p.o.), FRUT B (1 mg/kg), vehicle (control), or prednisolone (PRED, 3 mg/kg, p.o.); and 1 h later, an intraplantar injection of Zymosan was administered. (**A**,**B**) represent the evaluation of the mechanical hyperalgesia at 4 and 6 h, respectively, after Zymosan injection. (**C**,**D**) represent the evaluation of the knee edema at 4 and 6 h, respectively, after Zymosan injection; graph (**E**) represents the evaluation of the total leukocyte counts, and (**F**) represents nitric oxide measurements after 6 h after the stimulus. The letters "a", "b", and "c" indicate significant differences among groups according to Tukey's multiple comparison test.

2.3. *Oral Exposure to FRUT B Reduced CFA-Induced Acute Paw Inflammation*

The oral exposure to 1 mg/kg, but not to 0.3 mg/kg, of FRUT B significantly diminished the mechanical hyperalgesia, leukocyte migration, and nitric oxide production 3, 4, and 24 h after CFA injection.

Three hours after the CFA injection, the mechanical hyperalgesia reduction was 94.6% for FRUT B (1 mg/kg), while for prednisolone (PRED), it was 91.9% (Figure 3A). Four hours after the CFA injection, the mechanical hyperalgesia reduction was 86.14% for FRUT B (1 mg/kg), while for prednisolone (PRED), it was 75.3% (Figure 3B). Twenty-four hours after the CFA injection, the mechanical hyperalgesia reduction was 88.12% for FRUT B (1 mg/kg), while for prednisolone (PRED), it was 87.17% (Figure 3C).

Three hours after CFA injection, allodynia reduction to cold was 77.11% for 1 mg/kg of FRUT B, while prednisolone (PRED)'s decrease was 66.12% (Figure 3D). Four hours after CFA injection, allodynia reduction to cold by FRUT B (1 mg/kg) was 64.15%, while prednisolone (PRED) diminished it by 68.12% (Figure 3E). Twenty-four hours after CFA injection, allodynia reduction to cold was 80.8% for FRUT B (1 mg/kg), while prednisolone (PRED) diminished it by 84.7% (Figure 3F).

The reduction in paw edema was 63.3% for FRUT B, while for prednisolone (PRED), it was 70.0%. The inhibition was 63.7% for FRUT B (1 mg/kg) and 84% for prednisolone (PRED) 4 h after CFA. Twenty-four hours after CFA, the inhibition was 51.5% for FRUT B (1 mg/kg) and 80.1% for prednisolone (PRED) (Figure 3G).

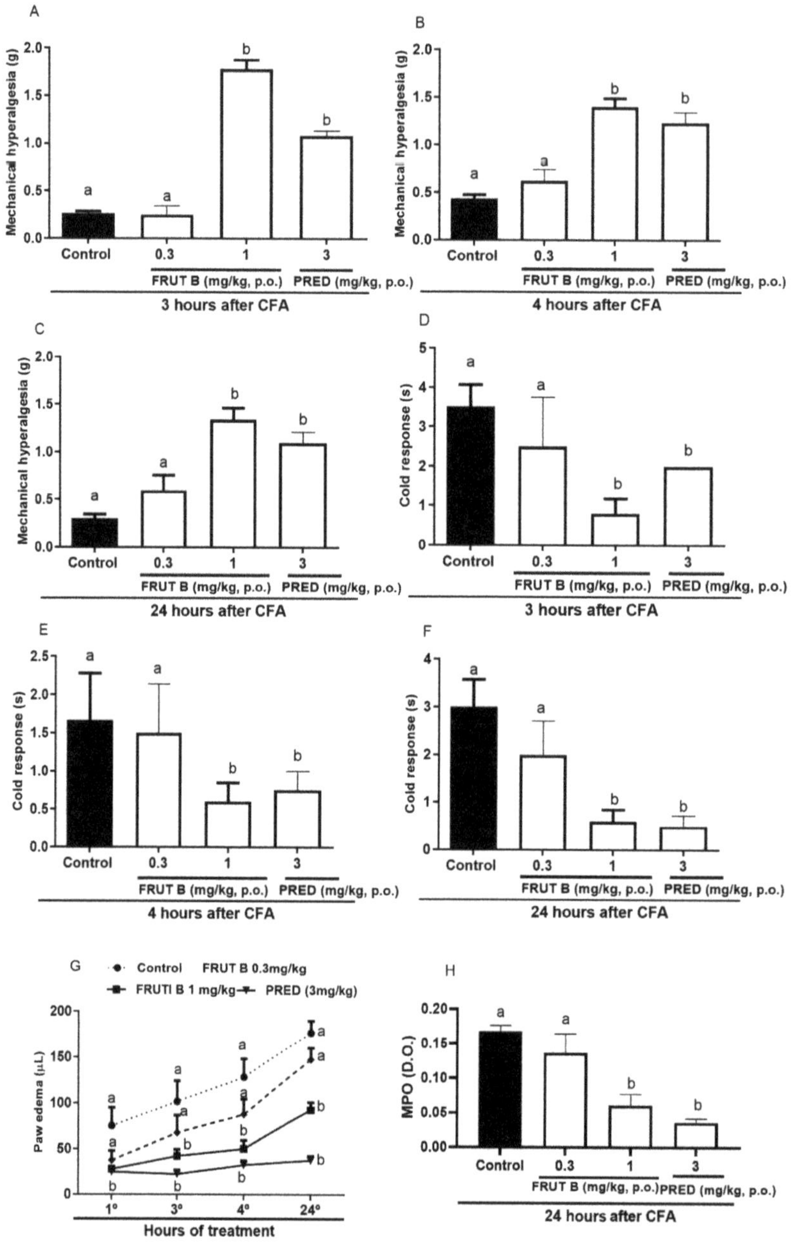

Figure 3. The effect of oral administration of FRUT B on the CFA-induced mechanical hyperalgesia, cold response, paw edema, and increase in myeloperoxidase in mice. The animals received FRUT B (0.3 and 1 mg/kg, p.o.), vehicle (control), or prednisolone (PRED, 3 mg/kg, s.c.), and 1 h later, an intraplantar injection of CFA was administered. (**A–C**) represent the evaluation of the mechanical hyperalgesia 3, 4, and 24 h, respectively, after CFA injection. (**D–F**) represent the analysis of the cold allodynia at 3, 4, and 24 h, respectively, after CFA injection. (**G**) represents the analysis of paw edema at 3, 4, and 24 h and (**H**) MPO activity measurements 24 h after the stimulus. The letters "a", "b", and "c" indicate significant differences among groups according to Tukey´s multiple comparison test.

The myeloperoxidase activity (measured 24 h after CFA injection) was 63.4% inhibited by FRUT B (1 mg/kg), while it was 76.9% inhibited by the prednisolone (PRED) group (Figure 3H).

2.4. The Oral Exposure to FRUT B Diminished Carrageenan-Induced Pleurisy

The evaluation of pleurisy induced by carrageenan showed a reduction in leukocyte migration of 89.1% for FRUT B (1 mg/kg), and for prednisolone (PRED), the reduction was 95.0% compared to the control group. There was a decrease of 50.3% in nitric oxide production for FRUT B (1 mg/kg), and for prednisolone (PRED), the reduction was 52.3%. The oral exposure of FRUT B and prednisolone (PRED) did not differ between themselves; however, they differed from the control group in relation to leukocyte migration or nitric oxide production (Figure 4A,B).

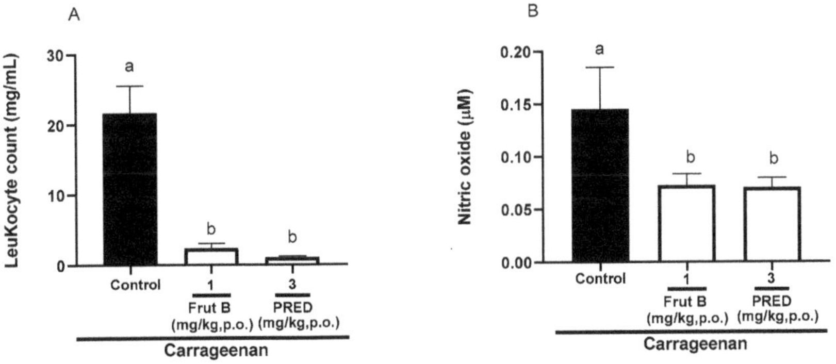

Figure 4. The effect of oral administration of FRUT B on the carrageenan-induced leukocyte migration and nitric oxide levels in pleura in mice. The animals received FRUT B (1 mg/kg, p.o.), vehicle (control), or PRED (3 mg/kg, p.o.), and 1h later, an intraplantar injection of carrageenan was administered. (**A**) represents the evaluation of leukocyte migration and (**B**) represents the evaluation of the nitric oxide levels in pleural exudate 4 h after carrageenan injection. The letters "a" and "b" indicate significant differences among groups according to Tukey's multiple comparison test.

2.5. The Oral Exposure to FRUT B Decreased Carrageenan-Induced Paw Inflammation

The oral exposure to FRUT B and prednisolone (PRED) diminished the mechanical hyperalgesia, paw edema, and response to cold 3 and 4 h after carrageenan injection. After three hours of carrageenan, the mechanical hyperalgesia was decreased by FRUT B in 77.0% (0.3 mg/kg) and in 82.0% (1 mg/kg) and by prednisolone (PRED) in 93.7% (3 mg/kg) (Figure 5A). After 4 h of carrageenan injection, the mechanical hyperalgesia was inhibited by FRUT B in 85.15% (0.3 mg/kg) and in 89.11% (1 mg/kg), and by prednisolone (PRED) in 93.7% (3 mg/kg) (Figure 5B).

After 3 h of carrageenan, the cold allodynia was inhibited by FRUT B in 71.21% (0.3 mg/kg) and in 79.9% (1 mg/kg), and by prednisolone (PRED) in 86.9% (3 mg/kg) (Figure 5C). After 4 h of carrageenan, the cold allodynia was inhibited by FRUT B in 88.1% (0.3 mg/kg) and in 82.12% (1 mg/kg), and by prednisolone (PRED) in 88.7% (3 mg/kg) (Figure 5D).

After 3 h of the stimulus, the edema was inhibited by FRUT B in 73.8% (0.3 mg/kg) and in 82.5% (1 mg/kg), and by prednisolone (PRED) in 64.3% (3 mg/kg) (Figure 5E). After four hours of the stimulus, the edema was inhibited by FRUT B in 68.7% (0.3 mg/kg) and in 65.8% (1 mg/kg), and by prednisolone (PRED) in 73.3% (3 mg/kg) (Figure 5F).

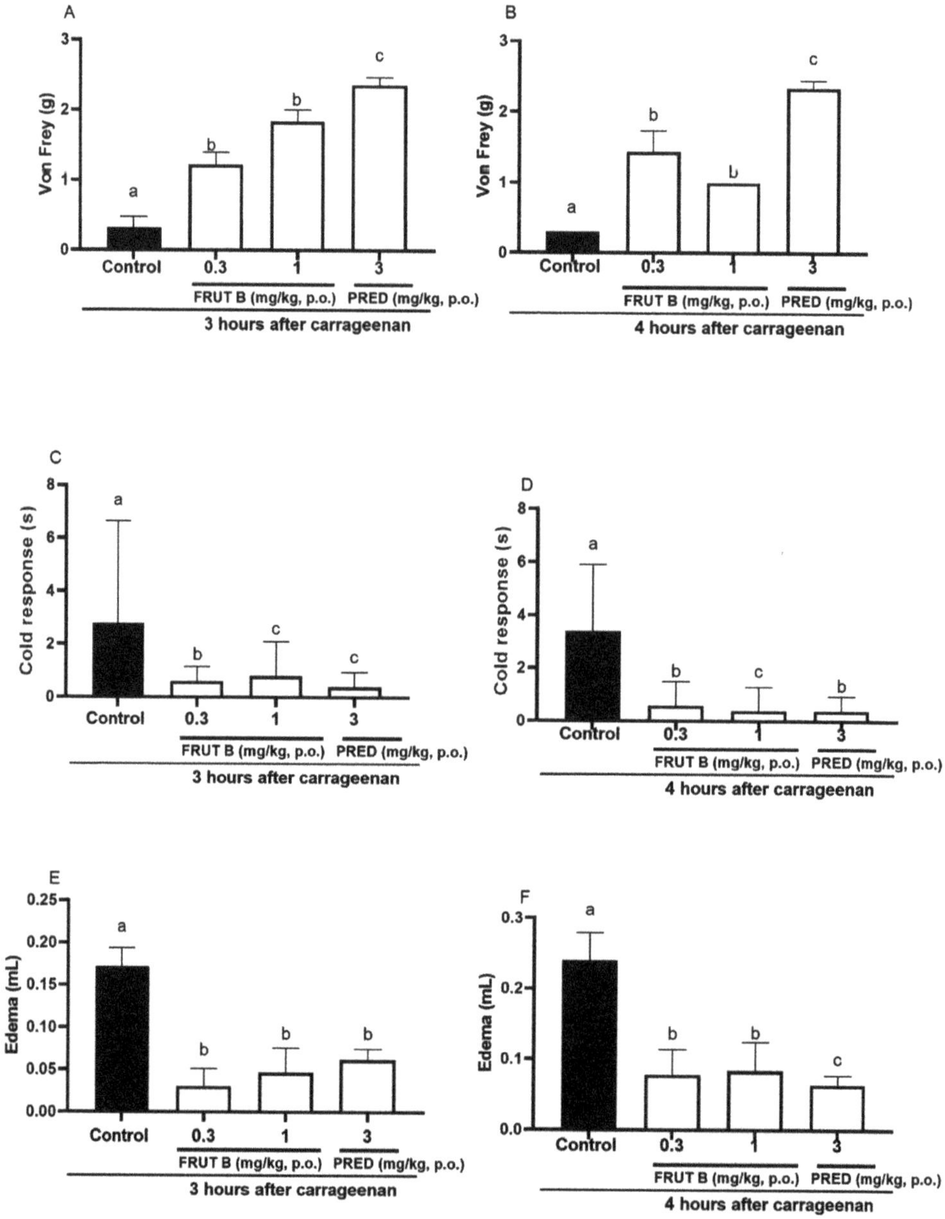

Figure 5. The effect of oral administration of FRUT B on the carrageenan-induced paw edema, mechanical hyperalgesia, and cold response. The animals received FRUT B (0.3 and 1 mg/kg, p.o.), vehicle (control), or prednisolone (PRED, 3 mg/kg, p.o.), and 1 h later, an intraplantar injection of carrageenan was administered. (**A**,**B**) represent the mechanical hyperalgesia 3 and 4 h, respectively, after carrageenan injection. (**C**,**D**) represent the cold allodynia at 3 and 4 h after carrageenan injection. (**E**,**F**) show the inhibition of edema at 3 and 4 h after carrageenan injection. The letters "a", "b", and "c" indicate significant differences among groups according to Tukey´s multiple comparison test.

2.6. FRUT B Did Not Present In Vitro Cellular Toxicity in the MTT Test and Did Not Present Alterations in Parameters of the Acute Oral Toxicity Test

In the MTT test, FRUT B at concentrations of 3, 10, 30, and 90 μg/mL presented cell viability of 82.0%, 89.3%, 90.9%, and 83.5%, respectively, indicating that this compound did not induce cellular toxicity in any tested concentrations.

The single oral exposure to EESL and FRUT B (doses of 500, 1000, and 2000 mg/kg) did not induce death and did not indicate alterations in the behavioral parameters of the acute oral toxicity test. The body weight, the amount of food consumption, and the weight of organs observed in FRUT B groups did not show significant differences when compared to the control group.

3. Discussion

FRUT B is an aromatic diterpene isolated from *S. lachnostachys* leaves and the results herein show, for the first time, the anti-inflammatory effects of this compound. Another compound found in *S. lachnostachys* is fruticuline A; however, the anti-inflammatory potential of fruticuline A, as well as the ethanolic extract of *S. lachnostachys* (EESL), was previously explored in animal models of inflammation. The oral administration of EESL, in a dose-dependent manner, inhibited parameters of inflammation [6,7,9]. Few studies have evaluated the anti-inflammatory effect and therapeutic potential of FRUT B, and it is important that the scientific investigation of FRUT B in relation to toxicity and pharmacology is carried out. The dose of 1 mg/kg of FRUT B was used to perform the biological evaluation since the yield of FRUT B in EESL was around 0.7%, and the effective dosage was 100 mg/kg. In the present study, FRUT B (1 mg/kg) also effectively inhibited the inflammatory parameters induced by Zymosan, CFA, and carrageenan.

The Zymosan articular inflammation model is used to analyze the effects of substances on parameters such as knee edema formation, mechanical hyperalgesia, and leukocyte migration. The oral administration of 100 and 300 mg/kg of EESL significantly reduced, in a dose-dependent manner, the mechanical hyperalgesia and decreased other Zymosan parameters analyzed. The EESL treatments (dose of 300 mg/kg) blocked the mechanical hyperalgesia 4 and 6 h after the intra-articular injection of Zymosan (Figure 1). Inflammatory mediators such as cytokines (IL-1 beta and IL-6), TNF, and endothelins are increased in the knee when animals are analyzed at 6 h after Zymosan knee injection in mice [18,19]. The oral administration of 300 mg/kg EESL, but not fruticuline B, was effective in inhibiting knee edema at 6 h (not 4 h), suggesting that the mechanism of action may involve mediators that increase at this time point (Figure 2C,D). In relation to edema, other compounds present in EESL may be involved in the mechanism of action of reduction in edema in this model. The inhibitory efficacy of EESL on leukocyte migration was higher than prednisolone (PRED) (Figure 1). FRUT B (1 mg/kg) exhibited efficacy against mechanical hyperalgesia and inhibited leukocyte migration, showing anti-inflammatory properties. The present study was the first to show that EESL and FRUT B present anti-arthritic potential against Zymosan articular inflammation.

The inflammatory response induced by CFA in mice is another inflammatory model used to efficiently evaluate new products. The hyperalgesia, edema, and leukocyte migration to the paw are inflammatory parameters induced by CFA [18,20,21], and the oral administration of 1 mg/kg of FRUT B was able to inhibit all these parameters. The oral administration of EESL (100 mg/kg) for 21 days to mice showed anti-hyperalgesic and anti-edematogenic properties in the CFA model of inflammation [8]. The present study also verified the anti-arthritic potential of FRUT B in CFA-induced acute paw inflammation.

The EESL showed anti-inflammatory efficacy in the pleurisy model induced by carrageenan (Figure 4). Models of pleurisy induced by carrageenan are important to study the influence of new products on phenomena such as migrating cells and exudate formation [22]. In the pleurisy model, the literature showed that the highest neutrophil accumulation was observed 4 h after the intrapleural injection of carrageenan [23]. The doses of 1 mg/kg of FRUT B caused a significant inhibition of leukocyte migration and nitric oxide production induced by carrageenan administration into the pleural exudate (Figure 4A,B), showing the anti-inflammatory properties of FRUT B. EESL and fruticuline A exhibited anti-hyperalgesic, antidepressant, and anti-nociceptive effects in the nerve injury (SNI) in rats and nociceptive behavior induced by formalin [9]. EESL and fruticuline A display anti-inflammatory and analgesic properties in paw edema and pleurisy induced by carrageenan injection [6]. FRUT B was also analyzed in the carrageenan-induced paw inflammation model and the parameters analyzed were mechanical hyperalgesia, cold allodynia, and edema (Figure 5). The oral exposure to FRUT B reduced all analyzed parameters (Figure 5). These results showed for the first time the potential of FRUT B as an anti-inflammatory agent and showed the inhibition of mechanical hyperalgesia, cold response, edema, leukocyte migration, and nitric oxide induced by carrageenan.

The safe oral administration of EESL and fruticuline A was shown by Santos Radai and coworkers (2018) [8]. Fruticuline A and B are secondary metabolites with a diterpene skeleton, so far only found in species from the *Salvia* genus. Fruticuline A has shown to be promising for cancer treatment because it causes cellular death in vitro, and in in vivo assays, the cells suffered necrosis [13].

This study has some limitations; for example, because of the small quantity of fruticuline B, it was not possible to test this substance in various animal toxicity models. Future studies are needed to evaluate other properties of fruticuline B and to better understand its mechanism of action. Another limitation is the use of only one genus of mice and only a few doses of the extract and isolated compound in the experimental models, but the ethics of the use of animal experimentation restrict the use of animals.

Two studies [7,10] showed that fruticuline A and isofruticuline A had the highest cytotoxic activity against several cancer lines; however, fruticuline B had low cytotoxicity against all cell lines tested [7]. Therefore, fruticuline B was evaluated in the MTT assay. The MTT assay also showed that FRUT B has no cellular toxicity. These preliminary evaluations showed, for the first time, that FRUT B did not show potential toxicity. No toxicity was observed in the acute toxicity assay when animals were treated with an ethanolic extract of *S. lachnostachys* leaves [7]; however, this plant has been described as a cytotoxic agent in the literature. According to Santos Radai et al. [8], the ethanolic extract of this plant has no genotoxic effect in male Swiss mice treated at a dose of up to 1000 mg/kg.

4. Materials and Methods

4.1. Plant Material

Leaves of *Salvia lachnostachys* Benth. were collected and identified in Curitiba, Paraná State, Brazil (25°30′44.6″ S, 48°18′7.13″ W), in May 2010 by Élide P. Santos. A voucher specimen was deposited in the Herbarium of the Federal University of Paraná (UPCB 85285). This study of this species was registered in the National System for the Management of Genetic Heritage and Associated Traditional Knowledge (SISGEN) under the code A19F875.

4.2. Extract Preparation and Isolation of FRUT B

Leaves of *Salvia lachnostachys* (415.3 g) were dried and powdered, and subsequently, this material was submitted to a successive extraction process with hexanes (Hex, mixture of isomers) and EtOH (2.0 L, three times each solvent at room temperature). The solvents were removed under reduced pressure, yielding extracts of Hex (11.3 g) and EtOH (EESL, 47.6 g). An aliquot (2.6 g) of the EESL was reserved, and the remaining (45.0 g) was submitted to vacuum liquid chromatography, eluted with Hex, yielding a fraction (A, 1.8 g) after the solvent removal. This fraction was fractionated by CC chromatography (silica gel), and eluted with several solvents in polarity order (Hex, Hex-CH_2Cl_2 (1:1, *v*/*v*), CH_2Cl_2–acetone (from 1:0 to 1:1, *v*/*v*), and finally with acetone), resulting in 14 subfractions (A1–A14), after a TLC analysis. Subfraction A6 (478.4 mg) was recrystallized in Hex, yielding a mixture of fruticuline A and FRUT B. An aliquot of this mixture (107.5 mg) was purified by semi-preparative HPLC (a Waters apparatus equipped with a PDA detector and a semi-preparative Nucleosil 100-5 C18 column, 250 × 10 mm), using MeOH-MeCN (50:50, *v*/*v*), isocratic mode (20 min), to obtain fruticuline A (58.8 mg, retention time = 9.2 min) and FRUT B (21.8 mg, retention time = 10.3 min). Compounds were identified by the comparison of their NMR data (Bruker spectrometer Avance 400, using deuterated chloroform, Bruker, Karlsruhe, Germany) with the literature [10].

4.3. Animals

The experiments were performed with female and male Swiss mice (aged between 8 and 10 weeks; males weighing from 33 to 39 g, females weighing from 28 to 32 g). The animals received food and water ad libitum. They were kept in an environment with a controlled temperature of 22 ± 2 °C, and 12 h of a light/dark cycle. The experiments were performed in the Pharmacology Laboratory of the Faculty of Health Sciences (FCS), after the approval by the Ethics Committee on Animal Use (CEUA) of UFGD under protocol CEUA 22/2022.

4.4. Zymosan-Induced Knee Inflammation

The animals (female mice) were randomly distributed in groups and were treated with a vehicle (saline solution (0.9%); negative control group), EESL (30, 100, and 300 mg/kg), FRUT B (1 mg/kg), and prednisolone (PRED, 3 mg/kg, positive group) one hour before Zymosan injection. The inflammation in the knee was induced by an intra-articular injection of Zymosan (500 µg per cavity with 25 µL saline) [17,24]. The mechanical hyperalgesia, cold response, and edema were measured 4 and 6 h after Zymosan injection. The animals were euthanized (ketamine—300 mg/kg, intraperitoneal (i.p.) + xylazine—30 mg/kg, i.p.) 6 h after Zymosan injection. Subsequently, the synovial cavities of the knees were washed with a solution of PBS/EDTA, and the synovial liquid was collected by aspiration 6 h after Zymosan injection. Total cell counts and NO were measured using a Neubauer chamber and Griess methods, respectively.

4.5. CFA-Induced Acute Paw Inflammation

In previous work of our research group, mice were subjected to prolonged treatment with an ethanolic extract of *S. lachnostachys* Benth. leaves and this extract exhibited anti-inflammatory parameters in the Complete Freund's Adjuvant (CFA) model [8]. For the study, the animals (male mice) were randomly distributed in groups and were treated twice (one hour before and 24 h after CFA injection) with a vehicle (saline solution, 0.9%; negative control group), FRUT B (0.3 and 1 mg/kg), and prednisolone (PRED, 3 mg/kg, positive control group). At time zero, 20 µL of CFA (suspension containing dead *Mycobacterium tuberculosis*, paraffin (85%), and monooleate (15%) oils) was injected into the right hind paw. The mechanical hyperalgesia [25], cold response [18], and edema [26] were measured at 3, 4, and 24 h after CFA injection. The animals were euthanized (ketamine—300 mg/kg, intraperitoneal (i.p.) + xylazine—30 mg/kg, i.p.) 6 h after Zymosan injection. Subsequently, the skin of the paw of each animal was removed for measurements of MPO and NAG activities.

4.6. Carrageenan-Induced Acute Pleurisy

One hour prior to carrageenan injection, Swiss female mice were distributed into three groups and treated orally with 0.9% saline solution (naive and negative control groups (p.o.)), prednisolone (PRED, 3 mg/kg, positive control group), and FRUT B (0.3 and 1 mg/kg). These groups received 100 µL of a solution of 1% carrageenan while the naive group received a similar volume of the saline solution by the intrapleural route. After 4 h, the animals were euthanized (ketamine—300 mg/kg, intraperitoneal (i.p.) + xylazine—30 mg/kg, i.p.), and the pleural cavity was washed with PBS/EDTA. The total leukocyte number and the level of protein were measured in the pleural exudate.

4.7. Cell Viability Assay by Colorimetric Method (MTT)

The cellular cytotoxicity test was performed using a colorimetric method with MTT (Sigma, São Paulo, Brazil) (Figure S4) [20]. The leukocytes were obtained from peripheral blood. The cells were plated with 5×10^5 cells/well (in 96-well plates) in a volume of 100 μL RPMI medium (supplemented with 10% fetal bovine serum (FBS) and penicillin at 100 U/mL + streptomycin at 100 mg/mL). After 90 min of exposure to FRUT B (3, 10, 30, 90 μg/mL), 10 μL of the MTT solution was added (5 mg/mL, Sigma) to each well. After 2 h of incubation at 37 °C, the supernatant was removed and 100 μL of the lysis solution was added to each well. The cells were incubated at 25 °C for 10 min, and subsequently, the absorbance was measured using a microplate reader at 540 nm. The values of the blank wells were discounted, and viability calculations were performed according to Silva-Filho et al. [22].

4.8. Statistical Analysis

Data are expressed as the mean ± SEM for each experimental group. The results were statistically analyzed by using a one-way variance analysis (ANOVA), followed by Tukey's post hoc test. The percentage of inhibition was calculated in relation to the control group prednisolone (PRED). Differences were considered significant when $p < 0.05$.

5. Conclusions

This study has demonstrated that the EESL and FRUT B reduced inflammation and hyperalgesia in Zymosan articular pain. Our study was the first to reveal the anti-hyperalgesic, anti-arthritic, and anti-inflammatory potential of FRUT B in experimental in vivo models. In the MTT test, no cytotoxicity was detected by the compound exposure.

Supplementary Materials: The following supporting information can be downloaded at: https://www.mdpi.com/article/10.3390/ph17091226/s1, Figure S1: ^{1}H NMR spectrum (400 MHz, CDCl3) of fruticuline B, Figure S2: HSQC spectrum (400 MHz, CDCl3) of fruticuline B, Figure S3: HMBC spectrum (400 MHz, CDCl3) of fruticuline B.

Author Contributions: Conceptualization, E.d.S.-P., N.d.M.B. and C.A.L.K.; Methodology, E.d.S.-P., N.d.M.B., C.S.O., M.H.V. and S.C.N.; Validation, E.d.S.-P., N.d.M.B., C.S.O., M.H.V. and S.E.S.-F.; Resources, S.E.S.-F., R.J.O., M.É.A.S. and C.A.L.K.; Writing—Original Draft Preparation, E.d.S.-P., N.d.M.B. and C.A.L.K.; Writing—Review and Editing, E.d.S.-P., N.d.M.B., C.S.O., M.H.V. and C.A.L.K.; Supervision, S.E.S.-F., R.J.O., M.É.A.S. and C.A.L.K.; Funding Acquisition, S.E.S.-F., R.J.O., M.É.A.S. and C.A.L.K. All authors have read and agreed to the published version of the manuscript.

Funding: This research was funded by CNPq (Conselho Nacional de Desenvolvimento Científico e Tecnológico), CAPES (Coordenação de Aperfeiçoamento de Pessoal de Nível Superior Brazil) (process 427859/2018-2—MEAS and process 310053/2023-4—CALK); and the Federal University of Mato Grosso do Sul—UFMS. The APC was funded by FUNDECT (Fundação de Apoio ao Desenvolvimento do Ensino, Ciência e Tecnologia do Estado de Mato Grosso do Sul) (process 59/300.112/2015; TO 136/2023; SIAFEM 33098) and the Federal University of Grande Dourados. ES, CSO, SCN, and MHV thank CAPES (Coordenação de Aperfeiçoamento de Pessoal de Nível Superior) for scholarships (funding code 001).

Institutional Review Board Statement: The animal study protocol was approved by the Institutional Review Board of the Ethics Committee on Animal Use (CEUA) of the Federal University of Grande Dourados (protocol number 22/2022).

Informed Consent Statement: Not applicable.

Data Availability Statement: Data is contained within the article and Supplementary Materials.

Acknowledgments: The authors thank Élide Pereira dos Santos for harvesting and identifying the species.

Conflicts of Interest: The authors declare no conflicts of interest.

References

1. Zarrin, A.A.; Bao, K.; Lupardus, P.; Vucic, D. Kinase inhibition in autoimmunity and inflammation. *Nat. Rev. Drug Discov.* **2021**, *20*, 39–63. [CrossRef] [PubMed]
2. Vieira, M.; Maalouf, G.; Hasan, M.; Le Joncour, A.; Karkeni, E.; Idir, M.; Amelin, D.; Salem, J.E.; Gougis, P.; Lacorte, J.M.; et al. Cytokine profile as a prognostic tool in coronavirus disease 2019. Comment on "Urgent avenues in the treatment of COVID-19: Targeting downstream inflammation to prevent catastrophic syndrome" by Quartuccio et al. *Jt. Bone Spine* **2021**, *88*, 105074. [CrossRef] [PubMed]
3. Alvarez-Nemegyei, J.; Pacheco-Pantoja, E.; González-Salazar, M.; López-Villanueva, R.F.; May-Kim, S.; Martínez-Vargas, L.; Quintal-Gutiérrez, D. Association between Overweight/Obesity and Clinical Activity in Rheumatoid Arthritis. *Reumatol. Clin. (Engl. Ed.)* **2020**, *16*, 462–467. [CrossRef] [PubMed]
4. Xu, J.; Eastman, A.J.; Flaczyk, A.; Neal, L.M.; Zhao, G.; Carolan, J.; Malachowski, A.N.; Stolberg, V.R.; Yosri, M.; Chensue, S.W.; et al. Erratum for Xu et al., Disruption of Early Tumor Necrosis Factor Alpha Signaling Prevents Classical Activation of Dendritic Cells in Lung-Associated Lymph Nodes and Development of Protective Immunity against Cryptococcal Infection. *mBio* **2018**, *29*, e01039-18. [CrossRef] [PubMed]
5. Mattos, G.; Camargo, A.; de Souza, C.A.; Zeni, A.L.B. Medicinal plants and herbal medicines in Primary Health Care: The perception of the professionals. *Cienc. Saude Colet.* **2018**, *23*, 3735–3744. [CrossRef]
6. Piccinelli, A.C.; Aquino, D.F.S.; Morato, P.N.; Kuraoka-Oliveira, A.M.; Strapasson, R.L.; dos Santos, E.P.; Stefanello, M.E.A.; Oliveira, R.J.; Kassuya, C.A.L. Anti-Inflammatory and Antihyperalgesic Activities of Ethanolic Extract and Fruticulin A from *Salvia lachnostachys* Leaves in Mice. *J. Evid.-Based Complement. Altern. Med.* **2014**, *2014*, 835914. [CrossRef]
7. Corso, C.R.; Stipp, M.C.; Adami, E.R.; da Silva, L.M.; Mariott, M.; de Andrade, S.F.; Ramos, E.A.S.; Klassen, G.; Beltrame, O.C.; Queiroz-Telles, J.E.; et al. *Salvia lachnostachys* Benth has antitumor and chemopreventive effects against solid Ehrlich carcinoma. *Mol. Biol. Rep.* **2019**, *46*, 4827–4841. [CrossRef]
8. Santos Radai, J.A.; da Silva, G.F.; Berno, C.R.; Leitão, M.M.; dos Santos, E.P.; Oliveira, R.J.; Kassuya, C.A.L. Genetic toxicological assessment and anti-arthritic effects of an ethanolic extract obtained from *Salvia lachnostachys* Benth leaves in mice. *Regul. Toxicol. Pharmacol.* **2018**, *92*, 239–244. [CrossRef]
9. Santos, J.A.; Piccinelli, A.C.; Formagio, M.D.; Oliveira, C.S.; dos Santos, E.P.; Stefanello, M.E.A.; Junior, U.L.; Oliveira, R.J.; Sugizaki, M.M.; Kassuya, C.A.L. Antidepressive and antinociceptive effects of ethanolic extract and fruticuline A from *Salvia lachnostachys* Benth leaves on rodents. *PLoS ONE* **2017**, *12*, e0172151. [CrossRef]
10. Oliveira, C.S.; Salvador, M.J.; de Carvalho, J.E.; Santos, E.P.; Barison, A.; Stefanello, M.E.A. Cytotoxic abietane-derivative diterpenoids of *Salvia lachnostachys*. *Phytochem. Lett.* **2016**, *17*, 140–143. [CrossRef]
11. Oliveira, C.S.; Alvarez, C.J.; Cabral, M.R.P.; Sarragiotto, M.H.; Salvador, M.J.; Stefanello, M.E.A. Three new diterpenoids from the leaves of *Salvia lachnostachys*. *Nat. Prod. Res.* **2022**, *36*, 5600–5605. [CrossRef] [PubMed]
12. Erbano, M.; Ehrenfried, C.A.; Stefanello, M.E.A.; dos Santos, E.P. Morphoanatomical and phytochemical studies of *Salvia lachnostachys* (Lamiaceae). *Microsc. Res. Tech.* **2012**, *75*, 1737–1744. [CrossRef]
13. Soriano-García, M.; Esquivel, B.; Toscano, R.; Estebanes, L.; Rodríguez-Hahn, L. Structure of fruticuline B: A new natural anthracene quinodimethide of abietanoid origin. *J. Crystallogr. Spectrosc. Res.* **1987**, *17*, 761–770.
14. Simmons, E.M.; Sarpong, R. Structure, biosynthetic relationships and chemical synthesis of the icetexane diterpenoids. *Nat. Prod. Rep* **2009**, *26*, 1195–1217. [CrossRef] [PubMed]
15. Corso, C.R.; Stipp, M.C.; Radulski, D.R.; Mariott, M.; da Silva, L.M.; Ramos, E.A.S.; Klassen, G.; Telles, J.E.Q.; Oliveira, C.S.; Stefanello, M.E.A.; et al. Fruticulin A, a chemically-defined diterpene, exerts antineoplastic effects in vitro and in vivo by multiple mechanisms. *Sci. Rep.* **2020**, *10*, 16477. [CrossRef] [PubMed]
16. Monticone, M.; Bisio, A.; Daga, A.; Giannoni, P.; Giaretti, W.; Maffei, M.; Pfeffer, U.; Romeo, F.; Quarto, R.; Romussi, G.; et al. Demethyl fruticulin A (SCO-1) causes apoptosis by inducing reactive oxygen species in mitochondria. *J. Cell. Biochem.* **2010**, *111*, 1149–1159. [CrossRef]
17. Hosseini, S.M. In-silico assessments of fruticulin-a and demethylfruticulin-a isolated from *Salvia* species against important anticancer targets. *Res. J. Pharmacogn.* **2023**, *10*, 31–41. [CrossRef]
18. Conte, F.P.; Barja-Fidalgo, C.; Verri Jr, W.A.; Cunha, F.Q.; Rae, G.A.; Penido, C.; Henriques, M.G.M.O. Endothelins modulate inflammatory reaction in zymosan-induced arthritis: Participation of LTB4, TNF-alpha, and CXCL-1. *J. Leukoc. Biol.* **2008**, *84*, 652–660. [CrossRef]
19. van de Loo, F.A.; Arntz, O.J.; van Enckevort, F.H.; van Lent, P.L.; van den Berg, W.B. Reduced cartilage proteoglycan loss during zymosan-induced gonarthritis in NOS2-deficient mice and in anti-interleukin-1-treated wild-type mice with unabated joint inflammation. *Arthritis Rheum.* **1998**, *41*, 634–646. [CrossRef]
20. Dixon, W.J. Staircase bioassay: The up-and-down method. *Neurosci. Biobehav. Rev.* **1991**, *15*, 47–50. [CrossRef]
21. Riss, T.L.; Moravec, R.A. Use of multiple assay endpoints to investigate the effects of incubation time, dose of toxin, and plating density in cell-based cytotoxicity assays. *Assay Drug Dev. Technol.* **2004**, *2*, 51–62. [CrossRef] [PubMed]
22. Kummer, R.; Fachini-Queiroz, F.C.; Estevão-Silva, C.F.; Grespan, R.; Silva, E.L.; Bersani-Amado, C.A.; Cuman, R.K. Evaluation of Anti-Inflammatory Activity of Citrus latifolia Tanaka Essential Oil and Limonene in Experimental Mouse Models. *Evid. Based Complement. Alternat. Med.* **2013**, *2013*, 859083. [CrossRef] [PubMed]

23. Dantas, L.B.R.; Alcântara, I.S.; Júnior, C.P.S.; de Oliveira, M.R.C.; Martins, A.O.B.P.B.; Dantas, T.M.; Ribeiro-Filho, J.; Coutinho, H.D.M.; Passos, F.R.S.; Quintans-Júnior, L.J.; et al. In vivo and in silico anti-inflammatory properties of the sesquiterpene valencene. *Biomed. Pharmacother.* **2022**, *153*, 113478. [CrossRef] [PubMed]
24. Rodríguez-Hahn, L.; Esquivel, B.; Sánchez, C.; Estebanes, L.; Cárdenas, J.; Soriano-García, M.; Ramamoorthy, R.T.T.P. Abietane type diterpenoids from *Salvia fruticulosa*. A revision of the structure of fruticulin B. *Phytochemistry* **1989**, *28*, 567–570. [CrossRef]
25. Penido, C.; Conte, F.P.; Chagas, M.S.S.; Rodrigues, C.A.B.; Pereira, J.F.G.; Henriques, M.G.M.O. Antiinflammatory effects of natural tetranortriterpenoids isolated from *Carapa guianensis* Aublet on zymosan-induced arthritis in mice. *Inflamm. Res.* **2006**, *55*, 457–464. [CrossRef] [PubMed]
26. Gupta, S.; Mishra, K.P.; Kumar, B.; Singh, S.B.; Ganju, L. Andrographolide attenuates complete Freund's adjuvant induced arthritis via suppression of inflammatory mediators and pro-inflammatory cytokines. *J. Ethnopharmacol.* **2020**, *261*, 113022. [CrossRef] [PubMed]

MDPI AG
Grosspeteranlage 5
4052 Basel
Switzerland
Tel.: +41 61 683 77 34

Pharmaceuticals Editorial Office
E-mail: pharmaceuticals@mdpi.com
www.mdpi.com/journal/pharmaceuticals